wm 35 ELD

2014

MENTAL HEALTH NURSING

Your textbook comes with a range of additional online resources

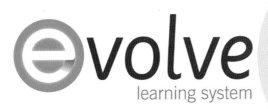

learning system

We have created a range of additional online resources specifically designed to expand the material in your textbook.

These include:

- Multiple Choice Questions
- True/False Questions
- Case Studies

The additional online resources are available on our **Evolve learning system**. For access, please go to **http://evolve.elsevier.com/Elder/mental/**, and follow the on-screen prompts.

Need help? For assistance with accessing your additional online resources, please visit **http://evolvesupport.elsevier.com/**

For Elsevier

Content Strategist: *Mairi McCubbin*
Content Development Specialist: *Catherine Jackson*
Project Manager: *Sukanthi Sukumar*
Designer: *Christian Bilbow*
Illustration Manager: *Jennifer Rose*
Illustrator: *Antbits Ltd*

Mental Health Nursing
A Manual for Practice

Original Australian Edition edited by

Ruth Elder BA(Hons), PhD, RN
Formerly Senior Lecturer, School of Nursing, Queensland University of Technology, Brisbane, Australia

Katie Evans BA, MLitSt, PhD, RPN, FACMHN
Freelance Educational Designer, Brisbane, Australia

Debra Nizette BAppSc, MNurStudies, DipAppSc, RN, Credentialled MHN, FRCNA, FACMHN
Mental Health Nursing Advisor, Nursing and Midwifery Office, Queensland Health, Brisbane, Australia

This UK Edition edited by

Steve Trenoweth BSc(Hons), MSc, PhD, PGDipEA, RMN, MBPsS, FHEA
Senior Lecturer, College of Nursing, Midwifery and Healthcare, University of West London, UK

Foreword by

Ian Peate BEd(Hons), MA(Lond), DipN(Lond), LLM, RN, RNT
Editor-in-Chief, *British Journal of Nursing*; Visiting Professor of Nursing, University of West London, UK

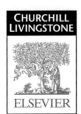

Edinburgh   London   New York   Oxford   Philadelphia   St Louis   Sydney   Toronto   2014

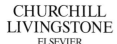

CHURCHILL
LIVINGSTONE
ELSEVIER

First UK edition 2014

First Australian edition 2005
Second Australian edition 2009

ISBN 978-0-7020-4493-9

British Library Cataloguing in Publication Data
A catalogue record for this book is available from the British Library

Library of Congress Cataloging in Publication Data
A catalog record for this book is available from the Library of Congress

Notices
Knowledge and best practice in this field are constantly changing. As new research and experience broaden our understanding, changes in research methods, professional practices, or medical treatment may become necessary.

Practitioners and researchers must always rely on their own experience and knowledge in evaluating and using any information, methods, compounds, or experiments described herein. In using such information or methods they should be mindful of their own safety and the safety of others, including parties for whom they have a professional responsibility.

With respect to any drug or pharmaceutical products identified, readers are advised to check the most current information provided (i) on procedures featured or (ii) by the manufacturer of each product to be administered, to verify the recommended dose or formula, the method and duration of administration, and contraindications. It is the responsibility of practitioners, relying on their own experience and knowledge of their patients, to make diagnoses, to determine dosages and the best treatment for each individual patient, and to take all appropriate safety precautions.

To the fullest extent of the law, neither the Publisher nor the authors, contributors, or editors, assume any liability for any injury and/or damage to persons or property as a matter of products liability, negligence or otherwise, or from any use or operation of any methods, products, instructions, or ideas contained in the material herein.

ELSEVIER   your source for books,
journals and multimedia
in the health sciences

www.elsevierhealth.com

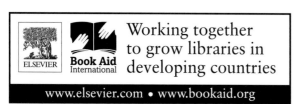

Working together
to grow libraries in
developing countries

www.elsevier.com • www.bookaid.org

The
Publisher's
policy is to use
paper manufactured
from sustainable forests

Printed in China

Contents

Foreword

Mental health is everybody's business; a clear recurring theme in this adapted text. At any one time, roughly one in six of us is experiencing a mental health problem. This is a staggering figure in itself; mental health problems are estimated to cost the UK economy over £105 billion per year. Good mental health and resilience are central to our ability enjoy physical health, the relationships we are in and those we would like to be in, our education, our ability to work and contribute to society and to succeed in reaching our potential and aspirations.

This book is timely, given the current Government's prioritization of mental health care and service provision. This adaptation is very closely aligned to and compliments the Mental Health Implementation Framework that sets out what employers, schools, businesses, local authorities, housing organizations, voluntary groups and health and care organizations can do to promote and enhance good mental health.

The way public services are designed and delivered is changing fundamentally in the NHS; new structures are emerging that signify an important shift towards a locally led system, with an increased accountability to local populations. The reform of the health and care system provides a significant opportunity to improve people's mental health and wellbeing.

This book will help nurses and other healthcare providers to improve people's mental health and wellbeing, with an emphasis on everyone playing their part. This text has the potential to empower those who are committed to improving the mental health and wellbeing of the whole population along with the life chances of people with mental health conditions. The book ensures mental health has equal priority with physical health, a principle to which the authors are clearly committed throughout.

This text is user friendly, adopting an adult learning approach that engages the reader. It offers a basis for undergraduate nurse education setting down the principles and practice that are essential for safe, high-quality and effective mental health nursing and providing the cornerstones and fundamentals of our practice. From this starting point students will be better prepared for the practice of mental health nursing.

I sincerely hope that you enjoy this text and that it helps you to develop mental health nursing skills and knowledge which are responsive and supportive to those people to whom you have the privilege to offer care.

Ian Peate

Preface

This book has been produced at a time of great change in mental health services in the UK. The Coalition Government's *No Health Without Mental Health* (Department of Health, 2011) strategy seeks to ensure the delivery of person-centred mental health care. Many Mental Health Trusts are embedding the principles of recovery in their service delivery while 'cost-improvement plans' brought about by austerity measures continue to bite. It is a time of considerable challenge but also an exciting time when mental health services can finally shake off a style of care that has not changed fundamentally since Victorian times. Nurses are in an excellent position to embrace new ways of working, such as helping people to achieve a personally acceptable state of mental and physical wellbeing.

However, this is merely the start of a great process of change, and new ways of working will inevitably take time to develop and embed in everyday practice. Mental health nurses have the opportunity to be at the forefront of this change process but in order to do that we will need to ensure that we consolidate our identity as an equal partner in the multiprofessional team: an identity and role which is often subsumed by the medical model by which our role may be relegated to the administration of medication and source of information on the clinical progress of 'patients'. The sort of nursing care that the authors describe in this book supports these new ways of working. The authors recognize that while the medical approach remains an important part of the care package for people experiencing mental distress, there are also different ways of working that seek to help and support people on their own personal journey to recovery.

This book has been designed to support the development of mental health nursing skills in the context of such change. Of course, no book can truly capture the complexity of mental health care and the full extent of mental health nursing skills. Our aim is more to help the reader to develop their appreciation and understanding of essential principles, knowledge, values and skills which underpin contemporary mental health nursing.

There are four sections in this book: in the first we explore preparing for mental health nursing, in the second we consider mental health and wellness, in the third we seek to understand mental health problems and in the final section we consider how to develop skills for mental health nursing. Each chapter gives a thorough overview of the topic, backed up with activities for critical thinking and nurses' stories and personal narratives that provide an important insight into what it is like to provide the sort of care described.

I hope that this UK edition of the best-selling Australian textbook will help and support you to deliver the sort of care that mental health service users frequently report as being the most helpful to their recovery.

London, 2012   Steve Trenoweth

REFERENCE

Department of Health, 2011. No health without mental health: a cross-government mental health outcomes strategy for people of all ages. <http://www.dh.gov.uk/en/Publicationsandstatistics/Publications/PublicationsPolicyAndGuidance/DH_123766>.

Contributors

UK CONTRIBUTORS

Kay Mafuba BA, MA, PGCertResearch, DipHE, RNT, RNLD, FHEA, CLTHE
Programme Leader, College of Nursing, Midwifery and Healthcare, University of West London, UK

11 Learning disabilities

Wendy Moyle BN, MHSc, PhD, DipAppSci, RN
Professor of Nursing and Director, Research Centre for Clinical and Community Practice Innovation, Griffith University, Brisbane, Australia; Visiting Professor, Northumbria University, Newcastle Upon-Tyne, UK

13 Mental disorders of older age

Reuben Pearce DipHE, PGCE, PGCR, FHEA
Senior Lecturer, College of Nursing, Midwifery and Healthcare, University of West London, UK

24 Psychopharmacology and medicines management

Alicia Powell BSc(Psych), RMN(Hons)
Community Practitioner, West London Mental Health Trust, London, UK

21 Settings for mental healthcare

Helen Robson BSc, MA, PGCert, DPSN, RGN, RMN, RM
Lecturer Practitioner, University of West London and West London Mental Health Trust, UK

25 Physical health

Deborah Taylor DipAppSc, MSc(Ed), PGDip, PGCE, RGN
Senior Lecturer, College of Nursing, Midwifery and Healthcare, University of West London, UK

25 Physical health

Steve Trenoweth BSc(Hons), MSc, PhD, PGDipEA, RMN, MBPsS, FHEA
Senior Lecturer, College of Nursing, Midwifery and Healthcare, University of West London, UK

25 Physical health

ANZ CONTRIBUTORS

Gail Anderson Adolescent Mental Health Cert, RN, CM, MN, MCN, MRCNA
Clinical Nurse Consultant, Adolescent Health, Westmead Hospital, Sydney, Australia

18 Eating disorders

Peter Athanasos BA, BSc(Hons), RGN, RPN
Adjunct academic, Discipline of Psychiatry, Flinders University, Adelaide, Australia

15 Mood disorders

Murray Bardwell DipAppSc, RN(Psychiatric Nurse), MNst
Course Co-ordinator, Bachelor of Nursing and Bachelor of Paramedicine, School of Nursing and Midwifery, Australian Catholic University, Melbourne, Australia

14 Schizophrenic disorders

Patricia Barkway BA, MSc(PHC), RN, CMHN
Senior Lecturer, Mental Health Nursing, School of Nursing and Midwifery, Flinders University, Adelaide, Australia

7 Theories on mental health and ill health

Jan Barling BA, DipAppSc, RN, MN, MRCNA, FACMHN
Lecturer, Mental Health Nursing, School of Health and Human Services, Southern Cross University, Australia

10 Assessment and diagnosis

Pat Bradley GradDipHealthEd, RPN, RGN, MMHN, MHN(C), FACMHN
Clinical Nurse Manager, Inpatient Unit, Top End Mental Health Service, Australia

6 Mental health and wellness

Christina Campbell BA(Hons), BN, MCert, PhD, RN, MHN
Senior Lecturer, School of Nursing, QUT, Australia

16 Personality disorders

Janette Curtis BA, PhD, DipPH, RN, MACMHN, FRCNA
Principal Fellow, University of Woollongong, New South Wales, Australia

19 Substance-related disorders and dual diagnosis

Ruth De Souza DipNurs, MA(Nurs), GradDipAdvNursPrac (Counselling)
Centre Co-ordinator/Senior Research Fellow, Centre for Asian and Migrant Health Research, National Institute for Public Health and Mental Health Research; Co-ordinator, Graduate Certificate/Diploma, Addictions, Community Health Development, AUT University, New Zealand

6 Mental health and wellness

Ruth Elder BA(Hons), PhD, RN
Formerly Senior Lecturer, School of Nursing, Queensland University of Technology, Brisbane, Australia

20 Somatoform and dissociative disorders
21 Settings for mental healthcare

Stephen Elsom PhD, RN
Associate Professor, Director, Centre for Psychiatric Nursing, Faculty of Medicine, Dentistry and Health Sciences, University of Melbourne, Australia

17 Anxiety disorders

Katie Evans BA, MLitSt, PhD, RPN, FACMHN
Freelance Educational Designer, Brisbane, Australia

3 Historical foundations

Gerald Farrell PhD, RN
Associate Dean, Division of Nursing and Midwifery, Faculty of Health Sciences, La Trobe University, Australia

16 Personality disorders

Kim Foster MA, BN, PhD, DipAppSc, RN, RPN, MRCNA, FACMHN
Senior Lecturer, Deputy Head of School, School of Nursing, Midwifery and Nutrition, James Cook University, Cairns, Australia

22 Person-centred approaches to managing risk
24 Psychopharmacology and medicines management

Mike Groome PhD, RN, MAPS
International Student Consultant, Victoria; Lecturer, School of Nursing and Midwifery, Australian Catholic University, Australia

12 Working with children and young people

Charles Harmon MN, DipTeach, RN, FACMHN
Lecturer, School of Nursing and Midwifery, Faculty of Health, University of Newcastle, Australia

11 Learning disabilities

Kristin Henderson BN, DipAppNursEd, GradDipScComm, RN, RM, RPN, MHlthSc
Team Leader, Access, Inpatient and Consultation Liaison Services, Child and Youth Mental Health, Royal Children's Hospital, Brisbane, Australia

12 Working with children and young people

Sue Henderson BAppScNur, MN, RN(PsychNurse)
Lecturer, School of Nursing and Midwifery, Monash University, Melbourne, Australia

17 Anxiety disorders

Debra Jackson PhD, RN
Professor of Nursing, School of Nursing, College of Health and Science, University of Western Sydney, Australia

1 The effective nurse

Lauretta Luck BA, MA, PhD, RN, MRCNA
Associate Head of School, School of Nursing, College of Health and Science, University of Western Australia, Australia

22 Person-centred approaches to managing risk
24 Psychopharmacology and medicines management

Jem Masters MM, GradDipNM, UTS, RN(RGN, RCSN, RMN UK), FACMHN
Lecturer, Mental Health and Health Service Management, Faculty of Nursing and Midwifery, University of Sydney, Australia

12 Working with children and young people

Phillip Maude BHSci, PhD, DipMHN, CertAddictions, RN, MN(Res), FACMHN
Associate Professor, Co-ordinator, Graduate Diploma in Mental Health Nursing, School of Health Sciences (Nursing and Midwifery), RMIT University, Australia

5 Professional and ethical issues

Paul Morrison BA(Hons), PhD, PGCE, GradDipCouns, RMN, RGN, AFBPsS, CPsychol, MAPS
Dean, School of Nursing and Midwifery, Peel Campus, Murdoch University, Perth, Australia

9 Crisis and loss

Eimear Muir-Cochrane BSc(Hons), GradDipAdultEd, PhD, RN, RMHN, MNS, Credentialled MHN
Chair of Nursing (Mental Health), School of Nursing and Midwifery, Flinders University, Australia

4 The politicolegal context
5 Professional and ethical issues

Debra Nizette BAppSc, MNurStudies, DipAppSc, RN, Credentialled MHN, FRCNA, FACMHN
Mental Health Nursing Advisor, Nursing and Midwifery Office, Queensland Health, Brisbane, Australia

8 Mental health across the lifespan

Anthony O'Brien BA, MPhil, RN, FNZCMHN
Senior Lecturer, School of Nursing, University of Auckland; Nurse Specialist, Liaison Psychiatry, Auckland District Health Board, New Zealand

4 The politicolegal context
5 Professional and ethical issues

Louise O'Brien BA, PhD, RN
Associate Professor, School of Nursing, College of Health and Science, University of Western Sydney and Sydney West Area Health Service, Australia

1 The effective nurse

Christine Palmer DipAppSc(NEd), BAppSc, PhD, RN, RPN, MN, MHN(Private Practice), FACMHN
Mental Health Nurse in private practice

23 Therapeutic interventions

Philip B. Petrie BN, MEd
Executive Director, Allevia, Bankstown, New South Wales, Australia

11 Learning disabilities

Vicki Stanton BA(SocWel), GradDipPubHlth, GradCertMgmt, MA(SocSc), RN, RMRN, FACMHN
Clinical Coordinator, Aboriginal Mental Health, South Eastern Sydney Health District, New South Wales, Australia

2 The context of practice

Richard Taylor BEd, MEd, RN, RPN
Assistant Head of School, School of Nursing and Midwifery, Australian Catholic University, Melbourne, Australia

14 Schizophrenic disorders

Barbara Tooth BA(Hons), PhD, RN, RM
NSW Institute of Psychiatry, Sydney, Australia

2 The context of practice

Kim Usher BA, MNursS, PhD, DNE, DHS, RN, RPN, RMRN, FACMHN, FRCNA
Professor, School of Nursing, Midwifery and Nutrition, James Cook University, Cairns, Australia

22 Person-centred approaches to managing risk
24 Psychopharmacology and medicines management

Timothy Wand GradDipMHNurs, MN(Hons), DAS(Nurse), MHN
Nurse Practitioner, Mental Health Liaison, Emergency Department, Royal Prince Alfred Hospital; Senior Clinical Lecturer, Mental Health, Faculty of Nursing and Midwifery, University of Sydney, Australia

4 The politicolegal context

Pamela Wood GradDipEd, BANurs, RenalCert, RN, RPN
Lecturer, School of Health Science, Charles Darwin University; Renal Educator, The Top End Renal Services, Australia

6 Mental health and wellness

Part | 1 |

Preparing for mental health nursing

Chapter | 1 |

The effective nurse

Debra Jackson and Louise O'Brien

CHAPTER POINTS

- Mental health nursing is a challenging and stimulating area of practice that utilizes knowledge from both human and biological sciences.
- The development of therapeutic relationships is the key to effective mental health nursing.
- Mental health nurses and service users together develop therapeutic alliances as an arena for growth and recovery.
- Self-awareness, insight and reflexivity are fundamental skills for mental health nursing.
- Mental health nursing requires sustained and close engagement with people in highly charged situations, and this has the potential to cause occupational stress that can precede burnout syndrome.
- Burnout syndrome has three elements: emotional exhaustion, depersonalization and reduced personal accomplishment.
- Mental health nurses are required to develop therapeutic alliances while maintaining clear professional boundaries.
- Supportive collegial relationships can enhance the skills and confidence of mental health nurses at all stages of their careers.

KEY TERMS

- burnout
- burnout syndrome
- caring
- clinical supervision
- empathy
- ethics
- evidence-based practice
- healing
- hope
- mentoring
- preceptoring
- professional boundaries
- recovery
- reflection
- reflective practices
- self

DOI: http://dx.doi.org/10.1016/B978-0-7020-4493-9.00001-9

- self-awareness
- self-disclosure
- spirituality
- stress
- therapeutic alliance

LEARNING OUTCOMES

The material in this chapter will assist you to:

- describe the nursing skills needed to care for the spiritual needs of service users,
- describe the three components of empathy,
- define self-awareness and describe a strategy for developing self-awareness,
- discuss the three phases of reflection,
- list the factors that contribute to stress and burnout in nursing,
- explain strategies for managing stress and avoiding burnout,
- explain the importance of maintaining professional boundaries,
- describe the benefits of mentoring and preceptoring.

INTRODUCTION

Mental health nursing is one of the most interesting and challenging areas of nursing practice, and requires a fusion of professional knowledge, clinical and interpersonal skills and experiences. Although nurses in all settings care for the mental health and wellbeing of the service users in their care, those service users with acute or chronic mental health problems have complex and perhaps long-term needs. Service users with chronic mental health problems often engage in frequent and regular encounters with the healthcare system. The long-term and cyclic nature of some mental health problems means that the therapeutic relationships between mental health nurses and service users can last for long periods. They can also vary in intensity as service users move along a continuum between periods of high dependence at one end (in acute phases when they are experiencing symptoms of their health problem) and independence at the other (when their symptoms are less troublesome or their mental health problem is resolved).

Skilful mental health nursing requires more than a sound knowledge of human physiology, psychology, psychiatry and pharmacology. In order to practise effectively, nurses working in mental health need to be open-minded and reflective, and to have developed an understanding of esoteric concepts such as spirituality and hope. They also need to understand the nature and boundaries of professional and therapeutic relationships. Personal qualities such as responsiveness, self-awareness and insight are also essential. This chapter introduces some of the concepts and issues that are fundamental to the provision of effective and safe mental health nursing practice.

CARING

Caring is widely considered to be central to nursing theory and practice, and is frequently cited as a reason for choosing a nursing career (Jackson and Borbasi, 2006). Although the word 'caring' is used widely in the nursing and healthcare literature, as a concept it is ill defined. It is also controversial, and there are arguments for and against nursing adopting the concept of caring as the cornerstone of the discipline. Most of these arguments are concerned with:

- the 'fit' of a concept like caring in a discipline that is dominated by scientific biomedical discourses (Dunlop, 1986),
- the gendered nature of caring (Speedy, 2006),
- the care/cure debate (Jackson and Borbasi, 2006),
- ethical sensitivity and caring (Weaver, 2007),
- the inherent conflict between the concept of caring, and the economic rationalism and social privilege that control the provision of health services (Jackson and Borbasi, 2006),
- caring as resilient practice (Warelow and Edward, 2007),
- concerns with the dichotomy of professional nurse caring (what nurses do) and informal caring (the caring available to people through their own social networks and personal relationships) (Jackson and Borbasi, 2006).

Nurse scholars have invested much time and energy in trying to explain what it is that makes nurse caring special or different from informal caring and from the caring provided by other professionals (i.e. medical practitioners). There have also been many attempts to find a 'fit' between caring as a construct, and the biomedically dominated and efficiency-driven healthcare sectors within which nursing is situated.

From a mental health perspective there are even more issues to consider in relation to nurse caring. For example, there are special issues associated with caring for service users who are compelled (perhaps unwillingly) to accept professional care under the UK Mental Health Act 1983/2007 (see Ch. 4 for mental health legislation). Historically, mental health nursing has been associated with custodial care and control. Godin (2000) captures the current dilemma of mental health nurses when he raises questions about the dis-ease between the caring and coercive roles that mental health nurses assume.

Godin positions caring as 'clean' and constructs the coercive control elements of mental health nursing (a term he uses for forced treatment, community orders and so on) as 'dirty' (Godin, 2000, p. 1396). While Godin's argument is particularly focused on service users and nurses in the community, many of the issues he raises (related to forced administration of medication, seclusion and detention) are relevant to nurses in the inpatient setting as well. The absolute vulnerability of service users who can be detained against their will and subjected to various treatments that they may vigorously and robustly resist means that elements of the caring role, such as service user advocacy, are absolutely critical to skilful and compassionate mental health nursing practice.

Hope and spirituality

There is still much that we don't know about recovery, healing and how people manage chronic health problems. Why do some people pull through a disease, while others succumb? How is it that some people seem to cope very well with even very invasive treatments, while others suffer terribly? How do some people with chronic mental health problems function well in the community, while others are in and out of hospital in a revolving-door syndrome? We know that factors such as personality, resilience, social support, general health and access to acceptable (to the service user) health services all play a crucial role in service user outcomes (see Ch. 2 for more on service users, recovery and rehabilitation; Ch. 8 for resilience; and Ch. 23 for a discussion on instilling hope). But the importance and value of concepts such as hope, and the role it plays in the lives of service users and their families, are areas of increasing interest. Hope has particular relevance to mental health nursing practice (Cutcliffe and Koehn, 2007; Koehn and Cutcliffe, 2007) and there is growing recognition of the concept of hope and its relationship to health, wellbeing and recovery from mental health problems or traumatic life events.

'Hope' is a taken-for-granted term and although it is seen a lot in the literature, it is seldom clearly defined. It is considered essential in handling mental health problems and has been described as 'the act by which the temptation to despair is actively overcome' (Fitzgerald Miller, 2007, p. 13). We know it is a complex and multidimensional variable that has optimistic and anticipatory dimensions and involves looking ahead to the future. Daly et al. (1999, p. 43) refer to hope as 'a positive source of power' that individuals can find and foster. Their findings suggest that hope arises from suffering, adversity or misfortune of some sort (Daly et al., 1999). After undertaking a concept analysis of hope, Stephenson (1991, p. 1459) defined it as 'a process of anticipation that involves the interaction of thinking, acting, feeling and relating, and is directed toward a future fulfillment that is personally meaningful'.

In the literature, the concept of hope is consistently associated with spirituality and the belief systems that individuals hold (Daly et al., 1999). For example, Daly et al. (1999, p. 42) describe a theme they named as 'having faith in the primacy of a higher power' to capture the idea that spirituality is central to the meanings that can be drawn from major life events. Of course, spirituality does not only refer to religious issues. Goddard (1995) differentiates metaphysical spirituality, which she says focuses on the notion of God or a higher power, from existential spirituality, which relates to values, beliefs, ideologies and philosophies that provide individuals with guidance and direction throughout their lives. Furthermore, she states that spirituality is a way of understanding and making meaning of life, and is apparent in commonplace as well as unusual circumstances (Goddard, 1995).

The need for research to generate knowledge and enhance understanding about hope and spirituality in relation to mental health nursing is acknowledged in the literature (Cutcliffe and Koehn, 2007; Koehn and Cutcliffe, 2007). However, the biomedical model values things that can be seen, measured and quantified. Although they can be felt, hope and spirituality cannot be seen, touched or smelt and cannot always be clearly articulated, and so occupy what Crawford et al. (1998, p. 214) term 'an embarrassed silence'. However, if we recognize that spirituality underpins the meanings that people make of health problems and other life events, and that hope is a variable that has healing potential, then we cannot ignore the importance of spirituality in practice. Indeed, Thompson (2002) reinforces the importance of recognizing and responding to the spiritual care needs of service users, and calls for nurses to include spiritual care as a crucial aspect of holistic care.

This leads us to the question: what skills do we need if we are to care for the spiritual needs of our service users? The short answer is that we need to develop effective interpersonal skills. Being open to the belief systems of other people, active listening, being alert to the cues that tell us the things that matter to a person, self-awareness, spiritual awareness and reflective skills are considered crucial in the provision of spiritual care (Greasley et al., 2001; Thompson, 2002).

CRITICAL THINKING CHALLENGE 1.1

Colleen is a 37-year-old woman who has a 2-week history of becoming increasingly disorganized, thought-disordered, agitated and distressed. She reports hearing voices, and finds this very upsetting. She states that these voices are calling out to her and telling her things. While admitting Colleen to the ward you note that she is visibly distressed, appears to have difficulty concentrating and sometimes makes seemingly inappropriate responses to your questions, while at other times her responses are appropriate.

Colleen has no previous history of psychosis, although she does have a history of alcohol-related problems. She discloses that she has been drinking more than usual over the past month. Colleen tells you that her mother and uncle died 2 years ago in a car accident, and that her husband died of a heart attack 6 weeks ago.

♦ What are the main issues here?
♦ How might Colleen's recent social history be related to her current health status?
♦ How could the nurse respond to Colleen's distress?

ETHICAL DILEMMA

You are caring for Jack, a 22-year-old male with bipolar disorder who had been admitted to the psychiatric intensive care unit during a manic episode. In addition to a diagnosis of bipolar disorder, Jack is hepatitis B-positive. He has been detained under the Mental Health Act. Jack is observed attempting to initiate sexual activity with a couple of female service users. There is a 'no sex' policy in the unit and Jack has been reminded of this on several occasions. However, Jack tells you that he intends to form sexual relationships with some of the female service users.

Questions

1. What could the nurse do? List the options available.
2. Identify the potential risks and benefits of each option you have identified.
3. What ethical principles need to be considered?

THERAPEUTIC USE OF SELF

Therapeutic relationships are the central activity of mental health nursing. They are the foundation upon which all other activities are based. Mental health nursing is thus firstly an interpersonal process that uses self as the means of developing and sustaining nurse–service user relationships. Therapeutic use of self involves using aspects of the nurse's personality, life skills and knowledge to develop a connection with a person who has a mental health problem. Nurses intentionally and consciously draw on ways of establishing human connectedness in encounters with service users. The process is based on a genuine interest in understanding who the service user is and how they have come to be in their current situation.

The purpose of using self therapeutically is to establish a therapeutic alliance with the service user. Service users may not only be suffering from frightening symptoms or perhaps overwhelming mood changes, or out-of-control thoughts and feelings; they also suffer from alienation and isolation. Service users may be fearful of talking to others about their symptoms or difficulties because they fear being rejected and seen as 'crazy', or they may have had experiences of rejection because of their mental health problem that make it difficult for them to form relationships. Studies of service users' experiences of mental health services provide evidence that being understood and listened to in a thoughtful, sensitive manner confirms their humanity and provides hope for their future (Shattell et al., 2006).

In the process of using self therapeutically, the nurse develops a dialogue with the service user in order to understand the service user's predicament. Service users need to feel safe enough to disclose personal, difficult and distressing information. It is in the way in which the nurse can convey genuine interest, concern and desire to understand the service user that a therapeutic alliance can be established. How the nurse relates, and what prior understandings she or he brings to the encounter, will affect this relationship (Foster et al., 2006; Gallop and O'Brien, 2003).

Heifner (1993) used the term 'positive connectedness' to describe the therapeutic alliance that develops between service users and nurses in mental health settings. The therapeutic relationship is marked by recognition of a common humanity with the service user and feelings of reciprocity that result in connectedness between the service user and the nurse. A review of evidence for the necessity of therapeutic relationships when caring for people with severe mental health problems indicated that people who perceived a relationship as therapeutic had better outcomes (Hewitt and Coffey, 2005).

Therapeutic use of self is embedded in the theoretical frameworks of the interactionist nursing theorists Peplau, Travelbee and Patterson and Zderad (Meleis, 2007), who locate the focus of nursing in nurse–service user interactions and relationships. These theorists define health and illness as part of the human experience, and the goals of nursing as developing human potential to find meaning in the experience (Meleis, 2007). They stress the importance of self as a therapeutic agent.

Empathy and therapeutic use of self

The ability to empathize with service users is positively linked with the ability to develop therapeutic relationships. Studies have consistently shown that service users value empathic nurses highly (Forchuk and Reynolds, 2001; Geanellos, 2002; Hewitt and Coffey, 2005; O'Brien, 2000, 2001; Welch, 2005). Empathy is not merely a feeling of understanding and compassion for the service user. Empathy, as used in the therapeutic relationship, has a number of components. Firstly, empathy involves an attempt to understand the service user's predicament and the meanings that the service user attributes to their situation. This means that the nurse makes a conscious attempt to discuss with the service user their current and past experiences and the feelings and meanings that are associated with these experiences. Secondly, the nurse verbalizes the understanding that she or he has developed to the service user. The understanding that the nurse has of the service user's situation will be at best tentative; we can never really know what life is like for another. However, the process of seeking to understand, and of conveying to the service user the desire to understand, creates the opportunity for further exploration in a safe relationship. In addition, maintaining the stance of trying to understand rather than making assumptions averts the tendency to make judgements about service users and their behaviour. The third component of empathy is the service user's validation of the nurse's understanding. One of the most important aspects of the development of the therapeutic relationship through empathic understanding is that the nurse can convey to the service user his or her desire to understand. This level of empathic attunement allows the service user to participate in identifying those aspects of their mental health problem and healthcare experience that are problematic (see also Ch. 23).

Evidence-based practice and therapeutic alliance

The value of a therapeutic alliance, developed through therapeutic use of self, has been clearly identified from the perspective of nurses and service users in qualitative studies (Geanellos, 2002; Graham, 2001; O'Brien, 2000, 2001; Welch, 2005). Forming a strong, therapeutic, continued alliance has been linked with a reduction in admission rates and an improved quality of life for service users discharged from hospital (Forchuk and Reynolds, 2001) and in the enhancement of rehabilitation outcomes among people diagnosed with schizophrenia (Davis and Lysaker, 2007). In a review of the literature on therapeutic working relationships with people diagnosed with schizophrenia, Hewitt and Coffey (2005) concluded that the therapeutic relationship was greatly valued by people with a mental health problem. People who have a positive relationship with a clinician have better outcomes. However, a therapeutic relationship may not be sufficient to sustain health improvements, and so a combination of both therapeutic relationships and the technical skill of specific therapeutic approaches may provide the best outcomes.

that describes the core of our personality. Welch (2005, p. 164) found that nurses described 'congruency, genuineness, and authenticity' as ways of projecting 'the nurse's true self'. We use the concept of self when we want to convey our uniqueness as a human being. The self has consistent attributes that pervade the way we live in and experience the world. It is awareness of these attributes of self that can enhance the way we relate to others. A strong sense of self allows us to develop resilience in dealing with the difficulties and complexities of human communication and experience. Self-awareness is about knowing how you are going to respond to specific situations, about knowing your values, attitudes and biases towards people and situations, and about knowing how your human needs might manifest in your work.

The purpose of being self-aware is to know those things in our background and way of relating that might affect how we relate to service users. The way we view people is always subjective. The lens through which we look at the world is always our own. Although there can be no true objectivity, knowledge of the things that impinge on our subjective view of the world allows us to identify how they influence our thinking.

Nurses need to be aware of the belief systems and values that arise from their cultural, social and family backgrounds. Everyone develops biases that affect the way they view other people's behaviour. Behaviour that is understandable to one nurse might not be understandable to another. However, the self is not static but constantly evolving and sensitive to experience. We bring values, biases and beliefs to nursing and to our relationships with service users, and in turn those relationships offer the opportunity for self-development. It is through the process of self-reflection and the examination of particular experiences that nurses can learn.

Work in the mental health area requires the ability to listen to, respond to and empathize with people from a range of backgrounds. Unexamined belief systems can become obstacles to the development of a therapeutic alliance with a service user. Lack of self-awareness can cause nurses to respond to a service user's distress and behaviour in ways that may not be helpful. It may cause nurses to use their power coercively in the belief that this is best for the service user. Lack of self-awareness can lead to nurses being overly concerned, refusing to allow the service user choice or overwhelming them with advice in an attempt to protect them. Alternatively, nurses may avoid contact with particular service users, or fail to respond to distress.

SELF-AWARENESS

The process of understanding others begins with understanding the self (see also Ch. 2). 'Self' is a concept

REFLECTION

Reflection is 'a process of consciously examining what has occurred in terms of thoughts, feelings and actions against underlying beliefs, assumptions and knowledge as well as against the backdrop (i.e. the context or the stage) in which specific practice has occurred' (Kim, 1999, p. 1207). Reflection allows nurses to examine both their practice (actions) and the accompanying cognitions (thoughts) and affective meanings (feelings) in relation to values, biases and knowledge and in relation to the context in which the situation occurred. The purpose of reflection is to increase self-awareness, as well as to develop a conscious knowledge base for practice at both the macro and micro levels (Cooke and Matarasso, 2005). Johns (2001, p. 241) suggests that the purpose of reflection is to 'surface contradiction between what [the nurse] intends to achieve within any situation and the way she (*sic*) actually practices'.

Developing reflective practices

Most models of reflection involve three phases (Greenwood, 1998; Johns, 2001; Kim, 1999).

1. In the *descriptive phase*, nurses create descriptive narratives of specific clinical situations. The narratives include descriptions of actions, thoughts and feelings as well as descriptions of the situation and factors surrounding the situation. This process increases the nurse's ability to include self, and the context as well as the specific service user and health problem, in their understanding of the clinical experience. To some extent nurses do this in verbal handovers or in discussion of specific events. In these situations, however, nurses tend to be selective about their responses and the contextual factors.
2. The *reflective phase* involves the comparison of the narrative with the nurse's beliefs, biases and knowledge. This involves the identification of the nurse's knowledge base, as well as values and belief systems, and this allows the identification of gaps in knowledge, as well as previously unexamined beliefs about the service user and the situation, or the role and intentions of the nurse. The potential for further development of knowledge, clinical skills and self-awareness is enhanced by the reflective process.
3. The *critical/emancipatory phase* allows the nurse to identify differences between intentions and actions, thoughts/feelings and espoused values, values and practice, service user needs and the nurse's actions. This phase allows for self-critique, learning and change. It also allows for the development of greater understanding of the influence of the context on the nurse's actions.

PROFESSIONAL BOUNDARIES

Professional nursing boundaries are invisible yet powerful lines that mark the territory of the nurse (see also Chs 2 and 23). Professional boundaries define a role, and allow the nurse to say, 'This is what I do. This is the purpose of my presence here'. Professional boundaries are important in all areas of healthcare, but in mental health nursing they have an increased importance due to the nature of the work of mental health nurses and the vulnerability of the service user population. Over time there has been a decrease in formal divisions between staff and service users in mental health services, with the encouragement of friendliness and collaborative partnerships (Brown et al., 2000). Mental health nurses have to be able to maintain professional boundaries while simultaneously developing close therapeutic relationships with service users based on empathy and positive connectedness.

While many of the interactions and interventions of mental health nurses may appear social in nature (e.g. playing table tennis, cards or volleyball, going for a walk or having a coffee with a service user), it is the therapeutic intent and the conscious awareness of the purpose of the relationship that put them within the professional role. It is when interventions and interactions lose their therapeutic intent and are instead primarily for the benefit of the nurse that professional boundaries are breached. Any breach of professional boundaries has the potential to cause serious harm to service users, and is a violation of professional ethics (Campbell et al., 2005).

Professional boundaries are maintained by the nurse having a clear understanding of his or her therapeutic role, being able to reflect on therapeutic interactions and being able to document and narrate his or her interventions. Maintaining professional boundaries is always the responsibility of the nurse.

Self-disclosure

Mental health nurses use self-disclosure as a way of developing therapeutic relationships with service users. Many of the relationships that nurses have with service users are very long-term, either by repeated admissions to hospital or by continued contact in community settings. In a study of nurse–service user relationships between community mental health nurses and service users with long-term mental health problems, nurses described the use of self-disclosure. 'The nurses used their own experiences of living a life to: be seen as ordinary people; be credible; illustrate aspects of being-in-the world; allow the service users to identify with them; normalize the service user's fears and difficulties' (O'Brien, 2000, p. 188). The service users described the nurse as 'a friend—but different … not like other friends' (O'Brien, 2001, p. 180). The service users were able to identify that the therapeutic relationship was different even though they knew things about the nurse's life (O'Brien, 2001, p. 180). Similarly, Geanellos (2002) noted in a study of adolescent mental health nursing that there was a close relationship between nurses and the adolescent service users. Participants in her study commented that the nurse 'was more like a person than a nurse' (Geanellos, 2002, p. 178), and Welch (2005) also identified self-disclosure as part of the therapeutic relationship.

However, self-disclosure should be used consciously and carefully. The boundary issue is not whether disclosure occurs or does not occur. The issue is the nature of the disclosure and whether the nurse burdens the service user with his or her personal problems. The decision about what to disclose to service users about your life needs to be made in advance. Self-disclosure does not include unburdening one's personal problems. In the above studies these experienced nurse clinicians were able to use their own life experience to relate in ways that were beneficial to service users without overburdening them. The experienced clinicians in these studies also made decisions about what to share with service users according to the length of the relationship and what the service user could use productively.

ETHICAL DILEMMA: PROFESSIONAL BOUNDARIES

You are a newly qualified nurse working in an acute mental health inpatient unit. One evening you admit a 21-year-old woman (Kellie) to the ward. Kellie has been in a car accident and has several compound fractures to her right leg. She is in traction and so is to be nursed in bed. She has been admitted to the mental health ward because she has previously been diagnosed with paranoid schizophrenia. Though she is currently 'stable' from a mental health perspective, she has been admitted to the unit because the orthopaedic ward staff felt they could not give her adequate care.

Kellie settles into the ward well, and passes her time with knitting, watching television and enjoying the company of visitors and other inpatients in the unit. After a few days, when you are on afternoon shift, you notice that one of your colleagues is sitting at Kellie's bedside. On reflection you realize that this colleague has been spending quite a bit of time with Kellie since she was admitted, even staying and chatting to her well after the end of shift. At about 7 p.m. you approach the colleague (who should have gone off at 3.45 on completion of the morning shift) to ask if they know Kellie personally. The colleague replies, 'No, not personally, but we get on pretty well and my ex-girlfriend had mental health problems too'.

Questions

1. What are the main issues here?
2. Are any ethical issues involved? If so, what are they?
3. What could you do in this situation?

STRESS AND BURNOUT

Stress

Stress is a physiological response to any stressor or demand (Cohen, 2000) and a fact of life for everyone. When a person experiences a stressor, their homeostasis is disturbed and their body activates a stress response. Any foundational anatomy and physiology textbook can provide details of the stress response. For the purposes of this chapter it is enough to understand that the stress response involves the release of substances into the blood that cause a range of physiological changes including changes to heart rate, blood pressure and the gastrointestinal tract. Prolonged stress can be harmful and can have a negative effect on physical and mental health.

Stress can be experienced as negative (*distress*) or positive (*eustress*). A stressful event can have a positive effect, because it can be a catalyst for a person to make changes such as learning new skills, or a stimulant to some sort of positive action (Thorpe and Barsky, 2001). Individuals can respond differently to the same stressor. For example, say you and a friend need to travel from England to Jersey, and the only means of travel available is a light aircraft. You might find the thought of flying in a light aircraft stressful and anxiety-provoking, but your friend might find it exhilarating and exciting. Both you and your friend are experiencing stress reactions, but are experiencing them very differently.

Like other professions that involve close and sustained engagement with people, nursing is innately stressful (Coffey and Coleman, 2001). Mental health nurses frequently encounter situations that are tense and unpredictable, and these factors are known to increase stress levels (McGowan, 2001). In addition, therapeutic relationships can last for considerable periods of time and can be incredibly challenging at times. It is very important, then, to learn to monitor and manage your own stress, because unchecked stress can become chronic and can result in burnout syndrome (Melchior et al., 1996).

Burnout syndrome

The words 'burnout' and 'stress' are often seen together, because stress is seen as a precursor to burnout. However, stress is a feature of life and, when managed properly, does not lead to burnout. Unlike stress, which has some positive features (it can be a catalyst for effecting positive change such as learning a new skill), burnout has no positive aspects for the person experiencing it or for those around them. The term burnout was first seen in the literature in the mid-to-late 1970s, and burnout is widely considered to be a contributing factor to the current worldwide nursing shortage (Haddad, 2002).

Burnout is used to describe a pattern of emotional exhaustion, depersonalization and decreased personal accomplishment: together these three components are sometimes called 'burnout syndrome' (Melchior et al., 1996). While the effects of emotional exhaustion will vary from person to person, feelings of depression, irritability, a sense that one has nothing more to give and of being emotionally overwhelmed by work are commonly described (Barling, 2001; Haddad, 2002). Depersonalization can lead to unkind, indifferent, uninterested, deprecating, belittling and/or distant responses to service users (Barling, 2001; Haddad, 2002). It is not difficult to imagine how distressing it would be for a service user to be nursed by someone who responded to them and their situation in a cold and unfeeling way rather than with the warmth, caring, empathy and respect we ourselves would wish for if we were sick and needing care. The third element of burnout syndrome – reduced personal accomplishment – describes feelings of ineffectiveness, ineptitude, low satisfaction and a perceived lack of success in work (Barling, 2001).

It can be seen that burnout syndrome is an undesirable state, not only because of the detrimental influence it has on nurse–service user interaction, but also because of the negative effects on the affected nurse and his or her immediate colleagues. It has also been associated with diminished work performance, increased staff turnover and misuse of drugs and alcohol (Ewers et al., 2002). From the perspective of the affected person, there is nothing worse than going to work when feeling unhappy and distressed. Working with colleagues who are irritable, depressed and exhausted adds to everyone's stress. When people are experiencing emotional exhaustion and reduced personal accomplishment, it is difficult for them to work effectively as a team member. They may feel too lacking in creative energy to perform properly in some areas. For example, irritability might compromise a nurse's ability to mentor and support a novice or inexperienced nurse effectively.

Nurses are considered to be particularly susceptible to burnout syndrome because of the nature of nursing work, which involves a high level of close contact with people who are often in emotionally charged situations (such as when they or a loved one are experiencing sickness, pain, anxiety or exhaustion) as well as factors such as lack of autonomy and high workload, which are also common hallmarks of the nursing workplace (Jackson et al., 2002). Mental health nursing involves long periods of working in intensely stressful situations, which may be exacerbated by the environment (e.g. secured areas), and the literature suggests that these factors make burnout an issue of particular concern to mental health nurses (Ewers et al., 2002; Melchoir et al., 1996). The task for nurses, therefore, is to develop strategies to avoid getting burnout syndrome. Haddad (2002) positions burnout syndrome as an ethical issue in nursing, and considers that all nurses have a moral imperative to reduce burnout by taking active steps to avoid burnout in themselves.

Avoiding burnout syndrome

Burnout syndrome has been repeatedly linked to the current shortage of nurses and so there have been many research studies and published research reports on ways in which nurses can reduce burnout syndrome or avoid getting it. Most of these reports acknowledge two main areas that can be manipulated to avoid burnout: aspects of the individual nurse, and the environment in which the nurse works. It is important that we each learn to know ourselves and our limitations. In nursing we are often encouraged to develop reflective skills, and these are very helpful in learning to understand ourselves and our own responses to stressors (Thorpe and Barsky, 2001). If we are aware that we are becoming moody, irritable or short-tempered, or that we are not feeling empathetic towards service users, then this can be an indication that it is time to step back and reflect on the situation (Haddad, 2002). Most healthcare facilities provide a range of measures to assist staff, and these include debriefing, counselling and other measures.

It is important to extend the same care to ourselves that we offer to those in our care. Nursing is a high-stress profession and therefore it is necessary to be active in managing stress. Several factors have been identified as protective against burnout and other negative sequelae resulting from workplace adversity, and these include hardiness, optimism, nurturing relationships and networks, emotional insight and achieving life balance (Jackson et al., 2007). Although it can be difficult to fit leisure activities around shift work and study, it is important to maintain a balanced and healthy lifestyle, and take the time to participate in enjoyable leisure activities. Continuing to learn and develop skills can also be effective. Ewers et al. (2002) undertook a study investigating whether psychosocial intervention training affected the levels of burnout in forensic mental health nurses. Their findings suggested that staff undergoing intervention training showed a significant decrease in burnout rates. Although individuals can do things to reduce their risk of burnout, institutional practices are strongly implicated in nurses' susceptibility to burnout syndrome, and Haddad (2002) clearly positions burnout as a systemic problem rather than an individual one. Therefore it is also important to ensure that institutions and managers adopt policies and practices that support nurses rather than contribute to stress and burnout.

PROFESSIONAL SUPPORTIVE RELATIONSHIPS

Clinical supervision

Clinical supervision is a process that focuses on the clinical work of the nurse. It provides an arena in which the nurse can reflect with another experienced clinician on their clinical interactions and interventions. Fowler and Chevannes (1998) note that there is a high degree of compatibility between reflective practice and clinical supervision. Johns (2001) suggests that the success of reflective practice in creating change depends on the relationship between practitioner and supervisor. The purpose of clinical supervision is professional support, education and professional development, and enhancement of the quality of clinical practice (Mullarkey et al., 2001). Clinical supervision is not limited to review of case work or of actions, but provides an opportunity for nurses to reflect upon the subjective experience of their work (Rafferty, 2000). In order to develop the nurse's capacity for empathy, acceptance, nurturing and honest reflection, the clinical supervisor needs to be able to model these capacities in their relationship with the supervisee.

Preceptorship

Preceptorship is a supportive, formative professional relationship developed between nurses (McCloughen et al., 2006) and is usually based in the clinical area. It is a '... period of structured transition for the newly registered practitioner during which he or she will be supported by a preceptor, to develop their confidence as an autonomous professional, refine skills, values and behaviours and to continue on their journey of life-long learning' (Department of Health, 2010, p. 11). Newly qualified nurses are routinely allocated a preceptor. The preceptor will generally be a nurse with considerable experience in a particular clinical environment, and will usually have completed specialized in-service training to prepare for the preceptoring role. They will understand the difficulties and challenges facing people who are new to the area, and they will assist you to develop skills and confidence, and facilitate your becoming part of the team in the particular area (Freiburger, 2002). Preceptorship also provides an additional avenue for debriefing and feedback that can help in dealing effectively with confusing or upsetting incidents. You will remain under the guidance of the preceptor for a set period of time (usually between 6 months and a year; Department of Health, 2010) or until you feel confident to take your place as a fully independent and functioning member of the team. Preceptors tend to be attached to particular services, so if you move to a new area you will likely be working with a different preceptor.

NURSE'S STORY: CLINICAL SUPERVISION

Marietta is working in an acute inpatient unit. She has 2 years' experience. She arrives at clinical supervision saying that she feels angry with one of her service users, a young woman with a diagnosis of depression who self-harms.

She had spent considerable time with the service user in the preceding days, and felt that she had developed a good relationship with her. Last night after she had gone home, the service user had cut her arms with a razor blade. Today the service user is belligerent, appearing to take delight in having 'fooled' the nurses. Marietta says that the other staff have reinforced her belief that she was 'sucked in' and she is now confused about how to proceed with this service user.

The supervisor asks Marietta to tell in detail the story of what happened. She then asks Marietta to outline her feelings about, and knowledge of, the service user before and after the incident. The supervisor listens attentively and empathically, encouraging further exploration of the incident and Marietta's feelings about it. Marietta admits to feeling guilty, and is concerned that she may have said or done something to provoke the incident. Together they consider how the service user might have been feeling and what possible triggers to self-harm might have existed. They go on to consider what Marietta saw as important in developing the relationship with the service user. The supervisor suggests some reading that Marietta can undertake to increase her understanding of self-harm-related behaviours. Together they identify what might be the goals of nursing interventions with this service user. Marietta resolves to talk to the service user about how the service user was feeling last night and what provoked the self-harm incident.

As with all relationships, certain qualities are needed by both parties, including commitment, honesty, integrity and effective interpersonal skills. Preceptors need additional skills, such as problem-solving, clinical currency and expertise, appropriate scholarly, administrative or research expertise, the ability to provide constructive criticism and other feedback, understanding of professional boundaries and relationships, and the ability to maintain confidentiality where appropriate.

CONCLUSION

This chapter has introduced some of the core concepts and ideas that shape and inform mental health nursing practice. To be effective and therapeutic in caring for others, nurses must understand such concepts as caring, hope and spirituality. Stress and burnout are hazards for nurses and others in the caring professions and therefore nurses must learn to recognize and manage their own stress. Therapeutic relationships lie at the heart of mental health nursing, and a clear understanding of professional boundaries is crucial to the development and ongoing sustainability of such relationships.

Mental health nursing is an exciting and challenging area of nursing practice. Effective mental health nursing requires the culmination of all your skills as well as your professional and life experiences, and it offers a stimulating and rewarding career path. As we strive to meet the complex needs of diverse communities, and provide care within increasingly restrictive economic environments, there are many challenges before us. Developing positive personal qualities such as self-awareness, and fostering productive and supportive collegial relationships, will help us to meet the challenges that lie ahead.

EXERCISE FOR CLASS ENGAGEMENT

An effective way of developing self-awareness is the use of questioning. To raise your awareness of some important issues, ask yourself the following questions, then discuss your responses with other members of your group or class.

♦ What kinds of values do I hold important as a framework for living? Where do these values come from? How do they inform my understanding of what it is to be a person in this world?

♦ How has my family of origin influenced how I view the world? What values did my family hold as important? What do I see as important in family life?

♦ What do I know about why I choose to be a nurse?

♦ What are the pervading social attitudes towards people in mental distress or with mental health problems? What are my beliefs about people in mental distress or with mental health problems?

♦ What experiences have I had that influence how I feel about people with mental health problems?

REFERENCES

Barling, J., 2001. Drowning not waving: burnout and mental health nursing. Contemp. Nurse 11 (2/3), 247–259.

Brown, B., Crawford, P., Darongkamas, J., 2000. Blurred roles and permeable boundaries: the experience of multidisciplinary working in community mental health. Health Soc. Care Community 8 (6), 425–435.

Campbell, J., Yonge, O., Austin, W., 2005. Intimacy boundaries between mental health nurses and psychiatric patients. J. Psychosoc. Nurs. Ment. Health Serv. 43 (5), 32–39.

Coffey, M., Coleman, M., 2001. The relationship between support and stress in forensic community mental health nursing. J. Adv. Nurs. 34 (3), 397–407.

Cohen, J., 2000. Stress and mental health: a biobehavioral perspective. Issues Ment. Health Nurs. 21 (2), 285–302.

Cooke, M., Matarasso, B., 2005. Promoting reflection in mental health nursing practice: a case illustration using problem-based learning. Int. J. Ment. Health Nurs. 14 (4), 243–248.

Crawford, P., Nolan, P., Brown, B., 1998. Ministering to madness: the narratives of people who have left religious orders to work in the caring professions. J. Adv. Nurs. 28 (1), 212–220.

Cutcliffe, J., Koehn, C., 2007. Hope and interpersonal psychiatric/mental health nursing: a systematic review of the literature, Part 2. J. Psychiatr. Ment. Health Nurs. 14, 141–147.

Daly, J., Jackson, D., Davidson, P., 1999. The experience of hope for survivors of acute myocardial infarction. Aust. J. Adv. Nurs. 16 (3), 38–44.

Davis, L.W., Lysaker, P.H., 2007. Therapeutic alliance and improvements in work performance over time in patients with schizophrenia. J. Nerv. Ment. Dis. 195 (4), 353–357.

Department of Health, 2010. Preceptorship framework. <http://www.rcn.org.uk/__data/assets/pdf_file/0010/307756/Preceptorship_framework.pdf>.

Dunlop, M., 1986. Is a science of caring possible? J. Adv. Nurs. 11 (3), 661–670.

Ewers, P., Bradshaw, T., McGovern, J., et al., 2002. Does training in psychosocial interventions reduce burnout rates in forensic nursing? J. Adv. Nurs. 37 (5), 470–476.

Fitzgerald Miller, J., 2007. Hope: a construct central to nursing. Nurs. Forum 42 (1), 12–19.

Forchuk, C., Reynolds, W., 2001. Clients' reflections on relationships with nurses: comparisons from Canada and Scotland. J. Psychiatr. Ment. Health Nurs. 8, 45–51.

Foster, K., McAllister, M., O'Brien, L., 2006. Extending the boundaries: autoethnography as an emergent method in mental health nursing research. Int. J. Ment. Health Nurs. 15, 44–53.

Fowler, J., Chevannes, M., 1998. Evaluating the efficacy of reflective practice within the context of clinical supervision. J. Adv. Nurs. 27, 379–382.

Freiburger, O., 2002. Preceptor programs: increasing student self-confidence and competency. Nurse Educ. 27 (2), 58–60.

Gallop, R., O'Brien, L., 2003. Re-establishing psychodynamic theory as foundational knowledge for psychiatric/mental health nursing. Issues Ment. Health Nurs. 24, 213–227.

Geanellos, R., 2002. Transformative change of self: the unique focus of (adolescent) mental health nursing?

Int. J. Ment. Health Nurs. 11, 174–185.

Goddard, N., 1995. 'Spirituality as integrative energy': a philosophical analysis as requisite precursor to holistic nursing practice. J. Adv. Nurs. 22 (4), 808–815.

Godin, P., 2000. A dirty business: caring for people who are a nuisance or a danger. J. Adv. Nurs. 32 (6), 1396–1402.

Graham, I., 2001. Seeking a clarification of meaning: a phenomenological interpretation of the craft of mental health nursing. J. Psychiatr. Ment. Health Nurs. 8, 335–345.

Greasley, P., Chiu, L.F., Gartland, M., 2001. The concept of spiritual care in mental health nursing. J. Adv. Nurs. 33 (5), 629–637.

Greenwood, J., 1998. The role of reflection in single and double loop learning. J. Adv. Nurs. 27, 1048–1053.

Haddad, A., 2002. An ethical view of burnout. RN 65 (9), 25–26, 28.

Heifner, C., 1993. Positive connectedness in the psychiatric nurse–patient relationship. Arch. Psychiatr. Nurs. 7 (1), 11–15.

Hewitt, J., Coffey, M., 2005. Therapeutic working relationships with people with schizophrenia. J. Adv. Nurs. 52 (5), 561–570.

Jackson, D., Borbasi, S.-A., 2006. Nursing care and nurse caring: issues, concerns, debates. In: Daly, J., Speedy, S., Jackson, D. (Eds.), Contexts of Nursing: An Introduction, second ed. Elsevier, Sydney.

Jackson, D., Clare, J., Mannix, J., 2002. Who would want to be a nurse? Violence in the workplace: a factor in recruitment and retention. J. Nurs. Manag. 10 (1), 13–20.

Jackson, D., Firtko, A., Edenborough, M., 2007. Personal resilience as a strategy for surviving and thriving in the face of workplace adversity: a review of the literature. J. Adv. Nurs. 60 (1), 1–9.

Johns, C., 2001. Reflective practice: revealing the [he]art of caring. Int. J. Nurs. Pract. 7 (4), 237–245.

Kim, H.S., 1999. Critical reflective inquiry for knowledge development in nursing practice. J. Adv. Nurs. 29 (5), 1205–1212.

Koehn, C., Cutcliffe, J., 2007. Hope and interpersonal psychiatric/mental health nursing: a systematic review of the literature, Part 1. J. Psychiatr. Ment. Health Nurs. 14, 134–140.

McCloughen, A., O'Brien, L., Jackson, D., 2006. Positioning mentorship within Australian nursing contexts: a review of the local and international literature. Contemp. Nurse 23 (1), 120–134.

McGowan, B., 2001. Self-reported stress and its effects on nurses. Nurs. Stand. 15 (42), 33–38.

Melchior, M., Philipsen, H., Abu-Saad, H.H., et al., 1996. The effectiveness of primary nursing on burnout among psychiatric nurses in long-stay settings. J. Adv. Nurs. 24 (4), 694–702.

Meleis, A.I., 2007. Theoretical Nursing: Development and Progress, fourth ed. Lippincott, Philadelphia.

Mullarkey, K., Keeley, P., Playle, J.F., 2001. Multiprofessional clinical supervision: challenges for mental health nurses. J. Psychiatr. Ment. Health Nurs. 8, 205–211.

O'Brien, L., 2000. Nurse–client relationships: the experience of community psychiatric nurses. Aust. N. Z. J. Ment. Health Nurs. 9, 184–194.

O'Brien, L., 2001. The relationship between community psychiatric nurses and clients with severe and persistent mental illness: the client experience. Aust. N. Z. J. Ment. Health Nurs. 10, 176–186.

Rafferty, M.A., 2000. A conceptual model for clinical supervision in nursing and health visiting based on Winnicott's (1960) theory of parent–infant relationship. J. Psychiatr. Ment. Health Nurs. 7, 153–161.

Shattell, M.M., McAllister, S., Hogan, B., et al., 2006. 'She took the time to make sure she understood': mental health patients' experiences of being understood. Arch. Psychiatr. Nurs. 20 (5), 234–241.

Speedy, S., 2006. The gendered culture of nursing. In: Daly, J., Speedy, S., Jackson, D. (Eds.), Contexts of Nursing: An Introduction, second ed. Elsevier, Sydney.

Stephenson, C., 1991. The concept of hope revisited for nursing. J. Adv. Nurs. 16, 1456–1461.

Thompson, I., 2002. Mental health and spiritual care. Nurs. Stand. 17 (9), 33–38.

Thorpe, K., Barsky, J., 2001. Healing through self-reflection. J. Adv. Nurs. 35 (5), 760–768.

Warelow, P., Edward, K., 2007. Caring as resilient practice in mental health nursing. Int. J. Ment. Health Nurs. 16, 132–135.

Weaver, K., 2007. Ethical sensitivity: a state of knowledge and needs for further research. Nurs. Ethics 14 (2), 141–155.

Welch, M., 2005. Pivotal moments in the therapeutic relationship. Int. J. Ment. Health Nurs. 14, 161–165.

Chapter | 2 |

The context of practice

Vicki Stanton and Barbara Tooth

CHAPTER POINTS

- The context of mental health nursing practice is dynamic and ever-changing, responding to new ideas about what people need to have a meaningful life.
- The ultimate goal of mental health practice is to value the worth and facilitate the capacity of all people to be active participants in society, and to provide the range of resources that will help them to remain active citizens in the community of their choice, even during periods of mental distress.
- The quality of a person's relationships is a key determinant of their quality of life.
- Theories of mental health and mental health practice aim to influence people's attitudes, values and beliefs.
- Mental health nursing practice is ultimately influenced by the attitudes, values and beliefs of the nurse, and is developed through general life experiences, education and interaction with people who experience mental distress.
- The ability to think critically and develop self-awareness is central to nursing practice.
- The recovery paradigm addresses the issues necessary for people to have a meaningful life and provides the context and guiding principles for all mental health practice.

DOI: http://dx.doi.org/10.1016/B978-0-7020-4493-9.00002-0

- The recovery paradigm reconceptualizes the roles of mental health professionals.
- National and international laws protecting people's basic human rights provide the legal context for recovery-orientated practice within the recovery paradigm.
- Mental health policy and plans provide the sociopolitical context for practice and the implementation of services that, ideally, are based on the recovery paradigm.

KEY TERMS

- citizenship
- community
- deficits
- dualism
- health and wellness
- holism
- illness
- multidisciplinary teams
- partnerships
- professional boundaries
- recovery
- rehabilitation
- resilience
- self-help
- service users
- stigma
- strengths
- third-sector and non-government organizations

LEARNING OUTCOMES

The material in this chapter will assist you to:

- demonstrate an understanding of the role that your attitudes, values and beliefs play as key factors in what you say and do when you work with people, and of the role of theories and life experiences in this process,
- begin to appreciate the complex interaction between the current contexts that influence mental health practice,
- identify the key differences in the way nurses conceptualize their role and their practice between the recovery and medical paradigms,
- describe the principles of recovery-orientated practice,
- explain the rationale for the shift in mental health to the recovery paradigm, which values the primary role of expert knowledge that comes from the lived experience of severe mental distress,
- identify the underlying concepts of dichotomous practices such as holism/dualism, wellness/illness and strengths/deficits,
- appreciate the value of reflective practice and continually developing self-awareness,
- understand the importance of maintaining a person's citizenship rights and the implications for recovery-orientated practice.

INTRODUCTION

This chapter discusses some of the fundamental concepts and principles underlying what nurses do and say when they work with people, particularly people with mental health needs. It builds on the previous chapter by reinforcing the importance of reflection in order for nurses to become competent practitioners, and it provides a context for the chapters that follow.

To make sense of mental health nursing practice requires an understanding of the factors that can influence it. These include mental health policy and plans, current theories about the various aspects of mental health and mental health practice, social and cultural factors, and the attitudes, values and beliefs that guide our thinking. People's thinking changes over time and this is determined by the experiences they have had and by changes in thinking about what constitutes appropriate practice. In mental health in the past few decades, the rate of change in thinking about practice has been significant. This chapter addresses some of the major shifts in thinking that influence our understanding of what mental health nursing practice entails, the rationale behind *why* it is approached in this way, *how* it is put into practice, and the settings *where* nurses are likely to practise.

It can be tempting to think that mental health nursing is a discrete area of practice of little value to the other fields of nursing (adult, child and learning disabilities), but this is far from the truth. The fundamental concepts and principles underlying mental health nursing are considered so important to general practice that they have been incorporated into all nursing courses in the UK with the intention of ensuring a holistic approach to nursing care. In addition, one in four people in the UK will experience mental distress severe enough to be diagnosed and warrant intervention from a mental health professional. Physical illness exacerbates such distress and people cannot isolate parts of themselves in their interactions with general health professionals. It stands to reason therefore that general nurses frequently work with people in mental distress.

THE RELATIONSHIP BETWEEN THEORY AND PRACTICE

To begin to make sense of professional nursing practice requires an understanding of the relationship between theory and practice.

What is a theory?

Theories provide the rationale for the actions that guide our practice.

- A theory is a set of constructs, hypotheses, principles and propositions about specific phenomena and how they relate to one another.
- A theory is not a statement of fact, nor is it the whole truth, because it excludes what it judges to be of little or no importance.
- A theory is therefore only one perspective.
- Theories can be either *formal* (written with detailed support and presented to others in the field) or *informal* (residing in people's conscious or subconscious thoughts).
- Theories generate hypotheses about specific phenomena that can be tested to determine the theory's usefulness, predictive ability or 'fit'.

The last point is important to understand because theories can be revised, built on by others or disproved as a result of applying the principles of the theory to practice and evaluating their usefulness and fit. For example, theories promoting *dualism* (mind and body as separate and independent entities) were dominant in medicine for some time but their limitations are now widely acknowledged. *Holism* (mind and body cannot be separated) now provides the best fit.

The concepts of dualism and holism will be discussed later, but the example illustrates the fact that theories are not static. They are time- and context-specific and tell the reader about the theorist's thoughts on a subject based on their comprehensive knowledge and experience in a specific topic at that time. Theories also give us insights into how individual theorists make sense of their world: behind every theory is the person who proposed it. Knowing something of the person's background and experience can help to put the theory into context and provide a framework for making sense of the range of theories about certain phenomena. This framework also helps to demystify theories and their role in practice.

In fact, we are all theorists (albeit informal theorists). Consciously or subconsciously we make hypotheses (propositions to explain specific phenomena) about ourselves, others, situations and larger world events, and we make predictions about what will happen in the future based on our past life experiences. Testing these hypotheses will either support our predictions or make it clear that we need to revise them. This also holds true in nursing practice, where nurses have been found to be theorizers of their everyday practice (Cox et al., 1991; Graham, 2000).

Which theory best guides practice?

How do newly qualified nurses determine which formal theory is most appropriate for their nursing practice? It is not a question of deciding which theory is right or wrong, but rather of appreciating that there can be a number of ways of understanding a particular phenomenon. Nursing is just one of a number of disciplines in the field of mental health. There is a general body of knowledge in mental health and each discipline draws on this to expand the understanding of practice issues. In turn there are discipline-specific theories that add to the existing body of knowledge. These various theories can complement or contradict each other, or express similar ideas but use different language to do so, but all theories expand our understanding of specific phenomena, and each has valid points. They can provide richness and depth that is invaluable in professional practice and life in general. However, theories and perspectives are time-limited because nothing is static and change is inevitable.

Nursing theorists

A significant number of nurses have written about nursing practice, beginning with Florence Nightingale. It is only recently, however, that nurses have moved from writing about *what* they do, to writing about *how* and *why* they do it. There are now a number of nursing theorists who provide a broad range of ideas, and this can be overwhelming for the student nurse. It is the application of these theories to practice that determines their usefulness. To help make sense of nursing theorists, Alligood and Tomey (2002) have outlined a method of ranking the different theorists into three categories.

1. *Philosophies*: this category uses higher-order constructs and propositions about the nature of nursing. An example is Rogers (1970), who defines nursing as a holistic science of human nature and development.
2. *Conceptual models/grand theories*: these theories are more practically derived and suppose an outcome. Examples are Henderson's theory (1966), which focuses on outcomes of nursing care, and Orem's theory (1971), which establishes the notion of self-care as integral to nursing.
3. *Middle-range theories*: these more closely describe practice issues for nursing (McEwan and Wills, 2002). Peplau's 1952 theory (reprinted in 1988) focuses on therapeutic interpersonal processes in the nurse–service user relationship, and has been very influential in mental health nursing.

The Tidal Model (Barker, 2001) draws heavily from the body of knowledge in the emerging recovery paradigm and is an appropriate theory to guide mental health nursing practice. It was originally developed for mental health nursing because of the need for a paradigm shift in mental healthcare. It now extends to all disciplines and areas of mental health. The Tidal Model acknowledges that the concept of 'mental illness' can be viewed in a number of ways, but asserts the value of seeing such phenomena primarily as problems of living rather than as the consequence of a mysterious illness (Barker and Buchanan-Barker, 2004). 'By emphasizing the centrality of the lived-experience, of the person and his/her significant others, the need for mutual understanding between nurse and the person in care is also acknowledged and the need for a personally appropriate, contextually bound form of care, established' (Barker and Buchanan-Barker, 2004, p. 7). Basically the Tidal Model is moving from solving problems *for* the person to finding solutions *with* the person. The Tidal Model develops Peplau's theory on the nurse–patient relationship, with emphasis on finding pragmatic ways in which people learn what works for them and why (Buchanan-Barker, 2004).

As mentioned previously, theories reflect the theorist's world view at the time of writing. So a comparison of Florence Nightingale with a recent nursing theorist would demonstrate the constantly evolving nature of theory within a dynamic social context and in response to reflections on nursing practice. Theorists have contributed to the body of knowledge that describes nursing practice, leading to improvements in the discipline of nursing.

Incorporating theory into practice: the personal context

How then do nursing students make sense of what they read and incorporate this into their practice? This requires the ability to:

- think critically,
- continually develop your self-awareness,
- identify your values, beliefs and attitudes and appreciate their origin,
- modify your values, beliefs and attitudes,
- tolerate and even embrace ambiguity,
- *actively* participate in the quest for knowledge,
- remain open to the need to modify your practice and your role in light of the above.

The ability to think critically is essential. Critical thinking is an ongoing process that requires an open mind on a whole range of views. Just as important as the ability to think critically is the awareness that we are more likely to favour those theories that provide the 'best fit' with our already developed world view. We do this to alleviate the anxiety we will experience if we choose a theory that is inconsistent with our already established thoughts. This

is a normal subconscious process but it can trap the nurse in a comfort zone that leads to lack of awareness, narrow and blinkered approaches to practice, and a reluctance to be open to new ideas and practices. This is an important concept to understand in the lifelong activity of becoming more self-aware.

The requirement to be self-aware and to think critically about the basis for practice can be frustrating for nursing students because there is no clear step-by-step 'cookbook'. Understandably, when nursing students come onto a course they want to be told what it is they need to learn and *do* in this new area so they can be effective and feel competent. It is not uncommon for students to want to collect a 'bag of skills' to prepare them for everyday practice. Nurses want to know what they can do to people so they can feel competent and alleviate the ambiguity about their practice and their own anxiety. Students can become impatient and disgruntled if these skills are not given up front, and the course can be seen as ineffective or even useless. This is more likely to occur in students who prefer to be passive recipients rather than active participants in their professional development.

Your attitudes, values and beliefs underlie what you do and say when you work with people. It is these personal informal theories developed through your life experiences, both personal and professional, that provide the foundation for practice and determine which formal theories are more appealing to you. It is only with increasing self-awareness, critical thinking and personal reflection that the continual process of construction and reconstruction takes place and competent professional nursing practices develop. This is a lifelong process.

The importance of reflection

Teaching skills by themselves will not improve clinical competence or performance. Reflection, also discussed in Chapter 1, is a professional requirement at all levels of clinical practice by the UK's Nursing and Midwifery Council. Reflective practice involves learning from our experiences and from others and developing our practice as a result (Jasper and Elliot, 2006). Reflection affects nurses' individual understanding of a range of practice issues, increases awareness and clarifies aspects of themselves and their role. It involves being open to new challenges and seeking new opportunities. This very much reflects a nurse's capacity and willingness to be open to change in attitude and thinking.

Within the emerging recovery paradigm, a significant amount of learning is gained from our interactions and relationships with people who have the lived experience of mental distress. Mental health professionals have much to learn from them about the nature of mental distress and the most important factors in helping them to get on with their lives in a way that is meaningful to them. We also learn about how we help, and frequently hinder, their self-directed recovery. Reflection, critical thinking and analysis are essential skills enabling all those involved in mental healthcare to evaluate and incorporate evolving knowledge into their practice.

Reflection is a personal activity. When reflection takes place in groups (reflexivity), important dialogue between nurses about what they have learned can affect the shared meaning of the group. It enables not only the development of tacit (unspoken) knowledge in the nursing student but also its articulation by experienced nurses. Welsh and Lyons (2001) found that if nurses were asked why they performed in certain ways they were able to provide a rationale. Intuition comes with exposure to a whole range of situations and people over time, and this tacit knowledge complements nursing knowledge. It is 'increasingly evident that it is far more than just theoretical knowledge that informs the practice of expert nurses' (Crook, 2001, p. 4). Articulation of experienced nurses' tacit knowledge allows it to be examined and verified (Welsh and Lyons, 2001). This helps validate more of what actually happens in practice and thereby complements evidence-based practice.

Putting theory into practice: the wider context

The implementation of practice based on theory is not straightforward. Practice settings can be complex because they require mediation between people with different views, philosophies, beliefs and ways of interpreting what is required for effective mental health practice. Added to this is the influence of political, social, cultural and environmental constraints. Some political imperatives are short-lived, while others are more embedded in the economic and social fabric of politics. These are more significant than management trends and far less open to modification. The current political imperative for evidence-based practice is one such trend. It has particular implications for mental health practice, and these are discussed here.

Demand for evidence-based practice

In most of the Western world there is a demand that only those practices that have been shown to be effective be sanctioned in the provision of healthcare. This is known as *evidence-based practice*. Although there is a valid argument for this and intuitively it makes sense, it can be problematic in the provision of truly effective and meaningful mental healthcare, and it raises a number of issues that warrant further discussion.

Issues for discussion

1. Evidence-based practice is based solely on observable practices validated using the scientific method.

The scientific method requires that practices, their rationale and the theories behind them be clearly identified and documented. The only form of practice (treatment) that meets this criterion is that which can be observed and measured (this is known as quantitative research). The 'treatment' must then be 'tested' (this is known as empirical evidence) and this is usually done through 'randomized controlled trials'. In such studies, users of health services are divided into two groups. The first group is known as the treatment group and, as the name suggests, they receive the treatment that is the object of the study. The second group is known as the control group: they are matched to the treatment group for factors such as age, gender and status but they do not receive the treatment. Both groups are monitored for changes in exactly the same way, usually by various types of well-defined outcome measures. Only that which can be 'objectively' observed or measured is considered valid and reliable. The measures for the two groups are then compared to determine whether the treatment has been effective.

Although there is a valid argument for this approach, there is an equally strong argument that interpersonal relationships, intuition and tacit knowledge (unspoken knowledge), which are ignored by the scientific method, are invaluable in improving the quality of mental healthcare and nursing care in particular. For example, the nature of the interactions between nurses and the people with whom they work is very important in determining outcome. This has not been comprehensively studied within nursing but it has in research on the outcomes of psychotherapy, which is very similar in nature. This research has consistently found that the 'non-specifics of psychotherapy' (genuineness, respect, being human, using non-possessive warmth and unconditional love) are the most important in determining outcome (Hubble et al., 1999). These findings are important for the following reasons.

- It is not the (measurable) techniques that the professional uses, but factors to do with the nature of the relationship between professional and person, that are critical.
- In their relationships with people, professionals do use their intuition and unspoken knowledge base (tacit knowledge).
- What appears to be the key factor in determining a good outcome is the ability to use our humanness in a way that is healing.
- The above cannot be measured using the quantitative scientific method required for evidence-based practice as described above.

2. Evidence-based practice comes from the validated expert knowledge of professionals.

Evidence-based practice is derived from the expert knowledge of professionals and what they believe to be important in treatment. Professionals decide what is important to study and they also devise the treatments used in research. Evidence-based practice does not come from the expert knowledge of people with the lived experience of mental distress and what works for them.

In contrast, phenomenological researchers suspend this expert position and are more interested in exploring and describing individual meanings about phenomena, or their narratives about experience. In similar contrast to the reductionism of the quantitative scientific method, qualitative researchers tend to cast a much broader net to help in understanding the much bigger picture of all the complexities that make up people's lives within a social and cultural context. Unfortunately it is all too common for 'professional experts' to discount people's lived experience as unimportant because it is subjective and cannot be validated, and therefore it is omitted. Yet there is strong evidence (Roberts, 2000) that valuing people's stories is essential to improving outcome, and this is the essence of the narrative approach in mental health.

3. Resolving the tension.

There is no debate about whether people have the right to interventions/practices that have been shown to be effective. There is debate about what constitutes sound methodology, appropriate areas of research and types of interventions/practices to be studied. In reality there has always been tension between those who support the quantitative scientific method and those who support qualitative methods and believe that, due to the complexity and uniqueness of what it means to be human, such experimental research is meaningless. Qualitative research is the predominant methodology in recovery research.

Rather than arguing for the benefit of one approach over the other, it is more useful to acknowledge the tension between the two approaches and then move on to appreciating how they may complement one another. For example, there is a wealth of information in first-person accounts of people's recovery that has led to a consensus about the values and principles of service delivery that promote recovery. Farkas et al. (2005) argue for evidence-based practices to be implemented in a manner that is compatible with recovery, by researching the dimensions of recovery practice – including the programme's mission, policies, procedures, record keeping, staff selection, training and supervision, quality assurance, physical setting and network – to determine whether it is recovery-orientated. Such dimensions could be the subject of quantitative research, while qualitative research of people's experience of such services would provide a more complete overview of the service and its impact.

The following section outlines some of the major changes in thinking about mental health practice and continues the theme of providing a context for understanding nursing practice issues.

CHANGING BELIEFS ABOUT THE FOCUS OF NURSING PRACTICE

From dualism to holism

Dualism is derived from the Cartesian idea (Rene Descartes 1596–1650) that there is a mind–body duality, the body being a passive agent or vehicle with an immortal soul separate and absolutely distinct from the body. The concept of dualism has made the body the domain of medicine, and the soul or moral features (mind) of the individual the domain of religion and philosophy.

Failure to see the interdependence (holism) of the mind and body has led to the view of the body as a machine, with technical advances in science considered the necessary interest of medicine. This view suggests that only scientifically observable phenomena and technical knowledge are valued (Short et al., 1994). This view forms the basis of the argument for evidence-based medicine. Within this paradigm medicine, including psychiatry, has increasingly focused on the person's symptoms to the exclusion of most other things.

Dualism: issues for mental health practice

In a dualistic approach to mental health practice:

*   health professionals are taught to look for *illnesses* and *syndromes* (a collection of symptoms) and to value only that which can be observed (the basis of evidence-based practice),
*   the focus is on deficits within the functioning of the brain, and this objectifies the person and their problems,
*   the mind is not seen as influencing the physical body and vice versa,
*   traditionally, professionals have not been taught to value the meaning of the symptom(s) for the person or to understand the impact of the symptom(s) on the person's life,
*   meaning and purpose are considered to be within the realm of the mind, subjective and therefore of no scientific value because they are difficult to measure and standardize.

This dualistic position is no longer tenable because people with lived experience of mental distress have not found the focus on symptoms and problems helpful. What helps is an understanding of the meaning people make of their experience of mental distress, and the impact of this on their lives (Tooth et al., 2003). It is important to assist people to get on with their lives in a way that is meaningful to them and to participate fully in community life.

Holistic practice within nursing has as its main goal the healing of the whole person, recognizing the importance of the interrelationships between biological, psychological, social and spiritual aspects of the individual.

Holism: issues for mental health practice

According to a holistic approach to mental health practice:

- it is meaningless to separate out the 'parts' of a person as if they were discrete entities. A fundamental tenet is that the whole is greater than the sum of its parts (for example, a person's social needs cannot be separated out for treatment, but must be considered in relation to all aspects of the person),
- attention is paid to all aspects of the individual and the interrelationship between them,
- holistic practice attends to the person's relationships with themselves, others, society and their citizenship within the greater cultural context of the community,
- principles underlying such practice include trust, hope, respect for individual freedom and allowing people to exercise their rights as citizens,
- a person's rights include their civil, social and personal rights, including the right of choice and the 'dignity of risk'; that is, the right to fail and the right for self-determination.

The significant shift in thinking away from dualism towards an acceptance of holism has brought with it a much richer nursing experience that validates the complexity of life and cultural experience. Yet even our understanding of holistic practice has changed over time. In the past decade, holistic practice was promoted under the banner of biopsychosocial care. However, the increasing emphasis on recovery-orientated practice has outdated this concept by focusing on the more inclusive citizenship agenda that moves the debate beyond the medical versus social model. Bracken (2003, p. 2) states that 'being a citizen is about being regarded as a full human being, entitled to expect the same from life and the society in which one finds oneself as everyone else. On a basic level it involves being free from discrimination, exclusion and oppression … it means being able to define one's own identity and to celebrate this identity in different ways'. As citizens, people who have the lived experience of mental distress want what we all want. Within the recovery paradigm, a primary focus is maintaining people's engagement in meaningful work that fulfils a whole range of a person's needs.

NURSE'S STORY: THE LIMITATIONS OF DUALISTIC PRACTICE

When the authors of this chapter began mental health nursing (in the 1970s), which at the time was undertaken predominantly in large psychiatric institutions, our tasks were to observe people's signs and symptoms and document them in the person's file so the extent of the deficits could be noted and treated by the psychiatrists. The basic aim was to alleviate symptoms, primarily through medication, so the person could return to their home environment. People often stayed in the institutions for many years. During this time, the meaning and impact of these symptoms for the person were considered irrelevant. In fact, conversations along such lines were actively discouraged because it was believed that this would make the person's condition much worse.

One of the authors has a very vivid recollection of working in a 'back ward' (a ward for people with supposedly chronic and disabling illnesses requiring long-term care over many years) where one of the patients had exhibited a fixed delusion since she was admitted at the age of 17. At the time she was 24 years old and the 'delusion' was still just as distressing. The woman believed that her stepfather was the devil; she would become highly distressed whenever he visited with her mother, and the distress continued long after he left. The staff believed it was a delusion because they perceived the stepfather to be very caring and concerned about the woman's welfare. A young female doctor new to the ward decided to take up this woman's case because the delusion had not responded to medication. She went through the woman's file since admission and found that no one had actually talked to the woman about the content of the delusion (what it meant for her). When the doctor finally asked, the woman told her that she had been sexually abused by her stepfather from a very young age, and that for her he represented the devil.

Although this is a dramatic example, it illustrates the need for holistic practice and the need to include the meaning of the experience for the person and not limit practice to the observation of signs and symptoms.

Internationally, mental healthcare is moving to embrace the recovery paradigm, yet tensions still remain between the medical profession and nurses about having the now well-accepted complementary therapies included in people's healthcare choices. This is an expression of the tension between different theories discussed above. Therapies that are commonly used within mainstream society include massage and a range of other body therapies, counselling, acupuncture, therapeutic touch, homeopathy, imagery and spiritual healing, to name a few. Respecting the individual's right to choose what type of healthcare they receive, and exploring the range of available options with them, fully informs the individual not only of options but also of their consequences, and is empowering practice. Far beyond this, people want to get on with leading 'normal' lives following experiences of mental distress, just like every other citizen.

Challenges arise for the mental health nurse practising a holistic approach within the mainstream health system as the latter is based primarily on a medical, scientific approach geared to dualistic thinking rather than holistic thinking. In many practice settings, workforce shortages and pressure within health systems may present challenges to implementing holistic practice.

From deficits to strengths

Just as there has been a shift from dualism to holism as a result of the failure of dualism to provide an adequate basis for practice, so there has been a shift from focusing on deficits to working with strengths. As we have already stated, practice based on the medical model focuses on identifying signs, symptoms and what the person cannot do, so that a diagnosis can be made and a treatment plan devised to redress these areas of weakness or deficit.

Working with strengths was first used in education and is not a new concept. Educationalists found that focusing on a person's deficit and trying to fix it was likely to make the person feel more anxious, blocked or even immobilized: the problem would often be exacerbated rather than alleviated. The inability of the person (and the professional) to solve the problem led to a sense of failure, and a downward spiral was not uncommon.

The strengths model (see p. 23) proposes that all people have goals, talents and confidence, and that all environments contain resources, people and opportunities. However, we usually do not see these and instead focus more on people's limitations, dysfunction, pathology and the many barriers. The strengths model provides a new perception of possibilities rather than problems, options rather than constraints, and wellness rather than sickness; once this is seen, achievement can occur (Rapp and Goscha, 2006). It supports Deegan's assertion (1988) that people who have experienced mental distress are more interested in focusing on what they can do in order to move on with their lives and live as normally as possible within their community.

In a deficits-based approach, when mental health professionals think there is little hope of overcoming the difficulties the person is experiencing, there is a tendency to want to protect the person from experiencing further failure and this then becomes problematic for the person. The person might be counselled to avoid stress, for example, by stopping work or stopping study, but this protective behaviour can result in a person being denied the dignity of risk. We all have the basic human right to attempt what we choose, to succeed or fail and to learn from the experience: this is how we develop and grow. In practice, nurses should not advise against a person undertaking a particular activity, but instead work with the person to explore the advantages, disadvantages, required steps and possible consequences of an action so they can make an informed choice and appropriate plans.

The focus on a person's deficits also reinforces the notion that the problem resides within the individual rather than as a problem of living. Unfortunately, it has been common to blame the person for not responding to the clinician's intervention. In these circumstances pessimism rather than optimism prevails for all concerned, with a consequent stripping of hope. It is important to keep in mind the old adage that people don't fail, interventions and programmes do.

In contrast, focusing on strengths values and promotes a person's resilience, aspirations, talents and uniqueness, and what the person can do, and how these strengths can be mobilized and built upon to overcome current difficulties. A key therapeutic practice is reframing from a pessimistic world view to an optimistic one that instils hope. For example, the nurse would want to know what the person has done in the past to overcome life's difficulties and how they could use the strength they used then to overcome their current problems. The nurse encourages the person to think of ways that will work for them. The nurse does not impose his or her ideas but may offer suggestions, and works with the person to explore and create options. Nurses use the knowledge gained from a variety of sources to help in this exploration. The nurse works in partnership with the person: the nurse's role is to reinforce the person's plan and remind them of it if they do become unwell.

An illness-focused approach is based on the belief that overcoming a problem merely returns the person to the status quo. A strengths-based approach, on the other hand, is inherently person-focused, and opens up a whole range of possibilities. People overwhelmingly talk about the experience of mental distress as a transformative process where the old self is let go of and a new sense of self emerges (Deegan, 2001). The intense struggle leads to positive outcomes and a sense of personal agency that moves the person beyond where they would have been if they had not had the experience.

Focusing on strengths does not mean that mental health problems are ignored, but they are not the primary focus. Problems tend to resolve once the person starts to get on with their life in a way that is meaningful for them. An example of assisting in the management of symptoms would be to encourage the person to understand their signs of becoming unwell and to devise a plan of action they believe would work for them. For some people with severe mental health problems these plans can be formalized and are called 'advance directives'. These spell out the person's wishes with regards to treatment and who they would like to advocate on their behalf should they be mentally unable to do so. In this way a strengths focus allows the practitioner to respect the person's abilities, beliefs, values, support systems, goals, achievements and resources even when they are acutely unwell.

There is evidence that although both traditional treatment and the strengths-based approach led to improvements, people receiving strengths-based practices had their symptoms reduced by half (Barry et al., 2003), spent fewer days in hospital and were more satisfied with the services they received (Bjorkman et al., 2002). Daniel Fisher (1994), a psychiatrist with lived experience of psychiatric disability (his term), highlights the importance of a strengths focus.

I no longer search for the sickness in myself or in those I grew up with as an explanation for my woes. Instead I search for the strengths in myself and those close to me which propel me through my version of the suffering we all share but seldom face.

(Fisher, 1994, p. 1)

Charles Rapp has been the leader in this strengths focus in mental health practice. He has written extensively on the subject and proposed the strengths model (Rapp, 1998). Comprehensive research on the strengths model has lead to a revision of the key propositions on which it is based. To help the nursing student who has not witnessed the evolution of this theory in practice, both the earliest and latest principles are presented below.

The initial principles of the strengths model (Rapp, 1998) are as follows.

- The aim of strengths-based practice is to focus on the person's strengths and not on pathology, symptoms, weaknesses, problems or deficits.
- The community (social interactions) is viewed as an oasis of resources, not as an obstacle to working with people. The wider community provides far more naturally occurring resources than those that can be provided by mental health teams. The emphasis is on engaging people in existing community services rather than creating disability-only services.
- Interventions are based on the principle of self-determination and nothing is done without the person's approval. The person determines their care and has the same right to make mistakes and learn from them as everyone else (this has also been referred to as the dignity of risk).
- The relationship between the person and the nurse is primary and essential. The nurse needs to be available and with the person when the going gets tough as well as in the good times.
- People with serious mental health problems continue to grow, learn and change.

Revised key propositions of the strengths model (Rapp and Goscha, 2006) are as follows.

- The quality of niches people inhabit determines their achievement, quality of life and success in living.
- People who are successful in living have goals and dreams.
- People who are successful in living use their strengths to attain their aspirations.
- People who are successful in living have the confidence to take the next step towards their goal.

- At any given time, people who are successful in living have at least one goal, one relevant talent and the confidence to take the next step.
- People who are successful in living have access to the resources needed to achieve their goals.
- People who are successful in living have a meaningful relationship with at least one person.
- People who are successful in living have access to opportunities relevant to their goals.
- People who are successful in living have access to resources and opportunities and meaningful relationships.

CRITICAL THINKING CHALLENGE 2.1

What stands out for you, from the principles and propositions of the strengths model, in relation to what you do when you work with people who have the lived experience of mental distress?

The critical nursing process of enhancing strengths in people who have relied on less positive ways of coping is demonstrated in the nurse's story, Moving from deficits-based to strengths-based practice.

NURSE'S STORY: MOVING FROM DEFICITS-BASED TO STRENGTHS-BASED PRACTICE

Lucy was referred to me by health workers from the community health centre. These workers had been called to see Lucy on repeated occasions over the years since she had left the children's home in which she was raised. Lucy presented with many health problems and had more recently been binge drinking and engaging in self-harm behaviour: taking overdoses and cutting herself.

When I began working with Lucy it was immediately apparent that her self-esteem had been shattered. She walked with her head bowed, felt great discomfort with eye contact, and felt people were judging her and that no one cared about her. Unfortunately, her experiences in the accident and emergency department after she had self-harmed reinforced her low self-esteem, because the nursing staff in the accident and emergency department had responded angrily to her behaviour.

Working with Lucy to identify her strengths was an extremely slow and involved process of gradual engagement, building up trust, exploring her issues of loss and trauma, and assisting her to consider options she believed could improve her mental health. One of these was searching for family members. Throughout this process, I actively reinforced every step Lucy took that demonstrated her ability to deal with life issues without resorting to binge drinking and self-harm behaviour. Lucy was encouraged to look at healthy ways of reducing stress, and started to focus on writing and playing music, two activities that had given her great pleasure when she was younger.

Several years into this process, Lucy had located many of her family members and dealt with the issues using healthy coping mechanisms. She is now employed as a musician and has a well-developed sense of self-esteem.

From patient to service user: a person with lived experience

Consistent with the shift in focus from deficits to strengths is the change in terminology from 'patient' to 'service user'. The term service user is commonly used in the UK and refers to people who have the lived experience of mental distress who have received care from mental health professionals. Generally people have challenged the use of value-laden terms because they can shape the interactions that arise between people. The term patient is considered too bound up with illness and the medical model, with deficits and with the disparity in status between patient and professional. Patient also implies a more passive role, with the person being the recipient of care. The term 'client' has similar connotations to patient. Service user implies a more active role, with the person having rights, responsibility and a more equitable relationship with the care provider. In Australia, the term 'consumer' has been considered the most acceptable to people, although some prefer the term 'survivor' (USA). More recently the terminology has changed to 'a person who has the lived experience of mental distress'. The connotations in this phrase are that of being a person first and that mental distress is just one of a range of many experiences, and this removes the stigmatization that can occur when someone needs to consume services.

Language and the use of labels can be harmful and can significantly influence the interactions between people with lived experience and those who work with them (Walker, 2006). Nurses are in a powerful position in being able to influence community attitudes towards people with mental distress. We need to take every opportunity to communicate in ways that combat stigma, promote people's dignity, deepen community understanding and contribute to interactions that are empowering.

Distinguishing rehabilitation from recovery

In the previous discussions on the shift from dualism to holism and from deficits to strengths, it was reasonably easy to identify the difference between the concepts. However, this is not always the case with rehabilitation and recovery. We have chosen to address rehabilitation, a component of mental health services in which nurses practise, in this section because of the tendency to talk about 'rehabilitation' as if it has been replaced by 'recovery'. The concept of recovery has not replaced rehabilitation but it has changed the way it is practised.

Rehabilitation aims to support people who experience severe and enduring forms of mental health problems to reintegrate into the community. Traditionally, rehabilitation aimed to optimize functional ability by focusing on deficits in a range of areas such as social, vocational, symptom management, activities of daily living (hygiene, cooking, budgeting, travel and so on) and accommodation. Professionals, including nurses, assessed the person's deficits to determine their rehabilitation needs and the person then attended a rehabilitation service where programmes (often run by nurses) would address these skill deficits. This approach to rehabilitation has been criticized by Deegan (1988) because it requires people to progress through predetermined skills-based training programmes regardless of individual needs.

Deegan makes a useful distinction between recovery and rehabilitation in mental health services.

> *Disabled persons are not passive recipients of rehabilitation services. Rather, they experience themselves as recovering a new sense of self and of purpose within and beyond the limits of the disability…. Rehabilitation refers to services and technologies that are made available to disabled persons so they may learn to adapt to their world. Recovery refers to the lived or real life experience of persons as they accept and overcome the challenge of disability.*

(Deegan, 1988, p. 11)

Hence there has been a significant shift away from highly prescriptive rehabilitation programmes to recovery-orientated rehabilitation, emphasizing service user-directed goals and outcomes, and maximizing options in the setting of the service user's choice.

Recovery begins the moment the person develops a serious mental health problem. It is both a personal act (something the person does) and an approach (how others facilitate the process). Recovery has been difficult to define but it focuses on the person being able to live well with or without the mental health problem. The following comprehensive definition by a leading Australian psychiatrist will be used for this chapter. It clearly articulates the many facets of recovery and provides direction for how others may assist in facilitating this personal experience.

> *Recovery is the uniquely personal and ongoing act of reclaiming and regaining the capacity to take executive control of life that is meaningful, satisfying, purposeful and believing in oneself as a valued citizen, after one or more encounters with a mental*

illness, despite the limitations and challenges imposed by the illness, its treatment and the personal and environmental responses to it.

(Kalyanasundaram, unpublished manuscript, 2004)

In practice the nurse's role is to help promote and facilitate a person's self-directed recovery. While changing attitudes, values and beliefs about practice are essential, Pearson (2004) argues that it is more important to change professionals' perceptions of their role and that this results in the paradigm shift. Mental health policies are meant to provide the guiding framework for such practice. Policies are based on current theories and knowledge in the field of mental health. Hence the philosophy of care is continually being revised and updated. In practice, there can be a time lag in the implementation of policies and this appears to occur in many countries. This delay is in part understandable because of the lengthy process of developing policies and plans, educating the workforce on their implementation, setting up the structures and then providing the necessary resources. In the fast-changing area of mental health there has been difficulty in keeping mental health practice, including nursing practice, current.

Recovery-orientated practice is guided by thinking about what you do and say when you work with people and how you perceive your role. This is influenced by your theoretical and experiential knowledge. We highlighted the centrality of the nurse's attitudes, values and beliefs in guiding practice at the beginning of this chapter.

Superimposed on the above is the mistaken trend to use the words 'rehabilitation' and 'recovery' interchangeably: this use of language creates additional confusion, particularly for nursing students. In some instances services that have been called 'recovery-orientated' continue to be based on old rehabilitation practices. The distinguishing features of all services will be the principles of practice that guide them and how these are implemented; that is, it will be the values, attitudes and beliefs of the service, and the professionals who make up that service, that will determine whether the practices are truly recovery-orientated. According to Jacobson and Curtis (2000) this necessitates a fundamental shift towards the sharing of both power and responsibility within the therapeutic relationship. The following section briefly addresses the current principles of recovery and their implications for practice.

CRITICAL THINKING CHALLENGE 2.2

How would mental health service provision be different if it was driven by service users and meeting service user's needs rather than the needs of mental health professionals?

ESSENTIALS OF RECOVERY-ORIENTATED PRACTICE

In the past decade, many service users have published their stories of recovery and experiences of care, providing the initial impetus for the recovery movement (seminal works include Deegan, 1988; Lovejoy, 1984; Unzicker, 1989) and the push for recovery-orientated practice. People who have the lived experience of mental distress can and do recover, and to a very large extent their stories indicate that this has occurred without the involvement of mental health professionals, and, unfortunately, in spite of them in some cases. In light of this feedback, it is time to determine how best to promote the social nature of recovery.

Our values and beliefs underpin our actions. Similarly, the values and beliefs of professionals and service providers underpin professional practice. Recent research (Mezzina et al., 2006; Onken et al., 2002) identifies essential values, beliefs and subsequent principles to inform recovery-orientated practice. The following list of principles is a composite of these authors' work.

- The mental health service moves from being a treatment provider and manager of symptoms to being a broader community resource that enhances people's access to opportunities, community life and resources.
- As well as facilitating the active role of individuals in their recovery, mental health services must also elicit and heed feedback and undergo modification to meet people's needs.
- To achieve the above requires the sharing of power, by demystifying knowledge and the therapeutic power of providers, removing barriers to people accessing information.
- Mental health services need to accept that citizenship is necessary for recovery, rather than thinking that recovery is a prerequisite for citizenship (as has been the case for the past 200 years).
- Psychiatric knowledge doesn't necessarily equip professionals to access the broad range of supports required by individuals within the community, but as individuals that is what we do every day as part of living in the community.

Mezzina et al. (2006) make the following points and these are considered in the context of nursing practice. At an individual practice level nurses need to be aware of the important social dimension of recovery. Recognizing, promoting and supporting this and people's relationships with others in the community and with oneself are essential. Such practices promote the person's sense of belonging and active participation in community life. Practice also needs to support the person learning how to manage their distress, and live a safe, dignified, productive and full life. Another key issue for practice is the need to focus on the person reestablishing a meaningful and purposeful existence in society where they feel included and can participate, and their civil rights as a citizen are promoted and protected.

The document entitled 'Making recovery a reality' (Shepherd et al., 2008) provides indicators of how recovery can be promoted through practice in mental health settings, and we encourage you to read it. In sum, everyone needs a home, employment, a living wage and genuine control over their life. It is important that services are orientated towards hope and emphasize positive mental health and wellness.

Personal characteristics of recovery

International research (for example, Onken et al., 2002; Ralph, 2000; Ridgeway, 2001; Sells et al., 2006; Tooth et al., 1997, 2003) has identified personal characteristics as the most important factor in aiding recovery. Drawing on the findings from the above research, service users identified the following as the most important factors in their recovery: self-determination; discovering a more active sense of self; valuing themselves as a person through their interactions with others; realization of the need to help themselves and take responsibility for their distress; seeing the potential for richer identities other than that of a person with mental health problems; reflecting on positive experience leading to consideration of other potentials; exploring experiences with reference to current and possible self; finding ways to monitor and manage the symptoms of their distress; optimism and spirituality.

To facilitate this process, nursing practice needs to promote rather than hinder the above. It is important to realize that the recovery process is fragile in the beginning and can be either stifled or enhanced. Perhaps the single most important focus to help people reduce their symptoms is to help them to build lives that are satisfying and fulfilling. First-person accounts of recovery also suggest that the total elimination of symptoms is rare; that the experience of symptom exacerbation is something of a roller-coaster in frequency, duration severity of episodes, but these are often reduced; that even with symptoms people still work, play and live full lives in the community (Rapp and Goscha, 2006).

Facilitating self-help and personal responsibility

Care is the basis of nursing practice, and this creates tension between doing something for someone and encouraging people to care for themselves. There are times when fostering dependency by doing tasks for the person is necessary, but in many cases it is counterproductive.

Box 2.1 'Being with' a person to promote self-help

Examples of questions the nurse can use:
- Can you help me to understand what the experience of ... means for you?
- What are you most concerned about at the moment?
- Have there been other times in your life when you have had similar feelings?
- How did you overcome these difficulties in the past?
- What do you think you need now to help with your current situation?
- What do you know about yourself that will help you in your current situation?

Self-help is closely related to personal responsibility. Not only do people realize the need to help themselves but they also realize the need to take responsibility for doing so. These are valuable strategies that we all employ in dealing with life's challenges. We are experts on ourselves, with our own knowledge base of how we have coped in the past and what strategies have worked for us in dealing with life crises. However, there are times when our past coping mechanisms no longer work and we need to find new ways of dealing with difficult situations. In times of crisis or personal distress, individuals can become overwhelmed and lose sight of their own capacity for problem-solving. At a practical level, the role of the nurse is to be with the person (listening to the person to understand their concerns, fears and experience) while at the same time helping the individual to tap into their own wisdom by reminding them that they have coped in the past, and reinforcing the value of their own self-knowledge. Nurses don't need to find the answers, but they do need to encourage the process of self-help, personal discovery and personal responsibility, and identify the person's strengths, so they can take effective control of their life. Such practice is important in building a sense of self-control and autonomy.

The list in Box 2.1 is not exhaustive but it illustrates the therapeutic use of questioning. You are encouraged to complete the class exercise on self-help at the end of this chapter.

Self-help can also involve seeking assistance and support from other people who have had similar experiences. Self-help groups are useful in assisting people to gain support, learn coping skills, tap into resources and find out information about healthcare options. In the UK a considerable range of service user organizations provide advice, advocacy, support and service delivery. Some of the major voluntary and charitable organizations focused on service user and carer issues are listed in Box 2.2.

Box 2.2 **Voluntary and charitable organizations and useful websites**

MIND: provides information and advice, and campaigns to promote and protect good mental health for everyone (www.mind.org.uk).

Rethink Mental Illness: the largest national voluntary-sector provider of mental health services. Offers a national advice line and information (www.rethink.org).

SANE: provides help and information to those experiencing mental health problems, their families and carers and undertakes research into the causes of serious mental illness (www.sane.org.uk).

The Samaritans: provides free, confidential emotional support around the clock (www.samaritans.org).

Mental Health Foundation: a campaigning charity focusing on research, policy development and service development in support of mental health promotion and care (www.mentalhealth.org.uk).

Promoting overall health and wellness

Consistent with a recovery orientation to service provision is a focus on promoting health, wellness and a healthy lifestyle. This focus on health and wellness needs to be considered by nurses in all practice settings where they enter into partnerships for mental healthcare.

The significance of supporting people with mental distress to access healthcare has been highlighted in research by Coghlan et al. (2001) that demonstrated alarmingly high rates of physical illness experienced by people with mental health problems. This research found that people with mental health problems had high rates of heart disease, cancer and other serious illnesses, did not receive healthcare for significant illnesses to the same extent as the rest of the population, and that when they did receive healthcare their outcomes were poorer: for example, lower life expectancy and poorer treatment outcomes. Major contributing factors to poor health were considered to be smoking, alcohol and drug use. Nurses have a key role to play in promoting health and wellness in their interactions with people with mental distress.

Wellness and its opposite, illness, have specific implications for practice within the recovery framework. Past practices in mental health focused on the illness to the exclusion of the person experiencing the illness. Kalyanasundaram (2007) describes the process as follows. A person would go to a health professional who would ask about 'the problem' (usually symptoms/illness), building a bigger and bigger picture of 'the problem'. This would lead to the person focusing more and more on 'the problem'. The problem would grow bigger and bigger and be added to by the person's family or others asking about it. Soon the person's identity would be taken over and consumed by 'IT', 'the problem'. Further contact with mental health professionals would reinforce this by almost exclusively focusing on asking questions about 'IT'. This is similar to the concept of 'problem saturation'. Clearly this scenario is unhelpful and disables the person.

In the recovery literature, emphasis is placed on the person's experience of the problem and the impact it has on the person's life. This promotes the 'ME' and not the 'IT' (Jacobson, 2000). Again, the importance of the language we use and what we say to people is emphasized. Asking questions about the person and their experience promotes understanding and a sense of agency, and puts 'the problem' in context. The person does not become the problem but retains a more robust sense of self.

RECOVERY-ORIENTATED SERVICE PROVISION

The community

Services need to facilitate people's active and meaningful participation in the community and it is clear from listening to service users that there is a need to consider a much broader range of options than has traditionally been available within the mental health system. In addition, people's needs change over time and therefore services must be comprehensive and flexible enough to cater for these changes. Most importantly, the options must not tie service users to mental health services, but rather promote options within the broader community (Anthony, 2000).

To assist the person requires services to be orientated towards recovery. In practice there is a complex interrelationship between services and agencies (public, private and third-sector; see the following sections), systems, policies, cultures and society. Mental health services provided by the NHS form a small but important part of the assistance people require. People are likely to also come into contact with social care services (for financial support), housing services and employment services; from the non-government sector through to general services provided for everyone in the broader community. Collaboration and coordination between these various players is essential. There are a number of mechanisms to ensure coordination of care across multiple agencies. The Care Programme Approach (CPA) is one of these mechanisms and is addressed elsewhere in the text (see Chs 4, 21 and 23).

The community of which the person is a member provides a wealth of resources that are essential to all people, not just those experiencing mental distress. Nurses now need to be able to extend far beyond previous traditional roles in their ability and creativity in finding and using what is available in the person's community.

The mental health service

Within the mental health service there are a number of settings in which a nurse may practice: for example, inpatient services attached to general hospitals and community mental health teams (see Ch. 21). Nursing practice in these settings will be aimed at:

- obtaining the services the person needs and wants,
- promoting the person's inner resources,
- activating supports to assist in the achievement of the person's goals,
- promoting the person's engagement in fulfilling and satisfying activities of their choice,
- advocating for the upholding of a person's rights,
- assisting them to advocate on their own behalf,
- facilitating access to the people, places and things the person needs to survive (e.g. shelter, meals, healthcare),
- facilitating self-help by encouraging the person to exercise their voice and make choices in their life,
- promoting a healthy lifestyle,
- alleviating distress,
- working with the person to ensure their own safety and that of others.

The focus of practice in the various settings will be determined by the person's needs and these change over time. The Nurse's story: What nursing can achieve in the community, illustrates how community mental health nurses can provide a range of supports for people to achieve outcomes that are not possible in a hospital-based treatment episode.

NURSE'S STORY: WHAT NURSING CAN ACHIEVE IN THE COMMUNITY

Johanna, a 26-year-old woman, had recently emigrated from Armenia with her husband Frank and 6-month-old son. Johanna was experiencing her second episode of major depression with psychotic features. Her previous mental health treatment prior to coming to the UK had been entirely hospital-based, and when community care was suggested for this second episode of depression, Frank was reluctant to take any risks until Johanna was completely well. Frank was at work during the day, they had no family or friends in the UK and he could not take leave to care for Johanna. Therefore he felt she would be safer being admitted in hospital. Johanna was afraid that if she stayed in hospital as long as she did on her previous admission she would not bond with her son. Frank was persuaded to support the option of community care when reassured that resources were available to provide support during the day. Home Treatment Team (HTT) staff were identified who were available to provide support in their home during the day. A small network of women from

Armenia who met at the local migrant resource centre also provided much-needed social support.

The nurse in this situation used existing local community resources to provide support. These supports enabled Johanna to remain at home with her son and facilitated her recovery. The nurse provided education to Johanna about depression, medication and early warning signs, as well as addressing issues of health and stress management. Johanna reported that this episode of depression was not as prolonged as her previous one where she was hospitalized. She felt less isolated and more in contact with family and other people, and wanted to get better because she was encouraged by the normal day-to-day activity around her. Johanna felt confident that with the support of the nurse she could explore her mental health problem and learn how to manage it.

Multidisciplinary teams

Multidisciplinary teams are considered routine in the provision of mental healthcare in the community. The standard mix of disciplines within mental health teams includes nurses, psychologists, psychiatrists, social workers and occupational therapists. This mix of disciplines is seen as necessary to provide a holistic approach to care. The different professional groups provide complementary approaches that honour the complexity of the service user. Each discipline has a body of knowledge and a framework for practice that emphasizes different aspects of how to work with people. The framework of each discipline involves theoretical underpinnings that shape the approaches adopted by professionals.

No single discipline can prepare workers with the range of knowledge and skills required for the diversity that is encompassed in mental health practice. It is necessary for all professionals to respect and understand each other's skills and orientation for working in different ways, and to work collaboratively and interdependently. The orientation and discipline of any worker should not be seen to categorize or limit the capacity of that individual to develop a broad range of practice skills within the multidisciplinary team. Service users frequently tell us that our credentials as human beings are the most important aspect of good-quality care.

In addition to the traditional multidisciplinary team, in the past decade there has been a rapid growth of other key workers in providing support for people who experience mental distress. These include third-sector and charitable organizations, youth services, organizations for black and ethnic minority groups and self-help groups, to name a few.

Third-sector organizations

Third-sector organizations include voluntary services, non-governmental agencies and charities, which play an important role in the provision of support to service users and carers affected by mental distress through direct service delivery, complementing existing public and private mental health services, and strengthening community supports and partnerships. This fundamental role in providing for the range of needs of people with mental distress is crucial in retaining people's citizenship. The role of the nurse is to be aware of the range of services offered by third-sector organizations so this knowledge can be passed on to the people with whom they work. Nurses can also work with these organizations in activities such as raising community awareness.

However, it is essential to remember that third-sector organizations are not whole-of-life services, but stepping stones for those people who choose to use them. The aim is for people to develop naturally occurring supports within the community, or other created supports that are used by all members of the community.

The range of services provided by third-sector organizations in the mental health sector include:

- practical and emotional support for service users and carers,
- research,
- advice about rights and legal issues,
- campaigning for issues relating to mental healthcare,
- advocacy, advice and information,
- public education,
- community development.

Partnerships, participation and empowerment

The concepts of partnerships, participation and empowerment are inextricably linked. A partnership between different service providers or other stakeholder groups as well as between service provider and service recipients necessitates participation that hopefully leads to empowerment, not just for service users but for all concerned.

Within primary healthcare settings, where most of mental health care should occur, empowerment would mean a focus on people actively participating in exercising control over and taking responsibility for their health, having universal access to resources to enable them to do this, and having meaningful interactions with health providers and policy makers. Essentially, empowerment refers to reinstating the power that has been inadvertently stripped from people due to past practices in mental health. It is a human rights issue and has become another buzzword in mental health in the past decade. However, for some service users the implied need to be empowered has been seen as condescending because it implies that the person does not have power in the first place. Clearly this is not the case and again highlights the need for caution in making general assumptions about the wide range of human

experiences and the meaning an individual makes of these experiences. Barker (2001) asserts that the most common form of disempowerment occurs when there is a failure to hear people's stories of their experiences and their problems of living; hence enquiring about these and listening to them is an empowering nursing practice.

Participation is enshrined in mental health policy documents nationally and internationally. It is mandated that people are active participants in their care, and in service system and policy development. This signals the shift in practice from people being viewed as passive recipients of 'expert' care, to people being viewed as active participants and directors of their care based on their self-identified needs. Again this comes back to the fact that service users and carers, who have been through the experience of mental distress and recovery from it, are the best experts on their needs. Unfortunately, most attempts to move to authentic participation by mental health systems at the national and international levels have been seen as tokenistic by most service users and carers. The principles and practices of the emerging recovery paradigm attempt to redress this.

The person must be at the centre of anything to do with their mental health needs. People can only effectively meet their needs by participating in their care. Logically this requires partnerships with the person and a range of supports such as family, significant others, friends, the wider community and any needed services. There is also a need for partnerships among the various supports. In the context of modern mental health practice, as previously discussed, it is necessary to extend partnerships beyond mental health, third-sector organizations and other disability/welfare supports, to include partnerships with the community as a whole. Ensuring that people who experience mental distress have the same opportunity to participate in all aspects of their community and the wider society, just like everybody else, requires effective partnerships. The responsibility for ensuring this extends beyond the mental health system to the wider society. Nursing practice that helps facilitate such participation and partnerships is empowering.

Another important factor in participation, partnerships and empowerment, especially in mental health, is the environments people inhabit, referred to as niches by Rapp and Goscha (2006). These authors point out that niches are either naturally occurring in the environment or created to meet people's needs. Further, these niches can either enable the person to get on with their life or inadvertently entrap them, depending on whether they include or exclude the person from their environment. Examples of a created entrapping niche are the large mental health institutions of the last century. Similarly, stigma, unemployment and so on are naturally occurring entrapping niches. In contrast, created enabling niches focus on improving people's quality of life, provide a wide range of choices and allow movement through services (that is, there is a clear exit from services) so people can live, love, work and play in the community of their choice. Naturally occurring enabling niches are such things as work and recreation opportunities, family involvement and community affiliation.

In working in partnership with people it is important to ensure that our practices or the environments we create are as enabling as possible. In reality all environments tend to fall somewhere along the continuum of being enabling or entrapping. It is easy to see how people are better off when they are in environments that form the fabric of everyday life, in contrast to being marginalized. To date, helping has inadvertently reinforced such marginalization through practices and programmes such as segregated work programmes, group homes and treatment programmes. Implied therefore is the need to develop partnerships that will enable access to the whole range of options that are available to everyone in the community. These concepts also go far beyond the concept of 'community integration' that is often spoken about in mental health. They are about social inclusion and citizenship.

Professional boundaries

The issue of professional boundaries arises because the nature of mental health work necessitates the development of therapeutic relationships. It can be confusing for novice nurses to navigate the complex issues that arise in relation to professional boundaries, given the nature of the relationships we develop with people. Boundaries in mental health practice are vital in light of the historical legacy of abuses in psychiatry, the vulnerability of many users of mental health services and the potential for harm inherent in the relationship between nurse and the people for whom they care. The behaviour that most clearly constitutes a boundary violation is sexual contact between mental health professional and service user, an unquestionably prohibited behaviour.

Many other areas within the relationship between mental health nurse and service user may constitute problematic behaviour; this may include physical contact, gift giving, self-disclosure and personal or social involvement, depending on the circumstances. Behaviour in any individual relationship between mental health nurse and service user is generally not bound in a fixed or rigid way, as this might inhibit the nurse's ability to respond to different individuals in whatever way is most relevant in a given situation.

People who have the lived experience of mental distress often say that when a professional has helped them it is important for them and their sense of self-worth to reciprocate in some way. After all, this is the basis of normal human interactions and forms an important part of the fabric of human life.

The Nursing and Midwifery Council refers to boundaries in *The Code: standards of conduct, performance and ethics for nurses and midwives* (Nursing and Midwifery Council, 2008). The Code requires nurses to maintain clear professional boundaries by refusing any gifts, favours or hospitality that might be interpreted as an attempt to gain preferential treatment; not asking for or accepting loans from anyone in one's care or anyone close to them; and establishing and actively maintaining clear sexual boundaries at all times with people in one's care, their families and carers. Similarly, confidentiality must be respected ensuring that information is only disclosed when the nurse believes that someone may be at risk of harm.

Nurses should familiarize themselves with the emerging literature on boundaries. (Professional boundaries are discussed in more detail in other chapters: see the index.)

CONCLUSION

We encourage you to reflect on how the principles of mental health practice are fundamental to all nursing practice regardless of setting. We hope we have encouraged you to think about how you can participate more fully in your practice by developing your awareness of the complexities and realities of the context in which practice occurs. More specifically, we hope you appreciate how your attitudes, values and beliefs play a crucial role in your everyday practice.

Mental health nursing practice is also influenced by an ever-evolving knowledge base; hence the principles informed by this knowledge base continue to change and evolve. Practice is time- and context-specific, making the ability to tolerate and incorporate change vital. Consequently, your thinking about your practice will be continually influenced by your developing self-awareness, your incorporation of new ideas into your practice and your increasing professional and personal experience.

The primary focus of mental health nursing practice is the service user and how nurses can help facilitate the service user's recovery. Nurses can assist in this process by working in partnership with service users to help them realize their potential and tap into a wide range of community resources and supports, of which mental health services are just one. Just as importantly, we hope you find the experience of mental health nursing as rewarding as we have.

EXERCISES FOR CLASS ENGAGEMENT

Imagine yourself in the scenarios below and, in groups, answer the questions.

SCENARIO 1

You have been hospitalized with an acute medical condition. Medical advice is that you have diabetes. You are being given instructions for self-management of insulin injections and monitoring of blood sugar levels before discharge from hospital.

SCENARIO 2

You have been hospitalized after an acute episode of depression. Medical advice to you is that there is a high likelihood that you have bipolar depression. You are being given instructions on the possible side effects of the antidepressant medication you have been prescribed, and advised that you will have to continue taking some form of medication indefinitely.

Questions

In groups of four or five, discuss your thoughts and feelings about the above scenarios. Use the following questions as discussion points. Note similarities and differences in opinion among group members as well as between the two scenarios.

♦ What are your immediate concerns?
♦ What information would you seek?

♦ What type of support would you wish to receive, and from whom would you wish to receive it?
♦ What would be the most important knowledge and skills for nurses in the different care units?
♦ What could your nurse do that would be helpful or unhelpful?
♦ What do you think will be important considerations for the rest of your life?
♦ Do you think you should take an active role in your present and future care?
♦ If so, how could this best be achieved?

SCENARIO 3

Emily is 36 years old and married to Grant, with whom she has two sons, aged 5 and 7. They have recently moved to London and have no local family supports. Emily is currently experiencing her second episode of bipolar disorder, and is in the hypomanic phase of her illness. Grant is very concerned about Emily's ability to be an effective parent but he also has longer-term fears about their relationship.

Question

♦ How could the principles of recovery-orientated practice be used to assist Emily? Focus on aspects of the client's recovery rather than symptom management.

REFERENCES

Alligood, M.R., Tomey, A.M., 2002. Nursing Theory: Utilization and Application. Mosby, St Louis, MO.

Anthony, W.A., 2000. A recovery-oriented service system: setting some system level standards. Psychiatr. Rehabil. J. 24 (2), 159–168.

Barker, P., 2001. The Tidal Model: developing an empowering person-centred approach to recovery within psychiatric and mental health nursing. J. Psychiatr. Ment. Health Nurs. 8 (3), 233–240.

Barker, P., Buchanan-Barker, P., 2004. The Tidal Model: psychiatric colonisation, recovery and the need for a paradigm shift in mental healthcare. <http://www.tidal-model.co.uk/New%20Colonisation.htm>.

Barry, K.L., Zeber, J.F., Blow, F.C., et al., 2003. Effect of strengths model versus assertive community treatment model on participant outcomes and utilization: two-year follow-up. Psychiatr. Rehabil. J. 26 (3), 268–278.

Bjorkman, T., Hansson, L., Sandlund, M., 2002. Outcome of case management based on strengths model compared to standard care. A randomised controlled trial. Soc. Psychiatry Psychiatr. Epidemiol. 37 (4), 147–152.

Bracken, P., 2003. Citizenship and psychiatry. Paper Delivered at the Inaugural Seminar of the Centre for Citizenship and Community Mental Health, University of Bradford, 26 June.

Buchanan-Barker, P., 2004. Uncommon sense: the value base of the Tidal Model. <http://www.tidal-model.co.uk/New%20Uncommon%20sense.htm>.

Coghlan, R., Lawrence, D., Holman, C.D.J., et al., 2001. Duty to Care: Physical Illness in People with Mental Illness. University of Western Australia, Perth.

Cox, H., Hickson, P., Taylor, B., 1991. Exploring reflection: knowing and constructing practice. In: Gray, G., Pratt, R. (Eds.), Towards a Discipline of Nursing Elsevier, Sydney.

Crook, J.A., 2001. How do expert mental health nurses make on-the-spot clinical decisions? A review of the literature. J. Psychiatr. Ment. Health Nurs. 8 (1), 1–5.

Deegan, P.E., 1988. Recovery: the lived experience of rehabilitation. Psychosoc. Rehabil. J. 11 (4), 11–19.

Deegan, P.E., 2001. Recovery as a self-directed process of healing and transformation. <http://intentionalcare.org/articles/articles_trans.pdf>.

Farkas, M., Gagne, C., Anthony, W., et al., 2005. Implementing recovery-orientated evidence-based programs: identifying the critical dimensions. Community Ment. Health J. 41 (2), 141–157.

Fisher, D.B., 1994. Hope, humanity and voice in recovery from psychiatric disability. J. Calif. Alliance Ment. Ill 5 (recovery issue), 13–15.

Graham, I.W., 2000. Reflective practice and its role in mental health nurses' practice development: a year-long study. J. Psychiatr. Ment. Health Nurs. 7 (22), 109–117.

Henderson, V., 1966. The Nature of Nursing. Macmillan, London.

Hubble, M.A., Duncan, B.L., Miller, S.D. (Eds.), 1999. The Heart and Soul of Change: What Works in Therapy American Psychological Association, Washington DC.

Jacobson, N., 2000. A Conceptual Model of Recovery. Recovery and the Mental Health Consumer Movement in Wisconsin. WDHFS, Recovery Task Force. Wisconsin Coalition for Advocacy, Wisconsin.

Jacobson, N., Curtis, L., 2000. Recovery as policy in mental health services: strategies emerging from the states. Psychiatr. Rehabil. J. 23 (4), 333–341.

Jasper, M., Elliot, P., 2006. Vital Notes for Nurses: Professional Development, Reflection and Decision Making. Blackwell Science, Oxford.

Kalyanasundaram, V., 2007. Facilitating Recovery Oriented Practice. Workshop notes, 22–24 August. NSW Institute of Psychiatry, Sydney.

Lovejoy, M., 1984. Recovery from schizophrenia: a personal odyssey. Hosp. Community Psychiatry 35 (8), 809–812.

McEwan, M., Wills, E.M., 2002. Theoretical Basis for Nursing. Lippincott Williams & Wilkins, Philadelphia.

Mezzina, R., Davidson, L., Borg, M., et al., 2006. The social nature of recovery: discussion and implications for practice. Am. J. Psychiatr. Rehabil. 9, 63–80.

Nursing and Midwifery Council, 2008. The code: standards of conduct, performance and ethics for nurses and midwives. <http://www. nmc-uk.org/Documents/Standards/ nmcTheCodeStandardsofConduct PerformanceAndEthicsForNurses And Midwives_LargePrintVersion. PDF>.

Onken, S.J., Dumont, J.M., Ridgeway, P., et al., 2002. Mental Health Recovery: What Helps and What Hinders?. National Technical Assistance Center for State Mental Health Planning (NTAC), National Association for State Mental Health Program Directors (NASMHPD), Alexandria, VA.

Orem, D.E., 1971. Nursing: Concepts of Practice. McGraw-Hill, New York.

Pearson, A., 2004. Recovery: challenging the paradigm (a consumer perspective). Presentation to VICSERV Conference, Melbourne.

Peplau, H.E., 1952. (reprinted 1988) Interpersonal Relations in Nursing. Macmillan Education, London.

Ralph, R.O., 2000. Review of Recovery Literature: a Synthesis of a Sample of Recovery Literature. National Technical Assistance Center for State Mental Health Planning (NTAC), National Association for State Mental Health Program Directors (NASMHPD), Alexandria, VA.

Rapp, C., 1998. The Strengths Model: Case Management with People Suffering from Severe and Persistent Mental Illness. Oxford University Press, New York.

Rapp, C., Goscha, R.J., 2006. A beginning theory of strengths. In: Rapp, C.A., Goscha, R.J. (Eds.), The Strengths Model: Case Management with People with a Psychiatric Disability, second ed Oxford University Press, New York.

Ridgeway, P., 2001. Restorying psychiatric disability: learning from first-person accounts of recovery. Psychiatr. Rehabil. J. 24 (4), 335–343.

Roberts, G.A., 2000. Narrative and severe mental illness: what place do stories have in an evidence-based world? Adv. Psychiatr. Treat. 6, 432–441.

Rogers, M.E., 1970. The Theoretical Basis of Nursing. F A Davis, Philadelphia.

Sells, D., Borg, M., Marin, I., et al., 2006. Arenas of recovery for persons with severe mental illness. Am. J. Psychiatr. Rehabil. 9, 3–16.

Shepherd, G., Boardman, J., Slade, M., 2008. Making recovery a reality. <http://www.centreformentalhealth. org.uk/news/2008_services_need_ radical_changes.aspx>.

Short, S.D., Sharman, E., Speedy, S., 1994. Sociology for Nurses: an Australian Introduction. MacMillan, Melbourne.

Tooth, B., Kalyanasundaram, V., Glover, H., 1997. Recovery from Schizophrenia: A Consumer Perspective. Report to Health and Human Services Research and Development Grants Program, Canberra.

Tooth, B., Kalyanasundaram, V., Glover, H., et al., 2003. Factors consumers identify as important to recovery from schizophrenia. Australas. Psychiatry 11 (1), 70–77.

Unzicker, R., 1989. On my own: a personal journey through madness and reemergence. Psychosoc. Rehabil. J. 13 (4), 71–77.

Walker, M.T., 2006. The social construction of mental illness and its implications for the recovery model. Int. J. Psychosoc. Rehabil. 10 (1), 71–87. <http:// www.psychosocial.com/IJPR_10/ Social_Construction_of_MI_and_ Implications_for_Recovery_Walker. html>.

Welsh, I., Lyons, C.M., 2001. Evidence-based care and the case for intuition and tacit knowledge in clinical assessment and decision making in mental health nursing practice: an empirical contribution to the debate. J. Psychiatr. Ment. Health Nurs. 8 (4), 299–305.

Chapter | 3 |

Historical foundations

Katie Evans

CHAPTER POINTS

- The medical writers of Greece and Rome were able to recognize and differentiate between the major categories of mental disorders.
- Graeco-Roman treatment methods for mental health problems were generally compassionate.
- Research into the ancient literature shows that superstition and the supernatural influenced views about and treatment of the people with mental health problems less than was previously believed.
- The family has traditionally cared for and nursed mentally unwell members of society for most of humankind's recorded history.
- Nursing has existed as a profession since Graeco-Roman times but references to nursing as a dedicated professional activity are sparse in the ancient literature.
- For most of recorded history, the function of mental health nursing is not distinguished from general nursing.
- Medical and nursing practices were less sophisticated during medieval times.
- Graeco-Roman knowledge was kept alive during medieval times in monasteries and in the East, and revived during and after the Renaissance.
- The asylum developed as a response to social conditions and the emergence of new, chronic mental health problems.
- Institutional care and/or hospitalization are relatively recent alternative treatment modes.

KEY TERMS

- asylum
- doctor

DOI: http://dx.doi.org/10.1016/B978-0-7020-4493-9.00003-2

- family
- gender
- Graeco-Roman
- Greece
- historical
- history
- hysteria
- medieval
- mental health problem
- mental illness
- midwife
- nurse
- nursing
- research
- Rome
- schizophrenia
- superstition
- witches

LEARNING OUTCOMES

The material in this chapter will assist you to:

- discern the different ways in which mental health problems have been constructed in past times,
- examine the ways in which literature delineates and defines mental health problems,
- understand the ways in which diverse societies adapt to people with mental health problems,
- appreciate the various approaches that have been used to treat people with mental health problems in the past,
- critique the hypothesis that care and treatment have improved progressively over time,
- discriminate between compassionate and inhumane nursing processes.

INTRODUCTION

This chapter examines mental health problems, the ways in which they have been regarded, and the ways in which they have been treated in past times. It traces the transition from individual family care to the emergence of organized care for people with mental health problems. The consequent professionalization of the people who treat and care for sufferers of mental health problems is described, and it will become clear that it is difficult to distinguish between the activity of nursing the physically ill and that of nursing people with mental health problems when such problems are seen as a physiological

'illness'. We will establish what constituted a mental health problem in past times and societies, and how such problems were regarded, and consider how these perceptions differ from those of today.

Each generation and society blends new knowledge with the inherited scholarship of the past. Occasionally the progression falters, as it did during the Middle Ages when the vast scholarship of the Graeco-Roman period was for centuries barely kept alive by the diligence of monastic orders in the West, and by Eastern scholars. Fortunately, Graeco-Roman discoveries in science and medicine, literature and the arts were recovered during the Renaissance and thereafter.

Winston Churchill believed that studying history gave the modern politician a practical advantage, saying: 'The farther back you look, the farther forward you can see' (Howells, 1991, p. 1). An opportunity to reflect upon the historical precedents for prevailing mental health problems, and the ways in which they have been diagnosed and treated in the past, can enhance the richness and depth of contemporary clinical practice.

Mental health problems cannot be discovered by archaeology, or by any other means than written sources, and sometimes the terminology cannot be translated exactly. It is inevitable that in the millennia covered briefly in this chapter, attitudes towards mental health and the mentally ill, and even mental health problems themselves, will have changed over time. Also, as with our own society and culture, attitudes towards mental health problems probably would have varied within any society or culture at a given time. Both ancient and modern ideas about mental health problems and 'madness' are contextual and shifting. Sometimes the ancient world seems remarkably familiar, but there are moments when we realize how different is the world we inhabit now. We can learn from both the differences and the similarities. The history of a discipline or profession provides a common ground from which to evaluate clinical experience. We can learn from the mistakes of the past but we can also take pride in our predecessors' achievements.

THE VALUE OF HISTORICAL ANTECEDENTS

There is an increasing tendency to discount the historical antecedents of mental health problems and their treatment as health and medical education abandons its emphasis on the teaching of Latin and Greek. Sigmund Freud and his colleagues received a sound classical education, which included the study of Latin and Greek, legend and mythology (Richards, 1991). Just as the Greek language determined the nomenclature of most body parts and diseases, it also influenced the naming of early psychoanalytic phenomena such as *mania* and *melancholia*, *neurosis* and *psychosis*, the *ego* and the *id* and the Oedipal and Electra complexes.

Perhaps it is the need to believe that modern medical science holds the key to a better world that leads some writers to deride the achievements of the past, or to ignore them completely. However, in some cases medicine, culture and society have not changed dramatically. Sometimes the past can hold valuable lessons and precedents which have been lost and which, when rediscovered, can assist us to achieve the best possible outcome for ourselves as healthcare practitioners and for our clients. Suer (1995) says that modern French psychiatry is based on ancient medicine, and traces the survival in modern psychiatric care of ancient medical terminology, psychiatric terms (e.g. mania and melancholia), theories of aetiology (airs, climates and humours) and personality types.

Nursing is a genuinely ancient career with honourable credentials. Other professions use and even invent historical precedents to assist in the glorification of their own profession. For example, psychiatry as a profession has only slowly developed in the course of the past 150 years since the American Psychiatric Association was founded in 1844 with only 13 members. Yet the influential medical historian and psychoanalyst Bennett Simon boasts that what makes the medical model 'unique' is the unbroken line which joins ancient and modern practitioners (Simon, 1978).

Alexander and Selesnick, in their classic and much-reprinted psychiatry text, maintain that psychiatrists and psychiatry are the culmination of an intellectual and professional evolution which began with witch doctors and philosophers, and claim that: 'the precursor of the psychiatrist was any man who tended another in pain. The story of psychiatry thus begins with the story of the first professional healer' (Alexander and Selesnick, 1966, p. 3). It is clear that the possession of a lengthy historical pedigree is considered an advantage for a profession. For example, occupational therapists also claim that their chosen work has ancient Graeco-Roman origins in the treatment of mental health problems (Busuttil, 1992).

Some nurses have also wished to demonstrate that their profession has existed since ancient times. For example, Doona (1992) claims as 'nurses' three women from the ancient literature, Euryclea, Cilissa and Medea, but none of these characters can be said to be 'nurses' as we understand the term today. All three characters are aged women who had in their youth 'nursed' or suckled children. They would not have cared for ill or wounded patients as would their modern 'nursing' counterparts.

In the present climate, which emphasizes tertiary education, research and professionalization in nursing, if nurses were to investigate and to own their own true history they could lay claim to a very distinguished lineage.

Nurses do not need to invent or inflate the historical achievements of their ancient colleagues.

In an editorial Burnard (2007) laments the exclusive emphasis upon recent research in nursing education today and recommends that more historical research be performed by nursing scholars. That is, it is important to consider the originators of the Western medical knowledge base – the ancient Graeco-Roman medical writers – who are often omitted from mental health nursing textbooks.

Nursing scholarship in fact prides itself upon being present-centred in the belief that this is the same as being innovative and progressive. But Burnard (2007, p. 665) claims that in the 'clamour to cite only the latest papers … students are often citing older ideas without appreciating their genesis. Thus well known scholars' work is often attributed, inaccurately, to more recent workers in the field'. If we never use older works, how do we know if what we are reading is innovative or derived from some earlier, original thinker's work?

Mental health nurses are not well served by existing mental health nursing texts if they seek to find out more about the history of mental healthcare or mental health problems. McAthie (1999) states that 'Little is written about nursing in early historical accounts because the care of the sick was considered an ordinary event – it seems that it was not important enough to record'. This statement is debatable on many levels. It assumes that because no research is known to the author, none was undertaken, and it reveals a lack of awareness of the greatly enhanced 'visibility' of women in literature and society in recent years. The social context in which Western nursing takes place today has altered enormously. Today's professional nursing, undertaken outside the home in institutions removed from the family, is an exception in the historical sense compared with the millennia during which nursing was undertaken by the family and their peripheral members, neighbours, slaves and servants, or later by religious orders.

The origins of medical care are addressed by McAthie (1999, p. 4) in a brief and inaccurate statement using as the source a text written in 1938: 'Religion and medicine were united very early, with medicine men, and later physicians, becoming priests'. This chapter will illustrate how an over-simplification of this kind can be misleading. Another standard mental health nursing text provides a similarly confused and barren coverage of the centuries preceding the eighteenth century. Boyd (2002) asserts that mental health problems in the first century AD were believed to be caused by sin or demonic possession and that 'clergymen' often treated patients by exorcism, which, if unsuccessful, led to the patients' being excluded from the community or put to death. But as we will see, the Roman writer Celsus (25 BC–*c*.AD 79) lived and wrote in the first century AD, and the enlightened and humane methods he advocated for the treatment of the mentally ill could as well be used to great effect today.

Brief, inaccurate and negative appraisals of the historical precedents for the treatment of mental disorders are, sadly, all too common, as is the tendency to present the past in an inappropriately ethnocentric fashion. For example, Frisch (2002) and McAthie (1999)'s table of 'Significant events in nursing in the twentieth century' addresses only events that occurred in the USA.

Neither does Frisch (2002) differentiate between 'primitive cultures' which confused medicine, magic and religion, and 'early civilizations' such as the Graeco-Roman, wherein the vast *Hippocratic Corpus* is reduced to a statement that Hippocrates attributed melancholy to an excess of black bile and believed that a cure could be effected by bloodletting. Frisch represents mental healthcare in the millennia preceding the eighteenth century as exclusively custodial and restricted to the confinement of 'lunatics' who were thought to be evil, witches or heretics: a feared, criminal population.

The reverse was more often true. Having a mental health problem in past times was not necessarily an impediment to leading a productive and consequential life. Ancient societies did not acknowledge many of the manifold mental health problems which are assiduously identified and isolated today, and in some ways they were more compassionate and tolerant than many societies today. It seems that the aim of modern medical or psychiatric writers in propagating exaggeratedly negative notions about the past is to emphasize the belief that things have changed for the better, a belief that might be meaningful to the health profession but which does no justice to the past.

PAST IDEAS ABOUT MENTAL HEALTH PROBLEMS

The terms 'mad' and 'insane' are not acceptable medical terms for mental health problems today, but these general terms have in the past been used to describe a wide range of symptoms and behaviours. The Latin word *insana* means 'not of right mind' and the equivalent Greek term is *mania*. The term 'mad' is a middle-English, pre-twelfth-century word which is still used today to describe a loss of reason and judgement. Metallic mercury poisoning in the felt-hat industry produced toxic effects which gave rise to the expression 'mad as a hatter'.

The idea of 'madness' in the ancient world usually implied mania or psychotic illness. Medicine recognized and treated mainly those mental health problems which disrupted a person's normal functioning in society, or which threatened the social order. Violence, agitation or excitement, being overtly out of touch with reality, experiencing hallucinations or delusions, melancholia causing inertia and inability to carry out one's normal tasks, or epilepsy usually succeeded in attracting medical attention. As is the case in our own society, sometimes a person was called 'mad' because their behaviour differed from the usual societal norms.

There are some issues which we can examine to help us in understanding the ways in which mental illness might have been constructed in the past. The theory of the humours was a systematic hypothesis that sought to explain why some people were susceptible to certain kinds of illness, including mental illness. The humoural theory (see the next section) was still being applied in the nineteenth century, and has been correctly described as the first diagnostic classification system (Mack et al., 1994). Mental ill health has in the past been seen by some as a punishment from the gods or God, and we will examine the role of the supernatural, and the perceived influence of God/gods upon the minds of humankind. The survival of some mental health problems across different times and cultures will also be considered with the assistance of vignettes and case studies collected from primary source literature. Finally, the different meanings of 'madness' and the mental state which it implies will be assessed.

The 'humours'

Early Greek medical texts tended on the whole to view mental health problems as a physiological illness. This is generally the case in the earliest of these, the *Hippocratic Corpus* (*c.*469–399 BC), a collection of works that were not all written by a doctor named Hippocrates, but by a variety of authors. The humoural theory was based on the belief that the body contained within it four humours – blood, phlegm, yellow bile and black bile – which were produced in various organs of the body. Each humour intrinsically possessed a basic quality such as heat, cold, dryness and moistness. Disease developed when internal or external factors disturbed the balance of the humours, and the imbalance produced injurious effects such as madness. Black bile and phlegm in particular caused mental illness, and an individual might be predisposed to mental ill health because of hereditary factors. These theories are explained more fully in the *Hippocratic Corpus*: *The Nature of Man*, *Regimen I* and *The Sacred Disease*.

Some words which are still used to describe a person's personality derive from humoural theory. The description of a person as 'phlegmatic' (cold and sluggish) retains the ancient meaning, that the person suffered from an excess of 'phlegm'. The 'melancholy' person was believed to have too much 'black bile' in their system, which led to a form of depression, and the person who could be described as 'choleric' possessed excessive yellow bile, which made them passionate and easily angered. In the 'sanguine' person, blood predominated over the other humours, and in both ancient and modern times to be sanguine is to be confident and hopeful.

Mental health problems were believed to be especially prevalent in spring and at the beginning of winter when the humours were believed to be stirred into activity by changes in the weather. Each person was believed to have been born with a constitution in which 'dryness' and 'wetness', 'fire' and 'water' were mixed. Those with a preponderance of 'dryness' and 'fire' could be intelligent but also impetuous and inclined to more agitated forms of insanity, while those in whom 'coldness' and 'water' predominated were prone to fearfulness and depression.

Some aspects of the humoural theory are of a sophistication which is perhaps not appreciated by modern critics, but in fact the four-factor theory of temperament and body function has not only survived, it has been revived in the areas of personality assessment and the prediction of vulnerability to physical disease (Hawkins, 1982; Lester, 1990; Merenda, 1987). Research such as that currently being undertaken into the human genome similarly seeks to find some intrinsic yet individual factor which will explain why certain people are vulnerable to specific diseases, a continuation of the same quest that originally led to the devising of the humoural theory 2500 years ago.

Supernatural influences

The *Diagnostic and Statistical Manual of Mental Disorders* (DSM-IV TR; American Psychiatric Association, 1994, p xxiv) cautions against labelling behaviour that is based in the religious beliefs of another culture as pathological:

> *A clinician who is unfamiliar with the nuances of an individual's cultural frame of reference may incorrectly judge as psychopathology those normal variations in behavior, belief, or experience that are particular to the person's culture. For example, certain religious practices or beliefs … may be misdiagnosed as manifestations of a Psychotic Disorder.*

It has always been difficult in practice to differentiate religiously motivated behaviour from mental health problems. Research indicates that the more the religious beliefs of others deviate from the mental health professional's beliefs, the more liable the professional is to judge the others' beliefs as mentally unhealthy (Sanderson et al., 1999). Knowing this, the mental health professional needs to recognize their potential for making judgements based on erroneous religious or cultural assumptions.

CASE STUDY: CLEOMENES OF SPARTA

According to Herodotus's informants, Cleomenes could have suffered from a mild form of mental illness throughout his life, but towards the end of it he 'went quite mad' and his family had him confined to the stocks, bound and guarded. Cleomenes' subsequent suicide is reported in some detail.

As he was lying there, fast bound, he asked his jailer, when no one else was there, to give him a knife. At first the man, who was a serf, refused, but Cleomenes, by threats of what he would do to him when he recovered his liberty, so frightened him that he at last consented. As soon as the knife was in his hands, Cleomenes began to mutilate himself, beginning on his shins. He sliced his flesh into strips, working upward to his thighs, and from them to his hips and sides, until he reached his belly, and while he was cutting that into strips he died.

Herodotus, *The Histories*, vi.75

Greece and Rome

Herodotus (490–425 BC) wrote *The Histories*, the first prose work ever recorded. He is our primary source of information about Cleomenes the First of Sparta, who reigned between *c*.519 and 490 BC, so Herodotus could interview people who actually knew Cleomenes. Cleomenes' illness illustrates an instance of ancient mental illness which culminated in suicide. There are many factors that influence the decision to suicide and the ways in which the act is regarded. De Leo describes the vast differences in suicide rates that are found throughout history and across nations when one takes into account age, gender, socioeconomic status, ethnicity and religion (De Leo, 2002). Nurses still wrestle with the moral and ethical implications of intentional suicide and find that if they do not deal with them the unforeseen emotional implications can take them unawares (Rich and Butts, 2004).

Herodotus is personally unable to decide between a superstitious cause and a rational one for Cleomenes' madness and death. He includes contemporary opinions about the cause of Cleomenes' illness and suicide. Some Greeks said he was being punished by the gods for his impiety, but his fellow Spartans believed that 'heaven had no hand in Cleomenes' madness, but by consorting with Scythians he became a drinker of strong wine, and thence the madness came' (vi.84). The Spartans were a pragmatic people, and they were better acquainted with the man, his behaviour and the events surrounding his death. Their attribution of Cleomenes' death to prosaic, organic causes, and their specific rejection of the theory that Cleomenes' madness was divinely inflicted, is proof that mental distress was not universally believed to be the result of divine punishment.

In the case study below, Plutarch (*c.*AD 50–120) relates that Alexander the Great acted upon religious convictions and advice when he put to death a person who was deluded and hallucinating.

CASE STUDY: ALEXANDER THE GREAT

[Alexander] was playing at ball, and when it was time to dress again, the young men who were playing with him beheld a man seated on the king's throne, in silence, wearing the royal diadem and robes. When the man was asked who he was, he was speechless for a long time; but at last he came to his senses and said that his name was Dionysius … and for a long time had been in chains; but just now the god Serapis had come to him and loosed his chains and brought him to this spot, bidding him put on the robe and diadem and sit on the throne and hold his peace. On hearing this, Alexander put the man out of the way, as the seers directed….

Plutarch, *Life of Alexander*, LXXIII–LXXIV

Alexander the Great was harsh upon this man because he believed that if the god Serapis had instructed the man to wear Alexander's crown and robes, this could be an omen foreshadowing his own death. Perhaps it is scenarios such as this which lead many modern authors to believe that mental illness was always punished harshly, or regarded by ancient societies with superstitious dread (Blakemore, 1988; Devereux, 1970; Dodds, 1951; Hershkowitz, 1998; Parker, 1983; Roccatagliata, 1991; Rosen, 1968; Simon, 1978; Stone, 1997). This position is not wholly supported by the evidence. Perhaps there was a clear line of demarcation between the medical position on mental health problems and 'popular' attitudes and beliefs.

The Greeks seem generally to have differentiated between 'disease-induced madness' and 'divinely caused madness'. The *Hippocratic Corpus* states that the gods were more likely to purify and sanctify than to harm, and derides doctors who assigned a supernatural cause to epilepsy or mental health problems, denouncing them as charlatans who were at a loss because they did not know how to treat the patient and 'sheltered themselves behind superstition' (*The Sacred Disease* II–IV).

The medical term *melancholia* was used by both the Greek comic playwright Aristophanes (*c.*457–385 BC) and the Greek politician Demosthenes (384–322 BC), evidence that medical terminology was in common usage by as early as the fifth century BC. In Plautus's (*c.*254–184 BC) *The Menaechmi* the doctor enquires as to whether a patient's disorder was due to possession or hallucinations, indicating that although possession was a recognized 'disorder', it was clearly able to be distinguished from hallucinations by the medical profession, popular playwrights and their audiences.

The *Hippocratic Corpus*'s disapproval of superstition was still shared by Roman society over five centuries later, when Soranus of Ephesis (AD 98–138) stated in his work on gynaecology that the best midwives were free from superstition, and did not 'overlook salutary measures on account of a dream or omen or some customary rite or vulgar superstition' (Book I.II.4).

Perhaps two different attitudes towards mental abnormality coexisted in classical antiquity: the traditional one, which was 'superstitious and magical' and attributed abnormal behaviour to supernatural intervention; and the other, which is found in the medical literature, which rejects the supernatural or the divine agency as an explanation. Medical terms were adopted and used by the public, and they coexisted with superstitious or religious beliefs about possession and divine punishment. This would be a similar situation to that in which we might believe in both medical technology and in 'the stars' or astrology, simultaneously.

The Christian era

The spread of Christianity did not eliminate the association in some quarters of mental illness with the influence of supernatural agencies. Instead, the belief that the old pagan gods caused mental illness was translated into a belief that the devil might be at work when a person experienced hallucinations or delusions. In the late thirteenth century the Inquisition began to deal with isolated cases of supposed witchcraft involving heresy, but it was not until the fifteenth and sixteenth centuries that mass persecutions took place, involving accusations of night-flying, intercourse with the devil, transformation into animals and malicious spells. Both the sufferers from mental illness and those associated with them, or believed to have injured them, could be the objects of suspicion and ill-treatment.

By the 1630s the tide was beginning to turn against the persecution of witches, and influential writers such as Robert Filmer denounced witch-hunting. The American colonies were slow to react to European trends, and in 1692 150 'witches' were tried and 19 were hung in Salem, Massachusetts. The cause of the bizarre behaviour of the adolescent girls involved has been hypothesized by modern scholars as being due to ergot poisoning or mycotoxin (Woolf, 2000). Whatever the cause, when the hysteria died down public revulsion resulted in the annulment of the convictions and the release of those of the convicted who had survived. This event marks the virtual end of witch-hunting.

During a period of around two centuries a number of so-called 'witches' were put to death, but the figures on 'wise women' killed as witches because they were healers seem to be greatly exaggerated in some sources. Perhaps the emergence of the women's liberation movement in the 1970s and its adoption by early nursing scholars contributed to a discourse wherein women's unrecorded and uncelebrated role as healers was being explored. The persecution of witches for practising inherited healing arts seemed to offer some explanation for the failure of women to be recognized as health professionals. However, it is difficult to locate research evidence to support assertions that 'millions' of witches or 'wise women' were killed in societies which were basically illiterate. Neither is there any indication that all of the witches who were persecuted were practising healers or that all healers were persecuted as witches.

MENTAL HEALTH PROBLEMS FOUND IN GRAECO-ROMAN SOURCES

What follows is the result of comprehensive research into mental health problems in the ancient Greek and Roman literature (Evans, 2000).

The *mood disorders* or affective disorders (see Ch. 15), consisting of mania and depression, alone or in combination, were found to exist in the ancient literature, although the term *melancholia* evolved in meaning over the centuries (Evans, 2007). Melancholia by no means always meant the equivalent of 'depression', in the way it is constructed today. The most convincing and earliest conclusive instance of major depression was that suffered by the prominent Roman lawyer, statesman, philosopher and author, Marcus Tullius Cicero (106–43 BC).

At his most despondent, Cicero tended to withdraw from the Roman society in which he was celebrated, and retire to the country, as his surviving letters testify. Cicero wrote to his friend Atticus on most of the days they were separated, and his copious correspondence clearly documents three diagnosable episodes of major depression (Evans, 2007). Cicero seems to have discovered for himself a self-help treatment method that really works and is recommended today to alleviate depression. Writing a daily journal that addresses emotional issues over a period of months has been found by modern researchers to lighten depression, as has writing about bereavement following the death of a loved one (Range et al., 2000). Paradoxically, it is only narrative writing that helps to alleviate depression: writing poetry does not seem to help (Kaufman and Sexton, 2006). Cicero experienced his last and most severe episode of depression after the death of his daughter Tullia. Latham and Prigerson (2004) find that bereavement complicated by depression frequently results in a very high risk of suicide. An excerpt of one of Cicero's letters is shown in this case study.

CASE STUDY: CICERO'S DEPRESSION

In this lonely place I do not talk to a soul. Early in the day I hide myself in a thick, thorny wood, and don't emerge till evening. Next to yourself solitude is my best friend. When I am alone all my conversation is with my books, but it is interrupted by fits of weeping, against which I struggle as best I can. But so far it is an unequal fight.

Cicero, *Letters to Atticus*, Astura 9 March, 45 BC

The *anxiety disorders* (see Ch. 17) as they were manifested in the ancient world have not previously been the subject of a great deal of critical attention in the modern secondary literature, but convincing examples of anxiety disorders are described in the classical texts. The case study from the *Hippocratic Corpus* describes two ancient examples

CASE STUDY: PHOBIAS

Nicanor's affection, when he went to a drinking party, was fear of the flute girl. Whenever he heard the voice of the flute begin to play at a symposium, masses of terrors rose up. He said that he could hardly bear it when it was night, but if he heard it in the daytime he was not affected. Such symptoms persisted over a long period of time. Democles, who was with him, seemed blind and powerless of body, and could not go along a cliff, nor on to a bridge to cross a ditch of the least depth, but he could go through the ditch itself. This affected him for some time.

Hippocratic Corpus, Volume VII, *Epidemics* 5.81–2

CASE STUDY: POST-TRAUMATIC STRESS DISORDER

[Cassander] had only recently come to Babylon, and when he saw some Barbarians doing obeisance to Alexander, since he had been reared as a Greek and had never seen such a sight as this before, he laughed boisterously. But Alexander was enraged, and clutching him fiercely by the hair with both hands dashed his head against the wall.... Cassander's spirit was deeply penetrated and imbued with a dreadful fear of Alexander, so that many years afterwards, when he was now king of Macedonia and master of Greece, as he was walking about and surveying the statues at Delphi, the sight of an image of Alexander smote him suddenly with a shuddering and trembling from which he could scarcely recover, and made his head swim.

Plutarch, *Life of Alexander*, LXXIV.1–4

of phobic avoidance, and that which follows from Plutarch describes an instance of post-traumatic stress disorder.

Both the anxiety disorders and the *personality disorders* (see Ch. 16) were acknowledged by ancient cultures to be serious, chronic mental irregularities which could influence the sufferer's life, but they were not considered to be illnesses which required treatment. A number of examples of personality disorders have been identified, but since the concept of a personality disorder is often culturally determined, particular care was taken to ensure that the subject of the case study was considered by their peers to have differed from societal norms (Evans, 2000).

There was in the ancient literature evidence which affirmed that *epilepsy* was believed to be related to mental illness. Epilepsy can exhibit psychiatric sequelae, but whereas it was considered to be a mental health problem in the ancient world, it is not so regarded today. The *substance-related disorders* (see Ch. 19) were, conversely, not in ancient times conceded to be mental health problems, although drunkenness might lead to socially unacceptable behaviour. Alcohol-related disorders proved to be a complex topic; examples of these health problems were located in ancient Greek and Roman literature. Indeed, although excessive alcohol consumption seems to have caused or complicated many medical conditions, ancient medical and societal opinion seemed to indicate that conditions such as alcohol abuse, dependence and withdrawal went largely unrecognized (Evans, 2000).

Some *psychotic disorders* (see Ch. 14) were documented and recognized as such in the ancient Graeco-Roman literature, but this author's research indicates that the full gamut of criteria which would justify a modern diagnosis of schizophrenia (early onset, hallucinations, delusions and a degree of chronicity) was not apparent anywhere in the ancient Greek and Roman texts (Evans et al., 2003). The reportage of symptoms for all the major mental health problems in the ancient literature was often inadequate to satisfy modern diagnostic criteria with reference to the duration and range of symptoms.

Mental health problems not found in the ancient literature

The case study of King Cleomenes of Sparta provided evidence that although his contemporaries might have considered Cleomenes to be chronically insane, and that he had a psychotic episode which was well documented, a diagnosis of schizophrenia could not be made. Indeed, although the anxiety disorders and major depression appear to have survived in the exact form in which they present nowadays, indicating that these mental health problems can be said to be stable across time and culture, schizophrenia appears not to have manifested in the same way, or perhaps not to have existed in classical times (Evans et al., 2003).

Historical perspective on schizophrenia

Michel Foucault, the French philosopher considered by many to have made a significant contribution to our understanding of the social construction of madness, commences his study with the fifteenth century (Foucault, 1967). Foucault had no medical background and does not describe his subjects with sufficient clarity to allow clinical diagnoses to be made. To Foucault, 'madness' encompassed a bizarre collection of mental health problems: melancholia with delusional guilt, melancholy allied with mania, nymphomania, delirium, vertigo, hysterical convulsions, hysteria and hypochondria.

Some of Foucault's subjects appear to suffer from a form of chronic, lifelong 'madness' which disabled them from undertaking productive work, so they are identified with 'the indigent'. They are represented as deluded, demented and hallucinated, reduced to an animal state in which they are inured to 'hunger, heat, cold, pain' (Foucault, 1967, p. 74). Frequent references to the ability of the 'mad' to endure physiological hardship suggest a degree of neurological damage. Perhaps they were the victims of syphilis, which Grmek (1991) believes had emerged in Europe by then. Perhaps they suffered from chronic schizophrenia, if indeed this disorder had evolved by the late Middle Ages.

Research into the origins of schizophrenia has led some to conclude that not only has schizophrenia changed in its manifestation within the past 50 years, but that it might exhibit such different symptoms in different cultures as to cause one to question whether the diagnostic criteria refer to the same condition (Ellard, 1987; Jeste et al., 1985). Other reputable researchers believe that schizophrenia appeared in recent centuries. H Fuller Torrey and colleagues have investigated the origins of schizophrenia, and they postulate that the disorder is the product of a genetic mutation which occurred in recent centuries. Supporting evidence has been collected of viral-associated sequences in the brains of individuals suffering from schizophrenia (Yolken et al., 1997). It has been hypothesized that urban birth, household crowding and/or the transmission of a virus from household cats could assist the spread of the virus (Torrey and Yolken, 1995, 1998; Torrey et al., 1997).

The state of medical knowledge at present can assist in tracking the development and dissemination of new or unfamiliar diseases, but if schizophrenia emerged in a less technical and literate society, its advent would have gone undocumented. Mental ill health leaves no trace on skeletal remains; it can only be traced in the surviving literature.

'Hysteria': a translation error

The familiar term 'hysteria' is not an ancient Greek word and does not appear in any Greek dictionary or lexicon of Greek words. A number of ancient passages which have been interpreted as referring to a mental affliction arising in the womb appear to refer only to physical gynaecological complaints. The problem resides in the translation. The evidence suggests that the translator has bestowed a modern and anachronistic meaning upon the Greek text that is not supported by the evidence (King, 1993).

It is a remarkably durable belief that 'hysteria' is a feminine mental health problem which has been recognized since the days of Hippocrates. This belief confers upon hysteria a spurious respectability, whereas it was proved conclusively over a decade ago that the term 'hysteria' was invented by Littre, the French translator of the *Hippocratic Corpus* in the late nineteenth century. Helen King's informative scholarship will be briefly summarized, because 'hysteria' is still considered to be one of psychiatry's most celebrated apparent legacies from the ancient medical literature, and once something passes into the inherited 'knowledge' associated with a discipline, it is hard to eradicate even if it is untrue.

Since Freud 'rediscovered' hysteria it seems that male therapists have been especially keen to reinforce the notion that women have always been prone to gender-specific ills, and that men can cure them. Bennett Simon (1978) described Freud's psychoanalysis of a female patient's 'hysterical expression of the thwarted sexuality of the recently widowed young woman' and added that 'Greek doctors knew that virgins and widows were most susceptible to those diseases of the womb called "hysterical"' (p. 25). In fact, Simon devotes an entire chapter in his book about mental illness in ancient Greece to hysteria and social issues, commencing with the statement that 'Hysteria, the disease of the "wandering uterus" was given its name by the Greeks' (Simon, 1978, p. 238). The respected psychiatric textbook, Kaplan et al.'s *Synopsis of Psychiatry*, attributes Hippocrates with having 'introduced the terms "mania" and "hysteria" as forms of mental illness in the fifth century BC' (Kaplan et al., 1994). But 'hysteria' is not a Greek word, and Hippocrates did not use it.

Acceptance of the fact that 'hysteria' was a mental illness typically found in women and first described in the *Hippocratic Corpus* is dependent upon the incorrect translation of the words *hysterike*, *hysterika* and *hysterikos*, words which translate as 'suffering in the womb'. King (1993) found that hysteria is in reality 'but a mare's nest,

a spurious entity' (Gilman et al., 1993, p xi). *Hysterikos* was not considered to have connotations of mental illness in the ancient literature. The Emile Littre (1839–61) edition of the *Hippocratic Corpus* translates *hysterikos* as 'hysteria', in French *hysterie* (King, 1993, p. 7). By examining the original Greek texts, King found that Littre's chapter headings, such as 'Hysterie', have no analogies in the Greek manuscripts; Littre freely transposes the medical categories of his own time. King concludes that Littre translated the *Hippocratic Corpus* in the mid-nineteenth century, when the psychiatric condition 'hysteria' had begun to be a debated ideology. He expected to find hysteria in the text, and of course he found it, and composed his headings accordingly. The diagnosis was therefore made by the translator (King, 1993, p. 8).

It is probable that Celsus's translator, Spencer, was similarly influenced. The error was perpetuated in Spencer's 1935–38 translation of Celsus. Spencer notes, for example, that in *De Medicina* 5.21.6 the woman's 'fits' would have been 'hysterical fits'. Similarly, Spencer appends a footnote to indicate that the *Hippocratic Corpus: Aphorisms* V 35 is 'a description of hysteria' when it is more properly translated as 'suffering from illness in the womb'. Freud collaborated with Joseph Breuer to produce *Studies in Hysteria* in 1895. If *hysterikos*, meaning in Greek 'afflicted with suffering in the womb', is translated as 'suffering from hysteria', it is clear that the translation is influenced not by the original language of the text but by the meaning which Charcot, Freud and Breuer attached to the psychiatric diagnosis of 'hysteria' in mainly female patients in the late nineteenth century (Evans, 2000).

King suggests that in 'hysteria' we do not hear 'the insistent voice of a fixed entity calling across the centuries':

> *Nineteenth-century hysteria, a parasite in search of a history, grafts itself by name and lineage onto the centuries-old tradition of suffocation of the womb, thus making Hippocrates its adopted father. It is time that father disowned his hybrid child.*
>
> (King, 1993, p. 64)

Unfortunately, the parasite hysteria remains attached to Hippocrates in the minds of many, despite being conclusively disowned, because historical research is too often ignored or disregarded.

GENDER AND HEALTHCARE

In Western countries we are now used to considering nursing to be a profession suited to either gender. Indeed, mental health nursing was predominantly the province of the male nurse, since asylums were created to confine the seriously 'mentally ill' who could not be accommodated in society before the development of neuroleptic medication in the 1950s, because males possessed an advantage in terms of strength.

In past centuries nursing was considered to be the natural province of women, an extension of the maternal, caring role, but the absence of women in the literature has made nurses and nursing difficult to trace. The classicist who wrote an early essay entitled 'Ancient nursing' wrestles with what he sees as the absence of nurses in the ancient world: 'so little is told us of nurses and nursing. The conclusion we are tempted to draw from this silence is that the task of nursing fell to the women, whether slaves or free, of the household' (Jones, 1923).

The usual attitude towards 'respectable' women in ancient male-dominated societies was conservative and patriarchal. Ancient ideas about how women should conduct themselves are encapsulated in Pericles' speech to the Athenian women in 430 BC:

> Perhaps I should say a word or two on the duties of women to those among you who are now widowed … the greatest glory of a woman is to be least talked about by men, whether they are praising you or criticising you.

(Thucydides, ii.46)

Women have traditionally been poorly educated, and little has survived of the writing that the educated few have accomplished. Most ancient authors wrote about their male, aristocratic peers, and because so much of the literary evidence from most centuries preceding the most recent two or three is limited by the writer's upper social class and male gender, much historical research cannot accurately report the incidence of any type of illness in the female gender. Where women are mentioned, whether in the medical literature, in the histories, in biographies of their menfolk, in fiction or in poetry, it is from the perspective of a male and any such account cannot be said with certainty to represent the authentic female experience.

Women usually appear in the ancient medical literature in their reproductive role, in relation to childbirth and any gynaecological disorders which might prevent or complicate childbirth. Most health problems a woman might have were attributed to the possession of a womb. The Roman poet Martial (c.AD 40–104) records that when male doctors were called in to treat 'women's complaints' both they and their female patient's true motives were probably sexual. Note that the modern, mistaken term 'hysteria' has been used by the translator instead of the more correct translation 'pain in the womb'.

> One day Leda announced to her aged husband, 'I'm suffering from hysteria. I'm sorry, but I'm told that nothing but intercourse will make me feel cheerier'.

(Martial, The Epigrams, 11.71)

'Leda' had been attended by female nurses, but they leave when the doctors arrive, whereupon the doctors 'hoist and prise open her legs' with the exclamation: 'Ah, serious medicine!'. The male doctors are depicted as eager to 'treat' this illness fabricated to procure the sexual services of younger lovers. In a society where medical practitioners were male, the ailments of women, being outside the experience of men, could be seen as counterfeit, even if the prevailing masculine ideas about the innate immorality of women did not intrude.

'Leda' was an upper-class woman, but in the course of their lives most women were unlikely to be treated by a male physician. In fact women probably received little medical attention that was unrelated to reproductive affairs, and they would have treated themselves and their dependants in the seclusion of the women's quarters.

CARING FOR PEOPLE WITH MENTAL HEALTH PROBLEMS

Graeco-Roman origins of Western care

In ancient Greek and Roman times the Greek hero and god of healing, Asclepius, whose staff wound about with a snake inspired the present symbol of medicine, was commemorated by temple healing centres called Asclepions. Treatment consisted of a combination of medical and priestly practices but the main ceremonial treatment practised there was the ritual of incubation (temple-sleep and the interpretation of dreams). In the *Hippocratic Corpus* it is said of dreams:

> For when the body is awake the soul is its servant, and is never her own mistress, but divides her attention among many things … but the mind never enjoys independence. But when the body is at rest, the soul administers her own household….

(Regimen IV, LXXXVI)

This recognition of the importance of the unconscious as expressed in dreams was surprisingly sophisticated, and the prominence given to dreams in the ancient world was not equalled until Freud's work in the area 2500 years later. Yet the Asclepion was not an infallible remedy. In his play The Wasps, Aristophanes, the Greek writer of comedy, depicted a case of dementia which was treated initially by purification rites and a stay in the Temple of Asclepius, but the only treatment which was effective in preventing the demented patient from leaving the house was putting the house under guard and having every opening covered with netting. Graeco-Roman medical science and theory were highly sophisticated, but medical treatment was predominantly the concern of the individual, with perhaps assistance from the medical practitioner if the family was prosperous.

When he showed signs of a violent mental disturbance, Cleomenes of Sparta, who reigned between c.519 and 490 BC, was confined to the stocks by his family, who kept him bound and guarded. Despite this, he managed to trick the jailer into giving him the knife with which he suicided. The Roman medical writer Celsus (25 BC–c.AD 79) wrote five centuries after the time of Cleomenes, but it is clear that the kind of treatment which was considered suitable for the person who was mad and violent in Roman society had not changed a great deal in the intervening centuries. First, Celsus differentiates between the several forms of insanity:

> some among insane persons are sad, others hilarious; some are more readily controlled and rave in words only, others are rebellious and act with violence; and of these latter, some only do harm by impulse, others are artful too, and show the most complete appearance of sanity whilst seizing occasion for mischief, but they are detected by the result of their acts.
>
> (Celsus, De Medicina, III.18.3)

Celsus prescribed distinct interventions for the fearful, the violent, the melancholy and those who exhibited 'untimely laughter' (III.18.10). He allowed that those who 'merely rave in their talk, or who make but trifling misuse of their hands' ought not to be constrained unnecessarily, but he recommends that it is best to fetter those who are violent 'lest they should do harm, either to themselves or to others. Anyone so fettered, although he talks rationally and pitifully when he wants his fetters removed, is not to be trusted, for that is a madman's trick' (III.18.4).

This description perfectly fits the treatment accorded to Cleomenes. The person with a mental health problem who was violent presented a challenge in the era before the advent of the major tranquillizers in the 1950s. There was little alternative to physical restraint as a means of preventing people from violently harming themselves or others, and physical restraint was, as it sometimes still is, the only means of preventing harm to the person or the environment.

ETHICAL DILEMMA

Now that those who merely rave in their talk, or who make but trifling misuse of their hands, should be coerced with the severer forms of constraint is superfluous; but those who conduct themselves more violently it is expedient to fetter, lest they should do harm, either to themselves or to others.

(Celsus, De Medicina, III.18.4)

The regulation that the patient be prevented from harming themselves or others is still regarded as a legitimate reason for restraining a patient under most mental health legislation. Celsus forbade restraint for any longer than was strictly necessary, saying: '[sometimes] there is nothing else to do but restrain the patient, but when circumstances permit, relief must be given with haste' (III.18.6).

Question

◆ Is physical restraint too primitive a treatment for the mental health service user who is violent? The forced ingestion of tranquillizers is often seen as a more humane alternative. Is chemical restraint a more humane or less humane alternative to physical restraint?

Yet Celsus was basically humane and he respected individual differences. He recommended that the patient not be frightened, that they be kept in an environment that was reassuring, either in the light or in the dark, whichever was the most 'quieting of the spirit' for the patient. 'It is best, therefore, to make a trial of both, and to keep that patient in the light who is afraid of darkness, and him in darkness who is frightened by light' (III.18.5). Celsus forbade restraint for any longer than was required, and recommended that the restraint be removed the moment it was unnecessary. Just as the prevention of harm to the patient or to others is still regarded as a legitimate reason for restraining a patient under the mental health legislation of many countries, it also remains a legal requirement that restraint be alleviated as soon as is practically possible.

Celsus outlines a medley of responses that can be helpful in treating various mental health problems. The variety and sophistication of his suggested interventions can be seen as the birthplace of counselling techniques that are used in mental health nursing to this day. In the examples which follow, the patient is depressed and/or anxious. He is at home, and the simple yet effective suggestions were meant to be followed by family or friends.

> Some need to have empty fears relieved, as was done for a wealthy man in dread of starvation, to whom pretended legacies were from time to time announced … in others, melancholy thoughts are to be dissipated, for which purpose music, cymbals, and noises are of use. More often, however, the patient is to be agreed with rather than opposed, and his mind slowly and imperceptibly is to be turned from the irrational talk to something better.
>
> (Celsus, De Medicina, III.18.10–12)

Reassurance was clearly used to good effect, and it is interesting that the invention of good news to enhance hopefulness was not considered unethical if it was effective.

The patient was to be entertained, distracted and amused. Other suggestions included reading to the patient, games and storytelling 'especially by those with which the patient was wont to be attracted when sane', and praising any work the patient was able to produce. People who the patient liked and esteemed were urged to eat with them to stimulate their appetite and to 'gently reprove his depression as being without cause' (Celsus, *De Medicina*, III.18.18).

In AD 331, around seven centuries after the *Hippocratic Corpus* was written, and two and a half centuries after Celsus wrote, the Roman emperor Constantine the Great decreed that the Church should take responsibility for the care of the sick after a plague (perhaps anthrax) devastated the Roman Empire. The first public hospital in Europe was founded by a Roman woman, Fabiola, at Ostia near Rome in AD 390. Europe has had a strong tradition of healthcare by religious orders which has continued across the centuries since that time.

Eastern medical care

It is Ceylon which holds the honour of establishing the world's first hospital in 437 BC. At around the same time one-third of the population of Athens died of the plague (typhus or smallpox) without the benefit of organized medical assistance. The first public hospitals in India were founded in 256 BC, and the medicines used were supplied by the ruler (Mellersh, 1999).

The Indian public hospital system had developed upon egalitarian principles and by AD 400 it offered free treatment to all regardless of wealth or rank. Indian hospitals had become the benchmark, and the idea was transferred to China, although in China hospitals were usually only available to the fee-paying elite. After AD 430 when the rebellious Christian sect, the Nestorians, had been exiled from Constantinople, taking Greek medical texts with them, India and Persia used the texts to make independent medical and scientific progress (Mellersh, 1999).

After the fall of the Roman Empire, the Greek and Roman medical texts survived, having been copied and kept by religious orders in the West. This knowledge was both adopted and enhanced by the Eastern scholars; by AD 660, Indian physicians had developed sophisticated bladder and digestive tract surgery. In the ninth century a hospital was established in Baghdad which by the tenth century had become the largest medical faculty in the world, with 24 physicians. Whereas Western medicine and healthcare stagnated until around the twelfth century, Muslim, Japanese and Chinese scholars developed extensive surgical, anatomical and pharmacological expertise (Mellersh, 1999).

Western developments

The East retained its scientific ascendancy as the Catholic faith gained control in Europe. Access to healthcare in Europe in the Middle Ages was limited to that provided by religious orders at hospices which could care for those few in society who did not have family to provide services for them. The Christian Church was instrumental in forestalling some forms of medical research by forbidding practices such as the mutilation of the dead. This tended to hamper the training of medical personnel, the study of anatomy and eventually surgical interventions of most sorts.

Indian physicians had developed sophisticated bladder and digestive tract surgery at much the same time as the Hotel Dieu was opened in Paris (AD 660). The Hotel Dieu was technically a hospital but was more concerned with treating the patient's soul than their ailments. In the fifteenth and sixteenth centuries the Renaissance had reawakened European scholarship and engendered advances in many fields, including healthcare. Flamel had established 14 new hospitals in Paris, St Thomas's hospital had been established in London and universities proliferated throughout Europe (Mellersh, 1999).

As time progressed, society changed and the healthcare needs of the population changed too. During the eighteenth and nineteenth centuries the Industrial Revolution caused rural societies to be disrupted due to many of their inhabitants deserting their rural homelands to seek work in the factories and manufacturing towns, thereby removing themselves from the traditional sources of societal and family healthcare. This coincided with an upsurge of diagnoses of schizophrenia in industrialized societies. Schizophrenia appears not to have existed in the ancient Greek or Roman worlds (Evans et al., 2003) and some researchers postulate that it evolved comparatively recently, sometime in the seventeenth century (Jeste et al., 1985), causing a crisis in the evolving healthcare systems and demanding the creation of new solutions.

The asylum

Chronically ill and displaced populations required the creation of institutions which could cater for their needs. For some time little distinction was made between people with mental health problems and other persons unable to exist independently in society. The dissolution of the monasteries in England in 1536 had restricted funding of hospitals by the Church, but previous to this many early hospitals and carers had been allied with the Church. People with mental health problems were confined with others most in need of care and detention: lepers, criminals, the indigent, the unemployed and the ill. Perhaps a vestige of the confusion this caused between mental ill health, indigence and wickedness can be found in the stigmatizing view of people with mental health problems which persists to this day in some societies, diminishing the client's self-esteem and interfering with the delivery of supportive mental healthcare (Corrigan, 2004).

By 1400 Bethlehem Hospital in London ('Bedlam') was devoted to the treatment, or more correctly the confinement, of the mentally ill, and in 1851 Colney Hatch in London was built, the largest lunatic asylum in Europe. It was desperately needed. At this time there were in the UK alone some 3579 'lunatics' in public asylums, 2559 in the 139 licensed houses devoted to the treatment of mental ill health and 8000 more in workhouses or at home. The asylums were characterized as 'warehouses for the unwanted', the aged, destitute vagrants, alcoholics and syphilitics. Europe and the USA followed suit (Mellersh, 1999).

Custodial care was for a long time the only option if a mental health problem followed a chronic, disabling course in the absence of modern psychotropic medications, which were only developed less than five decades ago. Macalpine and Hunter investigated the alleged mental health problem of King George III, which they attribute to the medical condition porphyria (Macalpine and Hunter, 1969). It is clear that some of the methods of treating perceived mental health problems had not altered significantly in the two millennia since Hippocrates. The king was cupped, bled and dosed with emetics and purgatives, secluded from family and friends, and physically restrained for the protection of himself and others (Macalpine and Hunter, 1969).

CRITICAL THINKING CHALLENGE 3.2

What would be some of the disadvantages, difficulties and changes for the service user, their family and society if those with mental health problems were cared for by the family?

What would be the advantages for the service user and for society if the service user's family were solely responsible for the care of people with mental health problems?

DOCTORS AND NURSES

The amount of medical knowledge that existed in ancient times could be learned by an educated person of average intelligence. The concept of role specialization in healthcare was less developed in the premodern eras, and the amateur was not sharply distinguished from the professional. Even where roles such as 'doctor', 'nurse' or 'midwife' existed, their areas of expertise would be quite different from what they are now. For example, the midwife could be employed for the birth by wealthier families, but she relied upon family members for assistance, and handed the baby to wet nurses, who assumed the care of the infant.

Furthermore, it is impossible to distinguish between mental health nurses and general nurses until relatively modern times, because the distinction between problems of the mind and disorders of the body is of relatively recent origin. In this respect, ancient nursing was more holistic than it is today, when the distinctions between the disciplines appear to be stressed more than the similarities.

Ancient Greece and Rome

There were instances noted as early as Homer (circa eighth century BC) of systematic nursing of patients. *The Iliad* (*c*.800 BC), which describes the Trojan War, depicts the wounded as being removed to tents dedicated to healing, and tended mainly by captured slave women under the direction of Greek surgeons, although on the battlefield the 'nurses' were more often men attached to the military force.

The Roman writer Celsus is an important source for the history of medicine, but it is doubtful that Celsus was a practising physician. The philosophers Plato and Aristotle, among others, wrote about medical subjects although they had no formal medical training. The Greeks formalized scientific medical training at recognized medical schools such as Cos, Cnidos and later Alexandria. The early Greek doctor had no special status but, like a craftsman, he travelled from town to town and most probably employed his pupils as nurses. There was no form of licensure, but pupils were bound by an agreement: the *Hippocratic Oath* is one early form of private contract (Hornblower and Spawforth, 1996).

In the *Hippocratic Corpus* it appears that in the absence of the doctor the patient was attended to by family members, slaves or medical students, who reported the patient's progress to the doctor. The following sensitive advice from the *Hippocratic Corpus* would be useful for any person who cared for an individual who was physically or mentally ill.

NURSE'S STORY

Kindnesses to those who are ill. For example to do in a clean way his food or drink or whatever he sees, softly what he touches. Things that do no great harm and are easily got, such as cool drink where it is needed. Entrance, conversation. Position and clothing for the sick person, hair, nails, scents.

Hippocrates, Volume VII, *Epidemics* 6.4.7

The Roman poet Martial probably exaggerated when he said that the doctor who attended him had 45 students with 90 hands who examined him, but there would have been some students in any case. We may assume that a great deal of the information given in the clinical histories such as the *Epidemics* is the result of their observations and those of the family or carers. The information gathered about the patient required an awareness of what was significant and what was not, which means that responsible and intelligent laypersons would have been satisfactory sources of information. This nurse's story warns the reader of the sensitivity required when 'the practitioner' approaches the patient. The exact role of 'the practitioner' is never specified.

NURSE'S STORY

The bath and exercise and fear and anger and any other feeling of the mind is often apt to excite the pulse; so that when the practitioner makes his first visit, the solicitude of the patient who is in doubt as to what the practitioner may think of his state, may disturb his pulse. On this account a practitioner of experience does not seize the patient's forearm with his hand, as soon as he comes, but first sits down and with a cheerful countenance asks how the patient finds himself; and if the patient has any fear, he calms him with entertaining talk, and only after that moves his hand to touch the patient. If now the sight of the practitioner makes the pulse beat, how easily may a thousand things disturb it!

Celsus, *De Medicina*, Vol I, Book III, 6.6

Mistrust of doctors was apparently widespread in ancient society. Compare the reflective and idealistic image of holistic healthcare conveyed in the Celsus excerpt below with the distrust the poet Martial, who was roughly contemporary with Celsus, exhibits.

I was unwell. You hurried round, surrounded

By ninety students, Doctor.

Ninety chill, north-wind-chapped hands then pawed and probed and pounded.

I was unwell: now I'm extremely ill.

Martial, 1972, *Epigrams*, 5: IX

In the Roman-occupied lands – that is, most of what we know today as Europe, as well as North Africa and the Middle East – there existed a lively alternative culture which could be xenophobic about doctors, who were usually Greek and foreign. These people often applied and further developed traditional folk remedies in treating families and large households.

Sometimes it was the male head of the household who nursed the sick or directed their treatment. The Roman senator Marcus Cato (The 'Censor') was suspicious of Greek doctors, so he wrote a book of prescriptions, recipes and regimens, and used it successfully to treat himself

and his family. Plutarch says: 'By following such treatment and regimen he said he had good health himself, and kept his family in good health' (Plutarch, *Marcus Cato*, XXIII, 3–4).

Midwives and nurses

One male author who offers posterity a glimpse of those previously invisible in the literature – women, infants and a whole array of health personnel including midwives, nurses and assistants of various kinds – is Soranus of Ephesus (c.AD 98–138), who wrote the earliest surviving text on gynaecology, building on some earlier sources that have not survived. Soranus was a renowned physician from the Greek city of Ephesus on the Mediterranean coast of what is now Turkey, who worked during the reigns of the Emperors Trajan and Hadrian. Most of the good medical schools were Greek, and their graduates travelled the world plying their trade. However, Soranus wrote for the benefit of the female midwife and for the wet nurse, who both fed the infant and treated childhood ills. Both appeared to be independent practitioners who were called in by the family when they were required.

The translation of *The Gynecology* in 1956 (Soranus, 1956) by Owsei Temkin, Professor Emeritus of the history of medicine and a former director of the Johns Hopkins Institute of the History of Medicine, is clearly a product of a time and culture in which the midwife had a role subordinate to that of the doctor, who made the command decisions as the natural leader of a 'medical team'. Culture-bound beliefs led Temkin to make unwarranted authorial comment about the text, in which he assumes that although the midwife herself is consistently addressed by Soranus, she must be 'working under the supervision of a physician'. This is incorrect.

This extract from *The Gynecology* describes the necessary attributes of a midwife, and this passage has a timeless quality. Soranus could be describing the ideal modern nurse (or nursing student) and it is significant that many of the skills she must possess, such as sympathy, reassurance and the sharing of secrets, would encourage a therapeutic relationship which would benefit the mental health of the client. Note that the midwife is required to be a female, whereas elsewhere in the work the doctor is presumed to be a male.

NURSE'S STORY: WHAT PERSONS ARE FIT TO BECOME MIDWIVES?

She must be literate in order to be able to comprehend the art through theory too; she must have her wits about her so that she may easily follow what is said and what is happening; she must have a good memory to retain the imparted instructions (for knowledge arises

---

from memory of what has been grasped). She must love work in order to persevere through all vicissitudes (for a woman who wishes to acquire such vast knowledge needs manly patience). She must be respectable since people will have to trust their household and the secrets of their lives to her....

She must not be handicapped as regards her senses since there are things which she must see, answers which she must hear when questioning, and objects which she must grasp by her sense of touch. She needs sound limbs so as not to be handicapped in the performances of her work and she must be robust, for she takes a double task upon herself during the hardship of her professional visits.

Soranus, *The Gynecology*, Book I.1.1–3

NURSE'S STORY: WHO ARE THE BEST MIDWIVES?

It is necessary to tell what makes the best midwives, so that on the one hand the best may recognize themselves, and on the other hand beginners may look upon them as models, and the public in time of need may know whom to summon. Now generally speaking we call a midwife faultless if she merely carries out her medical task; whereas we call her the best midwife if she goes further and in addition to her management of cases is well versed in theory ... trained in all branches of therapy (for some cases must be treated by diet, others by surgery, while still others must be cured by drugs ... able to prescribe hygienic regulations for her patients ... she will be unperturbed, unafraid in danger, able to state clearly the reasons for her measures, she will bring reassurance to her patients, and be sympathetic.... She will be well disciplined and always sober, since it is uncertain when she may be summoned to those in danger. She will have a quiet disposition, for she will have to share many secrets of life ... she will be free from superstition so as not to overlook salutary measures on account of a dream or omen or some customary rite or vulgar superstition.

Soranus, *The Gynecology*, Book I.II.4

The ancient Greek midwife was clearly well trained. The skills she was expected to master were many, and they included many which might be considered traditionally medical functions, such as independent practice, diagnosis, prescribing and case management. She also selected and supervised the wet nurse, who was also skilled in treating the ailments of childhood. The translator Temkin felt that it was 'more natural' to think that *The Gynecology* was addressed to physicians, who could then 'explain' it to the midwife, but Soranus's text is clear

that the physician was only called to assist the midwife in her duties if the labour had been obstructed and surgical intervention was required to extract the fetus by hooks and embryotomy (IV; III [XIX], 9 [61]).

To conceal the true role of the ancient Greek midwife as an independent professional practitioner is to remove her historical importance, while simultaneously consolidating the dominant role of the physician. The reader is furtively being instructed: this is the way it always has been; the midwife would be breaking with an age-old tradition should she (or he) seek more autonomy. Remarkably, Temkin's interpretation has not previously been challenged by nursing scholars, perhaps because of an indifference to the importance of historical research and enquiry in nursing.

The midwife has retained her importance in the lives of birthing women. Many centuries after Soranus, Charles Dickens incorporated the character of the nurse and midwife Sairey (or Sarah) Gamp in his novel *Martin Chuzzlewit* (1844) when the practice of nursing had begun to be reformed. In the exaggeration of her fondness for tea and strong liquor, Gamp is usually cited by nurses as an example of the type of nurse who was made obsolete by the Nightingale training system (Summers, 1997).

It is possible that a society could hold respectful and ribald views of midwives simultaneously. The Roman dramatist Terence (*c*.186–159 BC) wrote roughly simultaneously with Plautus, but his midwife Lesbia, summoned to attend a childbirth in *The Girl From Andros*, is a serious, sober and independent practitioner (Terence, 1976). Perhaps Gamp was meant to be a caricature in the tradition of the midwives in classical Graeco-Roman writers of comedy, in much the same way as nurses are depicted in modern television dramas, films, books and advertisements in roles that run the gamut from skilful professional to scantily clad temptress.

PIONEERS AND PROFESSIONALIZATION

To many nursing scholars Charles Dickens' fictional character Sarah Gamp represents the earliest, and one must say the worst, historical role model in nursing. There is an understanding that previous to that time nursing was the exclusive province of the religious orders, both male and female, or the domestic amateur, but, as this chapter has demonstrated, the roots of the nursing profession extend much further back than the nineteenth century, and for most of this time it is not possible to isolate mental health nursing from general nursing. The body of knowledge contained in the ancient texts delineates a competent practitioner, technically expert, systematic, professional and well respected. St Vincent de Paul formed the association later named The Sisters of Charity in 1617, and they combined general nursing with caring for the insane. The care delivered to people with mental health problems ('lunatics') in asylums was harsh; indeed, if the asylum was overcrowded, as was often the case, the jail was considered an appropriate alternative.

It often happens that a number of advances in an area are made almost simultaneously. This was the case with nursing, and nursing people with mental health problems in particular. Despite slower communication methods and transport, new ideas were shared and each advance fuelled further advances in key areas across the world. Each of the English-speaking countries has its own nursing pioneer who is credited with bettering the lot of people with mental health problems.

Unusually, in the days when women were relatively constrained in what they could achieve, the pioneer general nurses were predominantly women. Nightingale incorporated both religious and feminine attributes when she called nurses 'sister', spoke of nursing as a 'vocation' and dressed nurses in the nun-like uniform and coif (Chatterton, 2000). However, the establishment of the asylum system in the middle of the nineteenth century provided both the impetus for the evolution of mental health nursing as a profession distinct from general nursing (Hamblet, 2000) and a different gender balance from that which applied in general nursing. Asylums also ensured that mental health nursing developed along institutional lines in both the UK and its colonies.

In the asylums, more male attendants were employed initially for their strength, although photographs of asylums in the nineteenth century clearly show female nurses, dressed in the starched general nurse's garb of the period (Chatterton, 2000). Since the introduction of neuroleptic medications in the middle of the twentieth century, and with the increasing emphasis on professional qualifications, attendants became nurses, endowing this branch of the nursing profession with an enduring tradition of male practitioners.

The USA

Dorothea Lynde Dix (1802–87) is credited with responsibility for mental healthcare reform in the USA. Dix was not a nurse, but a teacher who ran a Sunday school class for the inmates of the local asylum, who were kept in uncomfortable and unsanitary conditions. From the mid-1840s she successfully lobbied states in the USA and Canada for better mental healthcare and state-run hospitals. During the American Civil War (1861–65) Dix was appointed Superintendent of Women Nurses. The USA was among the first to recognize that confining those with mental health problems to protect society from their 'derangement' was not necessarily of benefit to the client. The first training for psychiatric nurses in the USA was organized at McLean Asylum in 1882.

The UK

In the UK, Florence Nightingale (1820–1910) is usually credited with being the trailblazer for modern nursing, although Elizabeth Fry opened the first institute for the training of Protestant nurses in London. Accounts of the originality of Nightingale's work also tend to ignore the fact that she initially spent time in the Lutheran deaconess facility at Kaiserwerth, Germany, which was itself a product of the centuries-old European tradition of religious nursing.

In 1854 Florence Nightingale collected and trained a force of nurses to tend the English troops who were involved in the Crimean War, in Turkey. English troops in Scutari died more frequently from diseases due to unsanitary conditions than from battle wounds. The Nightingale School for Nurses was established in 1860 at the historic St Thomas's Hospital in London (founded in AD 1215) but she had already published *Notes on Nursing* in 1859, which addressed much that is also relevant to the nursing of people with mental health problems. Nightingale wrote 147 works in all, and she included philosophy, sanitation, administration, health and hospitals, emigration, discipline and women's rights among her range of subjects. The nurse who writes eloquently can have an enormous influence on the profession and on others.

After the Lunacy Act of 1845 the numbers of public asylums and nursing staff or attendants who worked in them burgeoned. In the asylums, both staff and patients were segregated on the basis of gender: males worked in the grounds or workshops under male attendants who were ex-army, prison warders or farmers; female patients performed domestic work indoors under female attendants or nurses (Chatterton, 2000). This state of affairs continued until the shortage of suitable males during World War I led to the employment of more females, even in male wards, a trend which continued thereafter despite lower wages for women. In 1922, at the first state registration exam, more female nurses passed ($n = 113$) than males ($n = 48$) (Chatterton, 2000).

New Zealand

The first premises were provided for the care of 'lunatics' in New Zealand in 1846, and six provincial asylums were built on the British model between 1854 and 1872, staffed by ill-educated 'attendants' who were more akin to warders than nurses (O'Brien, 2001). While general nursing rose in status, the asylum worker of the Victorian era in New Zealand and elsewhere shared the stigmatized status of their charges in the asylum, characterized as 'a warehouse of despondency and gloom' (Russell 1988, cited in O'Brien, 2001, p. 132). New Zealand and Australia have, by virtue of their proximity, similar colonial histories and multicultural backgrounds and shared a comparable agenda of training and professionalization in the twentieth century.

Australia

Australia benefited from associations with both the Sisters of Charity and Florence Nightingale's work. Sydney Infirmary (later known as Sydney Hospital) was built in 1811, and was staffed not by trained nurses but by convict women, who were paid in alcohol. In 1839 five Sisters of Charity arrived in the colony to minister to the poor, and by 1857 St Vincent's Hospital was built and staffed by the Sisters of Charity. Nightingale influenced the earliest nursing care in Australia, when in 1868 the Colonial Secretary requested that Australia be sent a contingent of the new Nightingale-trained nurses. Lucy Osborn was sent from England to establish the Nightingale system of nursing, and she instituted hospital-based training for nurses in Sydney Hospital. Nurses received a nominal wage and board during training, paying for their training by working in the hospitals and providing cheap labour. This system stayed in place for nearly a century, with little real change.

In Australia, although modern research has rediscovered the value of exercise in anxiety reduction and for aiding the improvement of cognitive function, depressed mood and lowered self-esteem (Callaghan, 2004), the belief that 'fresh air, space and the climate of the country would preclude madness' proved not to be the case, and it became essential for the maintenance of law and order to build and equip asylums modelled on similar establishments in the UK (Ash et al., 2001). The first 'lunatic asylum' was opened at Castle Hill in New South Wales in 1811. All the 'lunatics' in the new colony were sent there, and by 1825 this facility was overcrowded. Gladesville Hospital in Sydney was opened in 1837 to accommodate the surplus, and each State soon developed its own psychiatric services.

Although attempts were made to provide humane care, and numerous commissions and inquiries were conducted, overcrowding meant that custodial care was the usual strategy employed with the mentally ill. The medical model continued to see mental 'illness' as an organic process, and the psychoanalytic theories initiated by Freud in the latter part of the nineteenth century and the early twentieth century were slow to be adopted in Australia.

Specialized mental health nursing education was not introduced until after 1910 when the first Nurses Registration Board was formed to oversee and regulate training. The Australian Nursing Federation was formed in 1924, but it was not until 1974 that the first Congress of Mental Health Nurses was held, which led to the formation of a professional organization in 1978.

CONCLUSION

This chapter has provided an overview of the ways in which mental health problems have been experienced, treated and regarded in past eras. The health problems that have survived in the same form over two and a half millennia have been examined, as have those that appear to be of more recent origin. The interpersonal skills which were used to treat mental ill health have proved to be at times as refined and humane as any we would use today, but there have also been regressive episodes featuring incarceration of and brutality towards people with mental health problems.

The transition from family-based care to institutional care has been outlined, and the emergence and reemergence of mental health professionals has been described. The earliest documented role models for nursing are found in the Graeco-Roman era. These women were as professional and competent as the women and men who practise today. Ancient Greek nurses displayed a measure of independence in their practice that has not been equalled until the present era.

One of the important changes that the professionalization of nursing wrought was that nursing became a commercial undertaking, a respectable source of employment and independence for women as well as men, and an organized profession that displaced the traditional role of family members as carers for the ill. People with mental health problems had been considered the responsibility of the asylum, or state-run institutions, for somewhat longer than the physically ill, but their treatment tended to be more humane and better regulated from the end of the nineteenth century to the beginning of the modern era. Even so, there is clearly a long way to go before we achieve the ideal of humane, safe mental healthcare for all. Nearly half of the people who were surveyed after having been treated in the USA in public-sector psychiatric settings reported that they had no communication from staff when they were distressed, and that they would not want to return to a psychiatric facility (Grubaugh et al., 2007).

The historical account in this chapter stops short of documenting the changes that have occurred since the early twentieth century. These have been so great and so many that they would require another chapter to describe them fully. Mental health nursing has blossomed into a skilled profession. The challenges that concern a mental health nurse, transformed in less than a century from ignorant attendant to university graduate, can be traced in Chapter 5, which deals with professional nursing issues. But let us end this chapter with Burnard's plea that all nurses and nurse education should embrace the 'true spirit of trying to understand the unfolding nature of ideas, theories and research', a process that has taken centuries and not just the past few years (Burnard, 2007, p. 666).

EXERCISE FOR CLASS ENGAGEMENT

Discuss the following questions with your group or class members.

◆ What traditional remedies for illness or stress have you seen or heard used in your own family? Are they effective?

◆ Was there any alternative to the evolution of the asylum for the care of people with mental health problems, given the numbers of sufferers?

◆ In what sense is the term 'hysteric' or 'hysterical' used today? Would you still find that there is a relationship with 'health problems of the womb', or perhaps the possession of a womb?

◆ Which aspects of mental healthcare in the past would you like to see incorporated into present mental health nursing practice? How would you go about doing this?

REFERENCES

Alexander, F.G., Selesnick, S.T., 1966. The History of Psychiatry: An Evaluation of Psychiatric Thought and Practice from Prehistoric Times to the Present. Harper & Row, New York.

American Psychiatric Association, 1994. Diagnostic and Statistical Manual of Mental Disorders (DSM-IV TR), fourth ed. American Psychiatric Association, Washington DC.

Aristophanes, 1964. The Wasps, the Poet and the Women, the Frogs (D. Barrett, Trans.). Penguin, Harmondsworth.

Ash, D., Benson, A., Farhall, J., et al., 2001. Mental health services in Australia. In: Meadows, G., Singh, B. (Eds.), Mental Health in Australia. Oxford University Press, Melbourne, pp. 51–66.

Blakemore, C., 1988. The Mind Machine. BBC Books, London.

Boyd, M.A. (Ed.), 2002. Psychiatric Nursing: Contemporary Practice, second ed. Lippincott, Philadelphia.

Burnard, P., 2007. The heresy of the 'recent' reference. Nurse Educ. Today 27, 665–666.

Busuttil, J., 1992. Psychosocial occupational therapy: from myth and misconception to multidisciplinary team member. Br. J. Occup. Ther. 5512, 457–461.

Callaghan, P., 2004. Exercise: a neglected intervention in mental health care? J. Psychiatr. Ment. Health Nurs. 11, 476–483.

Celsus, 1935–38. (revised 1940, 1948) De Medicina, vol I. (W.G. Spencer, Trans. Loeb Classical Library). William Heinemann, London.

Celsus, 1935–38. De Medicina, vol III. (W.G. Spencer, Trans. Loeb Classical Library). William Heinemann, London.

Chatterton, C., 2000. Women in mental health nursing: angels or custodians? Int. Hist. Nurs. J. 5 (2), 11–19.

Cicero, 1978. Letters to Atticus (D.R. Shackleton Bailey, Trans.). Penguin, Harmondsworth.

Corrigan, P., 2004. How stigma interferes with mental health care. Am. Psychol. 58 (7), 614–625.

De Leo, D., 2002. Struggling against suicide. Crisis 23 (1), 23–31.

Devereux, G., 1970. The psychotherapy scene in Euripides' 'Bacchae'. J. Hell. Stud. XC, 35–48.

Dodds, E.R., 1951. The Greeks and the Irrational. University of California Press, Berkeley.

Doona, M.E., 1992. Judgment: the nurse's key to knowledge. J. Prof. Nurs. 84, 231–238.

Ellard, J., 1987. Did schizophrenia exist before the eighteenth century? Aust. N. Z. J. Psychiatry 21 (3), 306–314.

Evans, K., 2000. Representations of mental illness in the classical texts. Doctoral Dissertation, University of Queensland, Brisbane.

Evans, K., 2007. 'Interrupted by fits of weeping': Cicero's major depressive disorder and the death of Tullia. Hist. Psychiatry 18 (1), 81–102.

Evans, K., McGrath, J., Milns, R., 2003. Searching for schizophrenia in ancient Greek and Roman literature: a systematic review. Acta Psychiatr. Scand. 107 (5), 323–330.

Fontaine, K.L., 2003. Mental Health Nursing, fifth ed. Pearson Education, New Jersey.

Foucault, M., 1967. (reprinted 1999) Madness and civilisation: a history of insanity in the age of reason (R. Howard, Trans.). Routledge, London.

Frisch, N., 2002. Psychiatric nursing: evolution of a specialty. In: Frisch, N., Frisch, L. (Eds.), Psychiatric Mental Health Nursing, second ed. Delmar Thomson Learning, Albany, pp. 17–25.

Gilman, S., King, H., Porter, R., et al., 1993. Hysteria Beyond Freud. University of California Press, Berkeley.

Grmek, M., 1991. Diseases in the Ancient Greek World (M. Muellner, L. Muellner, Trans.). Johns Hopkins University Press, Baltimore.

Grubaugh, A.L., Frueh, B.C., Zinzow, H.M., et al., 2007. Patients' perceptions of care and safety within psychiatric settings. Psychol. Serv. 4 (3), 193–201.

Hamblet, C., 2000. Obstacles to defining the role of the mental health nurse. Nurs. Stand. 14 (51), 34–37.

Hawkins, D.R., 1982. Specificity revisited: personality profiles and behavioral issues. Psychother. Psychosom. 38 (1), 54–63.

Herodotus, 1921. The Histories, vol II. Books III & IV (A.D Godley, Trans.). William Heinemann, London.

Herodotus, 1922. The Histories, vol III. Books V–VII (A.D. Godley, Trans.). William Heinemann, London.

Hershkowitz, D., 1998. The Madness of Epic: Reading Insanity from Homer to Statius. Clarendon Press, Oxford.

Hippocrates, 1923a. The Hippocratic Corpus, vol I. (W.H.S. Jones, Trans. Loeb Classical Library). William Heinemann, London.

Hippocrates, 1923b. The Hippocratic Corpus, vol II. (W.H.S. Jones, Trans. Loeb Classical Library). William Heinemann, London.

Hippocrates, 1923c. The Hippocratic Corpus, vol VII. (W.D. Smith, Trans. Loeb Classical Library), Harvard University Press, Cambridge, MA.

Hippocrates, 1931. The Hippocratic Corpus, vol IV. (W.H.S. Jones, Trans. Loeb Classical Library). William Heinemann, London.

Hornblower, S., Spawforth, A. (Eds.), 1996. The Oxford Classical Dictionary, third ed. Oxford University Press, New York.

Howells, J.G. (Ed.), 1991. The Concept of Schizophrenia: Historical Perspectives American Psychiatric Press, Washington DC.

Jeste, D.V., del Carmen, R., Lohr, J.B., et al., 1985. Did schizophrenia exist before the eighteenth century? Compr. Psychiatry 26 (6), 493–503.

Jones, W.H.S., 1923. Ancient nursing. In: Hippocrates, vol II. Introductory essay IV. William Heinemann, London.

Kaplan, H., Sadock, B., Grebb, J., 1994. Synopsis of Psychiatry, seventh ed. Williams & Wilkins, Baltimore.

Kaufman, J.C., Sexton, J.D., 2006. Why doesn't the writing cure help poets? Rev. Gen. Psychol. 10 (3), 268–282.

King, H., 1993. Once upon a text. In: Gilman, S., King, H., Porter, R. (Eds.), Hysteria Beyond Freud. University of California Press, Berkeley.

Latham, A.E., Prigerson, H.G., 2004. Suicidality and bereavement: complicated grief as psychiatric disorder presenting greatest risk for suicidality. Suicide Life Threat. Behav. 34 (4), 350–362.

Lester, D., 1990. Galen's four temperaments and four-factor theories of personality: a comment on 'toward a four-factor theory of temperament and/or personality'. J. Pers. Assess. 54 (1/2), 423–426.

Macalpine, I., Hunter, R., 1969. George III and the Madbusiness. Penguin, London.

McAthie, M., 1999. The nature of contemporary nursing practice. In: Lindeman, C., McAthie, M. (Eds.), Fundamentals of Contemporary Nursing Practice. W B Saunders, Philadelphia, pp. 3–20.

Mack, A.H., Forman, L., Brown, R., et al., 1994. A brief history of psychiatric classification: from the ancients to DSM-IV TR. Psychiatr. Clin. North Am. 17 (3), 515–523.

Martial, 1972. The Epigrams. (J. Michie, Trans.). Penguin, Harmondsworth.

Mellersh, H.E.L., 1976. (revised 1999) The Hutchinson Chronology of World History: The Ancient and Medieval World. Helicon, Oxford.

Merenda, P.F., 1987. Toward a four-factor theory of temperament and/or personality. J. Pers. Assess. 513 (3), 367–374.

Nightingale, F., 1859. (reprinted 1969) Notes on Nursing: What it is and What it is not. Dover, New York.

O'Brien, A.J., 2001. The Therapeutic Relationship: Historical Development and Contemporary Significance. J. Psychiatr. Ment. Health Nurs. 8 (2), 129–137.

Parker, R., 1983. Miasma: Pollution and Purification in Early Greek Religion. Clarendon, Oxford.

Plautus, 1965. The Pot of Gold and Other Plays (E.F. Watling, Trans.). Penguin Classics, Harmondsworth.

Plutarch, 1914. Lives, vol II. Themistocles and Camillus, Aristides and Cato Major, Cimon and Lucullus (B. Perrin, Trans.). William Heinemann, London.

Range, L.M., Kovac, S.H., Marion, M.S., 2000. Does writing about bereavement lessen grief following sudden, unintentional death? Death Stud. 24 (2), 115–134.

Rich, K.L., Butts, J.B., 2004. Rational suicide: uncertain moral ground. J. Adv. Nurs. 46 (3), 270–283.

Richards, A. (Ed.), 1991. Breue J & Freud S Studies on Hysteria (J. Strachey, A. Strachey, Trans.). Penguin, Harmondsworth.

Roccatagliata, G., 1991. Classical concepts of schizophrenia. In: Howells, G.J. (Ed.), The Concept of Schizophrenia: Historical Perspectives. American Psychiatric Press, Washington DC.

Rosen, G., 1968. Madness in Society: Chapters in the Historical Sociology of Mental Illness. University of Chicago Press, Chicago.

Sanderson, S., Vandenberg, B., Paese, P., 1999. Authentic religious experience or insanity? J. Clin. Psychol. 55 (5), 607–616.

Simon, B., 1978. Mind and Madness in Ancient Greece: The Classical Roots of Modern Psychiatry. Cornell University Press, London.

Soranus, 1956. The Gynecology (O. Temkin, Trans.). Johns Hopkins University Press, Baltimore.

Stone, M.H., 1997. Healing the Mind. A History of Psychiatry from Antiquity to the Present. W W Norton, New York.

Suer, L., 1995. The survival of ancient medicine in modern French psychiatry. Hist. Psychiatry 6 (24/4), 493–501.

Summers, A., 1997. Sairey Gamp: generating fact from fiction. Nurs. Enquiry 4 (1), 14–18.

Terence, 1976. The Comedies (B. Radice, Trans.). Penguin, Harmondsworth.

Thucydides, 1954. History of the Pelopponesian War (R. Warner, Trans.). Penguin, Harmondsworth.

Torrey, E.F., Yolken, R.H., 1995. Could schizophrenia be a viral zoonosis transmitted from house cats? Schizophr. Bull. 21 (2), 167–171.

Torrey, E.F., Yolken, R.H., 1998. Is household crowding a risk factor for schizophrenia? Schizophr. Res. 29 (1/2), 12–13.

Torrey, E.F., Bowler, A.E., Clark, K., 1997. Urban birth and residence as risk factors for psychoses: an analysis of 1880 data. Schizophr. Res. 25 (3), 169–176.

Woolf, A., 2000. Witchcraft or mycotoxin? The Salem witch trials. J. Toxicol.: Clin. Toxicol. 38 (4), 457.

Yolken, R.H., Yee, F., Johnston, N., et al., 1997. Molecular analyses of brains from individuals with schizophrenia—evidence of viral infections. Schizophr. Res. 24 (1/2), 61.

Chapter | 4 |

The politicolegal context

Eimear Muir-Cochrane, Anthony O'Brien, and Timothy Wand

CHAPTER CONTENTS

CHAPTER POINTS

- Understanding the history of the care of people with mental health problems in Western cultures will help contextualize contemporary policy and legal developments.
- Mental health policy is based on the concept of human rights.
- Mental health nurses require an understanding of current mental health policy at both a global and a local level to ensure that their practice is consistent with ongoing changes in healthcare delivery.
- Mental health policy is subject to review and change.
- Mental health legislation is the legal framework that informs the involuntary treatment of individuals, defines their rights and ensures appropriate treatment.
- Nurses working in mental health need to learn to balance their caring and controlling functions.

KEY TERMS

- aggression
- community care
- dangerousness
- deinstitutionalization
- human rights
- involuntary treatment
- least-restrictive alternative
- mental health legislation
- mental health policy
- mental health standard
- mental health strategy
- partnership
- primary healthcare
- risk
- risk management
- service user
- stigma
- voluntary treatment

DOI: http://dx.doi.org/10.1016/B978-0-7020-4493-9.00004-4

The material in this chapter will assist you to:

- outline the historical, social and political developments that have occurred in the development of mental health services,
- discuss mental health policies,
- understand the importance of mental health law in mental healthcare,
- discuss the tension between the controlling and caring functions of mental health nursing practice.

INTRODUCTION

Nurses require a sound understanding of mental health policy and legislation in order to work effectively with service users in both community and hospital settings. This chapter describes national policies, the historical events that have served to shape them and the institutions and concepts guiding their implementation. It traces the shift from a focus on the care and treatment of people with mental health problems to strategic aims of improving the mental health of the whole population. The role of the law in decisions about the involuntary treatment of people and the rights of people is also discussed. Also presented are examples of how nurses can work most effectively with people under often challenging circumstances to ensure that their rights are protected.

HISTORICAL LANDMARKS

In order to gain a clear and critical understanding of how mental health services have developed it is important to briefly explore some historical landmarks over the past 500 years. A full exploration of the historical foundations of the care and treatment of people with mental health problems can be found in Chapter 3. As noted in that chapter, asylums arose in the Middle Ages as a means of controlling the 'mentally ill'. People with mental disorders were socially and physically excluded from 'normal' social life and frequently subjected to institutional brutality. In countries such as Australia and New Zealand asylums were established as part of the process of colonization (Ernst, 1991; Maude, 2001). Prior to the middle of the twentieth century, 'psychiatric' treatment was medically dominated and focused on confining people deemed to be 'mentally ill'. Pharmacological treatments at this time were extremely limited and, when used, often ineffective or dangerous. Most treatments were of a physical nature and often involved the use of restraints such as straitjackets and being subjected to

cold-water baths or showers. After World War II, pharmacological treatments of varying efficacy and toxicity began to emerge: antidepressants first, then antipsychotics. Chlorpromazine is often credited as being the first 'antipsychotic' medication of the modern era, being first synthesized in 1950. Its impact on the treatment of people diagnosed with schizophrenia was profound, but it was, and is, a controversial medication which was often difficult for people to tolerate and was associated with many unpleasant side effects. The 1960s was an era of antipsychiatry sentiment which saw an increasing emphasis on human rights (Symonds, 1995). Works by Goffman, such as *Stigma: Notes on the Management of Spoiled Identity* (1968) and *Asylums: Essays on the Social Situtaion of Mental Patients and Other Inmates* (1968), Foucault's *Madness and Civilisation: A History of Insanity in the Age of Reason* (1965) and Laing's *The Divided Self* (1965) cast a spotlight on the perceived nature of mental ill health and the presumption that such problems had a biological origin requiring medcial treatment. They were also critical of large Victorian psychiatric asylums as 'closed communities' and 'total institutions' to which people with mental health problems were seen to be 'banished' and within which individual freedom, personal choice and human dignity were often severely compromised. As this sentiment grew over the 1970s many institutionalized service users were able to leave hospital for the first time in decades, a process which sped up the closure of large Victorian psychiatric hospitals and reduced focus on custodial and long-term care in favour of care in the community. This practice was known as *deinstitutionalization* with the aim of 'normalizing' mental health problems and removing the stigma associated with them. In 1983 the UK Mental Health Act enshrined in law a set of rights for people who were detained in hospital, including appeals against their detention.

THE CURRENT GLOBAL PERSPECTIVE

In 1991 the United Nations established the Principles for the Protection of Persons with Mental Illness and the Improvement of Mental Health Care, reflecting an international understanding and awareness of the individual and unique needs of those with mental disorders and the responsibilities incumbent on the 'state and professional communities to respond adequately and ethically to these needs' (Singh, 2001, p. 43). An overarching statement of the fundamental human rights of those with mental illness guides the 25 principles (Box 4.1).

The World Health Organization (WHO, 2001b) also recommends that all mental health policies be anchored by the four guiding principles of access, equity, effectiveness and efficiency. A description of each of these principles is given in Box 4.2.

Box 4.1 Rights of people with mental health problems

Rights of people with mental health problems include:

- rights in regard to confidentiality of all information about the person with mental health problems in regard to their care,
- the right to live and work in the community (further reinforced by the document 'Mental health around the world: stop exclusion: dare to care', WHO, 2001a),
- protection of minors and others deemed not able to give informed consent,
- the right to voluntary treatment, wherever possible, by those specifically qualified to care for such individuals and in approved mental health facilities,
- the right to receive appropriate medical treatment including medication, prescribed by mental health professionals, but never as punishment or for the convenience of others,
- the right that no treatment shall be given without informed consent other than when held as an involuntary service user,
- the right that physical restraint or involuntary seclusion of a service user shall not be used unless as a last resort, to prevent imminent harm to the service user or others,
- the right that involuntary admission will only occur if authorized by a qualified mental health practitioner, that the person is suffering from a mental disorder, that treatment occurs in an approved mental health facility, that a second medical opinion is sought where possible and that appropriate treatment can only be given within a mental health facility,
- the right to make a complaint.

Reproduced by permission of Oxford University Press Australia and New Zealand, from Mental Health in Australia: Collaborative Community Practice, 2nd edn, Meadows G, Singh B, Grigg M, 2007 ©Oxford University Press.

Box 4.2 WHO principles for guiding mental health policy

- Access: the right to obtain treatment for mental health issues based on need, not on ability to pay.
- Equity: mental health resources should be fairly distributed across the population as indicated by need.
- Effectiveness: mental health services should be aimed solely at improving health for individuals and collectivities.
- Efficiency: resources should be distributed in such a way as to maximize gains for individuals and society as a whole.

Source: abridged from WHO (2001c).

effective care for those with perceived mental health needs; increased access to a full range of services; reduced suicide rates; and support for the carers and families of people with mental health problems. The NSFMH policy also increased the range of community-based services supporting people at home and during a time of crisis as an alternative to hospital admissions (Department of Health, 1999).

'User involvement' has become an increasingly important central point of many recent policy initiatives (Hewitt, 2005) and there has been an expectation and requirement that service users will be involved in all aspects of their care, including the ability to influence service delivery and commissioning. Charities and voluntary organizations (such as Rethink Mental Illness, MIND and so forth) have also been influential in representing the views of service users and influencing policy at local and governmental level. For example, the Future Vision Coalition (a coalition of organizations including MIND, Centre for Mental Health, Rethink and the Mental Health Foundation, among others) called for *A New Vision for Mental Health*, which argued for a broader public health and more holistic approach to mental healthcare, seeing that good mental health is important for everyone's overall good quality of life (Future Vision Coalition, 2008).

The importance of the service user's experience has also been stressed in the Coalition Government's White Paper *Equity and Excellence: Liberating the NHS* (Department of Health, 2010), which emphasizes the centrality of service user choice and experience and empowered healthcare staff delivering demonstrable quality, outcome-focused care. The White Paper seeks to ensure that the UK National Health Service (NHS) is more accountable to service users, including choosing what treatment and which provider will best meet their healthcare needs. The Coalition Government's mental health strategy for England, *No Health Without Mental Health* (Department of Health,

MENTAL HEALTH POLICY

In recent years there have been a number of policies which have changed the way in which mental health services deliver care in the UK (Kemp, 2008). The New Labour Government's (1997–2010) approach to mental healthcare emphasized the promotion of citizenship and the importance placed on an individual's participation in society. For example, the National Service Framework for Mental Health (NSFMH) (Department of Health, 1999) set out to modernize mental healthcare by establishing a set of national quality standards involving

2011), is '…both a public mental health strategy and a strategy for social justice' (Department of Health, 2011, 3). The strategy recognizes the economic, social and personal cost of mental ill health and proposes to improve the mental health of people with existing mental health problems and prevent mental ill health wherever possible. The strategy also recognizes the social inequalities (such as a lack of access to work, poor housing, isolation from communities and so forth) that contribute to mental ill health and ongoing mental distress.

In recent years there has been a recognition that people with severe and enduring mental health problems also have an increased risk of developing serious physical illnesses (Robson and Gray, 2007), such as coronary heart disease, diabetes and respiratory diseases (Mentality/NIMHE, 2004; Sainsbury Centre for Mental Health, 2003). Additionally, they tend to have poorer access to medical care and are less likely to be offered routine health checks, such as blood pressure or cholesterol monitoring (Disability Rights Commission, 2006; Sainsbury Centre for Mental Health, 2003) or to receive health promotion advice (Mentality/NIMHE, 2004). Recently, the policy *Choosing Health: Supporting the Physical Health Needs of People with Severe Mental Illness* (Department of Health, 2006) has focused attention on the need for ensuring appropriate referral and access to various medical and other healthcare services and health promotion for people with long-term and enduring mental health problems, citing examples of good practice within mental healthcare services, such as healthy walking groups, smoking cessation and dieting programmes.

There has also been an increasing focus on the provision of mental healthcare that is hopeful, optimistic and positive (Department of Health, 2001), where people are supported to live a meaningful life of personal value and worth (NIMHE, 2005). This is often referred to as a 'recovery approach' or 'recovery paradigm' (see Ch. 2). In recent years this has found expression in mental healthcare policies, which have emphasized:

- the importance of working in partnership within the context of a supportive and empathic professional nursing relationship,
- shared decision making between mental health service users and nurses,
- nursing care which reflects the service user's preference based on informed discussions,
- a recognition that individuals have personal strengths and assets as well as problems and needs,
- support to deal with the future and cope with the challenges that mental health problems may bring (Future Vision Coalition, 2008; NICE, 2009a, 2009b).

As such, recovery approaches represent a movement away from medical treatment (Faulkner and Layzell,

2000), which has historically been the focus of mental healthcare. Instead, recovery approaches stress the importance of developing meaningful professional relationships between nurses and service users that focus on enabling, facilitating and supporting individuals on their journeys to recovery.

The Care Programme Approach (CPA) policy was introduced in 1990 by the then Conservative Government, and has been central to all government policy since that time (Department of Health, 2008). The Care Programme Approach aims to ensure that vulnerable people with mental health problems who have been in contact with mental health services receive the ongoing care they need. The policy aimed to provide:

- systematic arrangements for assessing the health and social needs of people accepted into specialist mental health services,
- the development of a care plan which identified the health and social care documenting not only agreed mental healthcare and treatment but also plans to secure employment, occupational activity, accommodation and adequate housing entitlement to benefits,
- the appointment of a key worker (care coordinator) to keep in close touch with the service user, and to monitor and coordinate care,
- regular review and, where necessary, agreed changes to the care plan.

In 2008, a further refocusing of the Care Programme Approach policy was undertaken in the New Labour Government's *Refocusing the Care Programme Approach* (Department of Health, 2008) in response to concerns about its implementation. The policy sought to reemphasize the personalization of mental healthcare and active service user involvement, along with an emphasis on improving quality of life, reducing distress and promoting social inclusion and recovery.

Many people with chronic or ongoing mental health problems live with carers such as family and friends (Department of Health, 1999; NICE, 2009a). Unfortunately, the needs of carers have often been overlooked. Carers, for example, are twice as likely to have mental health problems themselves if they provide substantial care (Department of Health, 1999, 2001; Office of the Deputy Prime Minister, 2004). In recent years it has been recognized that to fulfil such an important role carers themselves may require help and support from health and social care services. This may include advice and assistance on benefit entitlements but also information about the care and treatment options available to their friend or relative and what to do, and who to contact, should a crisis arise (Department of Health, 1999).

CRITICAL THINKING CHALLENGE 4.1

What skills do you consider service users would bring to mental health services?

What do you think nurses can learn from service user participation in service delivery?

What are some of the barriers to involving service users in services?

What opportunities does your service area or education programmes provide for collaboration with service users?

MENTAL HEALTH LEGISLATION

Mental Health Act 1983 (amended 2007)

The Mental Health Act 1983 (amended 2007) is the law in England and Wales which is used to admit, detain and treat people, against their wishes and in a hospital setting, who are deemed to have a mental disorder. Compulsory or involuntary admission (detention in an approved psychiatric institution) is controversial because it involves the removal of an individual's freedom and autonomy under the auspices of the Act, raising complex legal and ethical issues about the role of the state in controlling individuals deemed to be 'mentally ill'. There are many sections of the Mental Health Act 1983 (amended 2007) but here we outline its main features.

Guiding principles

The Mental Health Act generally includes statements about the need to involve service users in all appropriate aspects of their care and treatment regardless of their status (voluntary or detained). An important part of the Act is the emphasis which is placed on supporting the person's recovery from mental health problems while promoting their overall health and wellbeing, including physical health, and at the same time protecting people from harm (Department of Health, 2008). This includes ensuring effective communication is maintained with service users and that everything is done to overcome barriers to communication, such as when a person's first language is not English, when they do not understand technical jargon or have trouble in reading and writing, or when they have a visual or hearing impairment. If an interpreter is used then this person should be appropriate to the patient's cultural background, gender, dialect, religion and age. Family members should not be routinely used as interpreters.

Further guiding principles include the following.

- Least-restriction principle: to keep to a minimum restrictions that impact on a person's liberty.
- Respect principle: that a person detained and/or treated under the Act must have their views, wishes and feelings respected as far as possible, and that there must be no unlawful discrimination. Respect for individuals includes recognizing an individual's race, religion, culture, gender, age, sexual orientation or disability.
- Participation principle: people must be given, wherever possible, the opportunity to participate in their care, including decision making with regards to planning and reviewing their care. Involvement of carers and family members should be encouraged where possible and where the service user wishes this, and service users have the right to nominate other people to be involved in or notified about decisions relating to their care and treatment.
- Effectiveness principle: that the treatment and care of service users is effective and efficient in meeting their needs

Definition of a mental disorder

A mental disorder, as defined by the Act, is '...any disorder or disability of the mind' (Department of Health, 2008, p. 19). However, the fact that someone may be diagnosed with such a disorder does not mean that a person automatically should be made subject to the Act. For example, the mental health *Code of Practice* (Department of Health, 2008) requires that consideration is given to a person's cultural and social background. It states that 'Difference should not be confused with disorder.... Beliefs, behaviours, or actions which do not result from a disorder or disability of the mind are not a basis for compulsory measures under the Act, even if they appear unusual or cause people alarm, distress or danger' (Department of Health, 2008, p. 20).

In broad terms, applications for detention and/or treatment under the Act can be made where there are grounds that:

- the person is suffering from a mental disorder of a *nature* or *degree* which warrants their detention in hospital for assessment and/or to receive medical treatment,
- the person ought to be detained in their interest of their own health and safety with a view to the protection of others.

By *nature* the Act is referring to a particular mental disorder for which the person has been diagnosed as suffering from while *degree* is taken to mean the current manifestation of the disorder, such as signs and symptoms. Under Section 3 of the Act, if the person is detained for medical treatment, the following additional criteria apply:

- that appropriate medical treatment is available,
- that medical treatment cannot be provided unless the person is detained (Department of Health, 2008).

If a person is to be detained for their own health and safety, criteria here should include:

- reliable evidence of risk of self-harm or suicide, self-neglect or behaviour (whether intentional or unintentional) which jeopardizes their own health and safety,
- reliable evidence which suggests that treatment is required to prevent mental deterioration,
- views of friends, carers and families about the course of the disorder,
- benefits of treatment weighed up against any adverse effects,
- the person's own skills and resources in managing their own mental health and ill health (Department of Health, 2008),
- whether there are any other means of managing risk.

Reliability of evidence may come from knowledge of the person's previous history and the course of their previous mental ill health.

If a person is to be detained for the protection of others, then criteria here should include:

- the nature of the risk to other people arising from a person's disorder and the likelihood and nature of the harm that may result,
- the reliability of available evidence (including previous clinical history and past behaviour, criminal convictions or cautions),
- the willingness and ability of those who live with and care for the person to support and cope with and manage a particular risk (Department of Health, 2008).

Dependence on alcohol and/or drugs is not sufficient grounds alone for detaining people under the Act. However, dependence may be accompanied or related to another disorder that may require care and treatment under the Act and '...can include measures to address alcohol or drug dependence if that is an important part of treating the mental disorder which is the primary focus of treatment' (Department of Health, 2008, p. 21).

Applications for detention in hospital

An application for detention can be made under Section 2 or Section 3 of the Act. Applications can be made by an Approved Mental Health Professional (AMHP) (see below) or a nearest relative, and must be supported by two medical recommendations. Section 2 is used where the nature and degree of a person's disorder or condition is unclear and there is a need to carry out a full assessment in order to arrive at a clear treatment plan. This will also include an assessment of a person's willingness to accept such a plan on a voluntary basis. This section lasts for a maximum of 28 days and is not renewable. Section 3 can be used when a person is already detained under Section 2, and where the nature and degree of a person's disorder have been established along with a subsequent treatment plan and there is concern that a person would not voluntarily follow the plan. Section 3 can last for a maximum of 6 months after which it can be renewed for a further 6 months and then renewed on an annual basis.

Section 4 of the Act can be used only in genuine emergency situations and allows a person to be admitted to hospital for an assessment of their mental health for a maximum of 72 h. Here it must be of an urgent necessity that someone is so detained and in the interests of their own health and safety or the protection of others. Applications are made by AMHPs or nearest relatives and must be supported by a medical doctor's recommendation (who must have seen the service user within the previous 24 h).

The police also have powers under the Act to remove a person who appears to be suffering from a mental disorder to a 'place of safety' such as a hospital or a police station. The latter should only be used in exceptional circumstances as it conveys the idea that the person concerned may have committed a crime. There are local policies in place in every hospital detailing the most appropriate place of safety. Section 135 allows a police officer to enter premises, by force if necessary, and to search for, and remove, a person to a place of safety for up to 72 h. This requires a magistrate's warrant and when this is served the police officer must be accompanied by an AMHP and a doctor. Section 135(2) allows a police officer to enter premises and search for, and return, a person who is already detained under the Act to the hospital from where they may have absconded. Section 136 allows a police officer to remove a person thought to be suffering from a mental disorder from a public place (or a place to which the public have access) to a place of safety where they can be detained for a maximum of 72 h.

Holding powers

Circumstances may occur where a person may have been admitted voluntarily and then asks to leave but may be deemed too unwell to do so. At such times, the person may be detained against their will pending further assessment. For example, an issue that can arise for nurses in inpatient settings is that a voluntary service user may experience a deterioration of their mental state to the point where a nurse considers that to allow that person to leave the inpatient facility would be a dereliction of their duty of care. In these circumstances, nurses (mental health and learning disability nurses who maintain an entry under subparts 1 and 2 of the Nursing and Midwifery Council register) are empowered under Section 5(4) of the Act to detain the person for a period of up to 6h, subject to the condition that a medical review of the person's mental state is arranged. It cannot be renewed. The Section 5(4) holding power recognizes the assessment skills of the nurse and the potential for crises to occur that require an immediate response. In considering whether to invoke Section 5(4) nurses should consider the amount of time it might take for an approved clinician (see below) or doctor to attend (Department of Health, 2008, p. 100), the outcomes of attempts to persuade the person to stay and:

- the service user's expressed intentions,
- the likelihood of the service user harming themselves or others,
- the likelihood of the service user behaving violently,
- any evidence of disordered thinking,
- the service user's current behaviour and, in particular, any changes in their usual behaviour,
- whether the service user has recently received messages from relatives or friends,
- whether the date is one of special significance for the patient (e.g. the anniversary of a bereavement),
- any recent disturbances on the ward,
- any relevant involvement of other service users,
- any history of unpredictability or impulsiveness,
- any formal risk assessments which have been undertaken (specifically looking at previous behaviour),
- any other relevant information from other members of the multidisciplinary team.

Once a Section 5(4) is invoked an entry must be made in the service user's notes.

Section 5(2) of the Act is the holding power for doctors and approved clinicians or their nominated deputies. It allows an inpatient, who was admitted on a voluntary basis, to be detained for a maximum of 72h so that an assessment can be undertaken with a view to detaining that person under Section 2 or Section 3 of the Act. It cannot be used for outpatients or people who present to accident and emergency departments.

Appropriate medical treatment test

Under the Mental Health Act (1983, amended 2007) medical treatment (which is also taken to mean nursing care) is given for the purpose of alleviating or preventing the worsening of a mental disorder and associated symptoms. The purpose of this medical treatment test is to ensure that only those who are actually offered medical treatment are detained. Treatment must be an appropriate response to the service user's condition and situation and does not necessarily have to include medication, and may only consist of nursing care in a safe and therapeutic environment.

Supervised community treatment and community treatment orders

The purpose of supervised community treatment (or SCT) is to allow service users to be treated safely in the community, and at home, rather than being detained in a hospital setting. It is seen as a way of promoting recovery among people who are at risk of relapse and associated harm (Department of Health, 2008). Supervised community treatments apply only to people detained under Section 3 of the Act (and to those unrestricted patients who are subject to Part 3 of the Act which is concerned with those who are subject to criminal proceedings). A supervised community treatment may be appropriate for people who are assessed as being at risk of not following treatment plans, which has led to previous relapse, and there is a risk that the patient's condition will deteriorate as a consequence. While there is no requirement for consent, as decisions for a supervised community treatment lie with the responsible clinician (see below) along with an AMHP, service users should be involved in decisions about the treatment that will be provided in the community. For people who are discharged from hospital into supervised community treatment there will be a need to follow a community treatment order (or CTO), which will include the clear conditions with which the service user is required to comply. Community treatment orders are specified by the responsible clinicians, and may include where and when the service user is to receive treatment in the community, and avoidance of high-risk situations, and may also include directions as to where the service user can live. Service users subject to supervised community treatments may be recalled to hospital if there is evidence of relapse or high-risk behaviour which may contribute to deterioration in their mental health, or if there has been a failure to comply with the conditions of the community treatment order that may lead to a risk of harm.

Roles

There are many roles of people defined by the Mental Health Act (1983, amended 2007) but it is beyond the scope of this chapter to offer an in-depth discussion of the various and diverse roles of professionals involved in the Act. However, key roles include the following.

- Nearest relatives: who have powers under the Act to apply for a section and to discharge their relative.
- AMHP: the 2007 amendments to the Mental Health Act 1983 allowed for a wider range of professionals, including nurses, being enabled to undertake roles previously undertaken by approved social workers (ASWs). These roles include making an application for admission to hospital (NIMHE, 2008).

- Approved clinicians (ACs): the AC is in charge of a service user's treatment and there must be an AC in charge of a service user's medication (NIMHE, 2008).
- Responsible clinicians (RCs): the RC is an AC who has overall responsibility for a detained service user's case. The RC reviews the service user's progress and has the power of discharge or to grant leave of absence (NIMHE, 2008).
- Hospital managers: under the Act hospital managers have the authority to detain service users and, in effect, it is to them that applications under the Act are made. Hospital managers have responsibilities to ensure that the legal requirements of the Act are followed.
- Independent mental health advocates (IMHAs): provide advocacy services for people detained under the Act. They help service users to understand their rights under the Act and to ensure that they obtain appropriate and relevant information, including details about their care and treatment. Service users should have access to a telephone on which they can contact an IMHA. IMHAs have the right to meet a service user in private and, where the service user consents, they should have access to the service user's notes or any clinical records.
- Second-opinion appointed doctors (SOADs): a suitably qualified SOAD to approve some forms of treatment for a particular service user.

Consent to treatment

As mentioned, medical treatment under the Act is taken to mean medical and psychological interventions and nursing care. Treatment of physical health problems only extends to interventions and care that are part of the treatment for mental disorder, such as wound care for a depressed person who has self-harmed. The Act does not apply to the medical treatment for physical health problems.

Consent means the '...voluntary and continuing permission of a patient to be given a particular treatment, based on sufficient knowledge of the purpose, nature, likely effects and risks of that treatment, including the likelihood of its success and any alternatives to it. Permission given under any unfair or undue pressure is not consent' (Department of Health, 2008, p. 189). The Act does allow some medical treatment without consent but it is still good practice to seek consent wherever possible. Sections 2 and 3 of the Act allow for treatment against a person's will. When a person is subject to the Act, consent is not needed for the administration of medication for a mental disorder within the first 3 months of its commencement. After this time, the approved clinician must certify that the person has the capacity to consent to treatment and has done so. Alternatively,

for treatment to continue beyond the initial 3 month period, a SOAD must certify that the person does not have mental capacity to consent (see below) or that the person does have mental capacity but has refused to do so. However, some treatments, such as neurosurgery and surgical implantation of hormones to reduce the male sex drive, cannot be given without a person's consent *and* a second opinion from a SOAD.

Section 58A of the Act applies to electro-convulsive therapy (ECT) and medications which are used as part of the ECT process. Here, if a person has not consented, treatment can be given only if a SOAD certifies that the patient lacks capacity to consent, that the treatment is appropriate, and does not conflict with an advance decision (see below). In all cases, the SOAD must consult with two professionals concerned with the care and treatment of the patient, one of whom must be a nurse, and they must stipulate the maximum number of administrations of ECT they are approving.

Section 62 allows for necessary treatments to be given urgently. This only applies when such treatment is believed to be necessary and beneficial in order to:

- save the patient's life,
- prevent or alleviate serious deterioration of the patient's condition, and the treatment does not have unfavourable physical or psychological consequences which cannot be reversed, or
- prevent patients behaving violently or being a danger to themselves or others, and the treatment represents the minimum interference necessary for that purpose, does not have unfavourable physical or psychological consequences which cannot be reversed and does not entail significant physical hazard (Department of Health, 2008, p. 207).

Treatment against a service user's wishes in an emergency situation is justified under the principle of urgent necessity (Hatcher and Samuels, 1998). In emergency situations, healthcare professionals must balance the necessity of emergency treatment and their duty of care against the service user's right to autonomy based on his or her mental capacity. Eldergill (2002) adds that the purpose of involuntary hospitalization is not to eliminate that element of risk in human life, which is a consequence of being free to act. Rather, it is to protect the individual or others from those risks that arise when an individual's capacity to judge risks, or to control the behaviour giving rise to such risks, is impaired by mental health problems or disorder.

Rights under the Act

Service users detained under the Act have a right to privacy and should wherever possible have access to telephones, where their conversations cannot be overheard, and access to e-mail and the internet. Consent for personal searches should always be sought and should be conducted by a same-sex member of staff and with the maximum of dignity. A comprehensive record of all searches must be undertaken.

Service users must be told about what the Act says about their care, treatment and detention. This includes information about:

- the provisions of the Act that apply to them,
- the rights of their nearest relative to discharge them,
- contacting a suitably qualified legal representative,
- when they can be treated without their consent,
- the role of SOADs and when they may be involved,
- the rules on the use of ECT where necessary,
- the effect of community treatment orders and the associated requirements and circumstances when they can be recalled to hospital.

Service users must also be informed of the role of the Mental Health Tribunal and their rights to apply to them, and how this process may be facilitated. Such tribunals are independent judicial bodies which review cases for people detained under the Act and are able to discharge service users from sections where criteria for detention are not met.

The monitoring of the use of the Mental Health Act is overseen by the Care Quality Commission (see http://www.cqc.org.uk/guidanceforprofessionals/mentalhealth/workingwithpeoplewhoserightsarerestricted/ourmonitoringoftheuseofthementalhealthact.cfm). Service users must be informed of how to contact the Commission and how to make a complaint to them. Service users must also be informed about the complaint's procedures for the services and hospitals at which they have been detained, and how to access them.

Advance decisions

Advance decisions are statements made by individuals with mental capacity about their preferences for care and treatment if a future situation should arise. The statements are concerned only with the refusal of specific treatment(s). Sometimes service users may also make advance statements about the future care and treatment they would like, the steps that should be taken in emergencies and what should be done if certain situations should arise. However, stating a preference for a particular treatment in advance is not legally binding, and professionals are not obliged to comply with such requests.

The Mental Capacity Act 2005 (or MCA; see next section) states that people aged 18 years or over, who have the capacity to do so, may make an advance decision to refuse a specified treatment at a time when they no longer have capacity to refuse or consent to that treatment (Department of Health, 2008). A prior valid advance decision has the same effect as if the patient has capacity and makes a contemporary decision to refuse treatment, and is legally binding. However, whereas it is good practice to consider the expressed advance decisions if a person is subject to compulsory detention and treatment under the Act, their prior expressed advance decisions may be overruled.

Mental Capacity Act (2005)

The Mental Capacity Act 2005 came into force fully on 1 April 2009. The purpose of the Act is to ensure that people aged 16 years or over who lack the capacity to make decision for themselves are protected under the law. The Mental Capacity Act clarifies what is meant by a lack of capacity and specifies how and when a person should be assessed and the duties and responsibilities of those who provide care to such people. Nurses have a duty to know about and follow the Mental Capacity Act's code of practice and to know how to comply with it (available at http://webarchive.nationalarchives.gov.uk/+/http://www.dca.gov.uk/legal-policy/mental-capacity/mca-cp.pdf). The Mental Capacity Act '...is intended to assist and support people who may lack capacity and to discourage anyone who is involved in caring for someone who lacks capacity from being overly restrictive or controlling. But the Act also aims to balance an individual's right to make decisions for themselves with their right to be protected from harm if they lack capacity to make decisions to protect themselves' (Department for Constitutional Affairs, 2007, p. 15).

The Mental Capacity Act has five important key principles (Care Quality Commission, 2010).

1. There is an assumption that a person has capacity unless the contrary has been established.
2. People must be helped to make decisions.
3. Unwise decisions do not necessarily mean lack of capacity.
4. Decisions must be taken in the person's best interests.
5. Decisions must be as least restrictive of freedom as possible.

The Mental Capacity Act applies not only to people with mental health problems, dementia and learning disabilities but also to people who may have a brain injury or who are under the influence of substances, anaesthetic or sedation. However, it is important to realize that if someone lacks capacity to make *some* decisions, this does not imply that they lack capacity to make *any* decisions about their life and that decision-making capabilities can vary over time, even during the course of a day (Care Quality Commission, 2010).

There are two stages to making a test of capacity:

1. considering if there is an impairment or disturbance in the functioning of a person's mind or brain,
2. judging if such impairment is sufficient to lead to a lack of capacity to make a particular decision.

A person may lack capacity if they are unable to:

- understand information relevant to the decision, or
- remember the information long enough to make the decision, or
- weigh up information relevant to the decision, or
- communicate their decision: by talking, using sign language or by any other means (Care Quality Commission, 2010, p. 5).

Acting in a person's best interests may, at times, lead to a nurse (or nurses) making a decision to use restraint. It is important to realize that it is a criminal offence under the Mental Capacity Act to use unnecessary or excessive restraint, or to ill-treat or willfully neglect, a person who lacks capacity. In deciding to use restraint nurses and the multiprofessional team must:

- believe that the restraint is necessary to prevent harm,
- ensure the restraint is reasonable and proportionate to the potential harm.

Any restraint which has been applied must be regularly reviewed.

Providing that nurses are working within the principles and code of practice of the Mental Capacity Act, the Act protects nurses from legal action when providing personal care for a person who lacks capacity (such as washing, dressing or attending to personal hygiene; eating and drinking; walking and assistance with transport).

CASE STUDY: MELISSA, AN INCIDENT OF SELF-HARM

Melissa is a 19-year-old woman who is admitted to the acute mental health unit one evening via the accident and emergency department following an act of deliberate self-harm (DSH). Melissa had had a fight with her boyfriend David, who decided to end their 2-year relationship. Melissa had made a laceration to her left wrist with a knife, which required sutures. Following medical intervention she is referred to the on-call duty doctor for assessment. On assessment Melissa is vague about the intent to self-harm and admits to having cut her wrist twice in the past under similar circumstances. She has previously been admitted to the mental health unit following a similar episode. Melissa is reasonably calm and, following discussion with the duty doctor, agrees to a voluntary admission.

However, soon after arrival in the unit Melissa approaches her nurse and states that she wants to be discharged. The nurse reviews the admission notes written by the duty doctor. The notes clearly state that while Melissa is admitted as a voluntary service user she is to be scheduled if she tries to leave. The nurse explains to Melissa that she is unable to leave the unit at this stage and that it would be preferable if Melissa waited until the morning to speak to her responsible clinician. Melissa is annoyed by this suggestion and asserts that she is a voluntary service user and simply wants to go home. She states that she is not willing to wait until the morning and insists that she has a right to leave.

RESPONSE TO MELISSA

It is important to understand that DSH is not necessarily synonymous with suicidal intent. Some individuals may initially state that their intentions were to die, but on further exploration it can often be established that suicide was not really the intended goal. The term 'DSH' is preferred in this scenario rather than 'attempted suicide' or 'parasuicide', as the motivations for this behaviour often involve nonsuicidal intentions. Although individuals who self-harm may state that they wanted to die, the motivation is usually more to do with an expression of distress or a desire to escape a troubling situation. Even when death is the outcome of DSH, this may not have been intended. Most self-harm inflicts little actual harm and does not come to the attention of medical services. Self-cutting is involved in many such cases and this appears to serve the purpose of releasing tension or of self-punishment (Hawton and James, 2005).

Lambert (2003) discusses the risk of suicide and DSH associated with personality disorders. Risk management is especially challenging for this group of individuals because they often make nonlethal gestures of DSH but are also at chronic risk for suicide. He cautions against labelling this group as manipulative in such a way that precludes them ever being admitted to a mental health unit. Individuals with personality disorder may present in a more difficult manner at one point in time and yet pose a serious suicide risk on subsequent presentation, especially if comorbid substance abuse is an issue. Brief hospitalization for people with personality disorders can be effective, as suicidal and self-harm urges tend to subside quickly in the security of a mental health setting.

There is little evidence, however, that hospitalization reduces the long-term suicide risk in personality-disordered service users. In fact, hospitalization can be regressive and countertherapeutic in some situations (Lambert, 2003). If not admitted to hospital, close follow-up should be a routine component of the management plan.

It would appear excessive if Melissa were to be detained in the mental health unit against her will. Documenting that she is a voluntary service user but that she should be scheduled if she decides to leave is essentially in conflict with the spirit of mental health legislation and is questionable practice. The role of the mental health nurse is therefore pivotal in avoiding an escalation of this situation, and arriving at a suitable compromise. Melissa's situation is not life-threatening and she is not in a state of distress that impairs her decision-making capacity. There is every possibility that with time and effective interpersonal skills Melissa could agree to stay overnight and have a review with the psychiatry team in the morning. However, offering choices may also help in defusing the situation. For example, following consultation with the on-call duty doctor, Melissa could be offered the alternative of going home and returning for a review the next day, especially if a relative or friend were prepared to stay with her.

Hospitalization for a mental disorder greatly increases risk of suicide and DSH, especially for those recently discharged from a mental health unit. Studies have shown that this risk is highest in the 28 days after discharge. Requesting that an individual agree to a 'no self-harm' or 'no suicide' contract is considered ineffective in reducing the incidence of DSH (Royal Australian and New Zealand College of Psychiatrists, 2004). Expecting an individual with related risk factors to 'guarantee their safety' is therefore an unhelpful approach and may only raise the individual's level of anxiety. Eldergill (2002) emphasizes that risk in healthcare cannot be avoided and that even a very low risk is at times inescapable. The evaluation of risk always depends on the situation, but the myriad situations in which the individual may find him or herself in the future can only ever be a matter of speculation (Szmukler, 2003). Rather than simply exploring risk factors it is recommended that clinicians also consider protective factors that reduce the level of risk, such as concerns for dependent children, religious beliefs, the person's motivation to avoid a particular behaviour and willingness to engage with services (Bouch and Marshall, 2005).

The quality of the therapeutic relationship is pivotal to influencing the service user in a positive, safety-enhancing manner. Clinicians need to be aware of their own thoughts, feelings and values in regard to suicide and DSH as these may affect clinical decision making. Clinical supervision and consultation is an important support to ensure that clinicians gain experience in managing such situations (O'Connor et al., 2004). On discharge, early follow-up is important to reduce the risk of repeat self-harm and to promote engagement with care. Melissa should therefore have some form of follow-up mental health support offered to her. Assisting service users and their relatives following discharge by providing them with clear information about follow-up plans and crisis services is highly recommended (Crawford, 2004, Mortensen et al., 2000). Longer-term therapeutic intervention is indicated for Melissa's condition, and mental health nurses should play a role in providing information on supports and services available to Melissa and her family in the community. Clear documentation of the interaction between the mental health nurse and Melissa and the consultation process with colleagues and significant others is extremely important, as is documenting the agreed plan for discharge and follow-up.

RISK MANAGEMENT AND THE CONCEPT OF DANGEROUSNESS

The use of control measures in mental health nursing practice must also be understood in the social context of mental health legislation and increasing focus on 'risk management' of individuals in society (those perceived to be 'mentally ill' or otherwise) deemed to pose a risk to the general public, including health professionals. This section briefly explores the notion of dangerousness and risk management as recent concepts in the care and treatment of people in health settings and, in particular, mental health service delivery.

The growth of the concept of risk in healthcare can be seen to be reflected by the perception of the general public that people with mental health problems have an increased capacity for violence and being a danger to others (Morgan, 1998). Although there are indications that service user violence is increasing in the inpatient setting (Whittington and Wykes, 1994) and the community (Fry et al., 2002), it is not known whether this is due to a real increase, previous under-reporting, a worsening level of risk in the workplace or an increased awareness of the subject of violence in society in general (Morgan, 1998).

Davidson (2005) states that epidemiological studies have demonstrated that people with acute mental health problems are more likely to be violent than community controls. This is attributable to acute psychotic symptoms (particularly paranoia and persecutory delusions) which indicate an elevated risk. The vast majority of people with a mental disorder, however, are not violent. Paterson et al. (2004) conducted an extensive review of the violence literature in relation to mental health populations. They conclude that a link between severe mental disorder and violence appears to have been established; however, the risk of violence is significantly increased when comorbid substance abuse and/or antisocial personality traits are present. Substance abuse greatly increases the risk of aggression and violence in the total population, and comorbid personality disorder independently increases risk (Davidson, 2005).

Hiday (2006) identifies numerous confounding factors that are minimized or neglected in studies undertaken to explore a link between mental disorder and violence. Once comorbid substance abuse and personality disorder are taken into account, the contribution of psychosis to violence in the community diminishes dramatically. Furthermore, people with mental health problems are also most likely to reside in violent neighborhoods and this could be a significant variable, rather than a psychiatric diagnosis. Multiple studies provide evidence that mental disorder, substance abuse and violence are frequently associated with 'socially disorganized communities', which are characterized by poverty, high unemployment, low education levels, resource deprivation, physical deterioration and breakdown into micro-institutions, especially families. People with a mental disorder who grow up in these communities learn to be violent, just as everyone else who becomes violent learns that behaviour.

The impact of the media in raising alarm about people with mental health problems being violent in the community is also a factor in negative perceptions about such people. More balanced debates about this emotive subject remind us that people living with mental health problems also have to bear the stigma and 'presumed guilty' label without a voice to present their view when fatalities in the community occur (Sayce, 1995). The concept of dangerousness has become commonly used to assess the behaviour of the service user in a healthcare setting, although historically it was used to describe the likelihood of a forensic service user reoffending when released into the community (Mason and Chandley, 1999). The term 'forensic service user' can be defined as a person who has committed or been charged with a crime while suffering from mental health problems and is remanded in custody in an approved mental health service, within a prison, remand centre or forensic psychiatric hospital. Mental health nurses working in forensic psychiatric facilities face unique challenges (Mason and Mercer, 1998). Mason and Mercer (1998) state that this group of nurses, like all nurses working in prisons, have contradictory responsibilities, namely that they exercise control over service users while maintaining ethical professional practice and protecting the public. 'Nursing practice in corrections is concerned with issues such as: mental illness, criminal acts, morality, treatment, containment and punishment' (Mason and Mercer, 1998, p. 85). In short, forensic mental health nurses must provide nursing care and obey the security requirements of the institution. Given the nature of some of the crimes committed by this group of service users, risk assessment is a core and vital component of their role.

Governments have responded to concerns about the occupational health and safety of health professionals in the healthcare setting by implementing policies to guide practice in the management of aggression and violence in the workplace, citing the increase in risk and violence as the driving force. However, the adoption of strategies such as refusing service to service users who exhibit agitated or aggressive behaviour suggests a draconian, zero-tolerance approach. This approach does not take into account the need for treatment for individuals who exhibit behaviours such as agitation, anxiety or extreme fear that are symptoms of their ill health. While the assessment of risk is imprecise, mental health nurses are required to be prepared with the skills and knowledge associated with this aspect of nursing care.

CRITICAL THINKING CHALLENGE 4.2

Have you ever felt at risk in a nursing setting?
What risk-assessment policies and procedures do you know of in nursing settings?
How would you respond to the statement that 'all "mad" people are dangerous'?

MANAGING BEHAVIOURAL EMERGENCIES

The unambiguous message from the nursing and medical literature is that early recognition and the use of sound interpersonal skills to defuse a volatile situation is the safest and most effective approach in managing aggression and violence. Deescalation, or talking a person down, involves the use of psychological techniques aimed at calming a distressed individual and redirecting them to a more comfortable emotional space. The components of deescalation involve an assessment of the immediate situation, verbal and nonverbal communication strategies designed to facilitate cooperation, and problem-solving skills. A clinician facing a potentially violent individual should convey the message that he or she is willing to work collaboratively and to seek alternative ways to solve the perceived problem (Davidson, 2005). Using deescalation techniques requires increased cognitive demands in an already demanding environment (Lee, 2001); however, there is considerable evidence to suggest that nurses can learn how to better manage an aggressor (Sains, 1999).

Violence rarely erupts suddenly. Aggression and violence often follow a period of mounting tension. In a typical scenario, the service user first becomes angry, then resists authority and finally becomes confrontational and overtly violent. While it is necessary to deal with aggression and violence, it is preferable to identify the signs of impending violence and to intervene before it manifests (Kao and Moore, 1999). Clinicians must be aware of circumstances where a potential for conflict exists. Negotiating openly for cooperation on initial contact with an individual greatly diminishes the potential for further difficulties. The risk of a personal battle, the 'dominance reciprocal', between the clinician and service user is particularly high with resistive individuals and must be consciously avoided (Shea, 1998). Wherever possible there should be an avenue for compromise in the management of challenging behaviour (Wand, 2004).

Pearson (1984) describes nurses in particular as the humanizers of the healthcare team. He suggests that service users expect nurses to be 'with them' emotionally and physically. Nurses support individuals as they try to make sense of and come to terms with the situation they face. It is therefore essential for nurses to work at developing effective interpersonal skills. Establishing trust and developing rapport should therefore be viewed as core business for nurses. Support, reassurance and gaining trust are especially important with people who are difficult or reluctant to accept treatment. Nurses need to be attentive listeners and respond calmly. A conciliatory manner and supportive statements are required, rather than condescension (Rallis-Peterson, 2001). Nurses must also be particularly mindful of their own nonverbal communication, avoiding vocal qualities that may convey sarcasm, frustration, anger or an overly authoritarian manner (Wand, 2004).

Garnham (2001) provides useful and practical advice on understanding and dealing with aggression and violence. He promotes the principle of early recognition and identifies the significance of well-developed nonverbal and verbal interpersonal skills. Some broader strategies to assist clinicians are also highlighted and summarized as follows: wherever possible, allow the person some time and space, as he or she may just need to 'sound off'. Demonstrate concern and an interest in providing help. Acknowledge the persons' feelings, even if you do not agree. Reassure the person in an attempt to manage anxiety and distress. If possible, make concessions. Make deliberately friendly approaches. Avoid provocative or threatening comments or gestures. Avoid being overly confrontational. Communicate your thoughts and intentions clearly. Personalize yourself by reminding the person of your role and relationship to them. Offer some alternatives or a range of solutions. Emphasize that their health is your concern, although providing access to good healthcare is difficult without cooperation.

Once a situation escalates to a critical point it is frequently referred to as a behavioural emergency. Expert consensus guidelines on the treatment of behavioural emergencies developed by Allen et al. (2001) recommend beginning with the least paternalistic approaches – verbal intervention, offering food, beverage or other assistance, or voluntary medication – before moving to more intrusive strategies. The authors state that the main difficulty with a behavioural emergency is that, although an intervention is required, there is often a standoff between the individual at the centre of the incident and those responsible for managing it (Allen et al., 2001). Physical restraint is a final response to imminent dangerous behaviour when less restrictive measures fail or are not appropriate (Karas, 2002). Many violent individuals back down when confronted by a coordinated team response. A demonstration of team unity protects individual team members from being singled out and also allows the aggressor an opportunity to back down and rationalize that they would have retaliated had the odds not been so overwhelming (Kao and Moore, 1999). Restraint is an emergency response to protect the person in imminent danger of harming themselves or others. The challenge is to employ an approach that ensures safety while maintaining individual dignity and avoids the inappropriate use of restraint.

In 2005, the National Institute for Health and Clinical Excellence (NICE) published guidelines on the short-term management of disturbed/violent behaviour in psychiatric in-patient settings and accident and emergency departments (NICE, 2005). Additional guidance is supplied by the *Code of Practice* for the Mental Health Act (Department of Health, 2008). Both documents stress the importance of prediction (by consideration of risk factors for violence and warning signs), prevention

(by observation and deescalation) and the development of a therapeutic relationship. The *Code of Practice* (Department of Health, 2008) identifies factors that may contribute to violent or aggressive behaviour. These include:

- boredom and lack of environmental stimulation,
- too much stimulation, noise and general disruption,
- excessive heating, overcrowding and lack of access to external space,
- personal frustrations associated with being in a restricted environment,
- difficulties in communication,
- emotional distress, such as following bereavement,
- antagonism, aggression or provocation on the part of others,
- the influence of alcohol or drugs,
- physical illness,
- an unsuitable mix of patients (Department of Health, 2008, p. 113).

Physical interventions (that is, rapid tranquilization, restraint or seclusion) should only be used when nonphysical interventions (such as deescalation) have failed. The NICE guidelines emphasize the need for organizational policies guiding the appropriate response to aggressive and/or violent behaviour and training for all staff in risk assessment and interventions for the violent person. Of vital importance is for staff who are involved in rapid tranquilization or restraint to be trained in basic life support (resuscitation). During restraint, the NICE guidelines recommend one member of staff ensuring that the head and neck is protected and supported, and taking responsibility for leading the team through ensuring that the airway and breathing are not compromised and that vital signs are monitored. At all times the level of force must be proportionate, reasonable and justifiable and the deliberate application of pain must be avoided, only being justifiable for the immediate and urgent rescue of staff or other service users (NICE, 2005).

An important consideration is that physical restraint and rapid sedation carry a significant risk of injury to staff and service users (Davidson, 2005). Clinicians may fail to appreciate the detrimental physical and psychological effects of restraint and sedation. Emphasis on immediate safety should not involve excessive force or injudicious use of medication. A heavy-handed approach may adversely affect perception of care and limit the chances of successful treatment (Currier, 2002). The use of restraint alone does little to reduce the level of agitation or aggression in a service user if the reason for that initial aggression has not been addressed. Restraint, both physical and chemical, can be seen as coercive, and may cause trauma and endanger both service users and staff (Duxbury, 2002; Kao and Moore, 1999; Lee, 2001; Wand, 2004). It is noteworthy that the aim of occupational health and safety legislation is to promote the health, safety and welfare of people at work and over-rides all other legal statutes and regulations. Restraining a service user without a prearranged and coordinated response is therefore ill advised, as it jeopardizes the safety of the service user and staff members. Nurses must therefore consider their own safety a priority and not place themselves at risk of becoming a casualty (Wand, 2004).

CASE STUDY: TOM, AN AGGRESSIVE AND DISTRESSED SERVICE USER IN THE ACCIDENT AND EMERGENCY DEPARTMENT

Tom is a 21-year-old man who presents one morning to the accident and emergency department with his mother. He has smoked cannabis on a regular basis (with occasional amphetamine use) for several years but decided to stop 1 week ago. Tom has always had a problem with aggression but since he has stopped smoking cannabis it has become worse. Several friends have distanced themselves from him recently because he has started fights with strangers while they were out. Tom has also been aggressive towards his brother, with whom he lives, and last night broke some furniture in their flat during an argument. During their argument he punched a wall and injured his hand, which is now swollen and very painful.

Tom is calm at triage and tells the nurse that along with his painful hand he has a drug problem and wants assistance. He states that cannabis controlled his aggressiveness to a degree and now without it he is much worse. He feels constantly agitated and restless. The accident and emergency department is busy this particular day and Tom and his mother are left in the waiting area for almost 2 h. Tom becomes increasingly agitated at having to wait and wants to leave on several occasions but his mother is able to persuade him to stay.

A junior doctor comes out to the waiting room to see Tom. He is abusive towards her over the extended delays and about the pain in his hand. She reacts by threatening to call security and have him restrained. This only seems to inflame Tom, who then stands over the medical officer in a threatening manner. His voice is loud and he is gesticulating wildly. His mother is tearful and upset, standing to the side of the commotion with one of the nursing staff. Other people in the waiting room are looking on in alarm at the escalating situation.

RESPONSE TO TOM

This situation highlights the importance of keeping people informed of delays. The most effective method to manage aggression and violence is to have minimization strategies in place that reduce its likelihood. Tom is highly distressed and clearly has the potential to be violent. The medical officer's response to call for security is understandable, given Tom's threatening manner. However, he has interpreted this as a challenge and an opportunity to fuel a conflict. When staff become aware of a potential or actual aggressive incident, it is strongly advised that a team approach be employed.

Therefore in this situation, the medical officer would stand back at a safe distance and wait until a number of people from the accident and emergency department could be summoned to provide assistance. A unified response should consist of both medical and nursing staff. On no occasion are staff expected to manage an aggressive incident alone. Ideally, a team approach is led by a suitably trained and qualified person, who attempts to engage the service user, making it clear that the staff want the service user to gain control of his or her aggressive behaviour in a safe manner.

In this situation, the service user is calmly asked to desist from their dangerous behaviour, in an attempt to offer the individual an opportunity to demonstrate control of their behaviour. It should be emphasized that the service user has a right to healthcare but this cannot be provided if staff feel under threat. Lengthy discussions or explanations regarding delays are not indicated; however, an offer to have Tom's hand attended to promptly and a willingness to move ahead with his treatment (provided he remain calm) should be the priority. At this point Tom could be offered pain relief or medication to calm him down.

It is important to avoid a dramatic scene. Security guards may in fact inflame a potentially volatile situation. A highly aroused person may feel further pressured if they are surrounded by people, noise, competing voices and instructions. This may exacerbate the service user's dangerous behaviour. The team should therefore stay together slightly behind and to the side of the team leader, continually observing the service user. Having more people in the response team than necessary should be avoided, as should circling or surrounding the person, as this may be perceived as more threatening.

There are occasions where a service user may be asked to leave the accident and emergency department, but this is a team, not an individual, decision and should be made only when senior staff members are satisfied that:

- the service user's condition is not life-threatening or medically urgent,
- the service user's aggression is not due to any organic pathology that requires intervention and treatment,
- attempts to establish a reasonable degree of cooperation have failed,
- the service user's continued presence in the department constitutes a threat to safety.

If Tom did not respond to attempts at defusing his anger and he continued to present a threat to staff he could be asked to leave the accident and emergency department. It should be explained that he may return for treatment if he re-presents in a more rational state. If Tom were to respond by becoming more aggressive then it may be appropriate for security staff to be summoned for assistance. It may also be advisable to isolate and evacuate the waiting room.

It should be noted that many service users who constitute a threat are still owed a duty of care and will need to be managed and treated. Physical restraint and/or sedation are measures of last resort; nevertheless, when there is imminent danger to people, restraint and sedation may be appropriate. If this is indicated, suitable recording of the event and outcomes for the service user as well as incident and accident forms should be documented. Finally, staff involved in an aggressive situation involving restraint and sedation should be offered an opportunity to discuss their experience and, if necessary, be offered formal follow-up. The adverse physical and psychological effects of sedation and restraint on the service user should also be considered in post-incident management.

CASE STUDY: JEREMY, A DISTURBED MAN AT HOME

Jeremy is a 37-year-old man who has recently caused concern to his neighbours because of his agitated behaviour. Neighbours have observed Jeremy pacing up and down the driveway of his house and on occasions yelling at passers by. He has refused approaches by his neighbours to talk things over, telling them that they are cursed by the breath of Satan, and warning them to stay off his property. Tonight the police have been called, after Jeremy threw a pot plant against the house next door. The police have contacted the on-call AMHP to assess Jeremy because they believe he may be mentally ill.

RESPONSE TO JEREMY

Mental health emergencies often occur in community settings, and may initially present as behavioural problems calling for a police response. AMHPs liaise with police and are available to advise about the possible mental health service response and, if necessary, to provide an assessment of a person who has been removed to a place of safety or is in police custody and who is considered to be mentally unwell. One aspect of the AMHP's response is to consider the use of mental health legislation to detain the person as an involuntary service user.

In cases like Jeremy's, mental health services follow the principle of the least-restrictive alternative in deciding on the response. It is possible that Jeremy is simply upset and worried about problems in his life and is expressing these anxieties in ways that concern his neighbours. Other possibilities are that Jeremy is under the influence of alcohol or other drugs, or is suffering from delirium, a physical condition that can cause confusion and agitation.

In responding to this emergency situation it is important to gain as much information as necessary, especially about Jeremy's usual pattern of behaviour. It may be that this behaviour is not unusual for Jeremy and that the neighbours have simply reached the limit of their tolerance. Establishing whether Jeremy has been physically unwell recently will be important in gaining a full understanding of his needs.

Mental health legislation contains explicit criteria that must be satisfied if Jeremy is to be treated as an involuntary service user (see above). The severity of mental disorder will influence this assessment, as will the risk that Jeremy poses to himself or to others.

It is not unusual for members of the public or the police to conclude that erratic or agitated behaviour is the result of mental disorder. However, if the criteria of mental health legislation are not met then Jeremy cannot be held against his will. Jeremy retains all the rights of a voluntary service user, including the right to consent to or refuse treatment.

If Jeremy meets the criteria for involuntary treatment then it is important that the process of admission to hospital is conducted with respect for Jeremy's feelings and perceptions of events, even where they are in disagreement with those of the clinical team. Although involuntary treatment involves significant restrictions on individual rights, service users have the right to be heard, to express choices and to fair decision-making processes. Service users who are being assessed under mental health legislation may wish to have a friend or family member to support them; or, alternatively, they may prefer not to have others involved. Establishing service users' preferences is important in mental health crises. Service users also have the right to legal processes of appeal and review. Nurses should support service users in accessing those rights, with an awareness that repeated explanations may be necessary if the service user's thinking is disorganized, or if they are acutely distressed. Finally, any involuntary treatment should be for the shortest time possible without compromising the person's recovery, with the aim of restoring the autonomy lost in the process of involuntary treatment.

CONCLUSION

This chapter has explored a number of contemporary legal and political issues associated with mental health nursing practice. There are many challenges facing mental health nurses, including changes to the role of the mental health nurse, ongoing policy developments in the provision of mental health services and the need to balance the caring and controlling functions of mental health nursing practice. Such challenges serve to facilitate opportunities for reform, practice developments and the development of new partnerships with those for whom we care.

Nurses must be familiar with the ethical and legal considerations relevant to service users who self-harm or are aggressive, and follow a logical approach between the duty of care and the service user's right to self-determination. Working effectively with difficult service users requires the establishment of rapport. This is especially true in cases where a potential for behavioural emergencies exists. Managing resistive service users requires flexibility, adept use of interpersonal skills and conscious control over the nonverbal messages that can be conveyed in human interaction.

REFERENCES

Allen, M.H., Currier, G.W., Hughes, D.H., et al., 2001. The expert consensus guidelines series: treatment of behavioural emergencies. Postgrad. Med. May (Suppl.), 1–88.

Bouch, J., Marshall, J., 2005. Suicide risk: structured professional judgement. Adv. Psychiatr. Treat. 11 (2), 84–91.

Care Quality Commission, 2010. The Mental Capacity Act 2005. <http://www.cqc.org.uk/_db/_documents/ RP_PoC1B2B_100563_20100825_ v3_00_Guidance_for_providers_ MCA_FOR_EXTERNAL_ PUBLICATION.pdf>.

Crawford, M., 2004. Suicide following discharge from in-patient psychiatric care. Adv. Psychiatr. Treat. 10 (6), 434–438.

Currier, G., 2002. Drug selection: management of psychotic agitation in the emergency service. Psychiatr. Issues Emerg. Care Settings 1 (1), 3–11.

Davidson, S., 2005. The management of violence in general psychiatry. Adv. Psychiatr. Treat. 11 (5), 362–370.

Department for Constitutional Affairs, 2007. Mental Capacity Act 2005 Code of Practice. <http:// webarchive.nationalarchives.gov. uk/+/http://www.dca.gov.uk/ legal-policy/mental-capacity/ mca-cp.pdf>.

Department of Health, 1999. National Service Framework for Mental Health: modern standards and service models. <http://www.dh.gov.uk/en/Publicationsandstatistics/Publications/PublicationsPolicyAndGuidance/DH_4009598>.

Department of Health, 2001. The journey to recovery: the government's vision for mental health care. <http://www.dh.gov.uk/en/Publicationsandstatistics/Publications/PublicationsPolicyAndGuidance/DH_4002700>.

Department of Health, 2006. Choosing health: supporting the physical needs of people with severe mental illness - commissioning framework. <http://www.dh.gov.uk/en/Publicationsandstatistics/Publications/PublicationsPolicyAndGuidance/DH_4138212>.

Department of Health, 2008. Code of Practice: Mental Health Act 1983. <http://www.dh.gov.uk/en/Healthcare/Mentalhealth/DH_4132161>.

Department of Health, 2010. Equity and excellence: liberating the NHS. <http://www.dh.gov.uk/en/Publicationsandstatistics/Publications/PublicationsPolicyAndGuidance/DH_117353>.

Department of Health, 2011. No health without mental health. <http://www.dh.gov.uk/en/Aboutus/Features/DH_123998>.

Disability Rights Commission, 2006. Equal treatment: closing the gap. <http://www.drc.gov.uk/library/health_investigation.aspx>.

Duxbury, J., 2002. An evaluation of staff and patient views of and strategies employed to manage inpatient aggression and violence on one mental health unit: a pluralistic design. J. Psychiatr. Ment. Health Nurs. 9 (3), 325–337.

Eldergill, A., 2002. Is anyone safe? Civil compulsion under the draft mental health bill. J. Ment. Health Law December, 331–359.

Ernst, W., 1991. The social history of pakeha psychiatry in 19th century New Zealand. In: Bryder, L. (Ed.), A Healthy Country. Essays on the Social History of Medicine in New Zealand Bridget Williams, Wellington.

Faulkner, A., Layzell, S., 2000. Strategies for Living: The Research Report. Mental Health Foundation, London.

Fry, A.J., O'Riordan, D., Turner, M., et al., 2002. Survey of aggressive incidents experienced by community mental health staff. Int. J. Ment. Health Nurs. 11 (2), 112–120.

Future Vision Coalition, 2008. A new vision for mental health: discussion paper. <http://www.newvisionformentalhealth.org.uk/>.

Garnham, P., 2001. Understanding and dealing with anger, aggression and violence. Nurs. Stand. 24 (16), 37–42.

Hatcher, S., Samuels, A., 1998. Medicolegal aspects of managing self-harm in the emergency department. N. Z. Med. J. 111 (1069), 255–258.

Hawton, K., James, A., 2005. Suicide and deliberate self harm in young people. Br. Med. J. 330 (7496), 891–894.

Hewitt, P., 2005. Speech at the Britain Speaks - Effective Public Engagement and Better Decision Making Conference, London, 23 June 2005.

Hiday, V.A., 2006. Putting community risk in perspective: a look at correlations, causes and controls. Int. J. Law Psychiatry 29 (4), 316–331.

Kao, L.W., Moore, G.P., 1999. The violent patient: clinical management, use of physical and chemical restraints, and medicolegal concerns. Emerg. Med. Prac. 1 (6), 1–24.

Karas, S., 2002. Behavioural emergencies: differentiating medical from psychiatric disease. Emerg. Med. Prac. 4 (3), 1–20.

Kemp, P., 2008. User involvement and the micro-politics of mental health care. In: Lynch, J., Trenoweth, S. (Eds.), Contemporary Issues in Mental Health Nursing. Wiley, Chichester.

Lambert, M., 2003. Suicide risk assessment and management: focus on personality disorders. Curr. Opin. Psychiatry 16 (1), 71–76.

Lee, F., 2001. Violence in the A&E: the role of training and self efficacy. Nurs. Stand. 15 (46), 33–38.

Mason, T., Chandley, M., 1999. Managing Violence and Aggression: a Manual for Nurses and Health Care Workers. Churchill Livingstone, Edinburgh.

Mason, T., Mercer, D., 1998. Critical Perspectives in Forensic Care: Inside Out. Macmillan, London.

Maude, P., 2001. From lunatic to client: a history/nursing oral history of the treatment of Western Australians who experienced a mental illness. Doctoral thesis, University of Melbourne, Melbourne.

Mentality/NIMHE (National Institute for Mental Health in England), 2004. Healthy body and mind: promoting health living for people who experience mental distress. <http://www.staffordshirementalhealth.info/ftp/document/pdf/shift-healthybody-workers.pdf>.

Morgan, S., 1998. The assessment and management of risk. In: Brooker, C., Repper, J. (Eds.), Serious Mental Health Problems in the Community: Policy, Practice and Research. Baillière Tindall, London.

Mortensen, P., Agerbo, E., Erikson, T., et al., 2000. Psychiatric illness and risk factors for suicide in Denmark. Lancet 355 (9197), 9–12.

NICE (National Institute for Health and Clinical Excellence), 2005. Violence: the short-term management of disturbed/violent behaviour in psychiatric in-patient settings and emergency departments. <http://www.nice.org.uk/CG25>.

NICE (National Institute for Health and Clinical Excellence), 2009a. Schizophrenia: core interventions in the treatment and management of schizophrenia in primary and secondary care. <http://publications.nice.org.uk/schizophrenia-cg82>.

NICE (National Institute for Health and Clinical Excellence), 2009b. Depression in adults. The treatment and management of depression in adults. <http://publications.nice.org.uk/depression-in-adults-cg90>.

NIMHE (National Institute for Mental Health in England), 2005. NIMHE guiding statement on recovery. <http://www.psychminded.co.uk/news/news2005/feb05/nimherecovstatement.pdf>.

NIMHE (National Institute for Mental Health in England), 2008. Mental Health Act 2007: new roles.

<http://www.nmhdu.org.uk/silo/files/mental-health-act-2007--new-roles.pdf>.

O'Connor, N., Warby, M., Raphael, B., et al., 2004. Changeability, confidence, common sense and corroboration: comprehensive suicide risk assessment. Australas. Psychiatry 12 (4), 352–360.

Office of the Deputy Prime Minister, 2004. Mental health and social exclusion: Social Exclusion Unit report. OPDM Publications, Wetherby.

Paterson, B., Claughan, P., McComish, S., 2004. New evidence or changing population? Reviewing the evidence of a link between mental illness and violence. Int. J. Ment. Health Nurs. 13 (1), 39–52.

Pearson, A., 1984. The essence of advanced nursing is being there. Nurs. Mirror 159 (8), 16.

Rallis-Peterson, D., 2001. When a patient turns violent. RN 64 (5), 32–35.

Robson, D., Gray, R., 2007. Serious mental illness and physical health problems: a discussion paper. Int. J. Nurs. Stud. 44, 457–466.

Royal Australian and New Zealand College of Psychiatrists, 2004. Australian and New Zealand clinical practice guidelines for the management of adult self-harm. Aust. N. Z. J. Psychiatry 38 (11/12), 868–884.

Sains, J., 1999. Violence and aggression in A & E: recommendations for action. Accid. Emerg. Nurs. 7 (1), 8–12.

Sainsbury Centre For Mental Health, 2003. Primary solutions an independent policy review on the development of primary care mental health services. The Sainsbury Centre For Mental Health, London.

Sayce, L., 1995. Response to violence: a framework for fair treatment. In: Crichton, J. (Ed.), Psychiatric Patient Violence: Risk and Response. Duckworth, London.

Shea, S., 1998. Psychiatric Interviewing. The Art of Understanding. WB Saunders, Philadelphia.

Singh, B., 2001. The global perspective in mental health. In: Meadows, G., Singh, B. (Eds.), Mental Health in Australia: Collaborative Community Practice. Oxford University Press, London, pp. 44–45.

Symonds, B., 1995. The origins of insane asylums in England during the 19th century: a brief sociological review. J. Adv. Nurs. 22, 94–100.

Szmukler, G., 2003. Risk assessment: 'numbers' and 'values'. Psychiatr. Bull. 27, 205–207.

Wand, T., 2004. Duty of care in the emergency department. Int. J. Ment. Health Nurs. 13 (2), 135–139.

Whittington, R., Wykes, T., 1994. The prediction of violence in a health care setting. In: Wykes, T. (Ed.), Violence and Health Care Professionals. Chapman & Hall, London.

WHO (World Health Organization), 2001a. Mental Health Around the World: Stop Exclusion. Dare to Care. Brochure. World Health Organization, Geneva.

WHO (World Health Organization), 2001b. Mental health: new understanding, new hope. <http://www.who.int/whr2001/2001/main/en/chapter4/Box> 5.1. Rights of the Mentally Ill.

WHO (World Health Organization), 2001c. Mental health, new understanding, new hope. <http://www.who.int/whr2001/2001/main/en/>.

Chapter | 5 |

Professional and ethical issues

Anthony O'Brien, Phillip Maude, and Eimear Muir-Cochrane

CHAPTER POINTS

- The regulation of nursing occurs through legislation and the professional body, the Nursing and Midwifery Council (NMC).
- Other professional nursing organizations have an impact on the delivery of nursing care.
- Nurses are prepared for professional practice by completing programmes approved by the NMC.
- Accountability in nursing is achieved through adherence to standards of practice.
- Authority to continue to practise is determined by declared competence.
- Mental health nurses are able to work in extended roles, including consultant nurse, nurse prescriber and approved clinician roles.
- As the largest single group within the mental health workforce, mental health nurses play an important role in the development of mental health services that protects the rights of service users and their carers and ensures that their needs are met.
- The claim to professional status requires nurses to practise within a code of ethics.
- Mental healthcare involves reflection on ethical issues and the use of principles of ethical reasoning.
- Codes of ethics guide members of the professions as to the nature of proper conduct and their obligations to the public.
- Mental health nurses are confronted with ethical issues on a daily basis.
- Diagnosing a person with a mental disorder has powerful and potentially detrimental consequences for that person.
- Nurses need to consider the ethical issues arising from their choice of intervention and from many of the treatments prescribed in psychiatry.

KEY TERMS

- code of ethics
- competency

- confidentiality
- ethics
- mental health nursing
- nurse prescribing
- nursing education
- nursing organizations
- professional standards and regulation
- reviews of mental health nursing
- standards of practice

LEARNING OUTCOMES

The material in this chapter will assist you to:

- outline the roles of professional organizations in mental health nursing,
- discuss the influence of education on preparation for practice in mental health nursing,
- discuss the extended roles in mental health nursing,
- identify common ethical issues in mental health nursing,
- apply ethical principles to the analysis of ethical issues in mental health nursing.

INTRODUCTION

This chapter discusses key issues related to the professional practice of mental health nursing. The past 20 years have seen the final devolution of mental health-care from predominantly hospital-based services to integrated hospital and community care, together with the development of a wide range of clinical specializations within mental health nursing. In parallel with that process of change has been the move within nursing education to degree-based preparation for practice. The scope of practice has been extended to include nurse consultancy, prescribing, Approved Mental Health Professional (AMHP) and eligibility for approved/responsible clinician status (see Ch. 4). At the same time that the profession has been developing its own structures and processes, it has developed responses to the complex ethical issues that the changing mental health context demands. This chapter explores the professional context of practice, including the roles of professional regulatory bodies and nursing organizations. It also outlines the principles of ethical conduct and discusses some ethical issues commonly encountered in mental health nursing.

REGULATION OF PROFESSIONAL PRACTICE

Mental health nurses practise in a complex professional environment that requires a clear sense of professional identity and clear frameworks for practice. Broad frameworks for professional practice are provided by legislation and by the nursing regulatory body: the Nursing and Midwifery Council (NMC). In addition, support and guidance on professional issues are also provided by professional nursing organizations and unions, the largest of which is the Royal College of Nursing (RCN), which also provides workplace representation and bargaining over salary and conditions of employment. Nationally, the Royal College seeks to influence health policies and to be the voice of the nursing profession.

This distinction between the regulatory body and professional organizations, however, disguises the overlap between these bodies, as conditions of employment have a direct effect on the ability to meet professional standards, and the realization of the expectations of professional bodies can affect conditions of employment. The issues of numbers of beds provided by a mental health service and the number of staff allocated to different sections of the service demonstrate the overlapping functions of professional organizations. While these may be primarily 'industrial' issues because of their immediate impact on nurses' conditions of employment, they also have the potential to affect standards of clinical practice. All professional bodies have an interest in quality-of-service issues.

The legal and professional regulation of the nursing profession began in 1919 with the Nurses' Registration Acts of 1919. The acts established the General Nursing Council (GNC) which survived until 1983, when changes to the law created the United Kingdom Central Council for Nursing, Midwifery and Health Visiting (UKCC), which was responsible for maintaining a register of UK nurses, midwives and health visitors, along with providing professional guidance to registrants and handling misconduct complaints. National boards for each country in the UK were also established at this time. These bodies were responsible for monitoring the quality of educational courses for nursing and midwifery. In 2002, the UKCC was replaced by the NMC (following the Nursing and Midwifery Order 2001), the role of which integrated the functions of both the UKCC and the national boards.

The NMC's primary role is that of safeguarding the health and wellbeing of the general public by:

- maintaining of register of all nurses and midwives, ensuring that registrants are properly qualified and competent to work in the UK;

- investigating allegations made against nurses and midwives who may not have followed the code;
- ensuring that nurses and midwives keep their skills and knowledge up to date and uphold the standards of the professional code;
- setting the standards of education, training and conduct necessary to deliver high-quality care.

NURSING EDUCATION

The early programmes of education in 'psychiatric' nursing were based in psychiatric institutions and were apprentice-style programmes with students spending the greater part of their time meeting the service needs of the institutions. While this had the benefit of providing nursing students with a great deal of exposure to the clinical practice of nursing, it provided limited opportunities to develop academic and theoretical skills.

Educational preparation for practice in mental health nursing underwent tremendous change in the latter half of the past century. From a service-based training based in psychiatric hospitals, mental health nursing came to be included in nursing diploma and degree programmes within the tertiary (higher) education sector.

Today, following the publication of the *Standards for Pre-Registration Nursing Education* (NMC, 2010a) all prequalifying nursing programmes will lead to a minimum of a bachelor's degree (of at least 300 academic credits, 60 of which must be at level 6). The standards for preregistration nursing education '…aim to enable nurses to give and support high quality care in rapidly changing environments. They reflect how future services are likely to be delivered, acknowledge future public health priorities and address the challenges of long-term conditions, an ageing population, and providing more care outside hospitals' (NMC, 2010a, 4). Furthermore, the standards aim to ensure public confidence in the nursing profession by ensuring that new registrants will:

- deliver high-quality essential care to all,
- deliver complex care to service users in their field of practice,
- act to safeguard the public, and be responsible and accountable for safe, person-centred, evidence-based nursing practice,
- act with professionalism and integrity, and work within agreed professional, ethical and legal frameworks and processes to maintain and improve standards,
- practise in a compassionate, respectful way, maintaining dignity and wellbeing and communicating effectively,

- act on their understanding of how people's lifestyles, environments and the location of care delivery influence their health and wellbeing,
- seek out every opportunity to promote health and prevent illness,
- work in partnership with other health and social care professionals and agencies, service users, carers and families ensuring that decisions about care are shared,
- use leadership skills to supervise and manage others and contribute to planning, designing, delivering and improving future services (NMC, 2010a, p. 5).

STANDARDS OF PRACTICE

The professionalization of mental health nursing is reflected in the development of standards of practice. The growing emphasis on accountability in mental healthcare means that development of standards has assumed increasing significance (Rodgers, 2000). The NMC establish a code of ethics embodied in standards, guidance and advice for nurse's professional behaviour and conduct as part of their statutory professional regulatory function. The standards cover the broad scope of professional practice and include a rationale for each standard, attributes related to each standard, and performance criteria.

The standards represent the commitment of mental health nurses to accountability in the professional practice of nursing. They are the professional benchmark in examining the quality of mental health nursing care (O'Brien, 2002/2003) and are used in professional conduct investigations. Continued monitoring of achievement of standards of practice is essential for any group claiming professional status, as regulation is recognized as a defining characteristic of professions.

Mental health nursing standards of practice describe the expected performance of nurses providing mental healthcare, but nurses also work within service standards, strategies and policies that govern the practice of all mental health professionals (such as *No Health without Mental Health* (Department of Health, 2011) and *Equity and Excellence: Liberating the NHS* (Department of Health, 2010); see Ch. 2). The coexistence of nursing professional standards and national service standards reflects the interdisciplinary nature of mental healthcare (Holmes, 2001) and the demand for nurses to meet the standards of their own profession as well as those of the service sector.

STANDARDS

In order to ensure a framework of safety that will protect the public, professions specify sets of competencies that describe the expected skills of all practitioners within a particular discipline. The NMC sets professional standards for registered nurses embodied in *The Code: Standards of Conduct, Performance and Ethics for Nurses and Midwives* (NMC, 2008a). The NMC emphasizes the importance of the general public being able to trust nurses and in this regard nurses must:

- make the care of people your first concern, treating them as individuals and respecting their dignity,
- work with others to protect and promote the health and wellbeing of those in your care, their families and carers, and the wider community,
- provide a high standard of practice and care at all times,
- be open and honest, act with integrity and uphold the reputation of your profession (NMC, 2008a, p. 2).

In this way, mental health nurses are legally and personally accountable for their practice (both actions and omissions) and they must be able to justify their decisions. The NMC also provides frameworks for practice involving the administration of medication (NMC, 2007) and nurse prescribing (NMC, 2006) (see below), raising and escalating concerns (NMC, 2010b), record keeping (NMC, 2009a), care of older people (NMC, 2009b) and guidance for student nurses's practice (NMC, 2010c).

Whereas renewal of annual registration was formerly a procedural matter involving documentation and payment of a fee (the annual retention), nurses are now also required to demonstrate continuing competency in order to retain their registration. This means that every 3 years nurses must renew their registration (the periodic renewal). This is achieved by completing a Notification of Practice (NoP) form which is confirmation by the nurse that they are of good health and good character, that they have met the appropriate standards for practice and that they have completed, in the previous 3 years, 450 h of registered practice and 35 h of learning activity (continuing professional development) (NMC, 2008b).

The NMC recommend recording continuing professional development activity in a personal professional profile (NMC, 2008b) and that the profile includes the following:

- description of one's role profile,
- nature of the learning activity undertaken: dates and duration of learning activity,
- a full description of the learning activity: the reasons for undertaking the learning activity, and what one expected to gain from it,
- reflection on the outcome of the learning activity. How did the learning relate to one's work? What are the effects of the learning on one's work and the way in which one intends to work in the future? What follow-up learning may be necessary for future practice?

The NMC conducts audits of compliance with the Prep standards in which nurses are required to produce descriptions of learning activities, and the relevance of this to their work, as evidence of continuing competence (NMC, 2008b).

CAREER PATHWAYS

When mental health nursing was located primarily in large psychiatric hospitals, the nature of those institutions provided some structure to the careers of nurses; typically, as one's career progressed, one's role became increasingly managerial in its function. However, with the devolution of care to community settings and changes to the role and function of the profession, mental health nurses have been able to access more opportunities for career advancement. Nurses wishing to gain career advancement have opportunities to develop their career along academic, practice development, nurse consultancy, research or senior clinical lines as well as management ones. This has challenged the profession to develop and advocate for career progression based on experience and clinical expertise.

Career pathways for nurses need to consider the diversity of nursing, and encourage nurses to pursue careers in clinical practice, education, management and research. All these choices require a sound foundation in clinical practice that is further enhanced by education and professional development. This has been accompanied by extension to the roles of mental health nurses in terms of their leadership of clinical multiprofessional teams (approved/responsible clinicians) and involvement in the application of the Mental Health Act (AMHP; see Ch. 4). Mental health nurses are also now able, on completion of the appropriate postregistration educational programme, to prescribe medication (see Ch. 24).

PRESCRIBING

Nurses have long influenced the pattern of medications prescribed to service users by suggesting to doctors specific medications and medication regimens, based on their knowledge of service users' preferences and responses, assessment of service users' clinical state and knowledge of the actions and interactions of psychotropic medications (Bailey, 1999). Advanced practice nurses in the USA have been licensed to prescribe since 1977 (Fennell, 1991), and currently 50 of those States extend prescribing authority to nurses (Pearson, 2003).

The intention of extending prescriptive authority to nurses is to fully utilize the capacity of nurses to provide healthcare (Bailey, 1999), and to make healthcare more accessible to service users. However, this has not occurred without controversy. Medical practitioners have not always supported extension of prescribing authority to nurses (Elsom et al., 2007), arguing that nurses do not have adequate educational preparation for this role (Maling, 2000), and there are questions within the profession about whether prescribing is a legitimate aspect of mental health nursing (Hemingway, 2003). Preparation for prescribing involves rigorous educational processes which focus on both pharmacological knowledge and prescribing practice (Lim et al., 2007). However, there are also complex legal, professional and clinical issues that need to be addressed.

Prescribing does not stand alone as a clinical skill, but is embedded in a body of skills in assessment, diagnosis and treatment (see Ch. 24). For a nurse to prescribe safely and competently they are required to demonstrate theoretical understanding and practical skills in health assessment, pharmacodynamics and pharmacokinetics (Lim et al., 2007). In addition to their *Standards for Medicines Management* (NMC, 2007), which details professional requirements for the administration of medication, the NMC also provides frameworks of proficiency for prescribing and approval for educational programmes for nurse prescribers: the *Standards of Proficiency for Nurse and Midwife Prescribers* (NMC, 2006). The standards require nurse prescribers to be able to:

- assess a service user's clinical condition,
- undertake a thorough history, including medical history and medication history, and diagnose where necessary, including over-the-counter medicines and complementary therapies,
- decide on management of presenting condition and whether or not to prescribe,
- identify appropriate products if medication is required,
- advise the service user on effects and risks,
- prescribe if the service user agrees,
- monitor response to medication and lifestyle advice (NMC, 2006, p. 5).

Development of prescribing authority for nurses requires close collaboration with existing prescribers (designated medical practitioners or DMPs) as nurses undertake the necessary clinical programmes in prescribing. There is some evidence that nurses' prescribing patterns are different from those of doctors (Latter and Courtenay, 2004), with nurses prescribing medication less readily and in lower doses (Avron, 1991; Safriet, 1992). Negotiation with service users about preferences in relation to medication will be an important aspect of nurse prescribing, as nurses seek to develop collaborative, service user-focused models of prescribing.

REVIEWS OF MENTAL HEALTH NURSING

The seeds of modern mental health nursing practice were sown in the 1994 review *Working in Partnership: A Collaborative Approach to Care* (Department of Health, 1994). It established the contemporary framework for mental health nursing practice in the UK. It sought to define the contribution that mental health nursing can make to the lives of people with mental health problems reflective of the changes in society, such as the emphasis placed on responding to the needs and wishes of service users. The review stressed the importance of developing person-centred, collaborative relationships with service users and the '…principle of choice for people who use services and their carers needs to be fully established as a basis for the practice of Mental Health Nursing' (Department of Health, 1994, p. 5). The review also recommended the use of the title *mental health nurse* (rather than psychiatric nurse) to reflect the emerging broader remit of nurses in meeting the needs of service users.

In 2006 the Chief Nursing Officer's review of mental health nursing, *From Values to Action* (Department of Health, 2006), made recommendations for good practice based on wide consultation with nurses, service users, employers and other organizations. It made three primary recommendations, as follows.

1. Putting values into practice. The broad principles of the recovery approach should be adopted by mental health nurses. In particular they should provide evidence-based nursing care and work towards goals that are meaningful to service users, collaborating with the service user in developing realistic individual care plans, while being positive about change and promoting social inclusion, equality in care and social justice for mental health users and carers.

2. Improving outcomes for service users. By developing and maintaining positive therapeutic relationships with service users, their families and/or carers. The practice of mental health nurses should be holistic, taking into account the person's physical, psychological, social, emotional and spiritual needs. The review acknowledges the need for nurses to develop skills of assessment, including risk assessment, and health promotion to improve service users' physical wellbeing. Nurses should also provide more evidence-based psychological therapies.

3. Developing a positive, modern profession. The review recommended that mental health nurses should use their skills effectively by working directly with service users with high level of needs, while supporting others to provide care to those with less complex

needs. The review encourages nurses to undertake extended roles, such as nurse consultancy and prescribing, as a way of contributing more positively to the experience of service users.

ETHICS AND PROFESSIONAL PRACTICE

Eliot Freidson, a medical sociologist, defined a profession as 'an occupational group that reserves to itself the authority to judge the quality of its work' (Freidson, 1989, p. 9). This asserts that an occupation earns the right to call itself a profession partly through the credibility and trust that is built with the people to whom it provides a service. For nursing to assert itself as a profession, ethics and identity are inseparable. This is because the identity of nursing, and the self-regulatory processes that ensure continued trust within the community, are inextricably interwoven. In other words, nursing and nursing practice are guided by the law, ethical principles (see Box 5.1) and the public image of the nurse as an ethical practitioner. The nurse must practise in accordance with the law and adhere to a code of ethical conduct.

Within the health professions there is a long history of debate concerning the professional codes of conduct and ethics required to guide practice and research. Many professional groups have developed their own codes of ethics, which provide guidance to their members as to the nature of proper conduct and their obligations to the public. Most of these professional ethical codes consider three principal areas:

1. standards of professional competence,
2. standards of professional integrity,
3. standards of professional etiquette.

These guiding ethical codes originate from ancient Greek thinking and have continued to influence ethical decision making to the present. The post-World War II Nuremberg Code of 1949 inspired the formation of a medical code of ethical conduct: the Declaration of Geneva. In 1964 the Declaration of Helsinki (extended in 1975) guided the development of codes of ethical conduct for health research (Plueckhahn et al., 1994).

Ethical issues in mental health practice

People experiencing mental health problems are, by the very nature of their disorder, possibly the most politically powerless and vulnerable group in society. The manifestations of mental ill health often include low self-esteem, withdrawal, self-doubt and distortions in thinking. Consequently, this population of people find autonomy difficult to achieve and have difficulty advocating for themselves. Ethical issues abound in mental health, and nurses practising in this area are confronted daily with the need for ethical decision making. This section considers the following areas of mental health nursing practice, taking into consideration the need for ethical decision making: psychiatric diagnosis, mental healthcare and treatment, psychopharmacology, electroconvulsive therapy, seclusion, suicidal behaviour, involuntary treatment, psychological therapy, professional boundaries and confidentiality.

Psychiatric diagnosis

Psychiatric diagnosis should be the most fundamental aspect of mental healthcare delivery under ethical examination. The effects of diagnosis on an individual may include loss of personal freedom, imposed treatment regimens and the possibility of being labelled for life as 'mentally ill'. Diagnostic labelling and hospitalization of people with mental health problems can often marginalize them from their community and thus jeopardize their chances of achieving or regaining social integration. Consider a service user who leaves the ward, steals a car and later returns to the hospital safely with the car and a six-pack of beer. When asked why he did such a thing, he advises that it was not something he would normally do, but since he was classified as 'insane' he might as well act that way. Now consider the person with a diagnosis of schizophrenia who drops a glass in a mental health unit compared to someone in a restaurant. The person working as a nurse may view the dropped glass as a symptom

---

Box 5.1 Principles of ethical conduct

- Autonomy: the person should have the right to make their own decisions, provided these decisions do not violate other people's autonomy. For people to be able to make autonomous decisions they must be free of the control of others and be informed of their options.
- Beneficence: beneficence in regard to nursing research or clinical care implies that what is conducted is good for the wellbeing of the person. Beneficence is the deliberate bringing about of positive action or intervention.
- Non-maleficence: this means above all to do 'no harm' and implies the duty of care both to avoid actual harm as well as to consider the risks of any potential harm.
- Justice: this refers to society's expectations of what is fair and right. The characteristics of justice imply that equality, access and no evidence of subordination exist.

Source: Hawley (1997).

or side effect and this may result in treatment, whereas the person at the restaurant would be assisted to clean up the mess. These examples demonstrate how labels can attract behaviour.

Diagnosis is a powerful tool. It has the capacity to label behaviour that is odd or objectionable, and also has been used to explain behaviour that is unlawful, such as acts of theft or violence. In the latter case, the law recognizes that 'mental illness' compromises a person's free will and can classify them as not legally responsible for their actions. Therefore, a diagnosis of 'mental illness' can, in some cases, benefit a person. However, the process of psychiatric diagnosis has been reported as being of poor or questionable reliability (Boyle, 2002). In mental health, objective signs of mental distress are not always evident, so diagnosis may be a difficult procedure. Service users may not always have sufficient trust in professionals to tell the full story, and some aspects of their history may be too painful to recount in full. Also, service users, like others, are influenced by processes such as denial and fantasy in describing their lives. A diagnosis is often made on subjective data and has been found to vary according to the psychiatrist's own bias (Boyle, 2002), or the impression the service user gives to mental health professionals. Diagnosis plays a powerful role in some people's lives, but it has its limits. People can be left with a lifelong label, and care must be taken not to identify cultural differences as signs of mental disorder.

A diagnosis of mental illness may label the service user as deviant from the normal population and result in predetermined clinical and social behaviours, in both the person diagnosed and the healthcare professionals caring for the service user. Illich (2001) first suggested in his classic 1977 text that people are transformed into service users by labelling and the disabling dependence that requires self-care, while individuals are transformed into clinicians by enculturation that attributes to them the power to diagnose and heal. If a service user is described to you as 'Mr Brown, the man who has been hearing voices and is afraid that others are talking about him', you will have certain expectations based on this description. However, if Mr Brown is described as 'the schizophrenic in room 4', how might your initial perceptions differ? There are strong messages in the words we use, especially when they become labels.

Some of the questions that need to be considered are: who has the right to decide which types of behaviour are considered to be mental illness rather than moral deviance? How do we classify people who become verbally abusive when drunk, who are addicted to psychoactive substances, antisocial, have sexual preferences different to our own, hold unusual religious beliefs or who gamble excessively? Some of these you may see as 'mental illness', but other people would disagree with you. We do have systems of classification that

differentiate normal from abnormal behaviour: for example, the *Diagnostic and Statistical Manual of Mental Disorders* (DSM-IV TR; American Psychiatric Association, 2000), but this manual reflects contemporary beliefs about behaviour rather than objective standards (Moorey, 1998). The cultural sensitivity of these diagnostic criteria and the disempowerment that the service user feels from the confusing terminology used have also been questioned.

CRITICAL THINKING CHALLENGE 5.1

PSYCHIATRIC DIAGNOSIS

Consider the current diagnostic label of 'borderline personality disorder' (BPD) and the clinical signs and symptoms of BPD (see Ch. 16). People with BPD often present in states of high arousal with varying degrees of self-harm. Clinicians can find these presentations stressful and difficult. They provide major challenges to the healthcare service. The label BPD often invokes feelings of helplessness in clinicians, who may respond by attempting to dissuade the person from accessing the health service. If we were to take into account the fact that many of these people have been invalidated in their life and that this has often been a result of sexual or physical abuse, and if this consideration persuaded us to view BPD as posttraumatic stress disorder, would this change our attitudes to working with people who are given this diagnostic label?

Mental healthcare and treatment

There is an increasing body of literature documenting service users' experiences of mental healthcare and treatment. Quirk and Lelliot (2001) usefully summarize research from the UK which indicates that nurse–service user relationships are considered a core component of inpatient care by service users as well as nurses, but this contact is often perceived to be limited. Furthermore, service users appreciate 'humane' qualities in nurses (Quirk and Lelliot, 2001). Service users are critical of the use of coercive practices such as restraint and seclusion, and perceive their use by nurses as punishment (Rogers and Pilgrim, 1994). Worldwide, service user length of stay has decreased, while admission rates have increased, resulting in changes to the overall milieu of inpatient units, where acute interventions and containment are the predominant care provided, and less attention is paid to rehabilitation and comprehensive discharge planning. Within this climate, service users report that being in hospital is often boring and that they do not always feel safe (Quirk and Lelliot, 2001).

Many studies also support increased service user and carer involvement in aspects of treatment such as medication management and discharge planning and more research is indicated to explore the experiences of service users and their expectations of care. As an example, a study by Johannsson and Lundman (2002) describes service users' experiences of involuntary care. Their findings revealed that service users perceive both supportive and controlling interventions which provide 'good opportunities for care as well as great losses' (Johansson and Lundman, 2002, p. 639). Controlling interventions resulted in service users feeling that their autonomy was restricted, that they had been violated by an intrusion on their physical integrity and were not receiving information about their care or not being involved in care. Conversely, caring interventions included being consulted about their care planning, being given freedom to go outside and nurses' flexibility about care. This resulted in service users feeling respected as individuals and protected (Johansson and Lundman, 2002, p. 642). Similar findings also emerged in an ethnographic study exploring the process of constant observation of service users deemed to be at risk of suicide (Fletcher, 1999). In this study both nurses and service users identified therapeutic and controlling categories of nursing interventions. Some differences in perceptions related to service users not recognizing nursing actions, such as assessment. Nurses' explanations of nursing care suggest the need to reflect carefully on the care they provide and on how nursing care is perceived by service users.

Other authors have written about similar service user experiences of care and control in relation to the compulsory administration of medication, a sometimes necessary function of mental health nurses in both the inpatient and community settings. Service users who experience forced medication report negative responses (Haglund et al., 2003). While a minority of service users gave retrospective approval of the forced administration, this was in fact a smaller number than that expected by nurses. All service users spoke of the need to be offered alternatives, for nurses to take more time in discussing the need to take the medication and to have the medication in a form other than injection.

CRITICAL THINKING CHALLENGE 5.2

MENTAL HEALTHCARE AND TREATMENT

Using the four principles of ethical conduct (see Box 5.1), consider when and if it is appropriate to administer an intramuscular injection of medication against a service user's will.

Psychopharmacology

The drugs prescribed for mental disorders are potent agents, often causing major side effects, creating problems with toxicity and, in the case of tranquillizers such as the benzodiazepines, causing dependence. Psychotropic medications can also interact with other therapeutic agents, and so need to be monitored closely. These effects counter the argument that these drugs have been the single most important development in the treatment of mental disorders (Krauss and Slavinsky, 1982).

With respect to drug treatment, a question that needs to be considered is: what are a person's rights when placed on psychopharmacological agents? These rights should include access to effective professional treatment, information concerning the drug prescribed (desired effects, side effects, contraindications, complications) and the freedom to accept or refuse treatment. These rights may be limited if the person is an involuntary service user under mental health legislation. However, all service users should have some voice and choice in the selection of drugs. If the side effects of a particular drug are difficult to live with, the person should be able to ask for a review and change of treatment.

Electroconvulsive therapy

Electroconvulsive therapy (ECT) is used mainly for major depression. A major ethical problem occurs when ECT is prescribed in order to reduce the risk of self-harm or harm through neglect, but the person does not give consent. The thought of having ECT can be traumatic to service users due to negative perceptions about this form of treatment. All treatments need to be carefully negotiated with the service user. In the case of the person experiencing symptoms of depression, their lowered mood and pessimistic outlook may mean that they are unable to see any solution to their depression. Some service users may say that they do not deserve help. In the case of refusal of consent, a second opinion is required before ECT can be administered without the service user's consent. Nurses need to ensure that these service users and their families have been informed of the nature of the procedure and of why consent has been provided by another source.

Seclusion

Seclusion is defined as '...the supervised confinement of a patient in a room, which may be locked. Its sole aim is to contain severely disturbed behaviour which is likely to cause harm to others' (Department of Health, 2008, p. 122). Seclusion is not deemed in law to be a treatment per se but rather a management tool enabling other treatments such as medication or counselling to be given (Muir-Cochrane et al., 2002). It should never be used as the sole treatment for self-harm and must not be used as punishment or threat, or to manage disturbed behaviour where there are staff shortages (Department of Health, 2008).

Seclusion is generally deemed lawful when: it is used for service users receiving treatment for mental disorders, or when it is necessary to protect the person or any other person from imminent risk to his or her health or safety or to prevent the person from absconding, and it has been approved by senior members of the mental health-care team. Seclusion can be instigated by a doctor, a suitably qualified approved clinician or the professional in charge of the ward (Department of Health, 2008). Once instigated, an initial multidisciplinary review of the need for seclusion should be carried out as soon as possible. If it is considered necessary for the seclusion to continue, it should be reviewed:

- every 2 h by 2 nurses or other suitably skilled professionals (one of whom was not involved directly in the decision to seclude); and
- every 4 h by a doctor or a suitably qualified approved clinician (Department of Health, 2008, p. 128).

If the seclusion lasts for more than 8 h consecutively (or for more than 12 h over a 48 h period) an independent review should be conducted by members of the multiprofessional team who were not involved in the incident or decision making that led to the seclusion (Department of Health, 2008). A service user in seclusion must be subject not only to regular review but also must be carefully observed and a '…suitably skilled professional should be readily available within sight and sound of the seclusion room at all times throughout the period of the patient's seclusion' (Department of Health, 2008, p. 125). A record of the service user's condition and behaviour must be made at least every 15 min and a full handover between observing staff must be undertaken.

The seclusion room must:

- provide privacy from other patients, but enable staff to observe the patient at all times;
- be safe and secure and should not contain anything which could cause harm to the patient or others;
- be adequately furnished, heated, lit and ventilated;
- be quiet but not soundproofed and should have some means of calling for attention (operation of which should be explained to the patient) (Department of Health, 2008, pp. 125–126).

Service users must always be clothed in the seclusion room.

Seclusion has been identified as constituting a unique form of restraint, which 'effectively removes all social contact' (Alty and Mason, 1994, p. 4). This must be viewed in light of Farrell and Dares' (1996, p. 179) warning that 'in an era of increasing focus on human rights' there will be demands for 'treatment which is more curative and supportive rather than disempowering and punitive'. The current focus on human rights paves the way for service users and their advocates to increasingly seek redress in litigation (Muir-Cochrane et al., 2002, p. 502).

The differences in relation to the prescription and practice of seclusion reflect the tension between the protection of service users when acutely unwell and the need to provide care within the least-restrictive environment. World Health Organization (1996) documents suggest that authorities should pursue the elimination of isolation rooms and the prohibition of the provision of new ones. It is recognized therefore that the legal requirements for seclusion attempt to protect the individual concerned and provide practical approaches to difficult situations.

Suicidal behaviour

Care of the suicidal service user is possibly the most challenging clinical situation a mental health professional must face. The problem of suicide is well documented but few realize that the number of unsuccessful attempts at suicide is 8–10 times the figure for actual suicide (Cantor and Neulinger, 2000). The high incidence of suicide makes this problem a significant issue for mental health nurses. The prospect of members of our community considering whether they wish to live at all destroys the image of life as cherished and worthwhile and makes us face the reality of our own mortality. The ethical debate about suicide largely centres on the justification for intervening in a person's choice to live or die. Healthcare workers have a duty to intervene by preventing the suicidal act or treating the person who has made an attempt on their own life. This duty arises from our need to abide by the law but also our professional obligation to do no harm.

Involuntary treatment

Guidelines for ethical conduct are particularly relevant to mental health nurses because involuntary status under mental health legislation places restrictions on the therapeutic nurse–service user relationship. Service users who feel that they have few rights and are restricted by legislation may be less likely to engage in a working relationship with a mental health nurse. In this situation, where the service user's actions are subject to mental health legislation, the nurse exercises social control over the service user. If the service user is hospitalized, the nurse can initiate PRN (as-needed) medication and restrain and seclude the service user subject to local policies and the Mental Health Act *Code of Practice* (Department of Health, 2008). Mental health is not an area where the nurse can always refer the service user to other members of the multiprofessional team for the answers, because the nurse is often the person delivering care, and it is often the nurse's actions that the service user is questioning.

While the relationships that mental health nurses form with service users are recognized as central to the provision of care (Forchuk, 1995; Peplau, 1994), inevitable dynamics within this relationship are power and control. Issues of power and control were first brought into the psychiatric literature with the work of Goffman (1961) in the famous text *Asylums*, which described the relationship between service users and nurses as being controlled by the organizational rules and rigid hierarchical structure of the psychiatric hospital. Mental health nurses are in a unique position through the type and duration of therapeutic relationships that they can establish with service users. However, it is important to recognize the dichotomy between the caring and controlling functions mental health nurses must undertake as part of their professional practice. This often places nurses in difficult situations, ones that are not common to other health professionals (Muir-Cochrane, 1998, 2000). The use of coercion is an uncomfortable component of nursing practice. It may be subtle ('encouraging', 'deciding for', 'trading off', 'persuading') and be seen as a weak form of paternalism justified by the goal of benefiting or avoiding harm to the person whose will is overridden (Morrall and Muir-Cochrane, 2002, p. 8).

When a person is involuntarily detained at a mental health facility, the major ethical debate centres on legal rights versus moral rights. When should a person be admitted involuntarily under mental health legislation? This question is usually answered by saying: 'When the person is a danger to themselves or others'. However, consider whether you would feel comfortable committing this person to a mental health facility if the person was a member of your family or a close friend.

A service user voluntarily seeking treatment for a mental health problem should be treated as fully competent and retain the right to give or withhold consent to treatment (Wallace, 1995). However, involuntary service users should also be treated as competent unless assessed otherwise (Department for Constitutional Affairs, 2007, Department of Health, 2008). The ethical principles guiding treatment of mental health service users are beneficence and non-maleficence. But are such paternalistic actions ethically justifiable? Paternalistic actions may be ethically justified when the person is being protected from harm and does not have the capacity to make decisions by themselves (Beauchamp and Childress, 2001). In the case of an emergency, consent is often implied because of the nature of the condition (for example, when an unconscious individual arrives at an accident and emergency department). A determination of mental incapacity requires that the person has a cognitive impairment that affects their judgement and ability to make sound decisions (see Ch. 4).

We can be advocates for a service user but we must ensure that we advocate in collaboration with them, or else we risk being paternalistic. Paternalism is when nurses believe that they know what is best for the service user, that they are most qualified to speak on the service user's behalf and that the service user is not sufficiently capable of doing so. Although the intention is good, service user autonomy is at risk. All service users should be treated with the same degree of respect that you would require and, whenever practicable, the person's autonomy should be maintained. This would ensure that the person maintains their integrity and does not feel so vulnerable and powerless.

CRITICAL THINKING CHALLENGE 5.3

INVOLUNTARY TREATMENT

Beth is 23 years old and is admitted to an acute mental health inpatient unit as an involuntary service user. She has been diagnosed with a drug-induced relapse of psychosis and it is expected that she will have a short admission. Beth remembers a past admission where a male service user came into her room in the night and rummaged through her things. She is having problems sleeping on the ward as she remembers this experience. Should Beth be prescribed PRN sedatives? Considering contemporary beliefs concerning gender equality and mixed-sex wards, is allocating beds on a needs basis always appropriate? What gender issues arise from having integrated ward environments with involuntary service users and what can we do about them?

Psychological therapy

Service users place trust in their therapists, expecting that the therapist will not exploit it. The relationship between therapist and service user is therapy's strength and weakness. The therapist gains recognition as a health professional, and also power within the relationship. The ethical issue is how to use this power. Does the power remain egalitarian or become authoritarian? And to what extent does transference within the relationship hinder the therapeutic process? The therapist may become the most important person in the service user's life and runs the risk of assuming priority over all others.

In general, the ethical guidelines for one-on-one therapy and group work are threefold: first, to protect the service user from exploitation, incompetence and pressure to perform; second, to uphold the right of the service user to be provided with information and make informed decisions concerning their life; and third, to foster personal growth and wellness (Bancroft, 1995). The first two goals protect the service user and promote the service user's rights. The third goal outlines the true goal of therapy. It is often taken for granted that therapy is beneficial to the service user. After all, to look at oneself or share beliefs during group or individual therapy should help us to grow and understand why our lives have evolved as they have. This aim is compromised when the therapy is focused on the needs of the therapist or institution, rather than on those of the service user. In extreme cases this can lead to unprofessional conduct, including sexual exploitation of the service user (Horsfall and Stuhlmiller, 2000).

CRITICAL THINKING CHALLENGE 5.4

THERAPY

Jenny has been seeing a therapist for 5 months and receiving cognitive behavioural therapy for panic attacks and self-harm. Jenny writes a book of poetry that has a dedication to the therapist as the person who has saved her and the most beautiful man she has ever met. On reading the book, the therapist notices that the poetry is largely about their relationship as service user and therapist; however, she has also drawn pictures of them holding hands, lying in a bed and eating a meal together. How could clinical supervision assist the therapist to address this gift in a therapeutic way and keep working in a therapeutic relationship? Should he have accepted the gift in the first place? If he removed himself from the relationship, what would be the benefits and costs to Jenny?

Box 5.2 **Examples of professional boundary transgression**

- Sharing confidential information with others outside the treatment team
- Taking service users to social events outside work hours
- Inviting a service user home
- Having a sexual relationship with a service user during or following treatment
- Conducting inappropriate or unnecessary examinations or interviews
- Physical, sexual or verbal abuse
- Entering into a business transaction with a service user
- Allowing personal matters to intrude on clinical work
- Inappropriately exempting service users from responsibilities
- Giving or receiving inappropriate gifts
- Disclosing personal feelings without therapeutic justification
- Making seductive comments about a service user's appearance or being flirtatious
- Having an ongoing social relationship
- Entering into a financial relationship with a service user
- Not disclosing relevant change within a relationship to other team members
- Using nursing procedure to engage in inappropriate contact or prolonging contact

Source: Horsfall et al. (1999).

Professional boundaries

The therapeutic relationship is a privileged relationship for both the service user and the nurse or therapist. However, responsibility for maintaining the required professional standards rests with clinicians, who need to have safeguards in place that will enable issues involving professional standards to be identified and appropriately managed. These include reflective practice, especially use of a cotherapist or supervisor to discuss service user care confidentially. At times when you are working closely with a service user you may notice feelings of friendship, wanting to save the service user from reckless behaviour, boredom with their lack of progress or a sense of knowing better than the service user what their needs are. These are all signs of potential counter-transference. The clinician needs to be aware of the boundaries needed to keep the therapy sessions therapeutic and service user-centred. When a nurse moves outside the therapeutic relationship and establishes a friendship or social relationship with a service user the professional boundaries between the nurse as therapist and the service user become confused. When professional boundaries are blurred the relationship can become nontherapeutic and potentially harmful to both the service user and the

nurse. Ethical decision-making principles are especially important to ensure that professional boundaries are not transgressed. Horsfall et al. (1999, p. 7) have identified examples of professional boundary transgression from the available literature (see Box 5.2).

Confidentiality

Service users often reveal personal information to nurses and ask that we keep that information secret. Confidentiality is a primary principle of the therapeutic relationship, but how can it be upheld if the service user reveals information that must be shared with the rest of the team? Nurses should never promise to keep a secret. Secrets are appropriate within a friendship, but never within a therapeutic relationship. It is paramount that the service user is made aware that all necessary information will be shared with the team and that this information will remain within the team. So, too, when commencing a discussion during group therapy it is always important to remind people that what they share with the group is for the group alone and not to be taken out of the room.

CONCLUSION

The future of mental health nursing seems likely to become more rather than less complex. Current issues of regulation of practice and graduate pre-registration nursing education look set to continue to occupy the profession in the foreseeable future. At the same time the development of extended roles represents a future in which mental health nurses will play an increasing role in the provision and development of clinical services. The increasing role of mental health nurses and the growing diversity of services challenge nurses to articulate their contribution to mental healthcare and service user outcomes. So, too, the complexities of the ethical and legal issues concerning the care of vulnerable populations, such as people with mental health problems, require constant scrutiny. Mental health nursing is fraught with ethical issues arising from classification of 'mental illness', diagnosis, treatment and working within the constraints of mental health legislation. While there are existing codes of ethics for nurses, a code of ethical conduct specific to mental health nursing is required to guide practice in the complex challenges of mental healthcare.

Mental health nursing will need a strong professional voice and organization to support practitioners in the services of the future. The profession has already responded to the challenge of deinstitutionalization by refocusing on community-based roles while still retaining an essential role in inpatient services. Growing recognition of the prevalence and burden of mental ill health will require similar resourcefulness and adaptability as mental health nurses work to maintain a profession that is both rewarding to practitioners and valued by service users.

EXERCISES FOR CLASS ENGAGEMENT

ETHICAL ISSUES TO CONSIDER

You could split into discussion groups or individually consider the following case studies. Read the case studies and consider appropriate responses to the questions that follow.

Case Study 1

A 33-year-old woman reports that she wants to die as she cannot get over the death of her husband and 6-year-old son in a motor vehicle accident 11 months ago. She has no family and has lost her home because she is on an unemployment benefit and was unable to pay the mortgage. She feels the pain is too great and just wants it to end.

Case Study 2

A 59-year-old male widower, who has been diagnosed with liver and bowel cancer, presents with considerable pain and distress. He advises the nurse that he has always believed in euthanasia and has decided that his time is now up. He does not want to be a burden on his daughter and wishes to die with dignity. He is open about his wish to die and has planned his suicide. All his affairs are in order. He believes that he will carry this out sooner rather than later, as the pain is now too great and he just wants it to end.

Case Study 3

An 84-year-old famous actor has refused food and fluid for 6 days as she does not want to live anymore. She has right-sided paralysis following a cerebrovascular accident. She wants to be remembered as young and beautiful. She feels that her life has been full and now wants it to end, as she feels that her future prospects are hopeless.

Questions

In the above studies, who is making a rational choice to die? What are our responsibilities in each case as health professionals? Do health professionals have the right to stop people when they wish to die?

REFERENCES

Alty, A., Mason, T., 1994. Seclusion and Mental Health: A Break with the Past. Chapman & Hall, London.

American Psychiatric Association, 2000. Diagnostic and Statistical Manual of Mental Disorders, fourth ed. American Psychiatric Association, Washington DC, (text rev).

Avron, J., 1991. The neglected medical history and therapeutic choices for abdominal pain: a nationwide study of 799 physicians and nurses. Arch. Intern. Med. 151, 694–698.

Bailey, K., 1999. Framework for prescriptive practice. In: Shea, C.A., Pelletier, L.R. (Eds.), Advanced Practice in Psychiatric and Mental Health Nursing. Mosby, St Louis, pp. 297–313.

Bancroft, J., 1995. Ethical aspects of sexuality and sex therapy. In: Bloch, S., Chodoff, P. (Eds.), Psychiatric Ethics, second ed. Oxford University Press, Oxford, pp. 215–242.

Beauchamp, T.L., Childress, J.F., 2001. Principles of Biomedical Ethics, fifth ed. Oxford University Press, New York.

Boyle, M., 2002. Schizophrenia A Scientific Delusion?, second ed. Routledge, London.

Cantor, C., Neulinger, K., 2000. The epidemiology of suicide and attempted suicide among young Australians. Aust. N. Z. J. Psychiatry 34 (3), 370–387.

Department for Constitutional Affairs 2007. Mental Capacity Act 2005 Code of Practice. <http://webarchive. nationalarchives.gov.uk/+/http://www.dca.gov.uk/legal-policy/mental-capacity/mca-cp.pdf>.

Department of Health, 1994. Working in Partnership: A Collaborative Approach to Care. HMSO, London.

Department of Health 2006. From values to action: the chief nursing officer's review of mental health nursing. <http://www.dh.gov.uk/en/Publicationsandstatistics/Publications/PublicationsPolicyAndGuidance/DH_4133839>.

Department of Health 2008. Code of Practice: Mental Health Act 1983. <http://www.dh.gov.uk/en/Healthcare/Mentalhealth/DH_4132161>.

Department of Health 2010. Equity and excellence: liberating the NHS. <http://www.dh.gov.uk/en/Healthcare/LiberatingtheNHS/index.htm>.

Department of Health 2011. No health without mental health: a cross-government mental health outcomes strategy for people of all ages. <http://www.dh.gov.uk/en/Publicationsandstatistics/Publications/PublicationsPolicyAndGuidance/DH_123766>.

Elsom, S., Happell, B., Manias, E., et al., 2007. Expanded practice roles for community mental health nurses: a qualitative exploration of psychiatrists' views. Australas. Psychiatry 5 (4), 324–328.

Farrell, G.A., Dares, G., 1996. Seclusion or solitary confinement: therapeutic or punitive treatment? Aust. N. Z. J. Ment. Health Nurs. 5 (4), 171–179.

Fennell, K.S., 1991. Prescriptive authority for nurse-midwives: a historical review. Nurs. Clin. North Am. 26 (2), 511–522.

Fletcher, R.F., 1999. The process of constant observation: perspectives of staff and suicidal patients. J. Psychiatr. Ment. Health Nurs. 6 (1), 9–14.

Forchuk, C., 1995. Uniqueness within the nurse–patient relationship. Arch. Psychiatr. Nurs. 9 (1), 34–39.

Freidson, E. (Ed.), 1989. Medical Work in America: Essays on Health Care. Yale University Press, New Haven.

Goffman, I., 1961. Asylums: Essays on the Social Situation of Mental Patients and Other Inmates. Penguin, London.

Haglund, K., von Knorring, L., von Essen, L., 2003. Forced medication in psychiatric care: patient experiences and nurses' perceptions. J. Psychiatr. Ment. Health Nurs. 10 (1), 65–72.

Hawley, G., 1997. Ethics Workbook For Nurses: Issues, Problems and Resolutions. Social Science Press, Wentworth Falls, New South Wales.

Hemingway, S., 2003. Nurse prescribing for mental health nurses: scripting the issues. J. Psychiatr. Ment. Health Nurs. 10, 239–245.

Holmes, C.A., 2001. Postdisciplinarity in mental health-care: an Australian viewpoint. Nurs. Inq. 8 (4), 230–239.

Horsfall, J., Stuhlmiller, C., 2000. Interpersonal Nursing for Mental Health. McLennan & Petty, Sydney.

Horsfall, J., Cleary, M., Jordon, R., 1999. Toward Ethical Mental Health Nursing Practice. Australian and New Zealand College of Mental Health Nurses, Greenacres, South Australia.

Illich, I., 2001. Limits to Medicine. Medical Nemesis: The Exploration of Health. Marian Boyers, London.

Johannsson, I.M., Lundman, B., 2002. Patients' experiences of involuntary psychiatric care: good opportunities and great losses. J. Psychiatr. Ment. Health Nurs. 9 (6), 639–647.

Krauss, J., Slavinsky, A., 1982. The Chronically Ill Psychiatric Patient and the Community. Blackwell, Boston.

Latter, S., Courtenay, M., 2004. Effectiveness of nurse prescribing: a review of the literature. J. Clin. Nurs. 13 (1), 26–32.

Lim, G., Honey, M., Kilpatrick, J., 2007. Framework for teaching pharmacology to prepare graduate nurses for prescribing in New Zealand. Nurse Educ. Pract. 7, 348–353.

Maling, T., 2000. Extended prescribing rights—a statutory right or hard-earned privilege? N. Z. Med. J. 113 (1119), 410–411.

Moorey, J., 1998. The ethics of professional care. In: Barker, P., Davidson, B. (Eds.), Psychiatric Nursing: Ethical Strife. Arnold, London, pp. 39–56.

Morrall, P., Muir-Cochrane, E., 2002. Naked social control: seclusion and psychiatric nursing in post-liberal society. Aust. e-J. Adv. Ment. Health 1 (2) <http://ausienet.flinders.eduau/journal/>.

Muir-Cochrane, E., 1998. The role of the community mental health nurse in the administration of depot neuroleptic medication: 'Not just the needle nurse'. Int. J. Nurs. Pract. 4 (4), 254–260.

Muir-Cochrane, E., 2000. The context of care: issues of power and control in community mental health nursing. Int. J. Nurs. Pract. 6 (6), 292–299.

Muir-Cochrane, E., Holmes, C., Walton, J., 2002. Law and policy in relation to the use of seclusion in psychiatric hospitals in Australia and New Zealand. Contemp. Nurse 13 (2/3), 136–145.

NMC (Nursing and Midwifery Council) 2006. Standards of proficiency for nurse and midwife prescribers. <http://www.nmc-uk.org/Documents/Standards/nmcStandardsofProficiencyForNurseAndMidwifePrescribers.pdf>.

NMC (Nursing and Midwifery Council) 2007. Standards for medicines management. <http://www.nmc-uk.org/Documents/Standards/nmcStandardsForMedicinesManagementBooklet.pdf>.

NMC (Nursing and Midwifery Council) 2008a. The code: standards of conduct, performance and ethics for nurses and midwives. <http://www.nmc-uk.org/Documents/Standards/The-code-A4-20100406.pdf>.

NMC (Nursing and Midwifery Council) 2008b. The prep handbook. <http://www.nmc-uk.org/Documents/Standards/nmcPrepHandbook.pdf>.

NMC (Nursing and Midwifery Council) 2009a. Record keeping: guidance for nurses and midwives.

<http://www.nmc-uk.org/Documents/Guidance/nmcGuidanceRecordKeepingGuidancefor NursesandMidwives.pdf>.

NMC (Nursing and Midwifery Council) 2009b. Guidance for the care of older people. <http://www.nmc-uk.org/Documents/Guidance/Guidance-for-the-care-of-older-people.pdf>.

NMC (Nursing and Midwifery Council) 2010a. Standards for pre-registration nursing education. <http://standards.nmc-uk.org/PublishedDocuments/Standards%20for%20pre-registration%20nursing%20education%2016082010.pdf>.

NMC (Nursing and Midwifery Council) 2010b. Raising and escalating concerns: guidance for nurses and midwives. <http://www.nmc-uk.org/Documents/RaisingandEscalatingConcerns/Raising-and-escalating-concerns-guidance-A5.pdf>.

NMC (Nursing and Midwifery Council) 2010c. Guidance on professional conduct: for nursing and midwifery students. <http://www.nmc-uk.org/Documents/Guidance/NMC-Guidance-on-professional-conduct-for-nursing-and-midwifery-students.PDF>.

O'Brien, A.J., 2002/2003. Judging care against standards in mental health. Kai Tiaki Nurs. N. Z. 8 (11), 22–23.

Pearson, L., 2003. Fifteenth annual legislative update. Nurse Pract. 28 (1), 26–31.

Peplau, H., 1994. Psychiatric mental health nursing: challenge and change. J. Psychiatr. Ment. Health Nurs. 1, 3–7.

Plueckhahn, V., Breen, K., Cordner, S., 1994. Law and Ethics in Medicine for Doctors in Victoria. Henry Thacker Print, Geelong.

Quirk, A., Lelliot, P., 2001. What do we know about life on acute psychiatric wards in the UK: a review of the research evidence. Soc. Sci. Med. 53, 1565–1574.

Rodgers, S.J., 2000. The role of nursing theory in standards of practice: a canadian perspective. Nurs. Sci. Q. 13 (3), 260–261.

Rogers, A., Pilgrim, D., 1994. Service users of psychiatric nurses. Br. J. Nurs. 3 (1), 16–18.

Safriet, B., 1992. Health care dollars and regulatory sense: the role of advanced practice nursing. Yale J. Regul. 9 (2), 417–487.

Wallace, M., 1995. Health Care and the Law, second ed. The Law Book Company, Sydney.

World Health Organization, 1996. Mental Health Care Law: Ten Basic Principles. World Health Organization, Geneva.

Part | 2 |

Mental health and wellness

Chapter | 6 |

Mental health and wellness

Pamela Wood, Pat Bradley, and Ruth De Souza

CHAPTER POINTS

- An appreciation of the prevalence of mental health problems will help the mental health nurse to understand the impact that such problems have on the healthcare system, the health outcomes of individuals and demands for services.

- The extent of disability associated with mental health problems can have a significant influence on an individual's ability to function in all aspects of their life.

- The outcomes associated with many mental health problems may be influenced by gender differences.

- Culture consists of a body of learned behaviours, passed on by role modelling, learning and lore, which is used by the individual to interpret experience and to generate social behaviour.

- An awareness of cultural factors can enhance the mental health nurse's ability to offer individualized, holistic care within a therapeutic relationship, and to value the contribution that cultural interventions can make to the therapeutic environment.

- Openness to diversity in cultures offers the mental health nurse the opportunity to reflect on his or her own beliefs and values about health, what it means to be healthy, and what he or she recognizes as mental wellbeing.

- The culturally competent mental health nurse will aim to 'enter' the client's experience, while maintaining a strongly rooted sense of his or her own lived experience and developmental learning.

- The culturally safe mental health nurse will aim to provide care that is deemed culturally safe by the client.

DOI: http://dx.doi.org/10.1016/B978-0-7020-4493-9.00006-8

- cultural awareness
- cultural competence
- cultural safety
- cultural sensitivity
- culture
- disability
- ethnocentrism
- gender
- incidence
- mental health
- mental health problems
- morbidity
- mortality
- prevalence
- stigma

LEARNING OUTCOMES

The material in this chapter will assist you to:

- develop an awareness of the prevalence of mental health problems and the impact this has on the community and society,
- understand the concept of disability in relation to mental ill health and how the levels of disability are determined,
- appreciate the negative influence of misconceptions and discrimination experienced by people with a mental health disorder,
- understand how individuals can positively influence mental health outcomes for service users, carers and communities,
- describe the relevance of culture and gender issues to mental health outcomes for the individual and their family, friends and carers,
- understand the importance of cultural diversity in negotiating healthcare strategies that achieve outcomes endorsed by the service user.

INTRODUCTION

This chapter explores two interrelated facets of mental health problems. The first section discusses the prevalence of mental ill health in the UK and its impact on the individual, family, carers and health systems. Other factors such as misconceptions, gender issues and perceptions of mental health problems will be shown to have the potential to contribute to the degree of disability experienced by a person who is perceived as ill or recovering from mental health problems. The role of the media in shaping opinions and ideas is also examined. The second section of this chapter deals with the impact of culture, including gender and ethnicity, on the way in which mental health problems are perceived and managed by individuals and communities. Issues of stigma and stereotyping are explored, models of cultural competence and cultural safety are introduced and the importance of self-reflection in mental health nursing practice is emphasized.

INCIDENCE AND PREVALENCE OF MENTAL HEALTH PROBLEMS

The worldwide burden of mental health problems is high and is expected to increase: for example, depression is expected to become one of the greatest health problems in the world by the year 2020 (Murray and Lopez, 1996). Mental health problems cause considerable personal, social and financial distress to individuals, and have a huge impact on healthcare funding, implementation of service provision and community resources. In order to gauge the full extent of the problem, many countries have conducted research into the prevalence and consequent impact of mental health problems on the individual, society and healthcare funds.

The cost of mental ill health to the UK economy in 2009–10 is estimated to have been £105.2 billion. This not only includes direct costs, such as those involved in the direct provision of care (for 2008–9 this was £10.4 billion or 11% of all gross National Health Service (NHS) expenditure) but also other indirect costs which impact on quality of life and are associated with a reduction in economic output (Centre for Mental Health, 2010).

In 2009, the NHS Information Centre for Health and Social Care (NHSIC) published the results of the Adult Psychiatric Morbidity Survey (APMS; NHSIC, 2009). This survey provided detailed information of mental health problems among people aged over 16 in private households in England. The survey found that:

- 15.1% of people had symptoms of depression and anxiety (common mental disorders, or CMDs) and of these 7.5% were of sufficient severity to require treatment,
- 24% of CMDs were receiving treatment, mostly in the form of medication,
- people aged over 75 were least likely to have a CMD,
- people living in the poorest households were more likely to screen positively for CMDs than those with higher incomes,
- 33.3% of people were found to have had experienced a traumatic event since the age of 16, and men are more likely to have experienced a trauma (35.2%) than women (31.5%),

- 3% of adults screened positively for posttraumatic stress disorder (PTSD), of whom 28% were receiving treatment,
- the overall prevalence rate for psychosis in 2006 was 0.4% (that is, four people per thousand),
- the mean age of onset for psychosis is earlier in men than in women and the highest prevalence was found to be in the 35–44-year age group,
- the prevalence of psychotic disorders were higher among black men (3.1%) than men from other ethnic groups, but there was no significant variation by ethnicity among women,
- 65% of people assessed as having had a psychotic episode were receiving treatment (counselling, medication or other therapy),
- 0.3% of people aged 18 and over presented with symptoms of antisocial personality disorder (ASPD),
- 0.4% of people aged 16 and over presented with symptoms of borderline personality disorder (BPD),
- 6.4% of people screened positive with an eating disorder whereas 1.6% of people felt that food had a significant negative impact on their lives,
- 19% of people with an eating disorder were receiving treatment,
- 24.2% were consuming alcohol at hazardous levels,
- 5.9% of people were assessed as being dependent on alcohol (5.4% of people having symptoms of mild dependence; 0.4% moderately dependent; 0.1% severely dependent),
- 14% of people who were dependant on alcohol were receiving treatment,
- 9.2% of people used illicit drugs in 2006, most (7.5%) having used cannabis,
- 3.4% of people were assessed as being dependent on illicit drugs.

Comorbidity

Comorbidity refers to the simultaneous presence of another health problem, illness or disease in addition to the primary condition which has been diagnosed. In the APMS (NHSIC, 2009), 23% of people surveyed met the criteria for at least one of the mental health problems studied. Of these, 68.7% met the criteria for only one of the mental health problems studied, while 19.1% met the criteria for two mental health problems. Some 12.2% met the criteria for three or more problems. The study also suggested that having one condition increased the risk of another mental health problem being present. In particular, psychosis and antisocial personality disorder seemed to be highly comorbid.

In addition, there is much evidence of comorbidity between mental health problems and physical disorder (Disability Rights Commission, 2006). People with mental health problems tend to have higher prevalences of several chronic physical conditions than people of the same age without mental health problems. People with chronic physical conditions are also more likely to experience mental health problems than those without physical conditions.

Suicidal behaviour

The APMS (NHSIC, 2009) found that 16.7% of people surveyed said that they had thought about ending their lives, and 5.6% said that they had made a suicide attempt. Of those who reported self-harm, 53% of women and 42% of men sought medical or mental healthcare as a result.

In the UK there were 5675 suicides in 2009, 31 fewer than those recorded in 2008 (5706) (Office for National Statistics, 2011). More males than females in all age groups commit suicide, although this is greatest for those aged 20–44 years. However, the overall suicide rate has declined over the past 10 years. In 2000 the male suicide rate was 19.9 per 100 000, declining to 17.5 per 100 000 in 2009. For women, the rates also show a downward trend, from 6.2 per 100 000 in 2000 to 5.2 per 100 000 in 2009 (Office for National Statistics, 2011).

GENDER DIFFERENCES

There are some gender differences in the prevalence of mental disorders. The APMS (NHSIC, 2009) found that among people with CMDs women are more likely to experience depression and anxiety than men (21.5% and 19.7% respectively). This rate peaked among 45–54-year-olds among women, whereas among men the highest rates were found in the 25–54-year-old age group. Men were more likely to experience a trauma but rates of PTSD were similar for both men (2.6%) and women (3.3%). The prevalence of psychosis was also similar for men and women (0.3 and 0.5% respectively).

With regards to personality disorders studied, the APMS (NHSIC, 2009) found that 0.6% of men and 0.1% of women had symptoms of antisocial personality disorder, whereas 0.3% of men and 0.6% of women screened positive for borderline personality disorder. Women were more likely to have an eating disorder (9.2%) than men (3.5%) with the prevalence reducing over time: 20.3% of women aged 16–24 screened positive for symptoms of an eating disorder compared to 0.9% of women aged 75 and over.

The prevalence of hazardous drinking appears to be higher among men (33.2%) compared to women (15.7%), with the highest prevalence among men being in the 25–34-year-old age group and 16–24-year-old age group for women. Alcohol dependence was found among 8.7% of men and 3.3% of women. With regards to illicit drugs, the study found that 12% of men and 6.7% of women studied used drugs in 2006.

The discussion of gender differences in mental health cannot be limited to the statistics alone; there are many factors involved, such as the acceptance of treatment and the amount of disability suffered by individuals. Women are more likely to report recent episodes of depression and anxiety disorders, and to seek treatment for mental health problems, whereas men tend to be more reluctant to seek professional help. Women are more than twice as likely as males to seek help from a counsellor at some point in their life. This difference is not necessarily an indication that women have a greater need for such services but is more likely to reflect gender differences in help-seeking behaviours (Clarke et al., 2007).

This delay in seeking assistance may be attributed to a number of things, such as the stigma associated with mental health services, or the belief that seeking help is a sign of weakness and therefore a threat to an individual's manhood; or, if a person is in full-time work, it may be difficult to attend clinics. This delay results in poor access to early intervention and prevention services, which may lead to increased disability caused by the disorder. In general, men have a stronger tendency to turn to alcohol and other drugs as a means of dealing with their emotional problems, which does little more than exacerbate the problem in the long term (Nielsen et al., 2001).

Although women access services, they may have concerns about taking medication for a diagnosed problem if they are pregnant, likely to become pregnant or are breastfeeding, for fear of the effects the medication may have on the baby. A pregnant woman or nursing mother may well be limited in the medications she is able to take (see Ch. 24), leaving her susceptible to relapse due to inadequate treatment. Women are more likely than men to discontinue successful treatment because of medication-related weight gain and adverse side effects. Women with severe mental health problems such as bipolar disorder and major depression are at increased risk for an episode after childbirth, with some women experiencing their first episode at this time (Fullagar and Gattuso, 2002; Meadows and Singh, 2001).

Because of the later onset of some severe mental health problems, some women may already be married/partnered and be mothers before the initial onset of their problem. Although a woman has support and security, ongoing severe mental health problems may have a detrimental effect on her relationships with her husband/partner and children, leading to family breakdown and long-term hardship.

Men diagnosed with a severe health mental problem, such as schizophrenia, generally have worse outcomes than females, as measured by early onset, cognitive disabilities and social impairments. The earlier onset usually prevents males from developing personal relationships, which leads to most remaining single, childless and with reduced employment prospects. Women with a diagnosis of schizophrenia seem to have an increased risk of relapse at times of rapid changes in their levels of oestrogen, such as at menopause or before the onset of menstruation (Fontaine, 2003; Fullagar and Gattuso, 2002).

CRITICAL THINKING CHALLENGE 6.1

Investigate some possible reasons why females have a higher incidence of anxiety and affective disorders. You should consider biological, psychological and cultural influences.

Why do you think men have a much higher incidence of substance abuse? It will help to make a list of your thoughts.

Do you think the statistics as stated in this chapter are a true indication of the prevalence of mental health disorders between the sexes? Give at least five reasons to support your answer.

MARITAL STATUS

The APMS (NHSIC, 2009) also revealed that marital status appeared to be related to the prevalence of mental health problems, but this also seemed to vary according to gender and age. For example, married or widowed men and women tended to have lower rates of CMD but those who were divorced or separated had particularly high rates. With regards to PTSD, the prevalence was observed to be lowest among married men and highest among divorced women. A similar pattern was observed among people who screened positively for psychosis: the lowest rates were found among married people and the highest were among those who were divorced. With regards to those who screened positively for an eating disorder the highest rates were observed among single men and women and the lowest rates were found among people who were widowed. The prevalence of substance misuse also seemed to vary according to marital status. For example, levels of alcohol dependence were lower in married men and widowers than in single, divorced or separated men. In women, those who were single were more likely to be alcohol-dependent. Drug dependence was also found to be highest among single men and women and lowest among people who were widowed.

The survey also confirmed observations and findings from other studies, namely that suicidal thoughts, suicide attempts and self-harm tend to vary according to marital status. Divorce, however, was found in this study to increase the likelihood of suicidal thoughts; in particular, divorced men were three times more likely, and women twice as likely, to have such thoughts compared to those who were married. Likewise, suicide attempts seem more common among divorced adults, and lowest prevalence rates seem to be among those who were widowed or married.

The likelihood of having two or more comorbid mental health conditions was also seemingly related to marital status. In particular, prevalence seemed to be lowest among those who were married or widowed and highest among divorced men and separated women. However, it should be noted that age may be a confounding variable in these findings as younger people tend to be single while those who are widowed tend to be older.

DISABILITY AND MENTAL HEALTH

Disability in mental health refers to an individual's impairment in one or more important areas of functioning. Mental health problems are a leading cause of disability and account for 11% of all 'disease' burden worldwide (Murray and Lopez, 1996). In 1990, five of the 10 leading causes of disability worldwide were mental disorders: unipolar depression, alcohol abuse, bipolar affective disorder, schizophrenia and obsessive–compulsive disorder. Among these, depression was ranked fourth, but the World Health Organization has predicted that depression will be the second leading cause of disability in the world by 2020 (World Health Organization, 2001). Mental health problems and chronic physical conditions are, on average, associated with similar degrees of disability, and the combination of the two is more disabling than either alone.

Although mortality rates from mental health problems are not considered high, the impact of chronic disability on an individual's life can be measured in days out of their normal role. The severity of an individual's disorder can be measured using the Disability Adjusted Life Year (DALY) tool developed by the World Health Organization Harvard School of Public Health and the World Bank (Meadows and Singh, 2001; Murray and Lopez, 1996). This tool measures lost productivity associated with disability due to an individual's altered health status and is based on the years of life lost through living with disease, impairment and disability (Meadows and Singh, 2001).

Mental health problems cause considerable distress for individuals, families and friends, as well as contributing to absenteeism from work or school and to the extensive use of community support services such as crisis lines and welfare groups. Mental health problems are more prevalent in the young, and therefore these people may become significantly disabled at a stage of their lives when they are completing education and establishing relationships and independence.

The type and length of a problem (as measured by DALYs) is a major factor when determining the effects of a particular problem on an individual's life. For example, people with a psychotic disorder may be socially isolated, unemployed and suffer considerable psychological and physical distress. Likewise, anxiety disorders have a profound effect on a person's work, social and family life.

People diagnosed with some mental health problems, such as psychotic disorders or severe depression, may well be unable to attend adequately to their hygiene needs, or shop and/or prepare meals, or to make sure their environment is clean and safe, thereby placing their physical wellbeing in jeopardy. Poor physical health places a huge burden on the sufferer, their family, the community and the healthcare system. A significant number of people with mental health problems are living below the poverty line, requiring assistance from welfare groups (government and nongovernment). In general, people with chronic and enduring mental health problems are more likely to experience a severe perceived lack of social support, to have financial problems and to be single, divorced or separated. They are also far more likely to be living in cramped, rented accommodation than the general population (Office for National Statistics, 2002).

Even with assistance, a number of people may not have the means to provide adequate nutritious food, heating, clothing, housing, electricity, telephone or furniture for themselves and their families. Some housing and accommodation is available through a number of agencies, but the demand is greater than the resources available (Pinches, 2002). A relatively small number have turbulent problems and often find that they are turned out of accommodation because of disruptive behaviour (Robinson, 2003). Local councils have a legal obligation to provide temporary, emergency accommodation to people who are homeless but have limited resources to deal with the complex needs of those with mental disorders.

In recent years there have been policy developments which have had a direct impact on the lives of people with mental health problems, particularly those with long-term conditions. For example, successive UK governments have had stated policies of reducing perceived dependence on welfare benefits with an aim of achieving an overall of 80% employment. For example, the New Labour Government's policies (such as Welfare to Work, New Deal and 'Flexible' New Deal) aimed to support people's return to work, by developing skills base. The UK Coalition Government has announced a reform of welfare payments as way of reducing the budget deficit.

Encouraging people to return to work after experiencing mental health problems has more than financial benefits. In employment there is a greater potential for social contacts, activities which offer a sense of fulfilment and achievement. For people with mental health problems, being in paid employment can assist their inclusion into local communities and promote a sense of citizenship. Many people with mental health problems do wish to work (Office of the Deputy Prime Minister, 2004) but approximately one-third are unemployed or not economically active and about three-quarters of those with a diagnosis of schizophrenia are unemployed (Office for National Statistics, 2002). For people with long-term mental health problems, finding work can be particularly problematic (Future Vision Coalition, 2009) perhaps due, in part, to the increased likelihood that such people are more likely to have left school at 16 with no qualifications (Office for National Statistics, 2002), which further compounds disadvantage.

MISCONCEPTIONS ABOUT MENTAL HEALTH PROBLEMS

There is evidence that people with existing serious and enduring mental health problems are stigmatized and discriminated against (Future Vision Coalition, 2009; Office of the Deputy Prime Minister, 2004) despite the Disability Discrimination Act 1995, which makes discrimination against disabled people an offence. Mental health problems cause considerable distress to individuals, their significant others and the community as misconceptions about mental health problems can lead to social exclusion which may, in turn, contribute to the maintenance of mental ill health and to possible relapse among those with existing problems (Jenkins et al., 2008). This is seen as a vicious circle in terms of difficulties they may experience with engagement and participation in communities (Office of the Deputy Prime Minister, 2004). Being diagnosed with any chronic health problem is distressing. When stigma, negative misconceptions and discrimination are all attached to the diagnosis, the problem can seem insurmountable to those concerned.

Misconceptions regarding mental health disorders have a negative impact on the perception of mental health issues. Some commonly held misconceptions are as follows.

- All people with mental health disorders are violent and dangerous.
- People who have mental health problems have an intellectual disability or brain damage.
- People with a mental health problem will never recover.
- People with a mental health problem should be locked up and kept away from society.
- People who have a diagnosis of schizophrenia have a split personality.

Unfortunately, misconceptions have influenced the general perception and treatment of mental health problems for centuries. *Attitudes to Mental Illness* surveyed 1741 adults (aged 16 years and over) in England in February/March 2011 (NHSIC, 2011). The study, which has been repeated frequently since 1994, sought to reveal current attitudes to people with mental health problems and how attitudes have changed over time. Specifically, the survey sought to reveal attitudes to:

- fear and exclusion of people with mental illness,
- understanding and tolerance of mental illness,

- integrating people with mental illness into the community,
- causes of mental illness and the need for special services.

The survey found that:

- 77% of people agreed with the statement 'mental illness is an illness like any other', an increase from 71% in 1994,
- 70% said that they would be comfortable talking to a friend or family member about their mental health, for example telling them they had a mental health diagnosis and how it affects them, an increase from 66% in 2009,
- 43% said that they would feel uncomfortable talking to their employer about their mental health compared to 50% in 2010,
- 17% of people felt that locating mental health facilities in a residential area downgrades the neighbourhood,
- acceptance of people with mental health problems taking public office and assuming concomitant responsibilities has grown, with 29% of people feeling they should be excluded from public office in 1994 to 21% in 2011.

However, opinions on integrating people with mental health problems into the community were mixed. For example in 2011:

- 81% felt that 'no-one has the right to exclude people with mental illness from their neighbourhood',
- 79% felt that 'the best therapy for many people with mental illness is to be part of a normal community',
- 77% agreed that 'mental illness is an illness like any other',
- 72% agreed that 'people with mental health problems should have the same rights to a job as anyone else'.

However, the survey respondents also felt that:

- 'less emphasis should be placed on protecting the public from people with mental illness' (36% agreed),
- 'mental hospitals are an outdated means of treating people with mental illness' (34% agreed).

The survey also revealed that many respondents had had contact with someone with a mental health problem. Thirty-three per cent of respondents said they had had a close friend with a mental health problem and 82% agreed that in future they would be willing to continue a relationship with a friend who developed a mental health problem. Some 72% would be willing to live near a person with a mental health problem, while 68% would be willing to work with such a person. In addition, 56% of people suggested that they would be willing to live with someone with a mental health problem. Finally, 85% of survey respondents felt that people with mental illness experience stigma and discrimination, with 50% feeling that they experience a lot of discrimination (NHSIC, 2011).

The high level of misunderstanding concerning mental health problems in the community may well contribute to the low numbers of people seeking help or those who wait until they are in crisis before seeking help. Poverty and the resulting inability to access healthcare in some instances, the inability to travel to services, poor social skills or lack of support all contribute to delays in seeking help.

People who develop mental disorders may have had their own preconceived ideas and prejudices in regard to mental health issues before becoming ill. Many people believe it is the end of their life and will grieve for the life they had and for the aspirations they held for their future. While people are unwell, work or study can be interrupted. Unemployment often leads to financial hardship, forcing people to live below the poverty line, thereby exacerbating the feelings of frustration, low self-esteem and entrapment. The potential for suicidal thoughts and behaviour is particularly high in this group of people (Fryer, 1995; Mathers and Schofield, 1998).

Parents and siblings will also have their own misconceptions and prejudices against people with mental health problems. Parents may blame themselves for their child's problem, or may be ashamed or embarrassed and try to hide the problem from extended family members, neighbours, friends and work colleagues. Siblings may also feel embarrassed and stop bringing friends home. They may be fearful that they too will develop a mental problem and may become afraid of their brother or sister. The acute phase of many mental health disorders, especially psychotic disorders, will cause major disruption to family life (Fontaine, 2003). Parents may need to take time out from work, which will have financial implications for the family, and siblings may find it difficult to function at school or in the workplace. Both parents and siblings may well go through the grieving process as a result of the changes in their lives. Children who grow up with a parent who has been diagnosed with a mental disorder are at higher risk of developing a mental health problem, such as depression, through either genetic susceptibility or gaps in parenting (Davies, 2002; Dean and Macmillan, 2002).

The new mental health strategy for England, *No Health Without Mental Health* (Department of Health, 2011), recognizes the economic, social and personal cost of mental ill health. The strategy proposes a number of policy initiatives to improve the mental health of people with existing mental health problems, while seeking to prevent mental ill health. The strategy also recognizes that social inequalities (such as those described above; lack of access to work, poor housing, isolation from communities and so forth) compounds mental distress. The UK Government therefore argue that the strategy is '… both a public mental health strategy and a strategy for social justice' (Department of Health, 2011, p. 3).

NURSE'S STORY

When I was a young girl growing up in the 1960s I lived with my parents and siblings in a suburb next to a large mental health hospital. The hospital consisted of many buildings, some double storey and some single, spread out on a vast expanse of land. I remember big fences at the front of the hospital, and the surrounding area being very dark due to the vacant land that surrounded the hospital.

People in the neighbourhood usually referred to the hospital as the 'nut factory' and the people in the hospital as 'nuts'. Sometimes the 'nuts' escaped and people were scared that their families wouldn't be safe. I remember my mother being afraid when my father wasn't home, for that very reason. Driving past the hospital at night was particularly scary, but at the same time you had to look so that you could tell the kids next door if you saw anything worth reporting. I too grew up afraid of 'those people' and didn't like walking near the hospital, even during the day.

Years later I was working as an enrolled nurse when I met and worked with a registered nurse who was also a mental health nurse. She used to talk to me about her experiences and to my surprise I became interested. I decided I would like to become a mental health nurse, so I rang the very same hospital near where I grew up, and arranged an interview!

I was successful in my application and so began my mental health nurse training in the mid-1970s. By this time the bars were off the windows and the high fences had been pulled down, but the stigma surrounding mental problems was rampant.

Can you imagine my family's response when I announced I was going to work in the 'nut factory'? I took along all of my preconceived stereotypical ideas, fears and misconceptions. On the first day, I remember being scared, but began to relax as I walked around the beautiful grounds, with its beautifully maintained lawns, garden beds, vegetable gardens and bird aviary, unharmed and intact. To my added surprise the patients (as they were called then) didn't look anything like what I expected; rather, they were all ordinary people who had a problem that needed to be treated.

I worked at that hospital for 15 years and I often look back and smile as I remember all the interesting experiences I had there. Most of the hospital has now been demolished to make way for a housing estate, but I will always remember the people I met while working there, as they taught me not to be afraid and to recognize that mental health problems are problems just like chronic physical illnesses, and that the sufferers are mere mortals, just like you and me.

Even working in the 'general' medical/surgical arena, the skills learned as a mental health nurse are used every day. I teach mental health to undergraduate nurses and, with the assistance of my colleagues, strive to demystify all aspects of mental health problems and provide students with a positive and fulfilling experience.

As well as the stigma attached to mental health problems, immigrants bear the added burden of their cultural difference and potential racial stigma. Language difficulties and culturally specific ways of expressing distress increase alienation from mainstream community groups and place this group of people at an increased risk of being misdiagnosed or receiving inadequate care and support.

CRITICAL THINKING CHALLENGE 6.2

Write a short list (bullet points) of what you think about people with a diagnosis of:

♦ diabetes,

♦ schizophrenia.

How do you think these problems would affect people's lifestyles?

What would you expect to see if you walked into a mental health ward today? For example:

♦ What would the service users be doing?

♦ What would the nurses be doing?

What influences your perceptions of people with mental problems?

How could you test your perceptions against reality?

The media and misconceptions about mental health problems

The media are very powerful in conveying information and influencing the community's attitudes and perceptions of social norms. Media representations of mental disorders can reinforce stereotypes of individuals with mental health problems in society (Kemp, 2008). The effect of such stigma is that people often find that they are socially excluded from communities (Future Vision Coalition, 2009). Therefore it follows that media coverage and reporting, be it through films, television, newspapers, magazines, posters or pamphlets, are critical when attempting to form and influence community attitudes to mental health and mental disorder and the people affected by it. Unfortunately, media coverage often reflects the widespread misunderstanding of mental health problems and mental disorders. This is particularly so in films.

To highlight the inaccurate portrayal of mental health problems in television and the media, a 1 year analysis of television drama programmes (serials, plays and films) was conducted in the USA and found that:

73% of people with a mental illness were depicted as violent, while 23% of people were portrayed as

homicidal maniacs. When the same study analysed media reports about mental illness on television and in newspapers, it found that nearly 90% of stories depicted people with mental illness as violent and usually homicidal. This is grossly inaccurate.

(SANE Australia, 2000)

Newspaper reporting has a tendency to sensationalize issues related to mental disorders at times, thereby perpetuating negative stereotypes and unnecessary fears in the community (Blood, 2002; Lindberg, 2001; Mitchell, 2003).

Just as the media can have a negative impact, it can also be used as a tool to educate and change public opinion by ensuring that accurate information is reported in a rational and sensitive manner. In order to achieve this, scriptwriters, journalists and newspaper editors need to be educated on mental health issues (Martin, 1998).

WHAT IS CULTURE?

Culture can be defined as a body of learned behaviours, passed on by role modelling, by learning and by lore, common to any given human society, which is used by the individual to interpret experience and to generate social behaviour (Spradley, 1991). Culture shapes individual behavioural, emotional and social responses within the human environment.

Within any society there will be subgroups, or subcultures, which define themselves by social norms that deviate to a greater or lesser extent from the given (mainstream) norm. Variation in acceptable behaviour, speech and dress may set apart social classes, religious organizations, secret societies and age groups within a society. Variations may exist between urban and rural populations within a given culture. Differences in acculturation between males and females exists in all societies, influencing behaviour and societal responses (Friedl, 1991).

As noted, culture is passed on by role modelling, learning and lore. The relationship between teaching and learning is not absolute because some of what is taught is lost, and new experiences and learning occur daily. Culture exists in a constant state of change. Today's youth-culture deviation is tomorrow's status quo.

Culture and health beliefs

No culture is universal or static within any given community. Although we speak of an 'Anglo-Celtic' (or more broadly a 'Western') culture as informing mainstream health beliefs, it is important to understand that this shorthand covers a multitude of cultural approaches to healthcare. As with so-called Western culture, there is no single 'African culture' or 'Eastern culture' for example. These are shorthand terms covering a broad spectrum of beliefs that may vary geographically or by age or status within the given community. An attempt to define a person's culture only in terms of race or geography gives rise to stereotyping, generalization and potential inaccuracies. It is strongly recommended that mental health nurses develop relationships with cultural intermediaries and ethnic support workers, because it is not possible to learn everything about all the cultures you will work with in your professional life (Fuller, 1995).

The Ethnic Minority Psychiatric Illness Rates in the Community (EMPIRIC) study, undertaken by the National Centre for Social Research (2002), focused on five of the main ethnic minority groups in England (Bangladeshi, black Caribbean, Indian, Irish and Pakistani people) with a comparison white group. Some differences were found between groups in terms of how they experience mental health problems. For example, white and Pakistani men and Indian and Pakistani women reported symptoms of a depressive episode most frequently. The highest rates of anxiety among men were found in the Irish group, and for women the highest rates occurred among Indian, Pakistani and Irish women. Overall, the prevalence of CMDs was lowest among Bangladeshi women, and highest in Indian and Pakistani women. The study found no evidence for misunderstandings about concept of 'mental health' among ethnic groups but did reveal some differences in the way that people expressed mental distress. For example, white British, Caribbean and English-speaking Indian respondents discussed having problems with daily functioning, such as not being able to go to work, to 'think properly', to attend courses or fulfil responsibilities at home. Other respondents described their feelings in both mental and physical ways. For example, migrant Bangladeshi and Pakistani respondents often described a wide range of physical symptoms, such as feeling weak, body being gripped by shaking or a feeling of restlessness, dizziness and breathlessness, which were interrelated with expressions of mental distress. People who migrated from South Asian countries described looking ill or changing colour or a feeling of paralysis. Another area where there were differences was in how religion influenced the expression of mental distress. For example, the survey found that some non-white ethnic groups had a religious orientation that involved 'making sense of ill fortune' and a perception that mental health problems were seen to be initiated by God and as a test. These views were seemingly absent from discussions with white (British or Irish) groups. As such, the study suggested that there may be some differences in the way that people from different ethnic groups perceive mental ill health.

You might want to enhance your knowledge by accessing reputable websites and publications to gain a deeper understanding of cultural diversity (such as Geert Hofstede™ cultural dimensions: www.geert-hofstede.com) and the individual nurse's responsibility to provide cultural care and respect diversity (see Box 6.1).

Box 6.1 Strategies in the provision of cultural care

- Become aware of your own ethnocentrism; that is, the belief that your own group is superior to others (Henderson and Primeaux, 1981). It has been well documented that counsellors are more likely to have good relationships with service users who fit the YAVIS client model, namely 'young, attractive, verbal, intelligent and successful' (Schofield 1964, cited in Sue and Sue, 1990). Service users from other cultures are often seen as having fewer of these qualities (D'Ardenne and Mahtani, 1989). Your ethnocentrism may be reflected back to the services, causing them to withdraw or be seen as noncompliant and resistive (D'Ardenne and Mahtani, 1989).

- Recognize that it is counterproductive to treat all people alike. There are characteristics that all people share, such as the need for food and shelter, characteristics that some people share, such as language, and some that are unique to a group; these include racial or ethnic historical conditions such as slavery (Henderson and Primeaux, 1981).

- Avoid creating stereotypes and generalizations.

- Recognize the limitations of your own expertise and enlist the help of culturally appropriate practitioners as requested or required.

- Allow service users to define themselves rather than attempting to erase the clients' lived experiences with categories, notions of dysfunction or simplistic theories (MacKinnon, 1993).

- Assist service users to optimally use the services available.

- Acknowledge with the service user that there is a difference of cultures and encourage the service user to be your teacher of what is culturally sensitive. Use photographs, books and articles of significance. Also try using other ways of communicating, such as music, drawing or painting.

- Sharing of cultural practices is by invitation. When you experience this, acknowledge it.

- Become knowledgeable, sensitive and aware of service users in their cultural setting (Wright, 1991).

- Recognize that there is diversity within groups as well as between groups (Charonko, 1992).

- Advocate for service users from ethnic minorities, particularly in regard to the way in which decisions are made in hospitals and the community (Wright, 1991).

Black and minority ethnic and culturally and linguistically diverse groups

Mental health nurses in the UK will encounter many people from other cultural backgrounds who will provide challenges to their own beliefs regarding mental health. The cultural variety of migrant and refugee groups is broad and it is not the intention of this chapter to describe them. Many people from different cultures have experienced the stress that accompanies separation from country, families and communities, as well as the trauma associated with forced removal or refugee status, torture and incarceration (World Health Organization, 2001).

Some factors suggested by Ferguson and Browne (1991) as affecting migrant health are listed in Box 6.2.

Some cultures predicate spiritual origins for mental disorder, including demonic possession or punishment for sin. Others place great importance on 'cursing', 'ill wishing' or 'the evil eye'. Some believe that current ill health is a result of bad karma in previous lives, or of bad deeds by ancestors. Other cultures may be predisposed to presentation with somatising complaints (see Ch. 20).

As mentioned above, the words and behaviours used to describe mental distress vary among cultures. It is important that the mental health nurse respects the value of other people's beliefs, and understands that these beliefs shape behaviour in response to problems or disease.

Cultural values and beliefs also shape the ways in which people decide to access services, and who is deemed an appropriate channel of communication between consumer and health service. Some cultures find mental problems so shameful that they will resist seeking any kind of help outside the family unit. In patriarchal cultures, the senior male family member may decide who is to seek attention and under what circumstances. Similarly, people from black and minority ethnic and culturally and linguistically diverse (or BME and CALD) groups tend to be particularly reluctant to seek assistance for health-related problems from mainstream services (Zysk 2002, cited in Delfabbro and LeCouteur, 2003). Zysk suggests that the factors that contribute to this low rate of help-seeking can include language difficulties, a lack of cultural sensitivity by service providers, inappropriate treatments

Box 6.2 Factors affecting migrant mental health

- Previous personality, emotional health and coping mechanisms
- The stress of migration
- Bereavement aspects of the migration process
- Reception and ease of settlement into the host country
- Support measures available and the size of the ethnic community
- Cultural differences between the country of origin and the adopted country
- Acceptability and availability of the adopted country's services
- Social class, including underemployment and unemployment
- Discrimination and racism

Source: Ferguson and Browne (1991).

including lack of family involvement, a lack of information or misinformation and a greater degree of stigma and shame associated with mental health problems and related problems. Studies of recent immigrant groups show that they experience low rates of use of many important social and health services, despite evidence of significant need (Reitz, 1995). The barriers most often identified include those related to language, lack of information about services, cultural patterns of help-seeking, lack of cultural sensitivity by service providers, financial barriers and lack of service availability (Reitz, 1995). Reitz identified that if services were not culturally appropriate then the research focus on rates of use may actually underestimate the barriers in access to service; that is, services are used but are not appropriate to the culture of a group and therefore equivalent benefits may not be derived.

A central tenet of cultural safety is the ability to examine one's own beliefs and values, and therefore the mental health nurse needs to be aware of his or her own cultural bias when seeking histories and making assessments of presenting behaviours. Flexibility in approach will ensure that due respect is accorded to the opinions and explanations of those bearing cultural authority. Involving families too can make care more effective, because the knowledge and expertise of family members can be drawn upon.

- What healthcare actions are taken within the family?
- Who makes decisions about when and how to seek healthcare outside the family?
- Are these decisions made individually or by group negotiation?
- How does your family's health culture influence your response to people with different health beliefs and values?

Culture and communication style

The essence of mental health nursing is the ability to communicate; to engage in meaningful interaction with others, aimed at therapeutic results. This means having an awareness of our own communication style, as well as that of our clients. The Anglo-Celtic communication style is described as direct, dyadic and contained. The medical, and perhaps most notably the psychiatric, interview shows this style refined to a degree that is intrusive and threatening, even within mainstream culture (Carroll, 1995; Dudgeon et al., 2000). Nonverbal expression and behaviours that appear self-injurious, aggressive or extreme to Anglo-Celtic health workers may carry a very different meaning in the culture of the individual concerned.

Culture and self-reflection

For the mental health nurse, culture is a vital element of therapeutic alliance. If we accept, as the basis of our human interaction, that all behaviour has meaning, then it is essential that we understand the cultural templates that shape behavioural and emotional responses. It is essential to reflect on our own beliefs and values about health, about what it means to be healthy, and what we recognize as mental wellbeing.

As mental health nurses we must also reflect on the assumptions of our adopted culture of healthcare professional. Health education, training and practice rely strongly on an assumption that all involved in health service delivery subscribe to 'Western' values concerning the application of scientific methods to everyday life and health behaviour.

The scientific or biomedical model of healthcare also assumes a power differential between professional and client, assigning the evaluation of healthcare services and outcomes to the professional. Mental health nurses must be aware of the power differentials inherent in social structures and service delivery models that marginalize or devalue the client's identity, beliefs and wellbeing, and actively reflect on their own professional actions in light of this awareness (Stein-Parbury, 2000).

As we have noted, all cultural groups, including mental health nurses, are made up of individuals whose lived experience places them subtly apart from even their closest peers, and influences their assigned and chosen behavioural styles within the peer group, with multidisciplinary colleagues, and in therapeutic interactions. We all bring our own cultural and subcultural background, beliefs and values with us to all of life's interactions, including our professional healthcare beliefs and practices as well as our position in the society in which we live. An example is when we are from a cultural position that has exploited or colonized the culture we are working with (Allen, 1999). Allen gives the following example: 'I have not individually (at least not intentionally) participated in the colonization of Guatemala. But the United States (following Spain) certainly has. So if I study Guatemala, I do so carrying with me cultural assumptions that are not merely *different* from, but potentially *exploitive* of, Guatemalan culture' (Allen, 1999, p. 228).

Each of us, in our practice, must maintain awareness of our own cultural and subcultural assumptions, and of our natural tendency to ethnocentrism; that is, the belief that our own cultural values constitute the human norm and that difference is deviant and wrong.

CRITICAL THINKING CHALLENGE 6.5

As health workers we work within a model that is often characterized as 'Western, scientific and patriarchal'. What implications may that characterization have for:

- a workforce that is overwhelmingly female?
- the concept of care?
- service users seeking healthcare?

How accurate is the characterization?

Cultural competence and cultural safety

'Cultural competence' is a term that arises from the transcultural nursing model of Madeleine Leininger. Transcultural nursing theory was an early attempt to describe the role of culture in nurse–patient dynamics; the theory encouraged nurses to study and attempt to understand cultures other than their own (Leininger, 1995).

Models of cultural competence involve some or all of the following elements:

- respect for other people's cultural and religious beliefs and values,
- respect for spiritual and religious influences on health beliefs,
- awareness of variations in verbal and nonverbal communication styles,

- increasing knowledge of cultural differences,
- respect for the individual's explanations of their experiences,
- delivering culturally sensitive care to diverse groups via negotiation and consensus,
- instilling a sense of cultural safety for individuals, families and groups (Betancourt et al., 2002; Campinha-Bacote, 2003).

A major criticism of the cultural competence model is that the client is not empowered to evaluate the appropriateness of service delivery or to assess health professionals' knowledge (Commonwealth Government of Australia, 2002).

Cultural safety goes beyond describing the practices of other ethnic groups, because merely learning about aspects of a culture does not make one fully cognisant of the complexities of that culture. Culturally safe nurses are those who look at learning about themselves rather than learning about the cultures of their clients. The emphasis is on what cultural attitudes and values nurses bring to their practice, and their understanding of the impact that these may have on power relations within a given context.

Ramsden (2002) describes a progression towards culturally safe practice as follows.

1. *Cultural awareness* is the first step and involves understanding that there is difference.
2. *Cultural sensitivity* alerts students to the 'legitimacy of difference' and to self-exploration.
3. *Cultural safety* is defined as 'an outcome of nursing and midwifery education that enables safe service to be defined by those that receive the service'.

A criticism of cultural sensitivity concerns the underlying assumption that a group can be considered homogeneous. That is, nurses as a homogeneous group encounter patients who are culturally different and exotic, but are also homogeneous, possessing a body of finite cultural content, customs and traditions based on kinship. Culture is therefore seen as static and monolithic, rather than something that is created by people, and does not allow for generational or diasporic differences. Furthermore, a nurse having knowledge of a client's culture could be disempowering for a client who is disenfranchised from their own culture, and could be seen as the continuation of a colonizing process that is both demeaning and disempowering (Ramsden, 2002) or appropriating (Allen, 1999).

APPROACHES TO CARE AND SERVICE DELIVERY

Mental health strategy strongly emphasizes the need for a recovery approach in service provision, with the assumption that most people will get better and can live well even if their symptoms recur or persist. The recovery approach states that services must empower consumers and their families, protect their rights, increase their control over their own mental health and enable their full participation in society. The task of effective mental health service delivery is to assist the individual (or group of individuals) to identify the meaning of behaviours, and to promote the choice of healthy action within the social environment. When caring for people of different cultures, the mental health nurse must be prepared to step away from the central, leadership role assigned in the Western medical model.

To minimize misunderstandings in cross-cultural communication, a service user-focused service will, if requested by the service user, involve culturally appropriate health professionals. This can also be a fraught strategy as there can be many variations or subcultures within a culture (McAvoy and Donaldson, 1990). For example, I (RD) am from Goa, which, although part of India, has a distinct and unique flavour. Further to this, I was born in Africa. This gives me, and others like me, a different perspective from those who have been born and brought up in Goa.

If language is an issue and comprehension is difficult, then 24 h access to trained interpreters is essential. Using family members as interpreters cannot be justified except in emergencies, and can cause irreparable damage to family dynamics in any culture.

Factors that could prevent black and minority ethnic and culturally and linguistically diverse clients using services

Sue and Sue (1990) suggest that the reason people from culturally and linguistically diverse groups underutilize services is that systems (people) are often insensitive, antagonistic and discriminating. They suggest that this is related to the training of mental health professionals, which is biased towards a white, middle-class perspective. A person who is not verbal or speaks with an accent may be at a disadvantage, particularly if there are no bilingual staff. The qualities valued by staff working in mental health services, such as self-disclosure, insight and self-responsibility, might not be valued in another culture.

In 2002, the Sainsbury Centre for Mental Health (2002) (now the Centre for Mental Health) conducted a review which sought to account for evidence which shows that black African and Caribbean people are over-represented in mental health services and appear to experience poorer outcomes than white service users. The review found that there were 'circles of fear' which discouraged African and Carribean communities from engaging with mental health services which were experienced as inhumane, unhelpful and inappropriate. Acute services were perceived negatively. Mental health services were felt to be inaccessible by this group, and not welcoming or relevant to their needs. As a consequence, African and Carribean people tend to come to mental health services too late by which time they are already experiencing a crisis, which reinforces these circles of fear. Different perspectives of mental health and mental ill health between mainstream services were described, with black groups' world views not being understood or acknowledged.

Model of care delivery

Most forms of counselling and psychotherapy available in mental health services have been developed from a white, middle-class, American, English-speaking milieu. This has then been applied cross-culturally (Wright, 1991). The intrapsychic model that is used predominantly sees difficulties as the result of personal disorganization, rather than in the wider context of an oppressive society. This 'blaming the person' approach tends to deny the existence of society's ills, and consequently differences are seen as deficits (Wright, 1991). A rejection of help offered by mental health services is seen as an indicator of the individual's failure to function adequately. The result is that mental health workers validate their own role and function within the cross-cultural relationship by blaming the victim (Wright, 1991). Instead, if we respond to the person *in* their cultural setting rather than just *to* their cultural setting, we might be successful in engaging our clients (Wright, 1991). There can be a great deal of stigma associated with receiving mental health services within a particular culture, as well as little faith in psychotherapy as a treatment option, and fear of institutionalization. It is important to note that different ethnic groups practise illness prevention and health promotion differently. Some prefer direct, practical and immediate assistance from the Western care system rather than long-term strategies (Fuller, 1995).

Alternative models of care delivery

The biomedical model has failed to legitimize the traditional healers and networks of many communities, labelling them as supernatural and unscientific (Sue and Sue, 1990). Black and minority ethnic and culturally and linguistically diverse clients may prefer support from their own community (Gauntlett et al., 1995), whether these are informal support networks or trusted folk healers, who share their beliefs about the role of religion or the supernatural, the role of the family in treatment and the context and process of treatment (Flaskerud, 1984). Mental health workers need to develop some openness to compromise between conventional psychiatry and people's cultural beliefs (Wright, 1991), particularly where cultural practices are preferred, such as massage or consultation with folk healers. There needs to be a broadening of our attitudes as to what constitutes legitimate mental health practice. Research into this could provide us with alternative frames of reference to Western definitions of mental health (Sue and Sue, 1990).

Definition of the problem and diagnosis

Stern and Kruckman (1983) point out that the defining criteria for depression may vary greatly across cultures and so cannot necessarily be resolved by applying a Western concept of depression to them. The diagnosis and treatment of clients from black and minority ethnic and culturally and linguistically diverse cultures may therefore be inaccurate, even discriminatory and punitive (Flaskerud, 1990). Referring to distress as depression can cause harm in cultures where discussion of mental health problems is stigmatized or taboo. However, Barnett et al. (1999) argue that having a diagnosis means appropriate treatment and social and psychological support can be obtained. Fitzgerald et al. (1998) state, firstly, that the real debate is not whether distress exists, but rather how it is expressed and categorized and, secondly, whether a particular explanatory model should be predominant and common human experiences and responses pathologized. According to Fitzgerald et al. (1998, p. 21), the key issue is: 'How can we best understand and respond to culturally influenced and contextualized experiences in meaningful and useful ways?'

Structural barriers

Healthcare practices by professionals continue to be predominantly monocultural despite recognition of the need to be responsive to culturally diverse populations. Durvasula and Mylvaganam (1994) suggest that a lack of awareness or knowledge of services, where they are located, and a scarcity of ethnically similar counsellors, or counsellors who are bilingual, provide barriers to black and minority ethnic and culturally and linguistically diverse people using mental health services.

Gender-appropriate service

Full attention must be given to the importance in many cultures of providing access to gender-appropriate healthcare professionals. Many groups have strong rules about what is and is not appropriate in male–female interaction. In some cultures, males may not be given any information about issues to do with sexuality, pregnancy or childbirth. In others, males may only speak to other males of comparable rank in discussing some issues of behaviour associated with spirituality.

Interview styles should also be flexible enough to allow the patient and family to contribute fully to negotiation of health management and treatment options. With the presence of cultural intermediaries, support workers and linguistic interpreters as needed, and the provision of an appropriate area, it is possible to make space and time for full discussion. This may involve providing a large area, often an outside area, where adults and children can move about freely, and where discussion will not be intruded on by outsiders, a possible source of family 'shame' in Asian cultures.

It is important to ensure that all stakeholders are consulted or appropriately represented, especially the group's key opinion formers. If necessary, and if acceptable to the client, provision of conference phones or videoconferencing can enable extended family and other community stakeholders to become involved in discussions.

INCORPORATING CULTURALLY SAFE PRACTICE

Mental health nursing is about people: people of all cultures, socioeconomic groups and walks of life. So it follows that to provide quality care we must acknowledge the lived experiences of our clients, how these shape their beliefs and the acceptability of treatments. To provide quality care we must acknowledge cultural diversity. A system that does not consider race, culture, gender or

social values does not serve the people it purports to (Speight et al., 1991). As professionals we need to be able to work with everyone (Kareem and Littlewood, 1992).

Services must be accessible to all, regardless of their culture and colour. However, we should not underestimate the effort involved in achieving this. For example, mental health nurses can be viewed by some as agents of social control (Wright, 1991). We need to develop practical and realistic ways of supporting those whose cultural roots are different from our own and avoid projecting our own cultural expectations of what is therapeutic onto our clients.

CONCLUSION

Mental health nurses have a responsibility to ensure that they are well informed on current statistics, trends, models and philosophies relating to all areas of mental health. They need to examine their own perceptions and belief systems in regard to mental health issues and behaviours, so they can function effectively in an unbiased manner. Reflective practice and commitment to the understanding of each individual as a person, taking into account and respecting cultural diversity, will enable mental health nurses to work with clients to establish supportive care strategies and valid outcomes.

EXERCISES FOR CLASS ENGAGEMENT

Make a list of the thoughts you currently have on all issues relating to mental ill health. Discuss your list with other members of your group or class, and then reexamine the list as you progress through your study. You should be able to dispel misconceptions and replace them with the facts about mental health and ill health.

List the most widespread social perceptions of mental health problems/people with mental health problems. Discuss the ways in which misconceptions about mental health problems originate and are perpetuated. Identify how nurses can influence social perceptions of mental health problems/people with mental health problems.

In a small group, identify the values that operate in the mental healthcare system (you might have an experience from clinical practice that can be examined in analysing the value system). Discuss how the underlying values of mental health services affect individuals from diverse cultures.

Use your library service or the internet to answer the following questions.

♦ What results do you get when you search using the key words 'stigma', 'culture', 'mental health' and 'consumer groups'?

♦ What variation in perceptions can you find? Is there variation between service users and mental health professionals? Between different mental health disciplines? Between countries?

♦ Is all the information useful? How do you discriminate?

♦ Make a list of useful websites.

♦ Share your results with your group or class members.

Considering cultural background as encompassing socioeconomic status, migrant/refugee status, gender and age, answer the following questions, and then discuss your answers with your group or class members.

♦ What is the 'cultural mix' of your area? City? University? Cohort or intake? Hospital catchment area? Home town?

♦ Think of the healthcare service you have worked in most recently (or the one with which you are most familiar). How does that agency manifest its culture and ethos? How does the agency's culture affect the ways in which healthcare is offered to clients? What is the 'fit' between the agency's cultural approach and the catchment area it serves?

♦ How do you define yourself culturally? How does this self-definition affect your nursing practice?

REFERENCES

Allen, D.G., 1999. Knowledge, politics, culture and gender: a discourse perspective. Can. J. Nurs. Res. 30 (4), 227–234.

Barnett, B., Matthey, S., Boyce, P., 1999. Migration and motherhood: a response to Barclay and Kent (1998). Midwifery 15 (3), 203–207.

Betancourt, J.R., Green, A.R., Carillo, J.E., et al., 2002. Cultural Competence in Health Care: Emerging Frameworks and Practical Approaches. <http://www.massgeneral.org/healthpolicy/cchc.html>.

Blood, W., 2002. A Qualitative Analysis of the Reporting and Portrayal of Mental Illness in the Courier Mail and Sunday Mail. Report prepared for the Public Advocates Office, Queensland.

Campinha-Bacote, J., 2003. Many faces: addressing diversity in health care. Online J. Issues Nurs. 8 (1) http://nursingworld.org/ojin/topic20/tpc20_2.htm.

Carroll, P.J., 1995. Aboriginal languages and effective cross-cultural communication. In: Robinson, G. (Ed.), Aboriginal Health: Social and Cultural Transitions. NTU Press, Darwin.

Centre for Mental Health, 2010. The Economic and Social Costs of Mental Health Problems in 2009/10. <http://www.centreformentalhealth.org.uk/pdfs/Economic_and_social_costs_2010.pdf>.

Charonko, C.V., 1992. Cultural influences in 'noncompliant' behavior and decision making. Holist Nurs. Pract. 6 (3), 73–78.

Clarke, D., Abbott, M., De Souza, R., et al., 2007. An overview of help seeking by problem gamblers and their families including barriers to and relevance of services. Int. J. Ment. Health Addict. 5 (4), 292–306.

Commonwealth Government of Australia, 2002. National Review of Nursing Education. Our Duty of Care. CGA, Canberra.

D'Ardenne, P., Mahtani, A., 1989. Transcultural Counselling in Action. Sage, London.

Davies, J., 2002. Trapped in the hell of their parents' suffering. National Network of Adult and Adolescent Children who have a Mentally Ill Parent/s. <http://home.vicnet.net.au/~nnaami/trapped.html>.

Dean, C., Macmillan, C., 2002. Serving the children of parents with a mental illness: barriers, breakthroughs and benefits. Australian Infant, Child, Adolescent and Family Mental Health Association. <http://www.aicafmha.net.au/conferences/brisbane2001/papers/dean_c.htm>.

Delfabbro, P.H., LeCouteur, A., 2003. A Decade of Gambling Research in Australia and New Zealand (1992–2002): Implications for Policy, Regulation and Harm Minimisation. Independent Gambling Authority of South Australia, Adelaide.

Department of Health, 2011. No Health Without Mental Health. <http://www.dh.gov.uk/en/Aboutus/Features/DH_123998>.

Disability Rights Commission, 2006. Equal Treatment: Closing the Gap. <http://www.leeds.ac.uk/disability-studies/archiveuk/DRC/Health%20FI%20main.pdf>.

Dudgeon, P., Garvey, D., Pickett, H. (Eds.), 2000. Working with Indigenous Australians: a Handbook for Psychologists. Gunada Press, Perth.

Durvasula, R.S., Mylvaganam, G.A., 1994. Mental health of Asian Indians: relevant issues and community implications. J. Community Psychol. 22 (2), 97–108.

Ferguson, B., Browne, E. (Eds.), 1991. Health Care and Immigrants: A Guide for Health Professionals. McLennan & Petty, Sydney.

Fitzgerald, M., Ing, V., Heang Ya, T., et al., 1998. Hear our Voices: Trauma, Birthing and Mental Health Among Cambodian Women. Ausmed, Paramatta.

Flaskerud, J.H., 1984. A comparison of perceptions of problematic behavior by six minority groups and mental health professionals. Nurs. Res. 33 (4), 190–192.

Flaskerud, J.H., 1990. Matching client and therapist, ethnicity, language and gender: a review of research. Issues Ment. Health 11, 321–336.

Fontaine, K.L., 2003. Mental Health Nursing, fifth ed. Prentice Hall, NJ.

Friedl, E., 1991. Society and sex roles. In: Podolefsky, A., Brown, P.J. (Eds.), Applying Cultural Anthropology: an Introductory Reader. Mayfield, CA.

Fryer, D., 1995. Unemployment. A mental health issue. Letter. The Jobs 24/9.

Fullagar, S., Gattuso, S., 2002. Rethinking gender, risk and depression in Australian mental health policy. Aust. e-J. Adv. Ment. Health (AeJAMH) 1 (3) http://www.auseinet.com/journal/vol1iss3/fullagar.pdf.

Fuller, J., 1995. Challenging old notions of professionalism: how can nurses work with paraprofessional ethnic health workers? J. Adv. Nurs. 22 (2), 465–472.

Future Vision Coalition, 2009. A Future Vision for Mental Health. <http://www.newvisionformentalhealth.org.uk/index.html>.

Gauntlett, N., Ford, R., Johnson, N., et al., 1995. Meeting mental health needs of ethnic minority groups. Nurs. Times 91 (42), 36–37.

Henderson, G., Primeaux, M. (Eds.), 1981. Transcultural Health Care. Addison Wesley, CA.

Jenkins, R., Meltzer, H., Jones, P., et al., 2008. Foresight Mental Capital and Wellbeing Project. Mental Health: Future Challenges. The Government Office for Science, London.

Kareem, J., Littlewood, R., 1992. Intercultural Therapy: Themes, Interpretation and Practice. Blackwell, Oxford.

Kemp, P., 2008. User involvement and the micropolitics of mental health Care. In: Lynch, J., Trenoweth, S. (Eds.), Contemporary Issues in Mental Health Nursing. Wiley, Chichester.

Leininger, M., 1995. Transcultural Nursing: Concepts, Theories and Practices. Blacklick, OH.

Lindberg, W., 2001. Interview: Warren Lindberg. <http://www.mediawatch.co.nz/archive>.

McAvoy, B.R., Donaldson, L.J., 1990. Health Care for Asians. Oxford University Press, Oxford.

MacKinnon, L., 1993. Systems in settings: the therapist as power broker. Aust. N. Z. J. Fam. Ther. 14 (3), 117–122.

Martin, G., 1998. Media influence to suicide: the search for solutions. Arch. Suicide Res. 4, 51–56.

Mathers, C., Schofield, D., 1998. The health consequences of unemployment: the evidence. <http://www.mja.co.au/public/issues/feb16/mathers/mathers.html>.

Meadows, G., Singh, B., 2001. Mental Health in Australia. Collaborative Community Practice. Oxford University Press, Melbourne.

Mitchell, N., 2003. Media Interrupted: Mental Health and the Media. http://www.abc.net.au/rn/science/mind/s788631.htm.

Murray, C., Lopez, A., 1996. The Global Burden of Disease: a Comprehensive Assessment of Mortality and Disability, Injuries, and Risk Factors in 1990 and Projected to 2020. World Bank, Harvard School of Public Health and World Health Organization, Geneva.

National Centre for Social Research, 2002. Ethnic Minority Psychiatric Illness Rates in the Community (EMPIRIC)–Quantitative Report. <http://www.dh.gov.uk/en/Publicationsandstatistics/Publications/PublicationsStatistics/DH_4005698>.

NHSIC (NHS Information Centre), 2009. Adult Psychiatric Morbidity in England, 2007: Results of a Household Survey. >http://www.ic.nhs.uk/webfiles/publications/mental%20health/other%20mental%20health%20publications/Adult%20psychiatric%20

morbidity%2007/APMS%2007%20(FINAL)%20Standard.pdf>.

NHSIC (NHS Information Centre), 2011. Attitudes to Mental Illness – 2011 Survey Report. http://www.ic.nhs.uk/webfiles/publications/mental%20health/mental%20health%20act/Mental_illness_report.pdf.

Nielsen, B., Katrakis, E., Raphael, B., 2001. Males and mental health: a public health approach. NSW Public Health Bull. December.

Office of the Deputy Prime Minister, 2004. Mental Health and Social Exclusion: Social Exclusion Unit Report. OPDM Publications, Wetherby.

Office for National Statistics, 2002. The Social and Economic Circumstances of Adults with Mental Disorders. TSO, London.

Office of National Statistics, 2011. Suicide Rates in the United Kingdom, 2000–2009. <http://www.statistics.gov.uk/statbase/Product.asp?vlnk=13618>.

Pinches, A., 2002. Recognising not only consumers' legal rights, but also their 'community entitlements'. From an Address to a Mental Health Legal Centre Workshop at the National Conference of the Federation on Community Legal Centres, Melbourne.

Ramsden, I.M., 2002. Cultural Safety and Nursing Education in Aotearoa and Te Waipounamu. Doctoral thesis, Victoria University, Wellington.

Reitz, J.G., 1995. A Review of the Literature on Aspects of Ethno-Racial Access, Utilization and Delivery of Social Services. Multicultural Coalition for Access to Family Services, Toronto, and the Ontario Ministry of Community and Social Services.

Robinson, C., 2003. Understanding Iterative Homelessness: The Case of People with Mental Disorders. For the Australian Housing and Urban Research Institute. UNSW-UWS Research Centre, New South Wales.

Sainsbury Centre for Mental Health, 2002. Breaking the Circles of Fear. <http://www.centreformentalhealth.org.uk/pdfs/breaking_the_circles_of_fear.pdf>.

SANE Australia, 2000. Better Health Channel. Mental Illness and Violence Explained. http://www.betterhealth.vic.gov.au/bhcv2/bhcarticles.nsf/Mental_illness_and_violence_explained?open.

Speight, S.L., Myers, L.J., Cox, C.I., et al., 1991. A redefinition of multi-cultural counselling. J. Couns. Dev. 70, 29–35.

Spradley, J.P., 1991. Ethnography and culture. In: Worsley, P. (Ed.), The New Modern Sociology Readings. Penguin, London.

Stein-Parbury, J., 2000. Patient and Person. Harcourt, Sydney.

Stern, G., Kruckman, L., 1983. Multi-disciplinary perspectives on post-partum depression: an anthropological critique. Soc. Sci. Med. 17 (15), 1027–1041.

Sue, D.W., Sue, D., 1990. Counselling the Culturally Different. John Wiley & Sons, New York.

World Health Organization, 2001. The World Health Report 2001. Mental Health: New Understanding, New Hope. <http://www.who.int/whr2001/2001/main/en/chapter2/002h4.htm>.

Wright, J., 1991. Counselling at the cultural interface: is getting back to roots enough? J. Adv. Nurs. 16, 92–100.

Chapter | **7** |

Theories on mental health and ill health

Patricia Barkway

CHAPTER POINTS

- The concepts of mental health and mental disorder are complex, distinct entities that are not necessarily mutually exclusive.
- Various subjective factors influence whether human behaviour is perceived as normal or abnormal.
- Community attitudes about mental health and mental health problems contribute to stigma.
- Although personality and human behaviour theories provide explanations for the way in which individuals think, feel and behave, no theory has universal applicability.
- Personality and human behaviour theories underpin psychotherapeutic interventions for mental health problems.

DOI: http://dx.doi.org/10.1016/B978-0-7020-4493-9.00007-X

- Psychological and sociological theories have influenced the development of nursing theories.
- The answer to the nature-versus-nurture debate is not simply 'either/or'. A more plausible explanation is that personality develops as a consequence of the interaction between nature and nurture.

KEY TERMS

- biomedical model
- mental disorder
- mental health
- nature-versus-nurture debate
- nursing theories
- psychological theories
- sociological theories

LEARNING OUTCOMES

The material in this chapter will assist you to:

- describe and critique biomedical, psychological and sociological theories of personality and human behaviour,
- outline how the theories explain both normal and abnormal behaviour,
- understand the concepts of mental health and mental disorder,
- identify a preferred theory of personality development,
- explain the nature-versus-nurture debate,
- describe the contribution of psychological and sociological theories to the development of nursing theories.

INTRODUCTION

Who are you? How have you come to be who you are? What influences how you think, feel and act? Are your personality and behaviour determined by your genetic make-up and biological events, by thoughts and feelings, by your experiences in the world or by an interrelationship between some or all of these? Why are some people seemingly more vulnerable to mental health problems, while others are resilient despite adversity? Most of us, at one time or another, have pondered these questions. Through attempting to understand why humans behave as they do, a further question arises: are personality and human behaviour determined by genetics and biology (nature) or shaped by one's upbringing, experiences and environmental factors (nurture)? This question has long engaged the interest and passion of philosophers, healers

and health professionals and, in more recent times, scientists. Investigation of these questions has resulted in various theories being proposed to explain normal and abnormal behaviour, and mental health and mental disorder. These concepts, the theories that attempt to explain them and proposed interventions will be examined in this chapter. The nature-versus-nurture debate will also be explored.

WHAT IS MENTAL HEALTH?

A succinct, universally applicable definition of mental health has long been elusive. Although contemporary definitions encapsulate the breadth of factors that contribute to mental health, they are wordy and jargonistic, for example:

> Mental health is a state of emotional and social wellbeing in which the individual can cope with the normal stresses of life and achieve his or her potential. It includes being able to work productively and contribute to community life. Mental health describes the capacity of individuals and groups to interact, inclusively and equitably, with one another and with their environment in ways that promote subjective wellbeing, and optimise opportunities for development and the use of mental abilities.

(Australian Health Ministers, 2003, p. 5)

In the 1980s, Doona suggested that the problem of defining mental health was derived from the fact that the concept of health is not a measurable scientific term; she concluded that 'health is probably a value judgement and more amenable to philosophical analysis' (Doona, 1982, p. 13). Her comment remains pertinent today. Two decades later, Sainsbury (2003) draws a parallel between mental health and happiness. Although this is a seemingly simplistic comparison, Sainsbury does not see happiness as an individual pursuit, but rather a consequence of political and social factors that, in the main, remain outside the direct control of the individual.

Defining mental health

Initial attempts to define mental health have focused on the individual's ability to incorporate external factors. Kittleson cited four major components, namely high self-esteem, effective decision-making, values awareness and expressive communication skills (Kittleson, 1989, pp. 40–41). Kittleson's depiction of mental health as a positive construct separate from mental disorder was welcome but limited. It was welcome because it enabled mental health to be viewed as more than merely the absence of the symptoms of mental disorder. It was limited because a focus on individual factors implies individual responsibility, which may lead to victim blaming (McMurray, 2007; Talbot and Verrinder, 2005). Furthermore, a definition in terms of the individual fails to acknowledge the contribution of social factors and the environment to mental health.

In 1993, Raphael drew attention to contextual and social issues that affect mental health, namely workplace factors, education and macroeconomic and other forces. These social forces are acknowledged as contributors to mental health, as are personal qualities such as resilience, coping, physical health and wellbeing (Raphael, 1993). Contemporary definitions of mental health include social determinants such as social connectedness, acceptance of diversity, freedom from discrimination, and economic participation (Vic Health, 2003; Wilkinson and Marmot, 2003). Recognition of social determinants is evident in Friedli's (2001) framework for mental health promotion, which aims to:

- develop people's coping and general life skills,
- promote social support networks ; for example, to tackle bullying, support bereaved families, facilitate self-help groups and increase opportunities to participate in the community,
- address structural barriers to mental health in areas such as education, employment and housing (Friedli, 2001).

The emergence of a definition of mental health that encompasses positive constructs, not just the absence of symptoms, is important because it enables mental health and mental disorder to be viewed as distinct from each other, and not as two points at opposite ends of a continuum. Significantly, it means that the two states are not mutually exclusive. A person can enjoy mental health regardless of whether or not they are diagnosed with a mental disorder if they have a positive sense of self, personal and social support with which to respond to life's challenges, have meaningful relationships with others and have access to employment and recreation activities, sufficient financial resources and suitable living arrangements.

'Mental health' as a euphemism for 'mental disorder'

Health professionals and the health literature have adopted the practice of using the terms *mental health* and *mental disorder* interchangeably. In 1989 Kittleson drew attention to this phenomenon following an examination of undergraduate mental health texts. He found that 'personality development and emotional illness make up the bulk of mental health coverage in the texts' (1989, p. 40). A recent perusal of contemporary mental health literature found that this practice is still prevalent in texts

and journals (Fontaine, 2004; Forster, 2001; Meadows et al., 2007; Morrison-Valfre, 2005, and journals such as the *International Journal of Mental HealthNursing* and *Issues in Mental HealthNursing*). Although these publications include 'mental health' in their titles, in the main they contain chapters or articles concerning assessment of, and treatments for, mental disorder or mental health problems.

The substitution of the term 'mental health' when referring to 'mental disorder' is a twentieth-century phenomenon that has been carried forward into the new millennium. The first references to 'mental health' being used as an alternative to 'psychiatry' occurred in the UK and the USA in the 1920s. Momentum was gained after World War II, when proponents such as Caplan advocated a shift from treatment of mental disorder to prevention (Evans, 1992, p. 55). In the USA Szasz (1961) argued that mental disorder was a societal ill and not an individual sickness. Amid this debate, legislators worldwide changed the term 'mental disorder' in the names of legislation to 'mental health'. However, this change is nominal because the content of worldwide legislation continues to be concerned with mental disorder, such as the UK Mental Health Act 1983 (amended 2007). However, despite the title of the Act it contains no reference to mental health as a positive concept.

Following legislative name changes, organizations that provided treatment and rehabilitation services to individuals diagnosed with mental disorders also changed their names, replacing words like 'psychiatric' and 'mental illness/disorder' with 'mental health'. Indeed, mental health trusts in the UK continue to use the term 'National Health Service' in their title. Nevertheless, despite the change of name there has been little shift in the focus of the services provided, as they continue to address the needs of people with mental health problems, with minimal focus on mental *health*. This is not to suggest that such services should not be provided; clearly there is a demonstrated need for them and they are not under scrutiny here. Rather, the assertion is that to call them mental health services is a misnomer.

A further consequence of using the euphemism 'mental health' when referring to mental disorder is that this practice may in fact be contributing to the perpetuation of stigma and may have broadened the application of stigma to now include mental *health*. While it is important to acknowledge that the avoidance of the term 'mental illness' might perpetuate the idea that it is something to be hidden or is shameful, describing mental health *problems* as a mental *illness* seems to reinforce the idea that mental distress or mental health problems have a biological origin and are therefore a disease or dysfunction requiring medical explanation and possible treatment. As we shall see from the proceeding discussion, this is but one theory which seeks to account for mental distress.

What is mental *health*? How does it differ from mental *illness/disorder*? How do these terms differ from the concept of mental *health problems?* What are the implications for mental *health* nurses?

THEORIES OF PERSONALITY

Personality theories that develop models to explain human behaviour have long been sought. In addition to curiosity and philosophical enquiry, particular emphasis is placed on identifying the causes of abnormal behaviour so as to develop models for understanding prevention or treatment of mental illness. Explanations can be broadly divided into three paradigms:

- biomedical or biological/physical models,
- psychological models, including psychoanalytic, behavioural, cognitive and humanistic approaches,
- sociological models.

Within these paradigms the following are the major viewpoints to offer a theory of personality development or an explanation of human behaviour:

- biomedical model: proposes that behaviour is influenced by physiology, with normal behaviour occurring when the body is in a state of equilibrium, and abnormal behaviour being a consequence of physical pathology;
- psychoanalytic theory: asserts that behaviour is driven by unconscious processes, and influenced by childhood/developmental conflicts that have either been resolved or remain unresolved;
- behavioural psychology: presents the view that behaviour is influenced by factors external to the individual. Behaviours are learned, depending on whether they are rewarded or not, by association with another event or by imitation;
- cognitive psychology: acknowledges the role of perception and thoughts about oneself, one's individual experience and the environment in influencing behaviour;
- humanistic psychology: focuses on the development of a concept of self and the striving of the individual to achieve personal goals;
- sociological theories: shift the emphasis from the individual to the broader social forces that influence people. This model challenges the notion of individual pathology.

Each of these seemingly disparate perspectives makes a substantial contribution to the understanding of how and why humans think, feel and behave as they do, and thereby identifies opportunities for prevention and treatment of mental illness. Nevertheless, as a comprehensive theory of human behaviour each also has major shortcomings. Let us now look at these theories in more detail.

Biomedical model

Also known as psychobiology or the neuroscience perspective, the biomedical model asserts that *normal* behaviour is a consequence of equilibrium within the body and that *abnormal* behaviour results from pathological bodily or brain function. This is not a new notion: in the fourth century BC the Greek physician Hippocrates attributed mental disorder to brain pathology. His ideas were overshadowed, however, when throughout the Dark Ages and later during the Renaissance thinking and explanations shifted to witchcraft or demonic possession (Alloy et al., 2005; Davison et al., 2004). In the nineteenth century a return to biophysical explanations accompanied the emergence of the public health movement.

In recent times advances in technology have led to increased understanding of organic determinants of behaviour. Research and treatment have focused on four main areas:

- *nervous system disorders*, in particular neurotransmitter disturbance at the synaptic gap between neurons: over 50 neurotransmitters have been identified, 4 of which are implicated in mental illness. These are acetylcholine (Alzheimer's disease), dopamine (schizophrenia), noradrenaline (norepinephrine; mood disorder) and serotonin (mood disorder);
- *structural changes to the brain*: perhaps following trauma or in degenerative disorders such as Huntington's disease;
- *endocrine or gland dysfunction*, as in hypothyroidism: this has a similar presentation to clinical depression, and hormonal changes are considered to be a contributing factor in postnatal depression;
- *familial (genetic) transmission of mental disorders*: twin studies reviewed by Gottesman found the following lifetime risks of developing schizophrenia: general population 1%, one parent 13%, sibling 9%, dizygotic twin 17%, two parents 46%, monozygotic twin 48% (Alloy et al., 2005; Cando and Gottesman, 2000).

Although genetic studies demonstrate a correlation between having a close relative with schizophrenia and the likelihood of developing the disorder, a shared genetic history alone is not sufficient. If genetics were the only aetiological factor, the concordance rate for monozygotic twins could be expected to be 100%. Gottesman's research is important because it supports the diathesis-stress model, a widely held explanation for the development of mental disorder which proposes that constitutional predisposition combined with environmental stress will lead to the development of mental disorders (Alloy et al., 2005).

Critique of the biomedical model

Among treatments that emerge from the biomedical model are medications that alter the function, production and reabsorbtion of neurotransmitters in the synaptic gap. However, evidence that a particular intervention is an effective treatment is not proof of a *causal* link with the illness. Consider a person with insulin-dependent diabetes mellitus, for example. Because this person lacks insulin to metabolize glucose, the condition is managed with regular insulin injections. However, the lack of insulin is a symptom of the disease, not the cause. Whatever caused the pancreas to cease producing insulin is not known, despite the treatment being effective. Similarly, with schizophrenia the relationship between the use of antipsychotic medications, dopamine levels and symptom management is correlational, not causal. Therefore, although antipsychotic medication affects dopamine levels and can be an effective treatment to manage the symptoms of schizophrenia, this does not provide evidence that elevated dopamine levels *caused* the disorder.

Psychoanalytic theory

Sigmund Freud developed the first psychological explanation of human behaviour – psychoanalytic theory – in the late nineteenth century. He placed strong emphasis on the role of unconscious processes in determining human behaviour. Central tenets of the theory are that intrapsychic (generally unconscious) forces, developmental factors and family relationships determine human behaviour. Mental health problems are seen as a consequence of fixation at a particular developmental stage or conflict that has not been resolved.

Sigmund Freud (1856–1939)

Freud was an Austrian neurologist who, in his clinical practice, saw a number of patients with sensory or neurological problems for which he was unable to identify a physiological cause. In the main these patients were middle-class Viennese women. It was from his work with these patients that Freud hypothesized that the cause of their maladies was psychological. From this assumption he developed a personality theory, which he called psychoanalytic theory.

According to Freud the mind is composed of three forces:

- the id: the primitive biological force comprising two basic drives, sexual and aggressive. The id operates on the pleasure principle and seeks to satisfy life-sustaining needs such as food, love and creativity, in addition to sexual gratification;

- the ego: the cognitive component of personality which attempts to use realistic means (the reality principle) to achieve the desires of the id;
- the superego: the internalized moral standards of the society in which one lives. It can be equated to a conscience.

Freud's theory proposes that personality development progresses through four stages throughout childhood. At each stage the child's behaviour is driven by the need to satisfy sexual and aggressive drives via the mouth, anus or genitals. Failure of the child to satisfy these needs at any one of the stages will result in psychological difficulties that are carried into adulthood. For example, unresolved issues at the oral stage can lead to dependency issues in adulthood, and problems in the anal stage may lead to the child later developing obsessive–compulsive traits. Freud's stages of psychosexual development are:

- oral: from birth to about 18 months, where the primary focus of the id is the mouth;
- anal: from approximately 18 months to 3 years, where libido shifts from the mouth to the anus and primary gratification is derived from expelling or retaining faeces;
- phallic: from approximately 3 to 6 years, where gratification of the id occurs through the genitals;
- genital: once the child passes through puberty, sexual urges reemerge, but now they are directed towards another person, not the self as they were at an earlier stage of development;
- latent: Freud proposed that from approximately 6 to 12 years the child goes through a latency phase in which sexual urges are dormant (Alloy et al., 2005; Bond and McConkey, 2001; Davison et al., 2004).

Defence mechanisms

An important contribution of psychoanalytic theory to the understanding of behaviour has been the identification of defence mechanisms and the role they play in mediating anxiety. Defence mechanisms were first described by Freud and later elaborated on by his daughter Anna (Freud, 1966). They are unconscious processes whereby anxiety experienced by the ego is reduced. Commonly used defence mechanisms include:

- repression: the primary defence mechanism and an unconscious process whereby unacceptable impulses/feelings/thoughts are barred from consciousness (e.g. memories of sexual abuse in childhood);
- regression: the avoidance of present difficulties by a reversion to an earlier, less mature way of dealing with the situation (e.g. a toilet-trained child who becomes incontinent following the birth of a sibling);
- denial: the blocking of painful information from consciousness (e.g. not accepting that a loss has occurred);

- projection: the denial of one's own unconscious impulses by attributing them to another person (e.g. when you dislike someone but believe it is the other person who does not like you);
- sublimation: an unconscious process whereby libido is transformed into a more socially acceptable outlet (e.g. creativity, art, sport);
- displacement: the transferring of emotion from the source to a substitute (e.g. a person who is unassertive in an interaction with a supervisor at work and 'kicks the cat' on arriving home);
- rationalization: a rational excuse is used to explain behaviour that may be motivated by an irrational force (e.g. cheating when completing a tax return, with the excuse that 'everyone does it');
- intellectualization/isolation: feelings are cut off from the event in which they occur (e.g. after an unsuccessful job interview the person says, 'I didn't really want the job anyway');
- reaction formation: the development of a personality trait that is the opposite of the original unconscious or repressed trait (e.g. avoiding a friend's partner because you are attracted to that person).

Critique of psychoanalytic theory

Although the notions of unconscious motivations and defence mechanisms are helpful in interpreting behaviours, Freud's version of psychoanalytic theory has not been without its critics. Fellow psychoanalyst Erik Erikson disagreed with Freud's theory of psychosexual stages of development and proposed instead a psychosocial theory in which development occurred throughout the lifespan, not just through childhood as in Freud's model (Erikson, 1963; Santrock, 2007).

The unconscious nature of Freud's concepts and stages renders them difficult to test and therefore there is little evidence to support Freudian theory. Feminists, too, object to Freud's interpretation of the psychological development of women, arguing that there is scant evidence to support the hypothesis that women view their bodies as inferior to men's because they do not have a penis (Alloy et al., 2005).

Behavioural psychology

Behaviourism is a school of psychology founded in the USA by J B Watson in the early twentieth century with the purpose of objectively studying observable human behaviour, as opposed to examining the mind, which was the prevalent psychological method at the time in Europe. The model proposes a *scientific* approach to the study of behaviour, a feature that behaviourists argue is lacking in psychoanalytic theory (and in humanistic psychology, which developed later).

Behaviourism opposes the introspective, structuralist approach of psychoanalysis and emphasizes the importance of the environment in shaping behaviour. The focus is on observable behaviour and conditions that elicit and maintain the behaviour (classical conditioning) or factors that reinforce behaviour (operant conditioning) or vicarious learning through watching and imitating the behaviour of others (modelling).

Three basic assumptions underpin behaviour theory. These are that personality is determined by prior learning, that human behaviour is changeable throughout the lifespan and that changes in behaviour are generally caused by changes in the environment. The following were prominent figures in the development of behaviourist psychology.

Ivan Pavlov (1849–1936)

Russian physiologist Ivan Pavlov was the first to describe the relationship between stimulus and response. Pavlov demonstrated that a dog could learn to salivate (respond) to a nonfood stimulus (a bell) if the bell was simultaneously presented with the food. His discovery became known as classical conditioning.

John B Watson (1878–1958)

Watson, who is attributed with being the founder of behaviourism, changed the focus of psychology from the study of inner sensations to the study of observable behaviour. In his quest to make psychology a true science, Watson further developed Pavlov's work on stimulus–response learning and experimented by manipulating stimulus conditions. Watson believed that abnormal behaviour was the result of earlier faulty conditioning and that reconditioning could modify this.

B F Skinner (1904–90)

Skinner formulated the notion of instrumental or operant conditioning in which reinforcers (rewards) contribute to the probability of a response being either repeated or extinguished. Skinner's research demonstrated that the contingencies on which behaviour is based are external to the person, rather than internal. Consequently, changing contingencies could alter an individual's behaviour. This is an underlying principle in treatment using an operant conditioning approach (Bond and McConkey, 2001; Skinner, 1953).

Critique of behaviourism

Behaviourism provided the first scientifically testable theories of human development as well as plausible explanations of conditions such as depression and anxiety. However, behaviourist explanations are less convincing when applied to psychosis or organic disorders. Furthermore, most behaviourist research has been conducted on animals under laboratory conditions, so to extrapolate findings from this research to humans is mechanistic and does not allow for intrinsic human qualities like creativity or the ability to love, think or solve problems. Finally, behaviourist theory falls short in explaining the success of an individual brought up in an adverse environment, or how mental health problems can occur in a person whose environment is apparently healthy and advantaged.

Cognitive psychology

Since the 1950s, interest in the cognitive or thinking processes involved in behavioural responses has expanded. Cognitive theory proposes that people actively interpret their environment and cognitively construct their world. Therefore, behaviour is a result of the interplay of external and internal events. External events are the stimuli and reinforcements that regulate behaviour, and internal events are one's perceptions and thoughts about the world, as well as one's behaviour in the world. In other words, how one thinks about a situation will influence how one behaves in that situation. The following are prominent figures in the development of cognitive psychology.

Albert Bandura (b. 1925)

According to Bandura it is not intrapsychic or environmental forces alone that influence behaviour. Rather, human behaviour results from the interaction of the environment with the individual's perception and thinking. Self-efficacy, or the belief that one can achieve a certain goal, is the critical component in the achievement of that goal. Bandura also proposed that consequences do not have to be directly experienced by the individual for learning to occur; learning can occur vicariously through the process of modelling or learning by imitation (Bandura, 2001; Santrock, 2007).

Aaron T Beck (b. 1921)

Problem behaviour, says Beck, results from cognitive distortions or faulty thinking. For example, a depressed person will selectively choose information that maintains a gloomy perspective. Depression is experienced when one has a negative schema about oneself or one's situation. According to Beck, depression is a behavioural response to an attitude or cognition of hopelessness, as opposed to hopelessness being a symptom of depression; and anxiety is experienced when one has a distorted anticipation of danger. Treatment within Beck's model involves changing one's views about oneself and one's life situation (Beck, 1972).

Martin Seligman (b. 1942)

Seligman first proposed his theory of learned helplessness as an explanation for depression. The theory suggests that if an individual experiences adversity and attempts to alleviate the situation are unsuccessful, then depression follows. Seligman later expanded his model to include learned optimism, a process of challenging negative cognitions to change from a position of passivity to one of control (Seligman, 1974, 1994).

Critique of cognitive psychology

The therapeutic techniques derived from cognitive (and cognitive behavioural) theory are practical and effective, and can be self-administered by the service user under the direction of a therapist. These therapies have an established record in changing problem behaviours such as phobias, obsessions and compulsions, and in stress management (Carson et al., 1996). They also make a contribution in the treatment of depression and schizophrenia (Johnston, 1998; Seligman, 1994). Nevertheless, cognitive theory is criticized as being unscientific (as are psychoanalytic and humanistic theories) because mental processes cannot objectively be observed and subjective reports are not necessarily reliable (Alloy et al., 2005, pp. 115–116). Additionally, the insight that one's thinking is the cause of one's problems will not in itself bring about behaviour change.

Finally, contrary to the proposal that thoughts cause feelings, which cause behaviour (a notion that underpins the cognitive approach), research conducted by Wishman suggests that, in the treatment of depression, cognitive changes follow changes in emotion and behaviour (Wishman, cited in Alloy et al., 2005, p. 116). Wishman's findings can be explained by the relational model of Ivey and Ivey in which thoughts, feelings and behaviour interact with each other and with meaning, in contrast to the linear unidirectional explanation of cognitive psychology. The thrust of the interactive model of Ivey and Ivey is that 'a change in any one part of the system may result in a change in other parts as well' (Ivey and Ivey, 2003, p. 253). So while cognitions play an integral part in behavioural outcomes, they may not necessarily be the initiating factor as proposed by cognitive theory.

Humanistic psychology

Following disenchantment with the existing psychological theories of the time, Charlotte Bühler, Abraham Maslow, Carl Rogers and their colleagues in the USA established the Association for Humanistic Psychology in 1962. Humanistic psychology has its intellectual and social roots in philosophical humanism and existentialism, which brought psychology back to a close relationship with philosophy (Bühler and Allen, 1972). This school of psychology, which became known as the Third Force, arose in response to dissatisfaction at the time with the mechanistic approach of psychoanalysis and behaviourism and the negative views that underpinned both these theoretical perspectives.

Humanist psychologists objected to the determinism of the two prevailing theories: psychoanalysis, with its emphasis on unconscious drives, and behaviourism, which saw the environment as central in shaping behaviour. Humanistic psychology rejected the reductionism of explaining human behaviour, feelings, thinking and motivation merely in terms of psychological mechanisms or biological processes. It also opposed the mechanistic approach of behaviourism and psychoanalysis for the way in which they minimized human experience and qualities such as choice, creativity and spontaneity.

Humanistic psychologists focused on the intrinsic human qualities of the individual, such as free will, altruism, freedom and self-actualization, qualities which, they asserted, distinguished humans from other animals. Humanistic psychology therefore differed from its predecessors in its emphasis on the whole person, human emotions, experience and the meaning of experience, the creative potential of the individual, choice, self-realization and self-actualization. The theory also opposed dualistic (subject/object, mind/body splits), deterministic, reductionistic and mechanistic explanations of human behaviour.

The humanistic movement also reflected a historical trend in Western industrialized cultures at that time, which was to be interested in the worth of the individual and the meaning of life, and to be concerned about the rise of bureaucracy, the threat of nuclear war, the growing emphasis on scientific/positivist paradigms, alienation of the individual and consequent loss of identity in mass society. This led to humanistic psychology being aligned with existentialism as well as being associated with the human potential movements of the 1960s and 1970s, the legacy of which can be seen today in individual and group counselling approaches. Humanistic psychology also played a part in the growing interest in qualitative research methods, which seek to understand the experience of the individual and the meaning of the experience, such as phenomenology (Crotty, 1996). The following were prominent figures in the development of humanistic psychology.

Charlotte Bühler (1893–1974)

Bühler distinguished her theory from Freudian psychoanalysis with the thesis that development was lifelong, goals were personally selected and that the individual was searching for meaning in life beyond one's own existence. She maintained that self-fulfillment was the key to human development and that this was achieved by living constructively, establishing a personal value system,

setting goals and reviewing progress to thereby realize one's potential. Throughout the lifespan, according to Bühler, individuals strive to achieve four basic human tendencies, which are to:

- satisfy one's need for sex, love and recognition,
- engage in self-limiting adaptation in order to fit in, belong and feel secure,
- express oneself through creative achievements,
- uphold and restore order so as to be true to one's values and conscience (Bühler and Allen, 1972; Ragsdale, 2003).

Carl Rogers (1902–87)

Rogers proposed a more hopeful and optimistic view of humankind than that of his psychoanalytic and behaviourist contemporaries. He believed that each person contained within themselves the potential for healthy, creative growth. According to Rogers, the failure to achieve one's potential resulted from constricting and distorting influences of poor parenting, education or other social pressures. Client-centred therapy is the counselling model that Rogers developed to assist the individual to overcome these harmful effects and take responsibility for their life (Rogers, 1951, 1961).

Abraham Maslow (1908–70)

As a frequently cited author in the nursing literature, Maslow is renowned for his theory of human needs. This is often presented as a triangular figure with physiological needs at the base and self-actualization at the apex. Maslow, like Bühler and Rogers, premised his theory on the notion that human beings are intrinsically good and that human behaviour is motivated by a drive for self-actualization. Maslow identifies three categories of human need:

- fundamental needs:
  - physiological (hunger, thirst and sex),
  - safety (security and freedom from danger);
- psychological needs:
  - belongingness and love (connection with others, to be accepted and to belong),
  - self-esteem (to achieve, be competent, gain approval and recognition);
- self-actualization needs:
  - to achieve one's innate potential (Gething et al., 2004; Maslow, 1968).

Critique of humanistic psychology

Intuitively, humanistic psychology appeals as a positive, optimistic view of humankind with its focus on personal growth, not disorder. However, this can also be a criticism, in that as a theory humanistic psychology is naive and incomplete. If humans are driven by a need to achieve their best and to live harmoniously with others, as Bühler, Rogers and Maslow suggest, how does this account for disturbed states like depression, or antisocial behaviour like assault? Humanistic concepts can be difficult to define objectively, thereby posing a challenge for scientific investigation of the theory. Finally, there is little recognition of unconscious drives in explaining behaviour, which limits the ability of the theory to contribute to an understanding of abnormal or antisocial behaviour.

Sociological models

Sociological theories differ from psychological theories in that they do not seek explanations for individual behaviour; rather, they examine societal factors for their influence on the behaviour of its members. Sociologists propose that the causes of abnormal behaviour lie not in the individual's mind, but in the broader social forces of the society in which the individual lives. Demographic factors for which patterns of mental ill health are observed include:

- age: younger people are more likely to suffer from eating disorders;
- gender: the suicide rate for men is higher than for women, although the rate for attempted suicide is higher for women than for men;
- socioeconomic status: poverty is associated with poorer physical and mental health outcomes;
- marital status: depression and alcohol problems are more prevalent in people who have never married or are divorced, than among people who are married.

The following social commentators propose interpretations of mental disorder that challenge the notion of individual pathology.

Emile Durkheim (1858–1917)

Durkheim's classic study of suicide led him to postulate a societal rather than an individual explanation for this phenomenon. He argued that suicide was not an individual act, but that it could be understood in terms of the bonds that exist between the person and society, or the regulation of the individual by social norms. Durkheim's analysis of suicide statistics found that suicide was more prevalent in groups where the bond between the individual and the group was overly weak or strong, or where the regulation of individual desires and aspirations by societal norms was either inadequate or excessive. According to Durkheim there are four types of suicide:

- egoistic, where the social bonds of attachment are weak and the individual is less integrated into the social group and therefore not bound by its obligations (for example, unmarried men);
- altruistic, where the social bonds of attachment are overly strong and the individual's sense of self is not distinguished from the group: the individual may be driven to suicide by a commitment to the group (for example, suicide bombers);
- anomic, where regulation of the individual's desires and aspirations is not adequate. This can occur in a society undergoing rapid change, which dislocates social norms, as has been the experience of manufacturing workers where a factory has been a large employer within a community who have had to adjust to the change in their social and economic circumstances as a result of the economic downturn;
- fatalistic, where there is overregulation by society, which renders a sense of powerlessness in the individual and predisposes the person to suicide (for example, deaths in custody) (Cheek et al., 1996, pp. 8–12).

Thomas Szasz (b. 1920)

Since the 1960s, prominent psychiatrist Thomas Szasz has challenged the concept of 'mental illness', arguing that disease implies a pathology which often cannot be objectively identified (Szasz, 1961, 2000). He attacks the biomedical model, claiming that its purpose is to give control over people's lives to psychiatrists, and argues that psychiatrists exercise coercive domination in the guise of protecting the public and the mad from their madness (Szasz, 2000, pp. 44–45). Contrary to the illusion that psychiatry is coping well with society's vexing problems, Szasz claims that social problems are in fact being obfuscated and aggravated by the disease interpretation of psychiatry (Szasz, 2000, p. 53).

Critique of sociological models

Sociological models identify vulnerable populations and also biases that influence diagnosis and treatment. It is important to note, however, that although social factors are associated with better or poorer mental health outcomes, the relationships are correlational and cannot be assumed to be in themselves causative. Nevertheless, the contribution of population statistics and social demographic data remains significant and as the World Health Organization (2002, p. 9) in its document *Prevention and Promotion in Mental Health* suggests:

> *The determinants of mental health include not only factors related to actions by individuals, such as behaviours and lifestyles, coping skills, and good interpersonal relationships, but also social and environmental factors like income, social status, education, employment, housing and working conditions, access to appropriate health services, and good physical health.*

By demonstrating links between protective factors for mental health and risk factors for mental ill health, potential areas for prevention and intervention are thereby identified.

CRITICAL THINKING CHALLENGE 7.2

Identify factors that influence whether a particular behaviour (e.g. hearing voices) would be considered normal or a symptom of mental ill health.

Compare and contrast two theories of personality development with regard to how each theory explains:

◆ mental health,
◆ mental ill health.

How do sociological theories differ from psychological theories of personality development and human behaviour?

Table 7.1 Production of a conditioned response

UCS	+ CS	= CR
Anxiety-producing event	+ Public place	= Anxiety response
	Public place	= Anxiety response

CR, conditioned response; CS, conditioned stimulus; UCS, unconditioned stimulus.

FROM THEORY TO PRACTICE

Psychological personality theories and sociological perspectives provide plausible explanations of human behaviour in specific situations. These theories inform therapeutic interventions and treatments of mental health problems. It must be noted, though, that in the main the theories outlined were developed in Western Europe and the USA, and therefore may not be applicable outside those contexts. Consequently, caution is recommended regarding the applicability of treatments derived from these theories to other populations, such as people of non-English-speaking backgrounds.

Nevertheless, theories have clinical application. For example, the development of agoraphobia (fear of leaving a safe environment) can be explained by classical or respondent conditioning as described by Pavlov and Watson. Consider a situation in which an anxiety-producing event or unconditioned stimulus (UCS) may have occurred in a public place alongside a conditioned (originally neutral) stimulus (CS). Pairing of the UCS and CS can lead to a situation in which the CS alone is sufficient to produce the conditioned response (CR). Hence the anxiety response is learned through the process of classical conditioning (see Table 7.1).

Maintenance of the anxiety response, however, cannot be explained by classical conditioning because the theory predicts that the repeated occurrence of the CS in the absence of the UCS will diminish or extinguish the behaviour (Bond and McConkey, 2001, p. 4.8). Nevertheless, learning theory in the form of operant conditioning does provide an explanation for the continuation of agoraphobic behaviours. Operant or instrumental conditioning predicts that behaviour is controlled by its consequences (Skinner, 1953). If a behaviour is rewarded (positive reinforcement) it is likely to be repeated. Also, if a behaviour leads to the removal of an aversive stimulus (negative reinforcement) then it is likely to be repeated. If, however, a behaviour is ignored or punished, the theory predicts that it will lead to extinction of the behaviour. For example, if an individual experiences anxiety in a public place and that anxiety is reduced by withdrawal to a safe environment (frequently the home) then negative reinforcement is in operation. The likelihood of withdrawal behaviour occurring again is thereby increased because the individual has been rewarded by a reduction in anxiety. This interpretation of agoraphobic behaviour suggests that the disorder is not so much a fear of open or public places, but a fear of the anxiety one might experience away from the safe environment.

Behavioural treatment of agoraphobia can use classical or operant conditioning strategies or both. An example of a classical conditioning strategy is the repeated exposure of the person to the anxiety-provoking situation with the goal of extinguishing the anxiety response. Operant conditioning involves the person being rewarded for engaging in activities that would normally produce a panic response for that person.

The biomedical model provides an alternative interpretation of agoraphobia and consequently its approach to treatment. This approach identifies the symptoms (anxiety and panic) as the problem. Hence, the focus of treatment from a biomedical perspective is to control the anxiety and panic attack experienced by the individual, with less emphasis on identifying the cause. Treatment would include the prescription of anxiolytic or antidepressant medications.

Cognitive theory poses yet another explanation of agoraphobia. It suggests that people who experience panic attacks interpret the physical symptoms of anxiety as catastrophic (palpitations are believed to be a heart attack) and respond accordingly (Bond and McConkey, 2001, p. 8.32). Intervention would focus on challenging and reframing these faulty perceptions.

In practice, though, behavioural, cognitive and biomedical interventions are generally used concurrently in what is referred to as an eclectic approach (Treatment Protocol Project, 2000).

CASE STUDY: KARIN

Karin is a 42-year-old woman who lives in an inner-city London borough with her partner Scott and their three children, Jordan (12 years), Sally (10 years) and Amelia (5 years). Following Jordan's birth, Karin continued to work half-time as an accountant. She has not worked since the birth of Sally 10 years previously.

Recently, Karin contacted an agoraphobic self-help phone counselling service to seek assistance. Her phone call was prompted by the prospect of the family relocating to Auckland, New Zealand, due to Scott being offered a promotion. Karin is terrified about moving because she has not left the family home for the past 3 years. Nevertheless, she wants to support Scott because he has unquestionably been her mainstay over the past 5 years since she developed agoraphobia.

Karin vividly remembers her first panic attack, although she did not recognize it as such at the time. It was early December, Amelia was a baby, and Karin was Christmas shopping at a large suburban shopping centre. Unexpectedly, she received a call on her mobile telephone informing her that her mother had been involved in a motor vehicle accident and was not expected to live. Karin remembers feeling cold, sweaty and as though her heart would jump out of her chest at the time; she immediately went home.

Karin's next visit to the shopping centre was during the January sales. On entering the crowded mall she was overwhelmed by a sense of foreboding and clamminess, and experienced extreme palpitations. She believed that she was having a heart attack and that she would die. A shopkeeper came to her assistance and called an ambulance. At the hospital accident and emergency department a doctor

explained to Karin that she had experienced a panic attack, not a heart attack. She was advised to breathe into a paper bag if this occurred again, and was prescribed oxazepam to take should her anxiety become extreme. Karin found that taking the oxazepam prior to an outing helped her to cope, so she continued to obtain prescriptions from her general practitioner.

Karin did not return to this particular shopping centre again. She began shopping at a nearby open mall complex where she knew she could quickly return to her car should the need arise. About 6 months after the first two panic attacks Karin experienced a further one at her local 'safe' supermarket. Her trolley was full of groceries, the queue was long and there was only one checkout open when, for no apparent reason, Karin suddenly felt she could not breathe and the palpitations returned. She departed immediately, leaving the trolley with the weekly shopping in the aisle. She has not shopped there since, telling Scott she was too embarrassed to return.

Following this event, Karin was selective about outings away from home. 'What if it happens again?' she worried. She needed to know that she could leave immediately, if necessary. Consequently, she limited outings away from home to places she knew and could leave quickly. Gradually, over the next 18 months, Karin stopped going out at all. Currently, Scott and Jordan manage the shopping, Jordan walks the younger children to and from school and Scott attends parent/teacher meetings and other events at the children's school. Their family and friends are always happy to socialize at Karin's and Scott's home because it is centrally located, and Karin is an excellent cook. Everything was fine until Scott was offered a promotion!

CRITICAL THINKING CHALLENGE 7.3

After reading Karin's case study, consider her experience in the light of cognitive and behavioural theory.

♦ How might other theoretical positions explain Karin's experience?
♦ What interventions to assist Karin would be indicated within each of these theoretical models?

Theories of psychology, sociology and nursing

During the 1980s and 1990s nursing education moved into universities following a similar move by American nurses in the 1950s. As a consequence, teachers of nursing were required to have graduate (and often postgraduate) education in addition to their nursing qualifications. Nurses undertook this study in the already established academic areas of anthropology, philosophy, education, psychology and sociology. Postgraduate study in these fields subsequently influenced the development of the thinking of many nursing theorists (Condon, 2000, pp. 104–105).

The first generation of nursing theories to emerge since the 1950s was a synthesis of ideas about nursing practice and psychological/sociological theory. For instance, Madeline Leininger integrated anthropological studies with clinical nursing practice to develop her theory of transcultural nursing (King and Averis, 2000, p. 181). In mental health nursing, Hildegard Peplau acknowledged the influence of the work of psychoanalyst Harry Stack Sullivan on her thinking and clinical practice (Peplau, 1988). Jocelyn Lawler developed her nursing theory about the body in nursing from her postgraduate studies in sociology (Condon, 2000, p. 122).

Also evident in the writing of nurse theorists is the influence of humanistic psychology. Maslow's human needs are embraced within models of care such as those proposed by Leininger, Parse, Orem and Watson (Greenwood, 2000; Marriner-Tomey and Alligood, 2002). So, too, are existentialist and phenomenological thought incorporated in Parse's theory of Human Becoming and Travelbee's model of Human-to-Human Relationship (Daly, 2000, p. 215; Travelbee, 1971). However, it is in the field of mental health nursing that the influence of psychological and sociological thought is most obvious, as seen in the theories of the following prominent mental health nurses.

Hildegard Peplau (1909–99)

Peplau is acknowledged as the mother of mental health nursing, and is also recognized as the first nursing author to use theory from other scientific fields in developing a theory of nursing (Marriner-Tomey and Alligood, 2002, p. 24). Peplau's Interpersonal Theory of Nursing is specific to practice, making it a mid-range theory, as distinct from a grand theory with broader applicability, like those of Orem and Roy, or a philosophy as espoused by earlier nursing writers such as Nightingale or Henderson (Marriner-Tomey and Alligood, 2002).

Peplau's seminal text, *Interpersonal Relations in Nursing*, was first published in 1952 and outlines the therapeutic relationship between the nurse and the service user. According to Peplau, the nurse does not perform therapy on the service user, but rather, the nurse *is* the therapy. This heralded a shift in nursing practice from *doing to* a service user to *being with* a service user (Doona, 1982, p. 9). Further legacies of Peplau's theory have been the valuing of teaching and learning about relationship skills in nursing curricula and practice, and a focus on the study of clinical phenomena as a nursing concern (Sills, cited in Werner O'Toole and Rouslin Welt, 1989).

In developing her theory, Peplau's thinking was influenced not only by the nursing discourse of her time, but also by several psychological clinicians, including the psychoanalyst Harry Stack Sullivan, humanistic psychologist Abraham Maslow and the social learning theorist Neal Miller. Sullivan's influence on Peplau's writing can be seen in her valuing of the individual, the intrapersonal (subjective experience) and the interpersonal (relationships). Peplau viewed utilization of the psychological model as enabling nurses 'to move away from a disease orientation to one whereby the psychological meaning of events, feelings and behaviours could be incorporated in nursing interventions' (Peplau 1996, cited in Howk, 2002, p. 381).

Joyce Travelbee (1926–73)

Travelbee's Human-to-Human Relationship model is underpinned by the assumption that the purpose of nursing is achieved through the establishment of a nurse–service user relationship (Travelbee, 1971, p. 16). Her theory extended the work of Peplau and Orlando on interpersonal relations in nursing and incorporated existential ideas concerning meaning, from the writings of Victor Frankl (Marriner-Tomey and Alligood, 2002, p. 419). Travelbee viewed the purpose of nursing as not only assisting the service user, family or community to prevent or cope with illness and suffering but also, if necessary, to find meaning in the experience (Travelbee, 1971, p. 7). Travelbee's emphasis on the emotional and psychological aspects of nursing, such as caring, empathy and rapport, is also consistent with the writings of humanistic psychologist Carl Rogers, in his model of client-centred therapy (Rogers, 1951; Travelbee, 1971) and is a contemporary influence in the field of palliative care nursing.

Phil Barker (b. 1946)

From his clinical research, mental health nurse and psychotherapist Phil Barker developed an interdisciplinary model of care, called the Tidal Model, which seeks to reveal solutions rather than solve problems. Central tenets of Barker's model include empowerment of the individual and humanistic notions of being human and helping one another. Underpinning the model are the key principles of:

- active collaboration between the mental health clinician, the individual and family in the planning and delivery of care,
- the development and use of a care plan which is centred on the individual's experience, thus empowering the person,
- the provision of nursing care in a multidisciplinary context,
- the use of narrative-based interventions, all of which form the basis of problem resolution and mental health promotion.

Barker acknowledges several influences in the development of the Tidal Model, including his studies of philosophy and psychology in the 1960s; an initial interest in psychoanalytic, then later behavioural, cognitive and family therapies; and the work of the radical psychiatrist R D Laing. Also significant in the development of the model were the seminal writings and mentorship of Annie Altschul and Hildegard Peplau from nursing. Together, these influences contributed to Barker's development of an enduring interest in humanistic approaches and ultimately to the development of the Tidal Model, with its focus on assisting the person to find meaning in their experience (Barker, 2000, 2001; Fletcher and Stevenson, 2001).

CRITICAL THINKING CHALLENGE 7.4

What role did psychological theories play in the development of mental health nursing theories?
What contribution do mental health nursing theories make to nursing practice?

PERSONALITY AND BEHAVIOUR: NATURE VERSUS NURTURE

Who or what is responsible for personality and human development: heredity or the environment? Philosophers have long debated this issue, though scientific interest is more recent, dating from the work of Galton, the nineteenth-century British pioneer in the study of individual differences. Galton is reportedly credited with proposing the immortal phrase, 'nature versus nurture' (Gottesman, 1997; Schaffner, 2001, p. 2). The ensuing debate resulted in a proliferation of philosophical discussion about, and scientific investigation into, the effects of biological phenomena and inheritance (nature) and the individual's environment and experiences in the world (nurture).

Theoretical perspectives on nature versus nurture

The theories discussed in this chapter place varied emphasis on whether hereditary or environmental factors play a more important role in personality development, human behaviour and mental disorder. Behaviourism and cognitive psychology advocate for the environment and factors external to the individual, as does the sociological perspective, though for different reasons. The biomedical model argues for a nature explanation, while psychoanalytic theory and humanistic psychology acknowledge the contribution of both. The psychoanalytic concept of the id, for instance, is biological but it interacts with the environment in personality development. In humanistic psychology the need to achieve one's potential is considered to be innate, but the eventual outcome is influenced by one's experiences in the world.

Nature *or* nurture?

There is an abundance of evidence to support an interactive explanation of nature and nurture rather than the answer being found in the 'either/or' proposal (Santrock, 2007; Schaffner, 2001). Despite this, some commentators and theorists continue to advocate for the relative importance of one over the other, notably exponents of the biomedical model for nature, and behaviourism for nurture.

Evidence to support a genetic or nature position can be found in family, twin and adoptee studies. Research over the past 20 years demonstrates that personality, behaviour and mental disorder do have a genetic component (Gottesman, 1991; Schaffner, 2001). Findings from studies into the heritability of intelligence (IQ) offer the most convincing nurture evidence. An American, British and Swedish study of 240 octogenarian twins found the heritability of IQ to be 62% (Gottesman, 1997). In the Colorado Adoption Project a correlation was found between the IQ of adopted adolescents and their birth parents, but no relationship was found between the IQ of adopted adolescents and their adoptive parents. The researchers concluded that the environment in which the young person was reared had little impact on cognitive ability.

In the case of schizophrenia, however, heredity accounts for less than 50% of the predictability of the disorder. Genetic inheritance is only a partial influence, with the environment accounting for the rest (Plomin, cited in Azar, 1997). Gottesman's research found that even when an identical twin had a diagnosis of schizophrenia, the likelihood of the other twin not having a similar diagnosis of schizophrenia was 52% (Gottesman, 1991). In addition, 63% of people diagnosed with schizophrenia do not have a first- or second-degree relative with the condition (Schaffner, 2001). It is clearly evident, therefore, that factors in addition to one's genetic inheritance influence whether the disorder manifests. Such factors, it is assumed, can be found in the environment.

Gottesman's research assumes that siblings reared together share the same environment. Schaffner (2001) recommends caution in presuming this, as different siblings in the same family do not necessarily experience exactly the same environment. Siblings do share many experiences such as the same parents, social class and home environment. However, other experiences are unique to the individual and not shared by siblings. This nonshared environment can include such experiences as birth trauma, illness and different schooling. Significantly, it appears that it is the nonshared environment that accounts for most of the environmental influence on a child's personality and mood (Santrock, 2007).

Nature *and* nurture

An individual's personality does not develop without a genetic inheritance, nor can it develop in the absence of influences from experience and the environment. How then can the nature-versus-nurture debate be resolved?

Gestalt psychology, founded by Fritz Perls (1893–1970) in the 1960s, comprises humanistic and existentialist elements, and offers a model for understanding the nature-versus-nurture debate: that is, to view personality development as a *gestalt*. There is no exact English equivalent for this German term, but it loosely translates as 'a meaningful, organized whole' that is more than the sum of its parts (Perls et al., 1973, p. 16). Consider a cake, for example: flour, eggs, milk and sugar are its basic ingredients, but the product or gestalt bears no resemblance to any of the original ingredients. Yet each of the ingredients is vital to the final product, as is the process of cooking. Leave out the sugar and it will not taste like a cake; omit the heating process and it will not have the texture of a cake.

Considering human development as a gestalt means that neither nature nor nurture can be considered in isolation from the other. The process of their interaction and the context in which they interact are significant. Attributing a relative value of one over the other serves no purpose. Both nature and nurture are vital, inseparable, interdependent components of personality development that also influence human behaviour and whether or not one develops mental health problems.

CRITICAL THINKING CHALLENGE 7.5

How useful is the nature-versus-nurture debate in understanding personality development and human behaviour, and why?

Investigate four contemporary psychotherapeutic interventions. Which theories inform these therapies, and how?

CONCLUSION

The theoretical perspectives discussed in this chapter provide complementary, overlapping and at times contradictory theories of personality development and human behaviour, and explanations for mental health and mental ill health. Yet despite individual theories being able to provide plausible explanations for specific behaviours in both normal and abnormal contexts, no theory alone is sufficient to explain all human behaviour, or a single behaviour in all circumstances. Some theories offer a nature, others a nurture, explanation, and yet others incorporate both. Even when a specific theory provides convincing evidence to support a nature or nurture explanation, such evidence is generally correlational, and therefore cannot be considered causative. Consequently, in seeking to identify factors that influence personality development and human behaviour, particularly in relation to mental health and mental disorder, it is evident that the answer will not be found in asking the nature-or-nurture question, but rather in investigating *how the nature is nurtured*.

EXERCISES FOR CLASS ENGAGEMENT

In small groups discuss the stigma associated with mental *health* and mental *ill health*.

- Identify factors that contribute to stigma.
- Consider how stigma might affect nursing care.
- Devise strategies to address stigma.
- Provide feedback to the rest of the class.

Students should complete Critical Thinking Challenge 7.1 prior to commencing a course of study in mental health.

- Compare and contrast pre- and postcourse responses in small groups.
- If attitudes have changed, identify influences that could account for the changes.
- Repeat this activity on completion of the course.

Reread the case study on Karin and debate the following statement: 'Behaviourist theory provides the best explanation of Karin's agoraphobia.'

In small groups discuss the following questions.

- What contribution can theories make to mental health promotion?
- What contribution can theories make to mental ill health prevention, early intervention, treatment and rehabilitation?

- What contribution do theories make to nursing practice? Provide feedback and debriefing to the rest of the class.

Prior to the tutorial, each student should interview either a registered nurse or a person with a mental health problem regarding their views on:

- what contributes to the development of their problems,
- what enables an individual to cope with or overcome their problems,
- what factors might hinder an individual's recovery from a mental health problem,
- what advice the person can give to nurses about caring for a person with a mental health problem.

Then, in small groups, discuss the following.

- What key issues emerged in the interview?
- Compare and contrast professional responses with that of the person who has experienced mental health problems.
- Discuss lay and professional interpretations of mental health problems in light of relevant theories.
- Identify students' learning with regard to nursing a person with a mental health problem.

Provide feedback and debriefing to the rest of the class.

REFERENCES

Alloy, L., Riskin, J., Manos, M., 2005. Abnormal Psychology: Current Perspectives, ninth ed. McGraw-Hill, New York.

Australian Health Ministers, 2003. National Mental Health Plan 2003–2008. Australian Government Department of Health and Ageing, Canberra.

Azar, B., 1997. Nature, Nurture: Not Mutually Exclusive. American Psychological Association. <http://www.snc.edu/psych/korshavn/natnur02.htm>.

Bandura, A., 2001. Social cognitive theory. Annu. Rev. Psychol. 52, 1–26.

Barker, P., 2000. Clan unity: mental health recovery and reclamation. <http://www.clan-unity.co.uk/philbarkerbiog.htm>.

Barker, P., 2001. The Tidal Model: the lived experience in person-centered mental health nursing care. Nurs. Philos. 2 (3), 213–223.

Beck, A., 1972. Depression: Causes and Treatment. University of Pennsylvania Press, Philadelphia.

Bond, N., McConkey, K., 2001. Psychological Science: An Introduction. McGraw-Hill, Sydney.

Bühler, C., Allen, M., 1972. Introduction to Humanistic Psychology. Brooks/Cole, CA.

Cando, A., Gottesman, I.I., 2000. Twin studies of schizophrenia: from bow-and-arrow concordances to star wars Mx and functional genomics. Am. J. Med. Genet. 97 (1), 12–17.

Carson, R., Butcher, J., Mineka, S., 1996. Abnormal Psychology and Modern Life. Harper Collins College, New York.

Cheek, J., Shoebridge, J., Willis, E., et al., 1996. Society and Health: Social Theory for Health Workers. Longman, Sydney.

Condon, J., 2000. Changing conceptions in nurse theorising: historical and social perspectives in the United States of America and Australia. In: Greenwood, J. (Ed.), Nursing Theory in Australia: Development and Application. Prentice Hall Health, Australia.

Crotty, M., 1996. Phenomenology and Nursing Research. Churchill Livingstone, Sydney.

Daly, J., 2000. Parse's human becoming school of thought. In: Greenwood, J. (Ed.), Nursing Theory in Australia: Development and Application. Prentice Hall Health, Australia.

Davison, G., Neale, J., Kring, A., 2004. Abnormal Psychology, ninth ed. Wiley, New York.

Doona, M., 1982. Travelbee's Intervention in Psychiatric Nursing, second ed. F A Davis, Philadelphia.

Erikson, E., 1963. Childhood and Society, second ed. WW Norton, New York.

Evans, J., 1992. Healthy minds: what is mental health and how can we promote it? Nurs. Times 88 (16), 54–56.

Fletcher, E., Stevenson, C., 2001. Launching the Tidal Model in an adult acute mental health programme. Nurs. Stand. 15 (49), 33–36.

Fontaine, K., 2004. Mental Health Nursing. Prentice Hall, NJ.

Forster, S., 2001. The Role of the Mental Health Nurse. Nelson Thornes, Cheltenham.

Freud, A., 1966. The Ego and the Mechanisms of Defense. International Universities Press, New York.

Friedli, L., 2001. Mental health promotion: coming in from the cold. Health Dev. Today 5, 9–11.

Gething, L., Papalia, D., Olds, S., 2004. Lifespan Development, second Australian ed. McGraw-Hill, Sydney.

Gottesman, I.I., 1991. Schizophrenia Genesis: The Origins of Madness. Freeman, New York.

Gottesman, I.I., 1997. Twins: en route to QTLs for cognition. Science 277 (5318), 1522–1523.

Greenwood, J. (Ed.), 2000. Nursing Theory in Australia: Development and Application. Prentice Hall Health, Australia.

Howk, C., 2002. Hildegard E Peplau: psychodynamic nursing. In: Marriner-Tomey, A., Alligood, R.M. (Eds.), Nursing Theorists and their Work, fifth ed. Mosby, St Louis.

International Journal of Mental Health Nursing, 2001–present. Blackwell Science, Melbourne.

Issues in Mental Health Nursing, 1978–present. Taylor & Francis Health Sciences, London.

Ivey, A., Ivey, M., 2003. Intentional Interviewing and Counselling: Facilitating Client Development in a Multicultural Society, fifth ed. Thompson Brooks/Cole, Pacific Grove, CA.

Johnston, B., 1998. Enhancing Recovery from Psychosis: A Practical Guide. Department of Human Services, Adelaide.

King, M., Averis, A., 2000. The application of Leininger's sunrise model to the culturally appropriate care of Indigenous Australians. In: Greenwood, J. (Ed.), Nursing Theory in Australia: Development and Application. Prentice Hall Health, Australia.

Kittleson, M., 1989. Mental health vs mental illness: a philosophical discussion. Health Educ. April/May, 40–42.

McMurray, A., 2007. Community Health and Wellness: a Socioecological Approach, third ed. Elsevier, Sydney.

Marriner-Tomey, A., Alligood, R.M., 2002. Nursing Theorists and their Work, fifth ed. Mosby, St Louis.

Maslow, A., 1968. Towards a Psychology of Being. Van Nostrand, NJ.

Meadows, G., Singh, B., Grigg, M., 2007. Mental Health in Australia: Collaborative Community Practice, second ed. Oxford University Press, Melbourne.

Morrison-Valfre, M., 2005. Foundations of Mental Health Care. Mosby, St Louis.

Peplau, H., 1988. Interpersonal Relations in Nursing. MacMillan Education, London.

Perls, F., Hefferline, R., Goodman, P., 1973. Gestalt Therapy Now: Experiment and Growth in the Human Personality. Pelican, London.

Ragsdale, S., 2003. Charlotte Malachowski Bühler, PhD (1893–1974). <http://www.webster.

edu/~woolflm/charlottebuhler. html> (30.07.07.).

Raphael, B., 1993. Scope for Prevention in Mental Health. National Health and Medical Research Council, AGPS, Canberra.

Rogers, C., 1951. Client-Centered Therapy. Houghton Mifflin, Boston.

Rogers, C., 1961. On Becoming a Person: A Therapist's View of Psychotherapy. Houghton Mifflin, Boston.

Sainsbury, P., 2003. The pursuit of happiness: the politics of mental health promotion. Aust. e-J. Adv. Ment. Health 2 (1) <http://auseinet. flinders.edu.au/journal/vol2iss1/ index.php>.

Santrock, J., 2007. Life-span Development, eleventh ed. McGraw-Hill, New York.

Schaffner, K., 2001. Nature and nurture. Curr. Opin. Psychiatry 14 (5), 485–490.

Seligman, M., 1974. Depression and learned helplessness. In: Friedman, J., Katz, M. (Eds.), The Psychology of Depression: Theory and Research. Winston-Wiley, Washington.

Seligman, M., 1994. Learned Optimism. Random House, Sydney.

Skinner, B., 1953. Science and Human Behaviour. Macmillan, New York.

Szasz, T., 1961. The Myth of Mental Illness. Harper & Row, New York.

Szasz, T., 2000. The case against psychiatric power. In: Barker, P., Stevenson, C. (Eds.), The Construction of Power and Authority in Psychiatry. Butterworth-Heinemann, Oxford.

Talbot, L., Verrinder, G., 2005. Promoting Health: The Primary Health Care Approach, third ed. Elsevier, Sydney.

Travelbee, J., 1971. Interpersonal Aspects of Nursing, second ed. F A Davis, Philadelphia.

Treatment Protocol Project, 2000. Management of Mental Disorder, third ed. World Health Organization Collaborating Centre for Mental Health and Substance Abuse, Sydney.

Vic Health, 2003. Together we do better. <http://www.togetherwedobetter. vic.gov.au/>.

Werner O'Toole, A., Rouslin Welt, S., 1989. Interpersonal Theory in Nursing Practice: Selected Works of Hildegard E Peplau. Springer, New York.

Wilkinson, R., Marmot, M., 2003. Social Determinants of Health: The Solid Facts, second ed. World Health Organization, Geneva.

World Health Organization, 2002. Prevention and promotion in mental health. <http://www.who. int/mental_health/media/en/545. pdf>.

Chapter 8

Mental health across the lifespan

Debra Nizette

CHAPTER POINTS

- An understanding of human development across the lifespan enhances mental health assessment and the provision of holistic care.
- Self-awareness assists the nurse to better understand the service user's experience.
- Mental health vulnerability increases at various times across the lifespan due to a combination of individual and contextual factors.
- The lifespan is generally conceived of as a linear concept, the time from birth to death. Paradoxically, development across this span is more appropriately conceived of as nonlinear, multidimensional and contextual.
- The concepts of attachment and resilience play a part in the attainment and maintenance of mental health.
- The promotion of mental health across the lifespan requires a primary healthcare approach to address the social and environmental factors that create vulnerability to mental ill health.

DOI: http://dx.doi.org/10.1016/B978-0-7020-4493-9.00008-1

- adolescence
- adulthood
- attachment
- childhood
- developmental psychology
- human development
- identity
- lifespan
- mental health
- mental health promotion
- older adulthood
- protective factors
- recovery
- resilience and thriving
- risk factors
- 'self'
- spectrum of prevention
- 'stage' theories

LEARNING OUTCOMES

The material in this chapter will assist you to:

- reflect on the relevance of lifespan concepts to your own experience,
- understand the relationship of developmental theories and concepts to mental health problems across the lifespan,
- apply these theories and concepts in all phases of the nurse–service user relationship,
- integrate prevention frameworks and strategies that promote mental health into clinical practice.

INTRODUCTION

This chapter provides a foundation for understanding mental health problems and psychopathology within the context of normal human development. It reviews the work of some theorists who have contributed to our understanding of human development, and presents emerging research and perspectives on mental health across the lifespan. The chapter also explores specific developmental issues at different stages of the lifespan and how they intersect with mental health, creating the potential for vulnerability and mental disorder. Concepts such as attachment, identity and resilience, which inform our understanding of development, are addressed in providing a holistic perspective on mental health issues across the lifespan. Strategies based on health promotion and a primary healthcare approach are described and proposed as a means of increasing protective factors and mental health across the lifespan.

A LIFESPAN APPROACH

If we consider the period from birth to our current age, we can in retrospect recall physical changes that we have experienced, such as changes in height, weight and appearance. We may also recall changes in our capabilities, skills, relationships, lifestyle and other aspects of our lives. In so doing, we acknowledge multifactorial aspects of ourselves that have evolved over time as a result of experience and change. Developmental psychologists have formulated theories to assist our understanding of how growth and change affect the personality and how we become 'ourselves'. Developmental theories aim to explain normal growth and development of the personality or 'self'.

A lifespan approach (lifespan developmental psychology) encompasses the sequence of events and experiences in a life from birth until death. Goals of the approach are to describe development, to explain how change occurs throughout the lifespan and to optimize development through the application of theory to real life (Peterson, 2004).

Recent conceptualizations of a lifespan approach emerge from the work of Baltes, who proposed a nonlinear theory emphasizing the multidimensional and nonintegrated nature of human development. A nonlinear model refutes the idea that there is a definite sequential pathway for development or an ideal end state or conclusion to development. Baltes challenges the idea that an ideal end state is ever achieved or desirable. He defines development as 'selective age related change in adaptive capacity' (Baltes et al., 1999, p. 476). Baltes' view supports the idea that development consists of a series of losses and gains. Losses and gains occur throughout the lifespan as new skills are acquired and the individual experiences certain benefits as a result; however, they may also experience a lack of continuity in other skills or abilities. For example, the older adult may not have the memory capacity of a younger person but they may develop pragmatic or problem-solving strategies (such as the use of mnemonics) which result in similar performance, thus compensating for age-related deficits (Baltes & Baltes, 1990). An additional gain of development is creativity. Creativity is perceived as essential in our ability to constantly develop new strategies, such as improved problem-solving, to compensate for age-related losses.

A lifespan approach to nursing practice

The nurse has an opportunity to provide information, resources and interventions for service users and families that will support and facilitate emotional development, cognitive growth and psychosocial wellbeing throughout the lifespan. The nurse's ability to use concepts related to development (e.g. attachment, resilience) will enhance his or her understanding of the service user and promote individually focused care. As well as equipping the nurse with knowledge to identify disruptions in development, developmental theories can increase the nurse's awareness of the service user, their perception of their problem and their responses to it. Moreover, knowledge of the lifespan can facilitate accurate assessment and communication, enhance empathy and promote the development of interventions that are specific and meaningful for the service user. It can be useful, for example, to understand why some adolescents and young adults have difficulty relating to others and regulating their own behaviour and emotions. See Box 8.1 and Box 8.2.

Box 8.1 A lifespan approach: key points

The tenets that guide an understanding of the lifespan approach include a belief that:
- the potential for growth and development exists throughout the lifespan,
- development is multidirectional, with no specific route or direction,
- patterns of development vary due to social, historical, cultural and gender variables,
- there are numerous dimensions to development and each may follow a different trajectory,
- dimensions to development include physical–motor, cognitive–intellectual and personal–social–emotional, and each interacts with the others,
- the individual and the environment influence each other,
- lifespan development promotes a holistic approach to nursing practice.

Box 8.2 A lifespan approach: role in practice

A lifespan approach in practice contributes to:
- communication, particularly development of rapport,
- establishment of empathy,
- interviewing,
- identification of service user concerns and general facilitation of therapeutic communication,
- risk assessment (self-harm and suicide),
- identification and implementation of appropriate interventions,
- appropriate referral,
- awareness of boundary issues.

CRITICAL THINKING CHALLENGE 8.1

Explain what is meant by 'the lifespan' and 'a lifespan approach for nursing'. Discuss how knowledge of lifespan theories and concepts contributes to nursing practice.

MENTAL HEALTH ACROSS THE LIFESPAN

The fundamental elements of mental health are acquired throughout a person's development. Developmental theories emphasize the importance of the early months and years of life in laying a foundation for sound mental health in adulthood. Mental health, like physical health, contributes to a person's quality of life. It enhances our functioning in all aspects of life – work, relationships and social situations – and also enables us to feel that we are worthwhile and acceptable just as we are. Mental health enables us to mediate and manage distress from external events in our life, to cope with the ups and downs, and to be hopeful about the future. Optimal personal development is related to and dependent upon an individual's mental health.

As well as describing normal development, developmental theorists propose a set of conditions or criteria necessary for optimal development and subsequent mental health. Each theorist sets out tasks, challenges or milestones that need to be achieved for normal development. Mental health problems can result when developmental tasks and challenges are not met due to some disruption in the internal or external environment. Internal conditions include inherited characteristics and personality characteristics. External conditions include parenting, nurturing in childhood and positive or negative life events. It is important for the nurse to be aware of the tenets of the lifespan approach (outlined earlier) when considering mental health issues throughout life, as many psychological issues recur repeatedly in different forms.

CRITICAL THINKING CHALLENGE 8.2

How would your own experience affect your ability to understand the significance of events and experiences in the lives of service users? Reflect on how differences in culture may influence your understanding.

'Ideal' development

Cognitive, perceptual, emotional and social functioning are dimensions of growth and development that are not well understood even though they are crucial to each individual's wellbeing and mental health. Development itself is difficult to define and hints that 'improvement' is part of a developing state. The literature on ageing (Baltes & Baltes, 1990; Bevan & Jeeawody, 1998) explores how we can age 'successfully'. The following outcome measurements are proposed:

- length of life,
- biological health,
- mental health,
- cognitive efficacy,
- social competence and productivity,
- personal control,
- life satisfaction.

These criteria demonstrate the multiple influences necessary for overall achievement of 'good ageing'. Multiple criteria take into account objective and subjective measures, so as to incorporate the individual's own definition of success.

'Good' outcomes of development proposed by Maslow (1968), Erikson (1963) and Allport (1961) all describe criteria that are normative; that is, they assume that everyone is the same and that there is a general standard which, if achieved, can lead to an ideal end state. As noted, this assumption has been challenged. It can be useful, however, to define development as an ideal state so that factors that are barriers to achieving this state can be explored, and ways of encouraging development can be addressed through health-promoting nursing interventions and a holistic approach to practice.

Abraham Maslow (1968) outlined a path of motivation to self-actualization (see Ch. 7) and outlined 15 characteristics of the self-actualized person. Gordon Allport (1961) defined the mature personality by describing six dimensions, and Erikson's theory (1963) identified 'wisdom' as the ideal end state of development, but acknowledged that positive outcomes of each stage were contingent upon meeting a challenge or completing a task.

These theorists share a similar philosophy of humanism, yet each has contributed unique insights into the process of development. Erikson's 'stages' differ from Maslow's and Allport's as they more clearly identify a process (stages) that needs to be undertaken whereby one may achieve mastery of the task of that stage. Erikson's theory suggests that a person may be unable to achieve mastery of one of the developmental tasks due to external factors, such as a loss, or injury, which may disrupt the person's development. Maslow proposed a set of preconditions for self-actualization that, if unmet, also interfere with development (see Ch. 7). Aspects of the human condition that are of interest to developmental theorists include personality as well as psychosexual, cognitive, psychosocial, moral and gender development. Each of these aspects affects the mental health status of the developing person.

The ideal outcomes of development (listed in Table 8.1) highlight the characteristics of optimal wellbeing and mental health, but the course of life and significant events can disrupt this ideal. Factors that can disrupt the path of normal development will be discussed further in this chapter.

Table 8.1 Ideal outcomes of development

Characteristics of the self-actualized person (Maslow, 1968)	Dimensions of maturity (Allport, 1961)	The 'eight stages of man' (Erikson, 1963)
Accurate perception of reality	Extension of the sense of self (having a life mission)	Basic trust versus mistrust (0–1 year)
Acceptance of self and others		→ Hope
Spontaneity	Warm relating of self to others	Autonomy versus shame and doubt (1–3 years)
Problem centering		→ Willpower
Detachment (emotionally self-sufficient)	Emotional security	Initiative versus guilt (4–5 years)
Autonomy	Realistic perception, skills and assignments (solves problems as required)	→ Purpose
Continued fresh appreciation		Industry versus inferiority (6–11 years)
Mystic or peak experiences		→ Competence and accomplishment
Unconditional positive regard for others	Self-objectification (insight or self-awareness)	Identity versus role confusion (12–18 years)
Characteristic interpersonal relations	Unifying philosophy on life	→ Fidelity
Democratic character structure		Intimacy versus isolation (early adulthood)
Definite moral standards		→ Love
Philosophical sense of humour		Generativity versus stagnation (middle adulthood)
Creativeness		→ Care and production
Cultural transcendence		Ego integrity versus despair (older adulthood)
		→ Wisdom

Stages and theoretical issues in human development

Theories of personality development such as the biomedical, psychological (psychoanalytic, behaviourist, cognitive and humanistic) and sociological (discussed in Ch. 7) assist us to understand human behaviour. Some theorists developed a lifespan approach and devised 'stages' to explain how changes occurred across the lifespan. Stage theories were initiated by the evolutionary perspective of Charles Darwin, who believed that human development could be understood through the study of childhood. Darwin's work was significant in introducing a scientific approach to the study of development. Stage theories support the idea that individual development can be measured and monitored according to a set of expected 'norms' at average ages when certain milestones are achieved.

Stages have different meanings depending on the variable being considered. For example, biological stage theories conceive of growth being completed by adulthood, followed by a maintenance period, after which physical decline results. A sociocultural/psychosocial conception of stages describes a series of roles and age- or development-related tasks throughout life (Erikson). Cognitive–structural stages (Piaget) are conceived of as an ascending staircase along the lifeline, with later stages integrating and building upon previous cognitive functioning. Stage theories require consideration of normative variables (age or historical influences shared by most people) and nonnormative variables (events unique to individuals). Nurses need to be able to use stage theories. During assessment, consideration of general and unique influences ensures that individuals and families are assessed holistically and that the range of issues affecting development can be examined. Theories help us understand why some people might be more vulnerable to mental health problems or at risk of developing mental illness than others.

Freud, Erikson and Piaget were twentieth-century theorists who, among others, were influential in contributing to a lifespan perspective of development.

Freud

Sigmund Freud (1856–1939) proposed three personality structures, which, if functioning in balance, help the person resolve the conflicts of different psychosexual stages of personality development. Maturation is the desired outcome of the individual successfully moving through four psychosexual stages (from infancy to adolescence). Chapter 7 outlines the stages and characteristics of each stage. The relevance of Freud's theory lies primarily in its ability to assist the nurse in understanding patient behaviours that appear inconsistent with age or the expected level of development, or behaviour and habits that are excessive or unexplained by other assessment frameworks. The concepts of regression and fixation are integral to this understanding.

Fixation refers to behaviours that indicate unmet needs or unresolved conflicts of a particular psychosexual stage. For example, the id is the dominant personality structure during infancy (oral stage, 0–12 months). If the infant failed to receive adequate oral gratification, frustration could result, and if over-attention was given to meeting oral needs the child may continue to have a preoccupation with their mouth as they grow, resulting in habits such as heavy smoking in adulthood. Similarly, any frustration or over-gratification experienced during the anal stage (1–3 years) could result in anal fixation and result in stubbornness, selfishness or slothfulness. According to this theory, parents have a significant role in ensuring the child's needs are met in a balanced and consistent manner.

Regression refers to behaviour that is inappropriate for a person's age. Regression is a defence mechanism that protects against threats and stress, such as thumb sucking in a school-age child in the first weeks of commencing school. Regressed behaviour often lessens when the threat or stress is withdrawn or weakens.

Criticisms of Freud's stages refer to the prominence given to sexual issues as a framework for development, and its lack of testing across cultures (Berk, 2001).

Erikson

Erik Erikson (1902–1994) envisaged successful personality development as an outcome of conflict resolution throughout eight 'psychosocial' stages. The relevance of Erikson's psychosocial theory for nurses is that it assists the nurse with increased interpersonal understanding of the individual's biological, psychological, spiritual and social dimensions. Stages highlight the central concerns of individuals at different times in their life and identify challenges that may contribute to vulnerability. Nurses are able to consider the tasks of each stage and integrate these understandings into appropriate assessment and planning. In addition, the nurse may convey an understanding to the service user of the importance of their concerns, increasing empathy in the nurse–service user relationship. A brief description of the conflicts and outcome of each stage is given in Table 8.1 and application of the theory to practice is outlined further in this chapter.

Evaluation of Erikson's work highlights criticisms that stage theories propose a 'normative' or standard recipe for development. Erikson has also been criticized for his optimistic view of people (Roazen, cited in Welchman, 2000) that negates the complexity and flaws in human nature. Welchman states: 'His affirmative view of human potential is a warning not to label antisocial behaviour as pathological' (Welchman, 2000, p. 120). Erikson used male subjects in his work, which led to criticisms that the male experience is understood as universal. Carol Gilligan, a student of Erikson, developed a critique of his work and proposed a need for a separate chart for women to account for differences in experience and challenges through life (Welchman, 2000). Gilligan developed theories of women's development being associated with relationships with others; her ideas are explored later in this chapter.

Piaget

Jean Piaget (1896–1980) proposed a theory consisting of four broad stages describing the development of thinking (cognitive–developmental theory). The relevance of Piaget's theory is that it assists the nurse to understand that in the early years infants and children require stimulation and an experience of the external world to learn ways of relating to their environment. Nurses can use play and concrete ideas to communicate meaningfully with children in healthcare settings. An awareness by the nurse that the ability to think abstractly or conceptually is necessary for problem-solving can assist the nurse with the facilitation of decision making with particular service users. Health teaching interventions with adolescents or young adults (assumed to be at the formal operations stage) would require nurses to be specific with information and not assume that they are able to apply health teaching information to a range of issues. Each issue would need to be addressed separately as some adolescents and young adults may be unable to generalize information.

There are several key concepts in Piaget's theory. Adaptation is the mechanism by which development occurs, as the structures of the mind 'adapt' to better represent the external world. According to this theory the individual develops 'schemas' or behaviour patterns. When a new item is incorporated into the existing schema, 'assimilation' occurs. 'Accommodation' occurs when the individual is unable to assimilate the new item into the existing schema. The schema is altered to accommodate the new item. An example would be when a baby reaches for and grasps an object (the baby will assimilate the action into a 'grasping schema'); the baby then accommodates as it modifies its grasp for a range of differently shaped objects. The aim of this process is to achieve equilibrium, thereby increasing the sophistication of thinking and understanding (Peterson, 2004).

Piaget was interested in how children think, reason and learn. He proposed a number of stages of cognitive development. At 0–2 years, the *sensorimotor stage*, Piaget saw that infants used their senses to explore and learn about the world. They are able to act on their world: for example, they can move an object (rattle) to make a noise. Next, at 2–7 years, children's thinking was illogical but they were able to use symbols to represent previous actions. This stage, the *preoperational stage*, was characterized by make-believe play and language development. During the next stage, the *concrete operational* (between 7 and 11 years), thinking is seen to be more logical and organized. Objects can be classified according to size and other hierarchies can be established. Finally, the *formal operational* stage (from 11 years onwards), children are increasingly able to think in abstract terms which defines this stage. Concepts and symbols can be used in advanced problem-solving (advanced mathematics). A variety of options can be generated to solve problems and generate creative thought (Peterson, 2004)

Long-held beliefs about the perceptual abilities of children have been challenged by research on the perceptual systems of infants, which reveals that neonatal behaviour encompasses goal-directed and spatially coordinated behaviours and is not merely reflexive, as previously understood through the work of Piaget. Bertenthal (1996) believes that further research is required to explore the development of infants' perception, action, object recognition and representation functions. Piaget concluded that cognitive development did not undergo significant change after adolescence. Recent enquiry and research into the postformal operations stages of adulthood demonstrate a further limitation of his theory (Berk, 2001).

Moral development

Piaget was concerned with moral as well as cognitive development. As he saw it, the maturing minds of adolescents experienced disequilibrium as a result of discussions with peers. Disequilibrium was seen as an opportunity for growth and development for the adolescent as they sought resolution of the particular dilemma (Golombok & Fivush, 1994; Piaget, 1932/1977). But as with Piaget's general developmental theories, recent researchers have found that morality begins at a much earlier age, although not always at such a sophisticated level (Darley & Shultz, 1990; Shultz & Wells, 1985).

Lawrence Kohlberg (Kohlberg, 1986; Kohlberg et al., 1983) developed a stage-based model in which people functioning at the higher levels were seen as being able to use a justice orientation in their moral decisions. A justice orientation emphasizes the need for reason and detachment in decision making. Kohlberg saw moral development as an internal process that happens as a result of increasing cognitive maturity with little external influence. His assessment of morality was based on people's responses to hypothetical moral dilemmas. Unfortunately, many nursing authors have tended to use his theory with no recognition of the many criticisms of his work. Critics have observed that his view of justice is limited to one theoretical perspective, and that his methodology was flawed and biased as it used only young male participants and ignored family influences. Others have pointed out that moral thoughts do not always result in moral behaviours (Bailey, 1986).

Carol Gilligan (Brown et al., 1991; Gilligan, 1982, 1987, 1998) emphasized a care orientation, where the relatedness of individuals to each other is seen as important in moral decision making. Initially she proposed that women used a care orientation, whereas men used a justice-based approach. This aroused much controversy at the time. Her current view is that males and females use either a justice or a caring 'voice', depending on the situation and the issue, although most males and females do appear to favour the style she originally proposed for each sex. Females are therefore not seen as inferior to men in their decision making, but different. Other findings have supported this view (Donenberg & Hoffman, 1988; Pratt et al., 1984).

Attachment, parenting and family factors

Eisenberg (2000) and Stilwell et al. (1997) carried out longitudinal research across various age groups from infancy to adolescence demonstrating how, through attachment, children and adolescents progressively develop a conscience. Research has often found that a bond between mother and child is the most significant factor (Garmon, 2000; Park & Roberts, 2002).

Research into parenting styles has also contributed to understanding moral development. In the 1960s Barbara Baumrind (1971) studied parents and their children. She described three parenting styles, which have since been studied extensively and are used frequently by child and adolescent workers.

- *Authoritative* parents had clear expectations, but were also warm, supportive, rational and reciprocating, willing to allow an interactive level of communication. Their children tended to achieve high levels of competent and responsible independent behaviour, with mature levels of morality.
- An *authoritarian* parent was dominant and detached, with a lower level of warmth than others, resulting in discontented, withdrawn and distrustful children. It is important to note the difference between this and the authoritative parenting style, as lay people as well as professionals can sometimes mistakenly use the two terms interchangeably.
- *Permissive* parents gave control to the child, were relatively warm, nondemanding and noncontrolling. Children of these parents were the least self-reliant, explorative or self-controlled, often with a poor social conscience (Baumrind, 1971).

White (1996) argues that moral development is more complex than simple developmental stage theories.

She sees family adaptability, cohesiveness and degree of family communication as critical factors (White, 1996). The early work of research scientist John Bowlby and Canadian psychologist Mary Ainsworth has generated a model of attachment known today as *secure-base phenomenon*. The notion of a secure base has moved beyond the parent–child dyad to include the significance of secure attachment in all relationships. It proposes that when an individual – child or adult – has a secure attachment to a stronger, supportive other, they are then capable of responding to the needs of others (Waters et al., 1995).

Implications for nursing practice

Moral development theories are useful in helping to understand the children and families with whom nurses work. Without making value judgements or blaming, one can sometimes understand, for example, that the individual who has become involved in antisocial or criminal behaviour may not have done so simply because of a 'deficient personality', but possibly because of suffering deficits in childhood. The person with severe anxiety, inappropriate guilt or poor self-esteem may be so due to authoritarian parenting. We as nurses might also be helped in understanding our own moral development and its influence on our ethical behaviour as professionals. The importance of a secure base, or a reliable relationship that encourages growth and exploration of the world, is important for us all.

Relationships and attachment were also researched by Bowlby and Ainsworth in developing the theory. Bowlby had a strong conviction that relationships influence who we become and how we relate to others into adulthood. Feminist perspectives criticize the notion of attachment because of the assumption that the primary relationship is always with the mother. Attachment theory is useful in helping us understand the role of risk and protective factors in early development and will be further discussed in this chapter. The concepts of thriving and resilience also help explain differences in outcomes between people who have experienced similar events in their lives. It is critical for nurses to acknowledge that identity is also important and that it has multiple meanings for people. In understanding this, nurses can support each person's self-concept and self-esteem, contributing positively to their mental health. These theories reinforce the importance of families, whatever style or structure, as supportive, nurturing sources underpinning development. It is always important, when interviewing service users, to gain a thorough understanding of their families and the influence they have had and continue to have on the person's mental health.

The complex nature of human development is reflected in the diversity of theoretical approaches to its study. Each of the aforementioned theories focuses on different dimensions of human development. Theories can be used eclectically in practice and integrated into a lifespan approach to help understand human development and behaviour. Additional concepts to assist in a more comprehensive understanding of the developmental process incorporate those already mentioned, which focus on the importance of interpersonal relationships in development, and those following, which highlight the interplay between the person and their environment, which Richard Lerner popularized as 'developmental contextualism' (Lerner, 1991).

VULNERABILITY, RISK AND RESILIENCE

Disruption in development can create vulnerability in an individual's mental health. Developmental crises, problematic attachments and environmental risks (e.g. poor parenting, poverty, violence) may result in a person being less able to manage and mediate distress. 'Mental illness' and 'mental disorder' are terms often used when a diagnosis is given to a person experiencing a mental health problem. Not all mental health problems are brought to the attention of a mental health professional and some problems may not meet the criteria for a diagnosis. The person who meets all the criteria for mental health at some stage of their life can nevertheless experience significant mental distress or mental disorder at some other stage. Strategies promoting mental health and resilience and reducing risk can be implemented at any time.

An individual is said to be resilient when they have had good outcomes 'in spite of serious threats to adaptation or development' (Masten, 2001, p. 228). Resilience and risk go hand in hand. Resilience helps to explain why some children with significant or numerous risk factors do not develop psychopathology when others do.

Resilience has been identified in a number of ways in the research over the past 20 years. Studies have examined people at all phases of the lifespan, some focusing on the variables that may put an individual at risk, others on factors that may offset risk. These variable-focused studies of resilience (Masten, 2001) have been useful in identifying interventions that can lessen the impact of adversity and threat, either by building assets and increasing protective factors (teaching parenting skills, decision making, coping) or by reducing risk (prenatal care to prevent premature births). For example, in high-risk individuals, poor parenting and cognitive skills are more likely to result in antisocial behaviour if a child is under threat or in adverse conditions. Alternatively, if the child receives positive, supportive parenting and has adequate cognitive skills (protective factors), it is more likely that more adaptive behaviour will result if the child is exposed to adversity or threat. These individuals are considered to be resilient.

Several additional factors have been associated with resilience: a positive sense of self, self-efficacy (competence), self-regulation of mood, cognitive abilities, perseverance, and relationships or contact with significant nurturing adults or a supportive community (Jacelon, 1997; Masten, 2001). In a study of homeless youths, resilience was represented by a sense of self-reliance (Rew et al., 2001). Youths with self-reported resilience were less likely to engage in life-threatening behaviours and experienced less loneliness and hopelessness. Antonovsky described 'generalized resistance resources' as contributing to resilience in children. Examples are 'adaptability on the biological, psychological, social and cultural levels; profound ties to concrete, immediate others; and formal or informal ties between the individual and family' (Antonovsky, 1979, cited in Werner & Smith, 1982, p. 160). Living in environments that support a sense of coherence, even if through one significant person, was found in resilient children (Werner & Smith, 1982).

Resilience can also be applied to families. Positive change can result in a family system despite adversity, such as a family member having a mental health problem. It has been found that resilient families take a problem-orientated approach when a diagnosis of mental disorder is made to a family member and they are quick to accept the reality of the disorder in their lives (Marsh et al., 1996). Deveson (2003), in describing her personal story, relates how a sense of coherence and meaning in life has mediated against illness, crises and death. Her book *Resilience* provides the nurse as reader with personal insights into resilience as a concept at work across the lifespan.

Resilience as a concept and tools which attempt to measure it continue to be researched. Critical evaluation of the research conducted to date suggests that it is a concept that assists us to understand not only the processes affecting people who are at risk (Luthar et al., 2000) but also its role in mental health throughout life.

The concept of *thriving* applies to both physical and psychological wellbeing and is a positive growth response by the individual to threat or danger (Bergland & Kirkevold, 2001). Unlike resilience, where the person's development continues along a predicted path, thriving means that the person is 'better off' after an adverse event than they were before, and may achieve better physical, social, cognitive and emotional development (Carver, 1998). This concept can help explain anomalies in expected developmental outcomes for certain service users. For example, some service users may experience disruption during their development, yet somehow thrive despite it. Others may suffer and fail to thrive from those same experiences, which can result in an increased risk for mental health problems.

Psychological thriving 'occurs when a person, after going through a traumatic situation, acquires new skills and/or knowledge that may promote mastery of similar situations in the future. This in turn leads to the belief that it is possible to cope with other difficult situations' (Bergland & Kirkevold, 2001, p. 247). The concept of thriving requires further research for application to mental ill health and lifespan development. The multidimensional nature of the concept suggests that it has relevance for examination of positive growth episodes throughout the lifespan.

Maturity, or a higher level of ego functioning, is achieved through adversity as a result of a person's adapting to an expectation not being met, or experiencing loss (King, 2001). The idea that difficult and challenging times are opportunities for growth is consistent with the literature on resilience and thriving. Baltes and Baltes (1990) contribute the idea of 'adaptivity' or 'behavioural plasticity' to explain how cognition, memory and coping skills work together to assist the individual to deal with life's stressful events.

Nurses can use resilience-promoting interventions focusing on the individual, family or community using the health promotion framework outlined in the next section of this chapter. These interventions can be regarded as primary healthcare approaches to mental health attainment across the lifespan.

Many of the concepts and ideas derived from observations and research, as outlined above, find support through application in everyday practice. Additional concepts such as optimism, pessimism and goal orientation derived from psychological theory (not discussed in this chapter) also play a part in explaining human development and understanding how it intersects with mental health and disorder. More research exploring these concepts in the context of lifespan stages and culture needs to be undertaken so that nurses and other healthcare professionals can use these important concepts in practice to enhance care. Chapter 10 provides information on the assessment of strengths and risk factors.

PRIMARY HEALTHCARE AND MENTAL HEALTH PROMOTION

The aim of mental health promotion across the lifespan is for the individual to achieve mental health through primary healthcare strategies targeting the whole population. A primary healthcare approach considers the broad contextual (social, family, cultural and environmental) variables that influence a person's health. The elements associated with primary healthcare as described in the Ottawa Charter for Health Promotion (World Health Organization, 1986) include:

- promoting supportive partnerships,
- creating supportive environments,
- developing personal skills,

- promotion of public policy,
- reorientation of health services delivery towards promotion, prevention and early intervention.

The Ottawa Charter recognizes that the achievement of better health outcomes requires internal and external risk factors to be ameliorated and sustainable and protective factors to be implemented (Table 8.2). The Charter identifies basic prerequisites for health, including education, peace, shelter and food, an ecosystem that is sustainable, income, social justice and equity. Importantly, health promotion aims to achieve better health outcomes through strategies that educate and enable people to have more personal control over their own health.

In the UK there has been an increasing awareness of the importance of primary care services being able to meaningfully respond to the needs of people with mental health problems. Standard 2 of the National Service Framework for Mental Health required health services to '...deliver better primary mental healthcare, and to ensure consistent advice and help for people with mental health

Table 8.2 Examples of risk and protective factors across the lifespan

Risk factors	Protective factors
Internal	
Delayed biological development	Optimal biological development and wellness
Genetic predisposition	Educational/learning ability
Stress	Temperament (calm)
Anger	Positive sense of self/self-esteem
Fragmented sense of self	Resilience
External	
Poor childcare	Quality childcare support (family and friends)
Ill or stressed family	Consistent 'significant other'
Inadequate parenting skills (insensitive/inconsistent)	Positive relationships
Abuse and neglect	Supportive school environments
Poverty	Peer-group involvement (positive)
Violence (family and culture)	Community networks and resources
Poor access/resources	Mental health services

needs, including primary care services for individuals with severe mental illness' (Department of Health, 1999, p. 28). More recently, the No Health Without Mental Health strategy requires primary care health services to not only respond to the needs of all local people, but also to tackle health inequalities within communities (Department of Health, 2011). This means that primary care services must ensure that people have their mental health needs assessed and, where appropriate, be offered effective treatment including onward referral (Department of Health, 2003a).

In primary care there is often a high demand for, but low capacity to provide, care and treatment to people with mental health issues. It is estimated that 25% of GP consultations involve mental health issues and 90% of mental healthcare is estimated to be provided in primary care settings (Department of Health, 1999). However, the recognition of common mental health problems, such as depression, in primary care is often poor (Department of Health, 1999) which can mean a delay in referral to secondary mental health services for specialist assessment and treatment. In order to improve capacity, graduate primary mental healthcare workers (Department of Health, 2003a) and community mental health (or 'gateway') workers (Department of Health, 2003b) have also been developed to provide information to, and liaise with, local communities about mental health issues, while offering assessment and interventions for people with common mental health problems. Guidance from the National Institute for Health and Clinical Excellence (for example, *Depression*, National Institute for Health and Clinical Excellence, 2009) also seeks to ensure that mental health needs in primary care are recognized, assessed and treated wherever possible, but also that timely referrals to secondary and specialist services are undertaken where a patient presents with complex or severe problems.

A framework that integrates primary healthcare principles is suggested by Lindsey and Hartrick (1996) for use by nurses. They propose listening to the service user, participating in dialogue with the service user, working with the service user to recognize patterns or themes that may be problematic in maintaining or eliciting health-directed behaviours and discussing and preparing for action and positive change through the identification of relevant strategies or processes. Nurses who are informed of a primary healthcare approach can access service users' strategies that are part of primary healthcare initiatives.

Primary healthcare approaches are based on sound principles that fit very well with mental health nursing practice. Primary healthcare principles applied to nursing practice facilitate a service user-focused approach that is holistic in that social, political and environmental issues are taken into account and placed in the ambit of the nurse's awareness. A primary healthcare approach also acknowledges the importance of culture in that strategies are generated through engagement with individuals and communities. Primary healthcare also aims to promote resilience, thriving and healthy, secure attachment in individuals. These concepts deepen our knowledge of development across the lifespan.

MENTAL ILL HEALTH PREVENTION AND RECOVERY

While mental health promotion aims to build strengths and promote resilience, mental ill health prevention aims to reduce the extent and severity of mental disorder through reducing risk factors and enhancing protective factors. Caplan (1964) outlined a model of prevention that is still used today:

- primary prevention: reduces the incidence of mental disorders,
- secondary prevention: reduces the prevalence of disorders,
- tertiary prevention: reduces the impairment caused by disorders.

The mental health intervention spectrum for mental disorders (Mrazek & Haggerty, 1994) identifies three levels of prevention strategies within a broader framework of prevention, treatment and maintenance/continuing care (Fig. 8.1). The levels of prevention in this framework are:

- universal: prevention aimed at the population,
- selective: prevention aimed at high-risk groups,
- indicated: prevention aimed at high-risk individuals and groups with some evidence of mental disorder.

Recovery from an episode of mental illness depends on health-promoting interventions. The 4 A's Framework (Rickwood, 2006) establishes a baseline for mental health promotion and relapse prevention, but further aims to reorient mental heath services towards recovery. It focuses on the *continuing care* dimension of the 'spectrum of intervention for mental health'. The 4 A's are:

- awareness: awareness of risks, vulnerability and protective factors,
- anticipation: future planning and self-management strategies in case of crisis,
- alternatives: availability of a range of holistic services and strategies to reduce risk and increase protective factors,
- access: early and appropriate access to a range of services for service users and families.

Rickwood (2006) notes that operationalization of the framework depends on action to be taken individually by the person, their family, carer and friends, with a range of service providers and at the macro level of the broader community.

Concepts within the framework reinforce the notion of recovery as a process undertaken by the person who

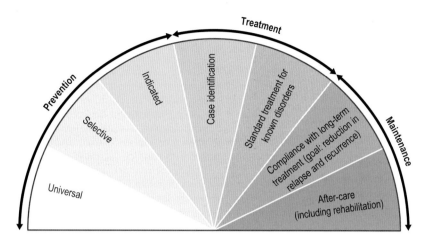

Figure 8.1 The spectrum of intervention.
From Mrazek PJ and Haggerty RJ, Reducing risks for mental disorders: frontiers for preventative intervention research. Reprinted with permission from the National Academies Press, Copyright 1994, National Academy of Sciences.

determines the nature and process of their recovery. Efforts have also been made to assess or measure the process of recovery using the key consumer-defined concepts of hope, identity, meaning and responsibility with the Stages of Recovery Instrument (STORI) (Andresen et al., 2006). Therefore the concept has limited utility in child mental health, where a more relevant focus for practice is on exploring ways to increase protective factors and resilience.

The application to clinical practice of strategies aimed at reducing risk and increasing protective factors is not disorder-specific. A broad application of both prevention strategies and mental health promotion acknowledges that risk factors can apply to a range of mental health problems and disorders, and that, similarly, strategies that promote mental health can be protective against a range of health problems. The following section gives an overview of major stages of the lifespan: it reviews developmental issues, risks specific to each life stage and relevant approaches to health-promoting interventions or illness prevention.

CHILDHOOD

Most theorists believe that the early years are the most significant in building a foundation for all future development. The most important outcomes of the infant–childhood developmental phases are the development of a positive sense of self, and the ability to trust others.

Development and theoretical issues

There is evidence that mental health in children and adults could be contingent on positive parent–child relationships (Barlow & Parsons, 2002; Licence, 2004). Dr John Bowlby's 1951 report, *Maternal Care and Mental*

Health, commissioned by the World Health Organization, documented his idea of the importance of 'attachment' in determining outcomes of childhood development (Bowlby, 1951). *Attachment* has been described as 'the strong affectional tie we feel for special people in our lives that leads us to experience pleasure and joy when we interact with them and to be comforted by their nearness in times of stress' (Berk, 2001, p. 190). The report noted that in the first 3–4 months of life infants are observed to recognize their mother among other figures, and respond differently to her by smiling and vocalizing. Attachment behaviour was also identified as occurring with others, usually fathers or family members, about a month after it was observed occurring with the mother. The behaviour of the mother (attentive or distant) and differences in the child (attractive appearance and settled behaviour or otherwise) determine how attachment behaviour occurs.

Attachment behaviour develops throughout the first 3 years of life. During this time the child protests when the mother is out of sight. However, when the child realizes that the mother will return, trust increases, and the child is later able to feel secure with subordinate attachment figures such as preschool teachers and relatives. Attachment to parents grows weaker throughout the lifespan, but it continues as we age and is transferred to other adults in our lives. Attachment behaviour is also directed to people outside the family, groups and organizations. Increased need for attachment is experienced when people are under threat or stress and a need for security is felt. Secure attachments in childhood are predictive of positive sociable behaviour towards others, higher self-esteem and greater achievement throughout the lifespan.

The quality of attachment can vary. It can be either secure or anxious (Karen, 1994). Less securely attached individuals are more likely to experience problems with self-esteem and socializing and be more vulnerable to mental health problems and psychopathology (Arbona & Power, 2003; Nakash-Eisikovits et al., 2002).

The achievement of secure attachment equates to Erikson's first stage and the ability to trust. The first four of Erikson's stages relate to infancy and childhood, as follows.

1. Basic trust versus mistrust (0–12 months). Resolution of the conflict at this stage requires the infant to compromise when his or her basic needs are not met, to develop acceptance and to cope with frustration until such time as these needs are restored. The outcome or strength the child acquires from this is hope.

2. Autonomy versus shame and doubt (1–3 years). Resolution of this conflict is the acquisition of autonomy, which is experienced as a growing feeling of self-control. The child is encouraged, with appropriate limits, to be independent, to explore relationships with others and to develop curiosity about their environment. Inhibition can result if the child is overly directed or limited, whereas defiance and problems with self-regulation can result when there is no guidance or limit setting.

3. Initiative versus guilt (4–5 years). A sense of purpose balanced with responsibility and initiative is the desired resolution of this stage. The child has mastered the previous stages and is capable of basic social functioning and self-regulation. However, parental guidance is still required, to direct the child's initiative into constructive endeavours.

4. Industry versus inferiority (6–11 years). A sense of self as competent in a range of unique abilities is the desired outcome of this stage. Children are prone to suffer from comparison with others once they attend school and can acquire a sense of inferiority in certain skills that may be valued in a particular context. In this stage, children's strengths can be optimized and their weaknesses nurtured so they can work cooperatively with others and learn that they have particular contributions to make to group efforts (Erikson, 1963; Welchman, 2000).

Mental health is evidenced by the child entering into and maintaining relationships with others, engaging in learning and play, understanding the concepts of right and wrong, developing psychologically and exhibiting behaviour that demonstrates an ability to regulate distress (Townley, 2002). All these behaviours and abilities need to be appraised in relation to the developmental level of the child as outlined in the stage theories, and the context in which the behaviour is observed.

The following behaviours occurring in a continuing pattern may be indicators of mental health problems in children: difficulties with sleep, feeding, mood, relating to others; bed wetting (enuresis) and soiling (encopresis); overly active behaviour; frequent tantrums and defiance; and somatic complaints such as 'tummy pain' without any identifiable cause (Townley, 2002). (Mental health issues in childhood are addressed in Ch. 12.)

Risk factors

A number of risk factors may predispose infants and children to mental health problems and mental disorder in childhood or adulthood. Longitudinal research identifies numerous developmental variables and risk factors: prematurity and serious medical illness; infant temperament (behavioural inhibition); attachment between infant and caregiver; psychopathology in parents; maternal depression; maternal substance abuse; marital quality and interactions (exposure to conflict can cause distress and problems in regulating behaviour); poverty and social class; adolescent parenting; family violence and physical, emotional or sexual abuse and death (Salmelainen, 1996; Townley, 2002; Zeanah et al., 1997). Additional risk factors such as homelessness, disaster, discrimination and poverty can affect the individual (Townley, 2002). The behaviour styles of children have been researched, and those who were undercontrolled and impulsive at 3 years of age were identified as being more likely to meet the criteria for antisocial personality disorder. Children who exhibited inhibited behaviour were more likely to meet the diagnostic criteria for depression (Caspi et al., 1996).

Research on risk and protective factors also suggests a nonlinear and nonspecific transmission of risk. This suggests that the total number of risk factors is more predictive of psychopathology in later life than any one specific factor (Zeanah et al., 1997). In summary, protective factors against mental health problems or mental illness include: an easy temperament, a high level of intelligence, positive relationships with a parent and early attachment to a parent, support from peers, a sense of humour, positive experiences at school, and positive relationships with another adult, reflection, and planning and decision-making skills.

Prevention and promotion

In terms of health promotion, parenting skills that demonstrate to parents ways in which they can 'attach', through increasing maternal or parental sensitivity with their newborn or toddler, are significant in developing trust, feelings of security and positive mental health in the developing child (Bakermans-Kranenburg et al., 2003; Licence, 2004). As a result, parenting skills programmes are on the increase. Programmes use a variety of theoretical approaches such as behavioural family interventions, in which parents are instructed in ways to increase positive communication and behaviour with children with conduct problems (Sanders et al., 2000). Behavioural approaches have been criticized because, although they may assist in reducing overall family distress from problem behaviours and vulnerability, they often fail to engage those families who most require support (Sanders et al., 2000). It is acknowledged that a broader primary healthcare approach to interventions is needed. Such an approach is more likely to target the vast range of variables that affect families. Ongoing research is needed in this area as much of the evidence from research on primary prevention programmes is patchy; however, there is evidence that programmes which aim to develop coping skills, manage stress, promote physical activity or change school cultures have a positive impact on mental health (Licence, 2004).

During assessment the nurse can carefully observe interpersonal variables and relationship patterns in the family group. The importance of attachment and relationships within the family and extended social group needs to be explored, as they may contribute to maintaining nonadaptive behaviour in children (Kearney, 1997). Interventions aimed at increasing protective factors, such as stress recognition and management in the family context, and resources and support groups, need to be explored with the family, school or carers. In summary, children who are nurtured and have secure attachments with family members and others have usually achieved a positive sense of self, can regulate temperament and have normal physical and psychosocial development and therefore have the potential for sound mental health. Children whose lives lack these elements are more vulnerable to mental health problems and possible illness. Mental health promotion strategies need to focus on increasing opportunities for the implementation and acquisition of protective factors.

CRITICAL THINKING CHALLENGE 8.3

Ellie is 3 years old. She lives with her parents in a block of flats in an inner-city suburb. Ellie's mother drinks a lot of alcohol and often has arguments with Sean, Ellie's stepfather. Maureen, a retired woman in her sixties, lives next door. Ellie loves spending time with Maureen, who has developed a close bond with Ellie.

◆ Discuss the risk and protective factors in Ellie's life.
◆ How could Ellie's relationship with Maureen affect her future relationships?

ADOLESCENCE

Development and theoretical issues

The main tasks of adolescence are the successful transition to secondary schooling, learning skills for later life, psychological autonomy (self-reliance and confidence in decision making), developing close relationships within and between genders and the formation of personal identity (Masten, 2001). The development of a sense of meaning and purpose in life are part of this major task of identity formation.

The ability of the adolescent to achieve these tasks will depend largely on the accomplishment of the earlier tasks of childhood. The stage of Erikson's theory that relates to adolescence is identity versus role confusion (12–18 years).

During this stage the acquisition of a relatively stable sense of self, or identity, resolves the confusion associated with this stage. The person is challenged to accommodate a range of 'self-schemas' into a comprehensive sense of self that will form a lasting identity (Welchman, 2000). Schemas are various perspectives of the self, received from others. In addition, the adolescent has his or her own multiple perspectives of self. This stage is particularly challenging as the adolescent can experience confusion about the various roles expected of them. Adolescents have a need for ideology and occupation. This makes them vulnerable to exploitation by organizations and groups offering a particular world view or truth. Tension is also created for the adolescent who is encouraged to select a career, but who may require an extended time between childhood and adopting an occupational identity (Erikson, 1963; Welchman, 2000). An absence of role modelling or poor role models makes it even more difficult to resolve this conflict, as does the complex nature of contemporary society.

Existentialism provides some guidance in understanding the conflicts faced during this stage of development as the world view of the child makes a shift into an exploration of the meaning of life and existence, and concerns of the transition to adulthood (Fitzgerald, 2005). Integrative models also help explain this complex stage of development. Research on physical changes, mood and behaviour, and social and relationship variables has been explored in an integrated manner, investigating the many influences on adolescent development (Compas et al., 1995).

Identity

Erikson's theory suggests that identity develops over time and is the part of our self-concept that contributes to our overall sense of self. Formation of identity begins in infancy, as children identify with role models they perceive as attractive and important. Children aspire to become like those they admire (Phinney, 2000). The concept of identity consists of both individual and group identity, and it changes over time.

Identity is most significant to the adolescent because of the risks taken as they trial their various schemas or perspectives of self. The acceptability and congruence of gender identity at a personal and social level is critical for the adolescent. Nonacceptance and incongruence of identity is acknowledged as a risk factor in adolescent suicide. Racial, ethnic, sexual and class identities may also challenge the 'sense of self' of an individual, depending on their environment (Frable, 1997; Fitzgerald, 2005; Phinney, 2000). Family interactions that encourage adolescents to express their point of view and to disagree and participate in problem-solving can contribute to the development of individuality and identity. Holistic care for adolescents requires nurses to listen to the service user's personal narrative and understand that the service user may have a number of ways of seeing and expressing themselves (multiple self-schemas), depending on their environment and relationships.

Integrative models research the 'fit' between the individual and the environment, and suggest that the feedback adolescents receive from others contributes to either problematic or positive development (Eccles et al., 1993). The peer group is proposed as the primary influence on adolescent behaviour, and it may be that culture has more impact on behaviour than parenting (Eccles et al., 1993). Research continues, but the importance of interrelatedness between the adolescent and family, peer, school and work needs to be acknowledged, and positive relationships fostered, in order to decrease stress and confusion and to facilitate decision making and autonomy for the adolescent.

Risk factors

The risks and protective factors of childhood influence adolescence, with risks increasing due to additional developmental and social challenges. Approximately one in 10 children and young people in the UK under 16 have been diagnosed with at least one mental health problem (including 4% diagnosed with an emotional disorder [3% anxiety disorders and 1% depression] and 6% with a conduct disorder). Among 11–16-year-olds, 13% of boys and 10% of girls are clinically diagnosed with mental disorders (British Medical Association, 2006; Office for National Statistics, 2005). Many opportunities exist to change the balance of risk and protective factors during this time because of the numerous influences the adolescent is exposed to. The risk-assessment profile sheet (Fuller, 1998) identifies the extensive factors that contribute to risk in this group. Among the risk factors identified are: community factors such as poverty, isolation and accommodation; school factors relating to performance and attendance; family factors including the adolescent's connectedness to family, and family violence; peer friendships and the nature of the peer association (for example, delinquent peers); and individual characteristics such as those discussed under Childhood, including temperament, intelligence, aggression and likeability. Suicide is a rare event in young people under the age of 15, accounting for less than 2% of all suicides in most societies, yet there is an increased potential for suicide in young people

from families where there is violence, abuse and neglect and with family histories of alcohol and drug abuse, suicide and depression (Beautrais & Mishara, 2006). Over the past 10 years the number of suicides among people aged 15 years and over in the UK have shown a downward trend. Men tend to commit suicide at higher rates than women. In 2009 the suicide rate was 17.5 per 100 000 for men and 5.2 per 100 000 for women (Office for National Statistics, 2011). Research is ongoing in identifying risk factors for specific mental health problems in attempts to prevent or intervene early and reduce mental health problems.

Prevention and promotion

Adolescence is a period of opportunity for prevention and intervention for mental health problems. The extensive number of factors that contribute to risk for the adolescent has been acknowledged previously. Adolescents who have been compromised in meeting earlier developmental tasks or who are at risk can be given opportunities to increase protective factors. Programmes that develop assertion skills, crisis management, suicide prevention, identity acceptance and safe sex are all protective against risk.

Skills-building in communication and conflict resolution for families are important in facilitating autonomy in the adolescent. The adolescent gains a sense of self through well-negotiated family conflict. 'Individuality without connectedness is not autonomy, but isolation, and connectedness without self–other differentiation is not interdependence but fusion' (von der Lippe, cited in Skoe & von der Lippe, 1998, p. 54). Families need skills to facilitate flexibility in problem-solving and open communication to manage family conflict. Negotiation and expression of conflict are important in developing coping skills as they provide opportunities for the adolescent to gain mastery of challenging situations.

One of the significant tasks of adolescence, the acquisition of self-confidence and decision making, can be encouraged in homes and schools. Decision making is undertaken by people at all stages of the life cycle. It is especially relevant during adolescence, with heightened risk behaviour including self-harm and suicide. Koshar (1999, pp. 134–135) proposes a decision-making model that can be used by nurses, families and mentor programmes with the adolescent to think through emotional issues. The following steps are proposed.

1. The problem confronting the adolescent is identified and the options to address it are proposed.
2. The consequences of each option are generated and then classified as either positive or negative. The service user lists what they anticipate or experience as outcomes of their choices.

3. The service user assesses whether the outcomes will be good or bad. The importance and desirability of the consequences are explored.
4. The likelihood of different consequences occurring is assessed and the adolescent makes this assessment according to their unique frame of reference.
5. The decision is outlined and the nurse/parent provides some input for the adolescent to consider.

In this model the focus is on listening to the adolescent and then providing them with input which they can consider (after they have explored the issue as they see it). The model provides a structure that the service user can use independently in other situations.

Health-promoting interventions, which acknowledge the adolescent in a holistic way, incorporating their family and community, may assist the adolescent in strengthening attachments (Fuller, 1998). Generally a system of care that includes a consistent connection with one or more people who provide structure, advocacy and mentorship is desirable (Fuller, 1998; Osterling & Hines, 2006). Other aspects of the system of care are a comprehensive assessment, coordinated decision making on managing behaviour and the creation of interagency linkages that assist the adolescent with support and resources.

CRITICAL THINKING CHALLENGE 8.4

Andrew loves sport and is on school teams for swimming and football. He likes spending time with his friends, music and going camping. Recently he has been spending increasing amounts of time with Sam, a friend who is in his swimming team. He is disconcerted by feelings that he has been experiencing towards Sam, and is fearful of talking to anyone about it.

Discuss the factors that would support Andrew in understanding his current situation.

ADULTHOOD

Development and theoretical issues

Adulthood can be conceived of as a series of changes that occur after adolescence until the final stages of life. Throughout adulthood there are changes to cognitive, social, psychological and physical development, although by early adulthood many of the brain's functions have stabilized.

Theories that relate to this stage of development include stages four and five of Erikson's theory, which describe early and middle adulthood. These will now be discussed.

Intimacy versus isolation (early adulthood)

A mutually satisfying relationship with another person in which individual identity is sustained is evidence of successful resolution of this stage. This stage also requires 'sacrifices or compromises' (Erikson, cited in Welchman, 2000) as a result of a commitment to another person. The risks associated with becoming a couple can be the loss of self-identity from domination of the other, or lack of assertion of one's own desires and needs. Similarly, feelings of aloneness despite being a 'couple' can result from incomplete commitment to the relationship. Early adulthood is a time of greater vulnerability to mental health problems than middle or late adulthood. Stresses associated with new roles at work and in relationships, accompanied by high expectations, are contributors to an increase in mental health problems and illness at this time (Bee & Boyd, 2002). The person aged 20 to 30 is struggling with issues of identity and adjusting to increased responsibility as they attempt to establish a career. This period of chaos and pressure to make good decisions for the future can create vulnerability, hence the use of the term 'crisis'. Neugarten (1979) suggested that family and work roles could create conflicts for young adults as they attempt to balance responsibility with possibility and change. Chaos, confusion and change present significant challenges for young adults. Many of the risks, in particular the suicide risk for males associated with alcohol and drug abuse and depression discussed in the previous stage (adolescence), emerge in early adulthood.

Generativity versus self-absorption (middle adulthood)

According to Erikson, the middle years are the most productive in terms of family, occupational and social contributions. Erikson identifies this stage as characterized by the individual having altruistic tendencies and energies directed at contributing to a better world. While 'generativity' relates to guiding and supporting the next generation, it is also about contributing to the enrichment of society. Resolution can be achieved through a realistic appraisal of strengths, limitations and opportunity, and identification of appropriate present or future achievements.

Feelings of frustration and unrealized goals and potentials can create dissatisfaction with life in this stage (stagnation), which can affect the next generation if adults place their unrealized expectations on the child (Welchman, 2000).

Daniel Levinson's writing on development in men and women (Levinson, 1978, 1996) stemmed from his desire to understand his own adult development. Biographical research on men identified stages or 'transitions' of 'early adulthood' (17–22 years), 'entering the adult world' (between mid-twenties and late thirties) and the 'age 30 transition' (ends at approximately 33 years), the tasks and issues of which resemble Erikson's sixth stage. The mid-life transition (for 5 years after age 38 or before age 43) is a period from early adulthood into middle adulthood requiring a review of the past and reevaluation of values and beliefs, which may result in changes to how life is lived. This phase involves evaluation of achievement of the 'dream' or expectations of life. Middle adulthood is a time in which a structure for the rest of life is made from the choices available during the transition. In his later study of women's lives, Levinson (1996) interviewed homemakers, women with corporate financial careers and those with academic careers, identifying that women's cycle of adult development mirrored men's in the stages and transitional ages and tasks. However, differences in resources and constraints led to life experience that was self-limiting for the homemaker group. He envisaged a future in society for men and women where differences in life because of gender were minimal, where adult development could focus on meaning and satisfaction from the diversity of experience in life.

Attachment, gender, identity and risk

Theories of women's development emphasize the importance of connectedness and positive relationships in maintaining women's mental health throughout the lifespan. An awareness of the work of Carol Gilligan (1982) assists nurses to understand relational issues for women. The concept that Gilligan has named 'voice' is central to this understanding. Gilligan asserts that voice is the 'core of the self' and that we use it to relate to others. Speaking and listening are ways of understanding another. She believes that women's voices need to be heard in order to enhance their personal and social development. Her book *In a Different Voice* asks questions about theories in which men's experiences stand for all 'human experience', excluding the experience of women (Gilligan, 1982, p. xiii).

Most developmental theories support separation, detachment and autonomy as desirable outcomes of development. Gilligan (1982) proposes that 'attachment' in relationships is integral to the successful development of identity in women and that the values of interdependence, nurturing and sensitivity need to be valued as well as independence and autonomy. Unlike boys, who need to separate from the mother as they grow in order to achieve a masculine identity, girls develop their identity in the ongoing relationship they have with their mother. Self-in-relation theory was developed by Jean Baker Miller, Judith Jordan, Jan Surrey and Irene Stiver from this early work. This group, from the Stone Centre of Wellesley College (in Massachusetts, USA), espouses

the importance of connection with others in developing a healthy sense of self (Jordan et al., 1991). Self-in-relation theory has been used to explain and understand the origins of mental health problems in women and also to guide appropriate interventions (Nizette & Creedy, 1998).

The attachment experience of childhood is important to both sexes, as early childhood experiences of attachment can affect one's sense of self and relationships in adulthood. Research proposes that secure, avoidant or ambivalent attachment in adulthood is associated with childhood relationships and the emotional styles of parents (Hazan & Shaver, cited in Karen, 1994). Hazan and Shaver found that people in a secure attachment were happy, and knew and accepted the negative as well as the positive characteristics of their partner. Avoidant people were found to suffer jealousy and fear intimacy, and ambivalent attachment led to obsessive involvement and 'ups and downs'.

In young women, sadness has been identified as a precursor to depression (Gramling & McCain, 1997). Sadness is explained as disillusionment with life. Disillusionment can occur in young adulthood (late twenties), as women perceive that life has failed to meet their expectations (Gramling & McCain, 1997; Levinson, 1996). Another study found that disillusioned women who were unable to draw on a 'childhood self' were vulnerable compared to women who were able to recall a positive sense of 'self' from a memory of childhood (Reinke et al., 1985). An intervention to address sadness and avert depression suggested by Gramling and McCain (1997) and Levinson (1996) is cognitive restructuring of the young woman's perception or world view.

Women's reproductive experiences of menstruation and menopause, and possibly pregnancy, birth or infertility, are significant lifespan markers. Psychosocial issues for women such as low self-esteem, poor coping skills and self-reported stresses are prevalent in women experiencing premenstrual syndrome (PMS) and menopause. For menopausal women, however, a stressful life context is more predictive of depression than the menopause event itself (Stanton et al., 2002), although there is some evidence of the protective role of oestrogen against mental disorder (Osterlund, 2002). Pregnancy, childbirth and infertility evoke unique responses in women to the psychological stress experienced. For some, depression, psychosis, post-traumatic stress disorder, postpartum depression, distress and anxiety are sequelae of these events (Brockington, 1997; Stanton et al., 2002). Models of assessment and intervention that focus on support, appraisal, coping and resources are most useful throughout women's lives.

In older women, deterioration in physical health accompanied by symptoms that contribute to decreased functioning and feelings of low self-efficacy have been related to negative self-perception and depression (Heidrich, 1998). The emotional and relational aspects of women are acknowledged as major contributors to mental health, but it is important that physical health status is also taken into account. In summary, women who have poor support networks, few or no attachments and poor physical health are vulnerable to depression and to mental health problems.

Prevention and promotion

The adult has a range of health promotion needs based on the events that typically occur during this stage. Premarital counselling, family planning information and relationship counselling all assist with skills-building and lay a foundation for family development.

During this time, events such as the death of parents, divorce, relationship breakdown, work pressure, redundancy/unemployment and, later, the 'empty nest' experience may require crisis counselling. Enhanced coping skills, stress management, assertion skills, vocational skills and general health teaching (alcohol and drug education) address risk factors of work pressure, conflict and lifestyle. Therapeutic communication strategies, especially listening, will facilitate the service user's clarification of their concerns. Teaching the skills mentioned would increase feelings of efficacy and control in a stage of increased responsibility. Nurses can assist service users to access appropriate resources for crisis care, ongoing skills development or risk management.

CRITICAL THINKING CHALLENGE 8.5

Vivian is a 44-year-old woman and mother who has spent the past 7 years at home being a full-time mum to her four children. Before she and her partner Dave had children she had enjoyed her work as a travel consultant in a local travel agency. She now wants to return to work but is concerned that her in-laws and other people might think she should just be a mum. Vivian feels torn: she knows she can be a good mum and have a career as well. She is hesitant to express her wishes to Dave and finds herself preoccupied with the need to get back to her career, which she enjoyed so much. She finds herself losing interest in her usual daily jobs and routines.

- ◆ What could be motivating Vivian to return to work?
- ◆ Which 'stage' challenges is she confronting?
- ◆ Discuss the different outcomes that may result.

OLDER ADULTHOOD

Development and theoretical issues

Development in older adults focuses on positive outcomes that relate to the final stages of life, such as feeling positive about one's contribution to society, having close and loving relations with family and others, maintaining a purpose in life and having a sense of autonomy and control over one's life. Erikson's stage of integrity versus despair relates to late adulthood. In this final stage, successful resolution is achieved when the person is able to transcend any feelings of guilt, self-absorption or regret for lost opportunities throughout their life. The person is able to understand and appreciate the part their life has played in society. It is a time of acceptance and reflection on the unique meaning a person may make of their life (Neugarten, 1979; Welchman, 2000). Despair can be identified as a fear of death. A change in time perspective occurs as the older adult's concerns relate to the time left to live rather than the years since birth (Neugarten, 1979). Feelings of dissatisfaction and despair may arise with the realization that life cannot be lived again (Welchman, 2000).

The theory of gero-transcendence (Tornstam, 1989, cited in Wadensten & Carlsson, 2003) focuses on the final stage of life as a period of redefining the self, relationships and one's view of the world. This theory on ageing differs from others in that disengagement in the older adult is explained as an increased need for reflection on the matters of life, not because of a loss of interest in life or the world. Gero-transcendence provides the nurse with a different way of viewing the older person and their needs, which could lead to nursing practices in caring for the older person that are more appropriate and holistic.

Risk factors

The older adult may face issues of retirement, loss of functional capacity and change in family and friendship networks and supports, additional stressors which may increase risk in this age group. Risks of depression and anxiety among older people can be attributed to the range of loss that is usually more commonly experienced by the older person. Risk factors for these problems in the over-55 age group include illness or death of a significant other or family member, premorbid personality factors, being female and self-perceived poor health (De Beurs et al., 2001). Despite the knowledge that loss is linked to risk of depression, it often goes undetected and untreated, as evidenced by high rates of suicide in this group (Bevan & Jeeawody, 1998).

For older women, poor physical health is a significant risk factor for depression because deterioration in physical health generally contributes to a person's inability to maintain relationships with others and to feel supported (Heidrich, 1998). This finding is consistent with developmental theories which propose that mental health is more likely if the individual has a positive self-perception of supportive relations with others, autonomy, purpose and personal growth (Cantor & Sanderson, 2000; Heidrich, 1998). Older people from non-English-speaking backgrounds suffer more from isolation and experience particular difficulties in accessing appropriate health services (Moore, cited in Bevan & Jeeawody, 1998). Isolation and loneliness can affect quality of life, as well as being significant risk factors for a range of mental health problems.

Prevention and promotion

It is important for the nurse to remember that the lifespan is dynamic and that personal growth and learning are significant needs of the older person (Heidrich, 1998). Barriers to health promotion exist in the attitudes of health professionals who feel that older people are resistant to change or will not benefit from interventions. Health professionals may also have styles of communication with older people that are not interactive or therapeutic, resulting in a relationship in which the older person's power and autonomy are disregarded. As a result of this view, older adults are often overlooked in health promotion programmes. However, when asked, older people are interested in health promotion activities that are likely to improve their functioning and overall health (Young, 1996) and therefore it is important that mental healthcare and medical care are coordinated (Sorocco & McCallum, 2006). Listening to service users and acknowledging and challenging stereotypes are important initial steps for nurses working with older adults. Practical interventions (Wadensten & Carlsson, 2003) are based on the need to accept the fact that reflection and redefinition (gero-transcendance) are normal in the older person. Secondly, nurses can reduce the older person's preoccupation with the body by using topics of conversation other than physical feelings or limitations. The nurse can focus on listening when the person wants to talk about death or dying. Additional communication 'microskills' of reflecting the feeling and content of the conversation may further assist with the person's reflections. Topics of conversation and activities that provide variety and challenge need to be offered, as well as opportunities for quiet time alone. All the interventions suggested may challenge current practices, which view this stage more as an extension of adulthood than a stage in which the person has specific and different needs.

NURSE'S STORY

I remember her as a quiet, white-haired women sitting on the edge of the bed. She had just been transferred to the mental health unit from a general ward. The patient had large cuts, more like gouges, to the inside area of her elbow joint. We discovered that she had done it with a bread knife. She had stayed in the surgical ward until the surgeon was satisfied with the integrity of the repair and sutures. I found out that her partner had died the previous year but even so I believe that I and the other nurses failed to take into account the significance of her actions and where she was 'at' in her life.

At the time, I couldn't understand how an elderly person could not cope with a partner's death. It's expected when you get old … isn't it? I suppose I believed that she should have been grieving 'normally' and that her interest would be directed to her grandchildren. I remember even feeling a little angry with her: it was as if I felt she should have had more sense at her age.

Now, with more knowledge and experience, I would be more empathic. I feel I would be better able to communicate with her, be therapeutic and make a difference. I've tried to use that experience as a learning one rather than beating myself up for making so many assumptions, stereotyping, and not hearing the patient's story. Finding out the patient's and their family's stories is now part of my everyday practice.

Health promotion can be an 'empowering' strategy: that is, a strategy that gives the service user choice and options for decision making about their own health. Interventions suggested by Wadensten and Carlsson (2003) and derived from gero-transcendence theory (as described above) are predicated on the older person as having wisdom, and are appropriate to working with older people in any setting. Services for non-English-speaking older people require policies that address and use culturally appropriate communication and consultation strategies (Moore, cited in Bevan & Jeeawody, 1998). Interventions aimed at reducing isolation, identified as a risk factor, also need to be built into policy.

CRITICAL THINKING CHALLENGE 8.6

What potential do nurses have to provide interventions aimed at increasing protective factors? How can nurses work towards mitigating risk factors?

CONCLUSION

Fluctuations in a person's mental health occur throughout the lifespan. Risk factors, both internal and external, can create vulnerability, exposing people to mental health problems and mental illness. Some of the vulnerability and risk can be mediated by health-promoting interventions. Health-promoting interventions that increase protective factors are appropriate at all times, even if risk is not apparent. Everyone is at risk or increasingly vulnerable at some stage during their life. Most importantly, the nurse works with the service user to identify and work with their strengths to build resilience and self-efficacy.

Knowledge of developmental psychological theories can assist the nurse to understand vulnerability and risk throughout the lifespan. Holistic assessment, including the establishment of a connection to health services through therapeutic communication, is a beginning step. During assessment, the nurse can identify risk, and access and connect individuals and families to culturally appropriate resources and services. Health-promoting strategies based on an understanding of theory and applied practically can become part of the nurse's practice in all settings with service users and their families. Some strategies have been described in this chapter.

A shift in our society and culture is required so that better mental health outcomes can be achieved throughout the lifespan. A primary healthcare approach incorporating changes in public policy will help resolve the transmission of violence, neglect, abuse, poverty and threat from generation to generation, a social phenomenon that contributes to the incidence of mental distress and disorder. Karen, in elaborating on the relevance of attachment in childhood, reports on studies demonstrating that 'social policy and social interventions can make a society more humane and give parents a better chance to raise secure children' (Karen, 1994, p. 420). Contextual issues, environmental and social, create and maintain the internal and external factors of risk for mental health problems and illness across the lifespan. Nursing practice that is holistic and focused on wellness (health-promoting interventions) can build awareness, skills, strengths and resilience, ultimately affecting a person's quality of life throughout their lifespan.

EXERCISES FOR CLASS ENGAGEMENT

Interview a family member or friend to record their 'life history'.

- Make notes and record events that the interviewee identifies as significant.
- Analyse the interviews and identify protective and/or risk factors from the person's story.
- In small groups, list the protective and risk factors and categorize them as internal or external.
- Can you identify an instance of increased vulnerability from the person's story and explain the contributing factors?

In small groups, identify what you consider to be the most critical time in a person's life. (Each group may identify different critical times.) Then devise a health promotion plan or strategy that includes:

- the target group,
- examples of interventions,
- types and content of information that may be needed,
- how the plan could be implemented.

Many of the developmental theories emerged from research undertaken on subjects who were white males.

Discuss and identify the issues in using these theories to understand people from different cultural backgrounds. Assign different cultural backgrounds to the critical thinking challenges in this chapter and discuss how risk and protective factors may vary (e.g. Vivian in Critical Thinking Challenge 8.5 may be an immigrant escaping war in a troubled part of the world).

ACKNOWLEDGEMENT

The author would like to acknowledge Michael Groome for his contribution on moral development.

REFERENCES

Allport, G., 1961. Pattern and Growth in Personality. Holt, Reinhart & Winston, New York.

Andresen, R., Caputi, P., Oades, L., 2006. Stages of recovery instrument: development of a measure of recovery from serious mental illness. Aust. New Zeal. J. Psychiatry 40, 972–980.

Arbona, C., Power, T., 2003. Parental attachment, self-esteem, and anti-social behaviours among African American, European American, and Mexican American adolescents. J. Couns. Psychol. 50 (1), 40–51.

Bailey, C., 1986. Kohlberg on morality and feeling. In: Modgil, S., Modgil, C. (Eds.), Lawrence Kohlberg: Consensus and Controversy. Falmer Press, Philadelphia.

Bakermans-Kranenburg, M.J., van Ijzendoorn, M.H., Juffer, F., 2003. Less is more: meta-analyses of sensitivity and attachment interventions in early childhood. Psychol. Bull. 129 (2), 195–215.

Baltes, P.B., Baltes, M.M. (Eds.), 1990. Successful Aging: Perspectives from the Behavioural Sciences. Cambridge University Press, New York.

Baltes, P.B., Staudinger, U.M., Lindenberger, U., 1999. Lifespan psychology: theory and application to intellectual functioning. Annu. Rev. Psychol. 50, 471–507.

Barlow, J., Parsons, J., 2002. Group-based training programmes for improving emotional and behavioral adjustment in 0–3 year old children. Cochrane Database Syst. Rev. 4, CD003680.

Baumrind, D., 1971. Current patterns of parental authority. Develop. Psychol. Monogr. 4 (1, Part 2), 1–103.

Beautrais, A.L., Mishara, B., 2006. World suicide prevention day—September 10, 2007. Suicide prevention across the lifespan. Crisis 28 (2), 57–60.

Bee, H., Boyd, D., 2002. Lifespan Development, third ed. Allyn & Bacon, Boston.

Bergland, A., Kirkevold, M., 2001. Thriving: a useful theoretical perspective to capture the experience of well-being among frail elderly in nursing homes? J. Adv. Nurs. 36 (3), 426–432.

Berk, L.E., 2001. Development through the Lifespan, second ed. Allyn & Bacon, Boston.

Bertenthal, B.I., 1996. Origins and early development of perception, action, and representation. Annu. Rev. Psychol. 47, 431–459.

Bevan, C., Jeeawody, B., 1998. Successful Aging: Perspectives on Health and Social Construction. Elsevier, Sydney.

Bowlby, J., 1951. Maternal Care and Mental Health. World Health Organization, Geneva, HMSO, London; Columbia University Press, New York. Abridged version 1965, Child Care and the Growth of Love, 2nd edn. Penguin, Harmondsworth.

British Medical Association, 2006. Child and adolescent mental health. <http://www.bma.org.uk/health_promotion_ethics/child_health/Childadolescentmentalhealth.jsp>.

Brockington, I., 1997. Liaison psychiatry: focus on psychogynaecology. Curr. Opin. Psychiatry 10 (6), 466–469.

Brown, L.M., Debold, E., Tappan, M., et al., 1991. Reading narratives of

conflict and choice for self and moral voices: a relational method. In: Kurtines, W.K., Gewirtz, J.L. (Eds.), Handbook of Moral Behavior and Development Theory 2. Lawrence Erlbaum Associates, NJ.

Cantor, N., Sanderson, C.A., 2000. Life task participation and wellbeing: the importance of taking part in daily life. In: Kahneman, D., Diener, E., Schwarz, N. (Eds.), Well-being: The Foundations of Hedonic Psychology. Russell Sage Foundation, New York, pp. 230–243.

Caplan, G. (Ed.), 1964. Principles of Preventive Psychiatry Basic Books, New York.

Carver, C.S., 1998. Resilience and thriving issues, models, and linkages. J. Soc. Issues 54 (2), 245–266.

Caspi, A., Moffitt, T.E., Newman, D.L., et al., 1996. Behavioral observations at age 3 years predict adult psychiatric disorders: longitudinal evidence from a birth cohort. Arch. Gen. Psychiatry 53 (1), 1033–1039.

Compas, B.E., Hinden, B.R., Gerhardt, C.A., 1995. Adolescent development: pathways and processes of risk and resilience. Annu. Rev. Psychol. 46, 265–293.

Darley, J.M., Shultz, T.R., 1990. Moral rules: their content and acquisition. Annu. Rev. Psychol. 41, 525–556.

De Beurs, E., Beekman, A., Geerlings, S., et al., 2001. On becoming depressed or anxious in late life: similar vulnerability factors but different effects of stressful life events. Brit. J. Psychiatry 179, 426–431.

Department of Health, 1999. National service framework for mental health. <http://www.dh.gov.uk/en/Publicationsandstatistics/Publications/PublicationsPolicyAndGuidance/DH_4009598>.

Department of Health, 2003a. Fast-forwarding primary care mental health: graduate primary care mental health workers. Best practice guidance. <http://www.dh.gov.uk/en/Publicationsandstatistics/Publications/PublicationsPolicyAndGuidance/DH_4005784>.

Department of Health, 2003b. Fast-forwarding primary care mental health: 'gateway'

workers. <http://www.dh.gov.uk/en/Publicationsandstatistics/Publications/PublicationsPolicyAndGuidance/DH_4006795>.

Department of Health, 2011. No health without mental health. <http://www.dh.gov.uk/en/Aboutus/Features/DH_123998>.

Deveson, A., 2003. Resilience. Allen & Unwin, Crows Nest, New South Wales.

Donenberg, G.R., Hoffman, L.W., 1988. Gender differences in moral development. Sex Roles 18 (11/12), 701–717.

Eccles, J.S., Midgley, C., Wigfield, A., et al., 1993. Development during adolescence: the impact of stage-environment fit on adolescents' experiences in schools and families. Am. Psychol. 48 (2), 90–101.

Eisenberg, N., 2000. Emotion, regulation and moral development. Annu. Rev. Psychol. 51, 655–697.

Erikson, E.H., 1963. Childhood and Society, second ed. W W Norton, New York.

Fitzgerald, 2005. An existential view of adolescent development. Adolescence 40 (160), 793–799.

Frable, E.S., 1997. Gender, racial, ethic, sexual and class identities. Ann. Rev. Psychol. 48, 139–162.

Fuller, A., 1998. From Surviving to Thriving: Promoting Mental Health in Young People. Australian Council for Educational Research, Melbourne.

Garmon, L.C., 2000. Relations between attachment representations and moral judgment. Doctoral thesis, Ohio State University. Dissertation Abstracts International, Section B: Sciences & Engineering DAI-B 60/11, p. 5811, May 2000.

Gilligan, C., 1982. In a Different Voice. Psychological Theory and Women's Development. Howard University Press, Cambridge, MA.

Gilligan, C., 1987. Moral Orientation and Moral Development. In: Kittay, E.F., Meyers, D.T. (Eds.), Women and Moral Theory Rowman & Littlefield, NJ.

Gilligan, C., 1998. Remapping the moral domain: new images of self in relationship. In: Gilligan, C., Ward, J.V., McTaylor, L. (Eds.), Mapping the Moral Domain. Harvard University Press, Cambridge, MA.

Golombok, S., Fivush, R., 1994. Gender Development. Cambridge University Press, Cambridge.

Gramling, L.F., McCain, N.L., 1997. Grey glasses: sadness in young women. J. Adv. Nurs. 26 (2), 312–319.

Heidrich, S.M., 1998. Older women's lives through time. Adv. Nurs. Sci. 20 (3), 65–75.

Jacelon, C.S., 1997. The trait and process of resilience. J. Adv. Nurs. 25 (1), 123–129.

Jordan, J., Kaplan, A., Miller, J.B., et al., 1991. Women's Growth in Connection. Guilford, New York.

Karen, R., 1994. Becoming Attached: Unfolding the Mystery of the Infant-Mother Bind and its Impact on Later Life. Warner Books, New York.

Kearney, J.A., 1997. Emotional development in infancy: theoretical models and nursing implications. J. Child Adol. Psychiatry Nurs. 10 (4), 7–17.

King, L., 2001. The hard road to a good life: the happy mature person. J. Humanist. Psychol. 41 (1), 51–72.

Kohlberg, L., 1986. A current statement on some theoretical issues. In: Modgil, S., Modgil, C. (Eds.), Lawrence Kohlberg: Consensus and Controversy Falmer Press, Philadelphia.

Kohlberg, L., Levine, C., Hewer, H., 1983. The current formulation of the theory. In: Kohlberg, L. (Ed.), The Psychology of Moral Development Harper & Row, New York, pp. 212–319.

Koshar, J.H., 1999. Helping adolescents make 'good' decisions. Am. J. Nurs. 99 (1) 24J–24L.

Lerner, R., 1991. Changing organism-context relations as the basic process of development: a developmental contextual perspective. Dev. Psychol. 27, 27–32.

Levinson, D., 1978. The Seasons of a Man's Life. Alfred A Knopf, New York.

Levinson, D., 1996. The Seasons of a Woman's Life. Alfred A Knopf, New York.

Licence, K., 2004. Promoting and protecting the health of children and young people. Child Care Health Dev. 30, 623–635.

Lindsey, E., Hartrick, G., 1996. Health-promoting nursing practice: The demise of the nursing process? J. Adv. Nurs. 23 (1), 106–112.

Luthar, S., Cicchetti, D., Becker, B., 2000. The construct of resilience: a critical evaluation and guidelines for future work. Child Dev. 71 (3), 543–562.

Marsh, D., Lefley, H., Evans-Rhodes, D., et al., 1996. The family experience of mental illness: evidence for resilience. Psychiatry Rehabil. J. 20 (2), 3–12.

Maslow, A.H., 1968. Toward a Psychology of Being, second ed. Van Norstrund, Princeton, NJ.

Masten, A., 2001. Ordinary magic: resilience processes in development. Am. Psychol. 56 (3), 227–238.

Mrazek, P.J., Haggerty, R.J., 1994. Reducing Risks for Mental Disorders: Frontiers for Preventative Intervention Research. National Academies Press, Washington DC.

Nakash-Eisikovits, O., Dutra, L., Westen, D., 2002. Relationship between attachment patterns and personality pathology in adolescents. J. Am. Acad. Child Adolesc. Psychiatry 41 (9), 1111–1123.

National Institute for Health and Clinical Excellence, 2009. Depression. <http://www.nice.org.uk/CG90>.

Neugarten, B., 1979. Time, age, and the life cycle. Am. J. Psychiatry 136 (7), 887–894.

Nizette, D., Creedy, D., 1998. Women and mental illness. In: Rogers Clark, C., Smith, A. (Eds.), Women's Health: a Primary Healthcare Approach Elsevier, Sydney.

Office for National Statistics, 2005. Mental health of children and young people in Great Britain, 2004. <http://www.statistics.gov.uk/downloads/theme_health/GB2004.pdf>.

Office for National Statistics, 2011. Suicide rates in the United Kingdom, 2000–2009. <http://www.statistics.gov.uk/statbase/Product.asp?vlnk 5 13618>.

Osterling, K.L., Hines, A.M., 2006. Mentoring adolescent foster youth: promoting resilience during developmental transitions. Child Family Soc. Work 11, 242–253.

Osterlund, M., 2002. The role of estrogens in neuropsychiatric disorders. Curr. Opin. Psychiatry 15 (3), 307–312.

Park, A., Roberts, C., 2002. The ties that bind. In: The 19th Report of British Social Attitudes, National Centre for Social Research, London.

Peterson, C., 2004. Looking Forward through the Lifespan: Developmental Psychology, fourth ed. Prentice Hall, Sydney.

Phinney, J.S., 2000. Identity formation across cultures: the interaction of personal, societal, and historical change. History Culture 43 (1), 27–31.

Piaget, P., 1977 (original work published 1932). Moral Judgement Development of the Child, tr. Gabain M. Penguin, Harmondsworth.

Pratt, M., Golding, G., Hunter, W., 1984. Does morality have a gender? Sex, sex role and moral judgement relationships across the lifespan. Merrill-Palmer Quart. 30 (4), 321–340.

Reinke, B., Ellicott, A., Harris, R., et al., 1985. Timing of psychosocial changes in women's lives. Hum. Dev. 28, 259–280.

Rew, L., Taylor-Seehafer, M., Thomas, N., et al., 2001. Correlates of resilience in homeless adolescents. J. Nurs. Scholarship 33 (1), 33–40.

Rickwood, D., 2006. Pathways to Recovery: 4 A's Framework for Preventing Further Episodes of Mental Illness. Commonwealth of Australia, Canberra.

Salmelainen, P., 1996. Child neglect: its causes and its role in delinquency. Contemp. Issues Crime Just. 33, 1–14.

Sanders, M.R., Markie-Dadds, C., Tully, L.A., et al., 2000. The triple p-positive parenting program: a comparison of enhanced, standard, and self-directed behavioral family intervention for parents of children with early onset conduct problems. J. Consult. Clin. Psych. 68 (4), 624–640.

Shultz, T.R., Wells, D., 1985. Judging the intentionality of action-outcomes. Dev. Psych. 21 (1), 83–89.

Skoe, E., von der Lippe, A., 1998. Personality Development in Adolescence: A Cross-National and Life Span Perspective. Routledge, New York.

Sorocco, K.H., McCallum, T.J., 2006. Mental health promotion in older adults: addressing treatment approaches and available screening tools. Geriatrics 61 (1), 19–22.

Stanton, A., Lobel, M., Sears, S., et al., 2002. Psychosocial aspects of selected issues in women's reproductive health: current status and future directions. J. Consult. Clin. Psych. 70 (3), 751–770.

Stilwell, B.M., Galvin, M., Kopta, S.M., et al., 1997. Moralization of attachment: a fourth domain of conscious functioning. J. Am. Acad.

Child Adolesc. Psychiatry 36 (8), 1140–1147.

Townley, M., 2002. Mental health needs of children and young people. Nurs. Stand. 16 (30), 38–47.

Wadensten, B., Carlsson, M., 2003. Theory-driven guidelines for practical care of older people, based on the theory of gerotranscendence. J. Adv. Nurs. 41 (5), 462–470.

Waters, E., Vaughn, B.E., Posada, G., et al., 1995. Caregiving, Cultural, and Cognitive Perspectives on Secure-base Behavior and Working Models: New Growing Points of Attachment Theory and Research. University of Chicago Press, Chicago.

Welchman, K., 2000. Erik Erikson: His Life, Work and Significance. Open University Press, Philadelphia.

Werner, E., Smith, R., 1982. Vulnerable, but Invincible: A Longitudinal Study of Resilient Children and Youth. McGraw-Hill, New York.

White, F., 1996. Parent–adolescent communication and adolescent decision-making. J. Family Stud. 2 (1), 41–56.

World Health Organization, 1986. Ottowa Charter—Achieving Health for all: A Framework for Health Promotion. World Health Organization, Copenhagen.

Young, K., 1996. Health, health promotion and the elderly. J. Clin. Nurs. 5 (4), 241–248.

Zeanah, C.H., Boris, N.W., Larrieu, J.A., 1997. Infant development and developmental risk: a review of the past 10 years. J. Am. Acad. Child Adolesc. Psychiatry 36 (2), 165–178.

Chapter | 9 |

Crisis and loss

Paul Morrison

CHAPTER POINTS

- Crisis is a normal part of life.
- A person's ability to cope with a crisis will depend on how much it is perceived as being beyond their ability to function.
- When a person is unable to deal effectively with a situation and the emotions associated with it, they may experience feelings of helplessness, anxiety, fear and guilt.
- Crisis nearly always involves significant losses (primary and secondary) for those involved, and a number of important tasks must be completed for adaptive grieving to occur.
- As people learn to cope effectively with life crises they build a repertoire of skills and competencies that can be used to manage crises that emerge later in life.
- If a crisis is not dealt with effectively it can lead to poor health.
- Nurses are frequently exposed to crisis in families and need to develop therapeutic approaches and skills to enable them to help service users.
- Helping people at times of personal crisis can be difficult and stressful for nurses and other health workers. It can raise issues and conflicts for the helper.
- Nurses need a strong commitment to cultural awareness and sensitivity when caring for service users and families from diverse backgrounds.

DOI: http://dx.doi.org/10.1016/B978-0-7020-4493-9.00009-3

KEY TERMS

- abuse
- adapting
- advanced training
- anger
- assessment
- assumptions
- attempted suicide
- conflict
- coping
- coping strategies
- crisis
- culture
- death
- disclosure
- distress
- emotional reaction
- feelings
- grief
- helping
- life crisis
- life events
- loss
- mourning
- nurse's role
- primary loss
- rape
- rapport
- resources
- risk
- secondary loss
- self-harm
- shock
- stress
- sudden death
- suicide
- support
- trauma
- uncertainty
- victim
- violent crime
- vulnerability

LEARNING OUTCOMES

The material in this chapter will assist you to:

- describe some of the types of life crisis that occur and the potential impact these may have on people's lives,
- understand how people deal with crisis by drawing on the resources available to them to adapt to the crisis situation, and be aware that a failure to cope may indicate a need for professional help,
- identify how nurses can help service users and families deal with the types of crisis that may present in a healthcare setting,
- describe nursing approaches and interventions that may be employed when caring for people and their families at times of crisis,
- acknowledge the importance of cultural sensitivity and understanding for professionals when working with service users from diverse cultures at times of crisis and loss,
- explain some of the vital constituents needed to establish a positive helping relationship with service users in crisis.

INTRODUCTION

A crisis in life often appears like a bolt out of the blue. The sudden onset of illness, the loss of a job or a death in the family can visit at any time. These events can throw stable lives into a chaotic state with no apparent positive solution. This chapter examines some of the crises that can erupt without warning. It considers the defining features of a crisis and the potential impact of a crisis on people's lives.

While two people can be exposed to the same stressful event, they are likely to construe the event differently; one may be able to adapt and cope well, while the other may feel anxious and 'crushed' by the experience. It is this personal appraisal process that is at the core of coping with a crisis.

When a person is unable to cope, even for a short time, some form of professional intervention may be required. A number of crisis events are broached here, including suicide, attempted suicide, self-harm, being a victim of crime and sudden death, with an emphasis on the important role that nurses can play in helping service users to deal with these effectively. There is also a strong focus on dealing with the loss that usually trails a life crisis. The need for a heightened awareness of cultural considerations in the helping process is also stressed.

The final section of the chapter deals with some of the helping attitudes and skills that are needed to assist people to deal with crisis and loss. These look straightforward enough on paper, but in the 'disordered' environment of a busy casualty department or an acute mental health admission unit they may be much more difficult to practise and sustain. These are nevertheless required competencies for high-quality nurse–service user relationships.

WHAT CONSTITUTES A CRISIS?

Most people can recall a crisis situation in their lives that made them feel out of kilter with the world, highly anxious and vulnerable, a sense of life being out of control and unpredictable. The death of a friend or parent, being the victim of a crime, physical assault or rape and being part of a natural disaster are examples of life crises. Some types of crisis are classed as 'situational' crisis (Aguilera, 1998): abortion, child abuse, rape, divorce, chronic physical illness, mental disorder, alcohol and drug abuse, suicide and attempted suicide. Others may be termed 'maturational' crisis and are linked to normal stages of development and ageing across the lifespan (Aguilera, 1998). Some life crises can be anticipated (natural death of a partner), while others are unanticipated (sudden death following a road traffic accident).

A crisis can be distinguished from a stressful event that may pass quickly, such as an exam. Parry (1990) summarized the most common defining features of a crisis as follows.

- There is a triggering stress event or long-term stress.
- The individual experiences distress.
- There is a loss, danger or humiliation.
- There is a sense of uncontrollability.
- The events feel unexpected.
- There is a disruption of routine.
- There is uncertainty about the future.
- The distress continues over time (from about 2 to 6 weeks).

CONSEQUENCES OF A PERSONAL CRISIS

A crisis will have a significant impact on the lives of those involved. It can produce great pain, distress and anguish. It can lead to feelings of unreality, uncertainty and isolation. A person in crisis will want to restore the general sense of balance in their life and feel able to cope with life again. The word 'crisis' also implies a sense of urgency, a turning point, a time for major decisions (Parry, 1990). People in crisis are often in a state of shock. It is a time when their thinking is muddled and their emotional reactions are characterized by feelings of loss, helplessness and hopelessness. They may try to cope with the situation by denial initially but they need to cope in a more effective way in the long run. The role of helpers is to enable service users to cope with the problem and with the feelings the problem has elicited. The type of support offered may be emotional support, practical help, companionship, advice and information (Parry, 1990).

A life crisis will stop people completing daily activities and routines. It causes a huge disruption in their lives and often the lives of those close to them. This usually means that the people involved in a crisis must make behavioural, social and emotional adjustments in their lives. These may be temporary or, in the case of a crisis brought about by the onset of chronic illness, enduring adjustments (Caltabiano et al., 2002). A crisis can change a person's life permanently. It can signal the end of a promising academic career, the end of a close relationship or the inability to get married and have children, or it can heighten personal vulnerability. A crisis brings much uncertainty into people's lives because they cannot foresee how it will unfold.

At a time of acute crisis the physical environment too, such as an emergency room, may be a frightening place for service users and their relatives. The level of noise, technical equipment and activity may be daunting. In accident and emergency departments, the service user who failed in their attempted suicide may feel guilty for wasting people's time. The rape victim may feel further exposed and violated. The abused child may be confused and scared and unsure of who to trust. These reactions are unlikely to be helpful at a time of acute crisis. On the other hand, strong supportive structures (families and friends) have been found to aid coping and adjustment following serious physical illness (Caltabiano et al., 2002) and are likely to play a role in adjusting following other types of crisis too.

Helping people in crisis is not about taking over (although on rare occasions this may be appropriate) and making them dependent. It is more effective to help them to use their own resources and to be supportive. It is about enabling, not disabling (Parry, 1990).

A FRAMEWORK FOR COPING AND ADAPTING TO CRISIS

How change is dealt with and the ways in which conflict and demands are handled are forms of coping. The ability to cope and tolerate these life events and incidents will be influenced by many factors that will shape feelings, thoughts, beliefs, values and actions as well as the responses of others. Crisis nearly always involves some form of significant loss for the person involved and these losses can come in many different forms: the loss of financial or personal security, sleep, appetite or the ability to think clearly, the loss of a sense of identity as a couple, a sense of trust or a sense of belonging.

The coping and adjustment effort required may be significant and people differ in how they respond to these circumstances. The upshot of a crisis will depend on how well the person copes, and the coping process will be influenced by the interaction of 'event' factors, background factors, physical and social environmental factors. For example, an illness can elicit new and distressing signs such as lack of interest in personal hygiene and an inability to communicate effectively with others. Feeling angry, depressed or guilty after surviving a suicide attempt can be stigmatizing for the service user and reinforces their desire to hide away from people. Sometimes the disabling effect of medication side effects (such as drowsiness and drooling mouth) can be very embarrassing (Morrison et al., 2000).

Some people just seem to possess an ability to find a sense of purpose or quality in their lives in spite of the awful things they come up against at a time of crisis. They can resist feeling 'helpless and hopeless' (Caltabiano et al., 2002). Other factors that are important include age, personal beliefs, gender, personal maturity, social class and the level of religious commitment that a person holds (Moos and Schaefer, 1986). These factors will shape the way individuals respond to crises (see also Ch. 7).

The complexity of issues, responses and settings in which crises and coping occur can be daunting. Holahan et al. (1996) devised a framework for coping as a process of adaptation by drawing on earlier research and bringing together the need to consider the person and the context in which coping happens. It takes account of the personal and situational issues that can affect coping. Panel 1 is made up of the constant stressors in life, such as illness, as well as the supports and aids available to the person, while Panel 2 contains the person's coping strategies and sociodemographic attributes.

These 'systems' influence the life crises and transitions that occur to all (Panel 3). The cognitive evaluation of these (Panel 4) has a direct impact on our health and wellbeing (Panel 5). According to Holahan et al. (1996), cognitive appraisal and coping responses play a critical role in responses to stress and crisis. It is also notable that the factors in each panel can provide feedback to earlier parts of the framework, giving it a dynamic quality.

Coping strategies have been described within this framework: people typically either 'approach' or 'avoid' stressful events. This illustrates the person's orientation. The approach or avoidance domains are also influenced by the methods of coping people can use. These are 'cognitive' or 'behavioural' methods. When combined, four basic types of coping response (cognitive approach, behavioural approach, cognitive avoidance, behavioural avoidance) are produced (see Holahan et al., 1996 for details).

Of particular importance here is the fact that the research literature indicates that consistent patterns of relationships have been found to occur using this framework. For example: 'people who rely more on approach coping tend to adapt better to life stressors and experience fewer psychological symptoms. Approach coping strategies such as problem-solving and seeking information, can moderate the potential adverse influence of both negative life changes and enduring role stressors on psychological functioning' (Holahan et al., 1996, p. 29).

In contrast, people who rely heavily on avoidance coping strategies like 'denial' and 'withdrawal' tend to suffer greater levels of distress after a period of crisis. A significant body of research exploring the relationship between approach/avoidance coping and a range of clinical issues, such as depression, physical illness, alcohol use and smoking behaviour, lends considerable support to this framework. It must be noted, however, that these trends might not apply across cultures.

Finally, Holahan et al. (1996) also noted that people exposed to crisis events often emerge stronger and with greater levels of competence. Their ability to cope with future crises may be enhanced. They may be more self-assured and assertive, have developed different views of themselves and their abilities, achieved a new sense of purpose in life and become more resilient, in spite of the fact that they have confronted significant life crises. The framework and the findings provide nurses and other care staff with some guideposts for working with people in crisis. They present a structure to ensure that staff consider the wider canvas of events, experiences, resources and coping styles that may be at the service user's disposal with appropriate support and guidance from the nurse.

EVENTS AND PERCEPTIONS THAT CAN LEAD TO PERSONAL CRISIS

Slaikeu (1990) described some of the common precipitating events that can spark a personal crisis, including pregnancy and the birth of a child, motherhood outside marriage, moving from home to school or from home to university, marriage, bereavement, relocation and migration, retirement, surgery and illness, natural disasters and rapid social and technological change. Other devastating events such as the death of a loved one or rape may elicit a crisis response. Events, even those that most are exposed to, can be interpreted as 'the last straw' after a crisis reaction (Slaikeu, 1990).

Some time ago Holmes and Rahe (1967) devised a useful way of considering how much stress a person may be exposed to, using the Life Events Scale. The scale lists 41 positive and negative common occurrences that require adjustment and can affect a person's risk of illness. Each occurrence is given a life-change unit score and these can be summed to reflect the level of life-changing events that have occurred in a particular person's life in the previous 12 months. Some examples include death of a spouse, 100; divorce, 73; marriage, 50; change in responsibilities at work, 29; Christmas, 12; and so on. When these are added together a total score can be arrived at; generally the higher the score the greater the risk of illness in the future.

Even if a person with a very high score seems to be coping with significant life stresses, a major crisis (anxiety, depression, suicide attempt, heart attack) can be imminent. Within this model a collection of life-change units that amount to more than 350 in a given year may lead to a crisis. It is also interesting to note how even positive events (such as a promotion or a marriage) can be stressful and lead to a crisis for some people.

There are no hard and fast rules about what may be deemed a crisis and what may not. A person's perception of events, their culture and life experience, the consequences and losses associated with these and their ability to manage effectively are primary. Scileppa et al. (2000, p. 87) commented: 'Allowing for personal differences in coping styles, it is fair to say that any situation or combination of life occurrence that taxes individuals beyond their typical ability to function can be viewed as a crisis'.

Levine and Perkins (1997) described crisis somewhat differently, as a time when a person's resources (material, physical, psychological) and those in the person's social network, are overburdened. The person is unable to deal effectively with the emotions surrounding the event. They may experience feelings of helplessness, anxiety, fear and guilt, and their behaviour is ineffective. Most people cope with crises but sometimes they can lead to other problems such as abuse of alcohol and drugs, or indeed to mental disorder.

The nurse's role is to help service users overcome this period in their lives, not to judge how bad things seem. Losing a pet is something most will deal with well but, for some, the loss can be followed by depression or a suicide attempt because that pet may have been the only companion in that person's life.

The nature of any nursing intervention at this time may be centred around giving comfort, helping the person to explore their intense feelings, helping to clarify events, options for the future and sources of support – physical, psychological and social – and trying to enhance the person's coping strategies. If these interventions are helpful then some common outcomes can be expected. The person will feel safe and well supported. Their view of the situation will be couched in reality and they will feel less vulnerable. They will be able to draw on the available sources of support and cope more effectively with the situation.

If the crisis is addressed effectively then this resolution may provide the service user with new skills and competencies that can help manage upcoming life crises. If, on the other hand, the crisis is not resolved successfully then this may lead to later problems and issues that have a negative effect on the service user's physical and psychological health. For example, unresolved issues may be the source of later problems in living for many victims of childhood sexual abuse who have been found to suffer from a range of negative consequences later in life, including depression, guilt, low self-esteem, feelings of inferiority, isolation, loneliness, distrust and poor-quality interpersonal relationships, promiscuity and sexual dysfunction (Johnson, 1998).

INTERVENING AT A TIME OF CRISIS

A crisis can present in many different ways and, if it is severe enough, professional helpers may be asked to intervene. Aguilera (1998) described two broad approaches to this process. The generic approach is based on the notion that certain common patterns emerge in most crisis situations and that these must be worked through if the person is to adapt in a healthy way. The intervention is aimed at achieving an adaptive resolution by focusing on the typical patterns of response in crisis rather than the distinctive ways in which individuals react (Aguilera, 1998). Hence the approach is a general one focusing on the usual steps and stages that might occur following, for example, the sudden death of a partner.

The individual approach is much more psychological and focuses on the service user's personal history, needs and responses. There is a greater focus on depth and human understanding, and greater levels of specialist training are required to practise in this way (Aguilera, 1998). Practical reality may dictate that professional helpers combine these two approaches. The typical steps in a crisis intervention scenario are outlined in Box 9.1 (see also Ch. 23).

While these steps may be typical, individuals do not always pass through them in a simple linear fashion. For example, the initial assessment of the problem may be revised as the helper learns more about the service user and their life over a period of time. This may change the focus of the intervention, making it more appropriate for the service user's needs. Sometimes the service user

---

Box 9.1 **Steps in crisis intervention**

Assessment: including assessment of the potential risk to the person and others.

Planning a therapeutic intervention: taking account of the impact on the person and the resources available to the person.

Intervention:

- help the person to understand what has happened,
- help the person to express feelings openly,
- explore coping mechanisms,
- reopen the social world.

Resolution of the crisis and future planning.

Source: described by Aguilera (1998).

may set a new direction as they regain a greater sense of personal control over their lives and the coping process. It is notable that a crisis might last between 4 and 6 weeks (Aguilera, 1998). In addition, many crisis situations are assessed by crisis teams. A fundamental orientation in psychological treatment has been emphasized by Schwartz (2000), who notes that however bizarre the service user's behaviour might appear, they are human beings first and foremost, which demands that they be treated with dignity, respect and compassion. The mental health problem is an important secondary consideration. This orientation is central to all forms of counselling and helping but it is especially important when helping very vulnerable members of society at times of crisis.

CRITICAL THINKING CHALLENGE 9.1

You are in charge of a Crisis Resolution Team, responsible for taking calls from people who may be experiencing a mental health crisis. Three calls come in almost simultaneously.

♦ The first call is from your very good friend. She tells you that she had an abortion this afternoon and can't stop crying now. You did not know she was pregnant.

♦ The second call comes from the local police, who ask for your immediate attendance at a local hospital where a 22-year-old man is threatening to shoot another resident and then himself.

♦ The third call is from Joan, a 38-year-old registered nurse who is well known to the service and has received treatment for depression in the past. She is obviously drunk but says she has taken 30 paracetamol tablets.

What course of action would you recommend in each of these cases?

CRISIS, LOSS AND GRIEF

Worden (2001) described mourning as the 'process which occurs after a loss', while 'grief refers to the personal experience of the loss'. Grief is an emotional response of distress, pain and disorganization. Mourning involves unravelling the previous bonds between the person and a deceased person (or object or part of the person). A process of mourning is needed to overcome grief.

Grief may be elicited by many different types of loss, such as a loss of self-esteem, loss of job, loss of financial status, loss of freedom, loss of physical abilities and loss of identity. Grief nearly always involves primary losses (death, job, relationship) and secondary losses or losses that result as a consequence of the primary loss (status,

security, self-esteem). Secondary losses may not be apparent to the service user, and nurses can assist in the grieving process by helping the service user to uncover these.

A number of key tasks of mourning have been described by Worden (2001) and these need to be accomplished if the service user is to return to a state of stability. These are:

Task 1 to accept the reality of the loss,
Task 2 to work through the pain and grief,
Task 3 to adjust to a world in which the deceased is not there,
Task 4 to relocate the deceased emotionally and move on with life.

When people are in mourning they experience feelings that are common. They may believe that these feelings are unique to them, but they are not. Acknowledging this commonality helps people to share the pain and may be facilitated through bereavement groups. Experiencing personal loss is part of what makes us human.

Grieving is a normal process after loss, and involves emotional (sadness, anger), physical (breathlessness, physical weakness) and cognitive (confusion, disbelief) sensations as well as behavioural changes (social withdrawal, crying). It can be helpful to let the service user know that these are normal and that it is helpful to express and share these facets of grieving to promote healing. Remembering and talking about the lost loved one can help people to feel stronger, and Hedtke and Winslade (2004) argue that this type of narrative remembering practice has a healing and inspiring effect on those grieving.

Conflict within a family about whether a dying relative should have been told they were dying may be a source of guilt and long-lasting family disharmony. Not to tell the person prevents them from getting their house in order and many things may be left unsaid. These types of family issues can complicate the grieving and healing process and create additional pressure for the nurse.

Resources are now widely available to ensure that counsellors, professional carers and service users are better informed about issues surrounding death and dying. People with internet access can now study a wide range of information about death and dying, arguments for and against legislation on euthanasia, and information about cancer, suicide and AIDS. In addition, there is growing recognition of the need for communities to be aware of the diverse ways of grieving that different communities need to undergo and experience. Nurses working with culturally diverse service user groups would be well advised to become familiar with some of these experiences.

SUICIDE AND ATTEMPTED SUICIDE

One crisis situation that most nurses will come across, in both mental health and general settings, is suicide and attempted suicide. Suicide is a significant mental health problem, especially in younger men (15–44 years) (Office for National Statistics, 2011).

People who are diagnosed with depression or who express feelings of worthlessness, guilt, anxiety and anger, and display severe agitation and irritability, may be at risk of suicide. It is important to note here, however, that 'not all suicides or attempted suicides are by individuals with a clinical diagnosis of depression. Stressful and negative life events can become triggers for suicidal ideation and attempts, such as drug or alcohol abuse' (Sharkey, 1999b, p. 92). Mann (2002) notes that alcohol and substance use increase the risk of suicide, as does the existence of a plan and a history of attempted suicide. Other disorders too, such as schizophrenia or bipolar mood disorder, can be prominent. Suicide is often a complication of mental health problems but it is usually accompanied by additional risk factors such as a genetic/familial link with someone who has committed suicide, access to lethal means, poverty, unemployment and social isolation (Mann, 2002). He also mentions the fact that some of the glossy media portrayals of suicide carry the risk of copycat suicides among young people.

The primary goal of crisis management is to reduce or eliminate the risk to the service users and/or to others (Doyle, 1999), whether in a hospital or a community setting. Schulberg et al. (2004) found that distressed people often visit primary care staff such as general practitioners in the weeks and months before a successful suicide. In a systematic review of suicide intervention strategies, Mann et al. (2005) found that the education of physicians in recognizing and treating depression, and removing or restricting access to lethal means, were the most effective interventions in preventing suicide. Professionals and lay people often explain suicide and attempted suicide differently, although there is a common perception that some form of crisis has occurred in the person's life. Zadravec et al. (2006) emphazise the need for health carers to acquire a clear understanding of the beliefs of the suicidal person, which may be incorporated into the treatment and management plan.

A key role here for the nurse is to recognize the potential risk and intervene beforehand. Sharkey (1999b) extracted a number of high-risk indicators from the literature in this area. These are outlined in Box 9.2.

If the healthcare team has identified a service user at risk of suicide, each team member will need to work with the service user at a time when the service user feels desperate and hopeless and sees no end to the darkness in their life (see also Ch. 23). Rapport can be established by heeding the advice offered by Wright (1993):

- Take a threat of suicide seriously. Individuals who have attempted suicide on a number of occasions can be ignored or dismissed as 'attention-seekers' and later found to have committed suicide.
- Try not to be judgemental. It is very easy to view the service user within your frame of reference

> **Box 9.2 High-risk indicators for suicide**
>
> - Deliberate self-harm
> - Following admission to a mental health unit, particularly during the first week
> - Following discharge from a mental healthcare setting, particularly during the first month
> - Drug or alcohol misuse
> - Recent major life event such as divorce or separation
> - Being unemployed
> - Nonadherence with treatment/medication
> - Rapid change in treatment type or in accommodation setting
> - Poor relationship with carers
>
> Source: Sharkey (1999b).

and assumptions and to judge their feelings and intentions accordingly, perhaps to think, 'What's he/she got to be depressed about with a lovely partner, family, home and a nice car?'

- Work with the feelings raised by the service user. Stay with the service user's feelings, not yours. Try not to steer the service user away from their feelings: 'It's not that bad – I'm sure you'll feel better in the morning'. Utterances like this may help you to feel better, but not the service user.
- Work with positives in a sensible manner. Even at times of great despair and desperation it may be possible to find glimpses of positive incidents, experiences or perspectives that might be helpful. Remind the service user how talking openly about their plans and intentions can be useful.
- Accept the service user's anger. The service user may release strong emotions such as anger and it is best if this is done in a quiet and private setting where others will not be disturbed. When you recognize that it is usual for a service user to express negative emotions such as anger or guilt at times of crisis, it can help you to understand and accept these uncomfortable emotional responses, even if they are directed at you.

The major challenge for the nurse is to provide a supportive relationship through which the service user's issues and perspective can be explored and fully understood by the healthcare team. This is a basis for establishing a safety framework for the service user that involves all the resources at the nurse's disposal while treating the service user in a respectful manner. This can be a challenge if the service user is not very communicative.

Caring for people at risk of suicide or self-harm is emotionally demanding and stressful. It is a source of major anxiety for inexperienced and experienced nurses alike. Despite a relatively common view that talking about suicide with someone at risk is likely to urge them into action, there is no evidence to support this view. In fact, people who are thinking about killing themselves are often relieved that the issue has been broached by staff. It brings it out into the open and allows them to share their sense of dread with another human being. It is okay to ask about their plans, the resources available to the service user (knives, ropes, tablets) and their intentions (Wright, 1993). A fuller understanding of the service user will help the team to be better able to care for them and decreases the likelihood of suicide.

Griever concerns following suicide

Loss through suicide can evoke certain types of concern in the griever (Cook and Dworkin, 1992) including psychological, social and personal concerns. The psychological issues may centre on the need to understand why it happened. They may feel guilty and display a sense of failure. They may blame others in an angry way and feel totally rejected. The taboo surrounding suicide can interfere with the grieving process and may lead people to withdraw socially, and patterns of communication in families can be disrupted (social concern).

Personal concerns can include the need to deal with a sense of betrayal or a reluctance to get close to people emotionally in the future. These fears will shape the helping process following suicide as the nurse attempts to help the service user complete any unfinished business with the deceased, use the support that other people and services provide, and avoid withdrawal from the social world.

SELF-HARM

Some people can harm themselves deliberately (inflicting injury with a sharp object resulting from delusional beliefs) or through neglect (e.g. lack of a proper diet). People with a diagnosis of schizophrenia tend to have a higher risk of self-harm, especially when their symptoms such as delusions and hallucinations are poorly controlled. These service users have a 10% lifetime risk of suicide (Hogman and Meier, 1995). Some of the key strategies for managing the risk of self-harming service users from this group and those with depression have been outlined by Sharkey (1999b) (see Box 9.3 and Ch. 22).

Sharkey (1999a) also makes the point that there has been a significant shift in the way in which risk in schizophrenia in particular is approached these days. There is a far greater emphasis on the service user's experience, community care, the use of formal and informal supportive

---

Box 9.3 **Managing the risk of self-harm**

Crises in community settings

Make frequent contact (home/day centre/outpatients).
Make rapid follow-up for failed contacts (establish an agreed team plan with clear roles and responsibilities).
Monitor medication and use optimum dose to lift mood with minimal side effects; avoid overmedication.
Build a therapeutic relationship.

Crises in hospital settings

Provide constant supervision through close observation.
Provide clear notes and communication.
Clarify responsibilities with team members.
Monitor medication and use optimum dose to lift mood with minimal side effects; avoid overmedication.
Use power of detention (if available and appropriate).
Build a therapeutic relationship.

Long-term management of risk

Work to an agreed plan for the future to identify stressors, building self-esteem and hope.
Work with family/carers to solve problems and increase or maintain coping strategies.
Develop structured, safe and meaningful daily activity.

Source: Sharkey (1999b).

---

networks and combination therapies, rather than a sole reliance on medication to control the disease within a constraining environment. Schwartz emphasizes that in a crisis:

> it is important to remember that, no matter how bizarre their behaviour, people with schizophrenia are human beings with the same feelings, fears, desires, and hopes as everyone else.
>
> (Schwartz, 2000, p. 371)

BEING A VICTIM OF CRIME

A person who has suffered some form of physical and/or psychological harm (rape, sexual assault, domestic violence, incest, assaults on children or old people) is a victim (Wright, 1993). In cases where it is obvious what has happened, the police and other agencies will be involved directly. In other cases, when staff suspicions are aroused that a crime has occurred (that a child is being abused, for example), the consequences of raising these suspicions may be devastating for the family and child.

If these suspicions are correct and can be supported by evidence, a child could be spared future episodes of abuse. If incorrect, the child could be removed in error from the home, causing great distress to the child and the family. In other cases a woman may be reluctant to press charges against a partner who assaults her routinely after drinking binges. She may believe that she has brought this abuse on herself through her own behaviour and fear that separation from her partner will result in her losing her children because she does not have a job or cannot support them alone.

Emotional and physical abuse are offensive to most people and it is sometimes difficult to imagine how some people can continue to live in these circumstances. Zink et al. (2004) note the particular problem of older women (those over 55 years) who are not identified as victims of partner violence by members of the healthcare team because this issue is often perceived by staff as a problem of younger women. They claim that older women may find it difficult to raise the issue with professional carers, highlighting the need for privacy and knowledge of appropriate helping sources of referral. Abuse can raise issues for staff, too, and trigger strong emotional responses (such as anger) that interfere with their ability to care in a professional manner. These personal responses may stem from the staff member's having been abused themselves, or being a child with an alcoholic parent, and being unable to deal with these events in an adaptive way.

In an exploration of the traumas that have been found to occur in the lives of children, Johnson (1998) noted that the professional helper may have to:

- identify specific crisis situations,
- recognize who is and who is not affected,
- decide who is at risk in a particular situation,
- devise options for managing the crisis,
- intervene appropriately,
- monitor postcrisis recovery,
- decide when and how to follow up.

This profile of the professional's role with respect to children is typical of all crisis work. In the case of children, the identification of a crisis poses additional problems and responsibilities. A child turning up at a nurse's clinic for a consultation about head lice may be a victim of assault, rape or incest but be unable to report this due to fear of, or emotional attachment to, the perpetrator. The identification process becomes crucial here. This is why a supportive team approach is vital, as a means of ensuring that assessments are thorough and accurate, and as a means of lending support to other team members. In such cases other agencies (such as the police and social services) are involved.

Abuse can occur in older people too. Kinnear and Graycar (1991, p. 1) reported that some '4.6% of older people are victims of physical, sexual or financial abuse, perpetrated mostly by family members and those who are in a duty of care relationship with the victim'. The abuse of older people has been found to occur in residential care settings as well as private homes (Kinnear and Graycar, 1991). An increase in the incidence of abuse in this vulnerable group is also likely to occur as older people comprise a growing proportion of the population as a whole. While most people in this group will live independently, an increasing minority will be dependent on relatives or residential care providers as their primary support, and in some instances conflict, power relationships and abuse will emerge.

As is the case with other vulnerable groups, the nature and extent of abuse of older people can be very difficult to uncover and validate. The initial contact with these service users may be coincidental (e.g. at a health centre or accident unit) and if the signs are very 'obvious' (bruising, fractures, severe agitation) then suspicions may be raised. However, an older, slightly confused person may be locked in a room all day by relatives to stop them wandering the streets, or not be allowed to drink after 4 p.m. in case of bed wetting. These restrictions too are forms of abuse and are much harder to spot unless, in the short time that a skilled and attentive nurse has with them, these older people can feel safe enough to voice some of their experiences. Then further exploration must follow.

Although the acute phase of the crimes may be seen to be 'sorted out' in a few short weeks, the aftermath may raise long-term issues requiring counselling and therapy over a period of time. A woman who has been raped may be seen by others (or herself) as a 'whore' and be ignored by her partner. A male victim of sexual assault might end up questioning his own sexual identity (Van der Veer, 1998). These violations raise significant issues and personal conflicts for the victims. In the UK there are many services for sexual assault and rape victims (such as Rape Crisis (England and Wales), http://www.rapecrisis.org.uk/, and Victim Support, http://www.victimsupport.org.uk/). Time and specialist counselling may be needed to come to terms with these significant events and their impact on all concerned.

It may be worth mentioning here that crime and violence and mental disorder tend to be strongly linked in many people's minds, giving rise to unwarranted fear and prejudice about people with mental health problems living in the community. This perception can influence healthcare staff too. However, most violent crimes occur between people who know each other. Nonmentally disordered offenders were five times more likely to focus on people not known to them and therefore present a greater risk to the community than those with a diagnosis of mental disorder. In 95% of cases where a mental health service user has been involved in a violent crime there has been previous contact with the victim (Pilgrim and Rogers, 2003).

In stark contrast, recent research from the USA and Denmark indicates that people diagnosed with a psychotic disorder are actually much more likely to become victims of murder. One-third of people with serious mental health problems were victims of crime. Of these, some 91% were violent crimes, including rape and assault. Drug users and people who were dependent on alcohol faced even higher risks (Cuvelier, 2002).

However, there will be rare occasions when a person who has mental health problems may try to harm others, and the risk must be assessed very carefully. A new mother diagnosed with severe postnatal psychosis may try to harm the new baby because she feels that the baby is trying to kill her, or an older man with delusions may try to harm his wife of 40 years because he thinks she is trying to poison him. While not common, these scenarios nevertheless highlight the tension instilled into the nurse's role in assessing and managing a potentially risky situation, and the need to protect potential victims as well as those who might commit such a crime.

While very few victims of crime do actively seek treatment, Hembree and Foa (2003) note the importance of establishing a helping alliance with victims of crime such as rape, abuse or violent attacks. A helper who provides compassion, understanding and a nonjudgemental attitude is likely to help in the healing process (Hembree and Foa, 2003).

SUDDEN DEATH

There will be times when a service user commits suicide, especially in mental healthcare, or when a service user suddenly dies, perhaps in the emergency room following a road accident. A sudden and perhaps unexpected death through suicide will be a source of great stress for staff if they have known the service user and then need to support the relatives in their grief. Within the staffing group, such events can give rise to strong feelings of guilt and self-blame, personal shame, failure and inadequacy. The shock of such events can be immobilizing (Wright, 1993). Relatives can be overcome by emotion following unexpected death. In these cases Worden (2001) recommends that the helper begin at the crisis scene (hospital or morgue) to offer help and direction there and then. At this time people may be in a state of shock and disbelief, unable to ask for direct help, and uncertain of what to do.

Nurses in accident and emergency departments and other settings may be called upon to: comfort a relative following the sudden death of a child, parent or partner; be an advocate for the relative; provide positive support when they appear lost and uncertain; and

help in breaking and accepting bad news. On occasions, the nurse may have to support the relative to view the body and just be there for them when strong emotions and naked human distress are given a free rein (Wright, 1993). Traumatic loss may be sudden and violent. It may involve bodily mutilation. It may be seen as preventable. It may be the grieving person's first encounter with a dead person.

While the circumstances of individual crises may vary – suicides, sudden unexpected deaths, accidents and trauma, children and infants, miscarriages and still-births – the pain experienced is traumatic and shocking for those who remain. They can be helped to begin to come to terms with this loss in a number of ways. Some of these are outlined in Box 9.4. Of course it is important to be aware that some cultural and religious practices may need to be observed. Nurses who lack experience should consult more senior and experienced colleagues and, if available, specialist helpers or advisors who know about the accepted customs of a particular cultural group.

It is also important to offer support for family members if possible because they too are often victims of social stigma because of the circumstances surrounding the service user's death (suicide, drink driving or drug-taking) (Lively et al., 1995).

Parental bereavement

Gillies and Neimeyer (2006) described how people attempt to construct meaning to help them adapt to bereavement, including attempts to make sense of the

---

Box 9.4 What is valued by relatives who have experienced a sudden death

Clear, unambiguous messages: 'The news is bad. Your daughter has just died'. People need to know the facts quickly.

Confirmation: you might need to verify the facts of the death several times.

Try to prepare yourself to answer difficult questions: Why now? Why us? Why could it not be prevented? Why could you not do more?

It will help if relatives and friends can spend time with the deceased to say goodbye. You might have to help by saying: 'Maybe you would like to see him/her one last time before you go home'. This helps to normalize the viewing.

Allow the relatives time and space to spend time with the body. Let them sit down. Encourage them to talk and touch the body.

Before they go home give them some time to go back over what has happened.

Source: Wright (1993).

death, exploring possible benefits and considering important identity changes that might evolve. This can be particularly difficult when a child dies. In a qualitative study of parental bereavement, Wheeler (2001) found that the death of a child led to a severe crisis of meaning in parents. Many reported that they had eventually found meaning after the death through connections with people, beliefs, values and engaging in routine activities of living.

Sudden death of a partner

In a qualitative study of people who had lost a partner suddenly, Rodger et al. (2006/2007) described some of the great difficulties people experience when trying to regain a sense of functionality in their lives, and the strain this event places on their coping resources. However, they also described the new life order that emerged eventually in their lives, which was more hopeful and optimistic and future-orientated. Somewhat surprisingly Carnelley et al. (2006) explored the experiences of people who had lost a partner and found that they continued to think and talk about, and to feel emotions for, the deceased person, even decades after their death. Hence grieving can take many years and it is very common for people to have conversations and emotional experiences many years later.

Furman (2007) described grief and loss as a brutal force which entails great suffering and which may be followed by positive life change.

If grief and mourning are brutal teachers, they can also be silent but empowering ones. Social workers and other health professionals should not minimise the supportive roles that they often play as facilitators and witnesses in the interface of religion/spirituality, death, dying and bereavement.

(Furman, 2007, p. 110)

Attitudes to death

Dealing with death can be problematic, as attitudes have changed over the years. Increasingly, people now die in hospitals and nursing homes, when in the past they died at home. In addition, in Western cultures professional services are hired to look after the dying and the death, and this is very different to how things were done years ago. Then, families played a much greater role in these processes. The attitudes of people and professional healthcare staff have changed too, with the growing emphasis on technology in the health system and changing lifestyle patterns. People live longer now, and fewer people are exposed to death or to dying relatives until later in life. Jalland (1997) suggested that the emphasis in medical teams these days is on avoiding death through scientific expertise rather than on providing comfort to the dying. Yet Kübler-Ross (1981) argued that dying can provide important lessons for professional staff and for the families of the deceased.

CRISIS, LOSS AND CULTURE

Dealing with the losses associated with a life crisis has been referred to as 'grief work' (Levine and Perkins, 1997). Moos and Schaefer (1986) described a number of tasks that need to be worked through to help people adapt effectively:

- to find meaning in the event and understand its significance for the person(s),
- to face up to the reality and manage the demands of the situation,
- to sustain interpersonal relationships,
- to preserve an emotional balance,
- to uphold a satisfactory self-image and keep a sense of self-efficacy.

Working through these tasks enhances a person's ability to cope. However, this process is made much more complicated (for carers and service users) when different cultural groups are involved. Culture refers broadly to patterns of attitudes, beliefs, values, behaviours and knowledge that are shared by people from particular social groups and which evolve over time. These become a general blueprint for people's actions and reactions to their experiences and to the crisis points in their lives. In some cultures, for example, community members will feed and support a recently bereaved person (Wright, 1993). In some societies, psychotic behaviour can be a sign of special powers and abilities (Helman, 1990). Cultural norms dictate how a particular situation or experience is defined and understood (Robbins, 1997) (see also Chs 6 and 7).

Being aware of the influence of culture in the person's life will enhance the nurse's ability to care effectively. Indeed, this is a responsibility of all professional mental health workers. If a person is labelled suicidal, depressed or anorexic by professional staff this label may become a badge of shame for the family, who might then hide away. That in itself is bad enough but if the family hail from other parts of the world and English is not their first language then this experience may further alienate them and make successful integration much more difficult and less likely.

Culture has many layers and levels, and nurses cannot be expected to get a good grasp on all the relevant aspects of different cultural groups. However, nurses need at least a heightened awareness of the complex nature of culture and an attitude of openness and commitment in order to learn about it from individual service users.

CRITICAL THINKING CHALLENGE 9.2

Complete the following questionnaire on personal vulnerability. Answer each question with Y (yes, I agree), P (perhaps, I'm not sure) or N (no, I disagree).

	Y	P	N
1. It's hardly worth working hard in your job since most times other people get the benefits of it.			
2. I like it when something unexpected happens to break up the routine of the working day.			
3. When someone in authority has made a decision there's not much you can do about it.			
4. I've found that most of my misfortunes have happened because of mistakes I've made.			
5. Life is an interesting adventure.			
6. It upsets me a great deal if other people get annoyed with me.			
7. If someone has it in for you there's not much point in trying to reason with them.			
8. Every problem has a solution.			
9. I often feel let down by people I thought I could trust.			
10. Most problems will go away if you ignore them.			
11. People can avoid problems by planning their lives.			
12. I think you can get most things you want if you try hard enough.			
13. I've found people are generally very ungrateful for things you do for them.			
14. You always have some freedom of choice, even in difficult situations.			
15. I enjoy listening to other people and hearing about their experiences.			

Score as follows:
Questions 2, 5, 8, 11, 12, 14, 15: Y = 0, P = 1, N = 2
Questions 1, 3, 4, 6, 7, 9, 10, 13: Y = 2, P = 1, N = 0

Results
Below 5: you are exceptionally resilient to crisis stress.
5–10: you manage to face most crises successfully.
11–15: you may find yourself knocked sideways by stress at times.
Above 15: you are probably very vulnerable to the effects of crisis.

Source: Parry (1990), p. 53.

NURSING INTERVENTIONS: ATTITUDES AND SKILLS

Developing enhanced cultural sensitivity

Lorion and Parron (1985) described a number of studies that showed that if helpers or counsellors display low expectations of success with ethnic service users, the outcomes will also be low. Hence it is important for the counsellor or nurse to expect the service user to be successful and to move forward. Also, for counselling to be effective, the boundaries for counselling need to be clearly established. These boundaries may come under close scrutiny when counselling any service user, but especially one from a different culture, who may expect a friendship outside the formal parameters of the helping relationship.

When counselling service users from a different culture, verbal and nonverbal communication signs may be a major source of misunderstanding. It is important, therefore, for the nurse to spend time checking the accuracy of his or her understanding rather than assuming that they know what the service user means. While the need to check for understanding is vitally important with service users from different cultures, it is also a core process in any helping situation. It is all too easy for the nurse to assume that they know what the service user means because they were both brought up in the same place.

The need to check for understanding should not be over-looked. Poor communication generally tends to be the major source of complaints against healthcare staff (Audit Commission, 1993).

A nurse from a similar cultural group to that of the service user might be a useful resource, or they might be perceived as a threat to confidentiality, and hinder the development of a trusting relationship in which the service user feels comfortable disclosing personal information (d'Ardenne and Mahtani, 1989). In time, a trusting rapport could be established and this may not be an issue for the service user, but if it continues to be problematic a different nurse should be invited to work with the service user. It is important to note, too, that the nurse being a member of a professional group may help service users and family members to talk. The professional relationship allows them the space to talk about issues that could not be broached with relatives or friends.

It is also important to remember to take account of cultural aspects of people's lives when providing end-of-life care. Shrank et al. (2005) explored the views of two culturally different groups in order to examine how cultural preferences influence decision making. They found that non-Hispanic white people tended to be 'exclusive' and limited end-of-life discussions to closest family participants, while African-American participants opted for a more 'inclusive' approach extending to family, friends and spiritual healers.

Helping service users deal with loss

A period of crisis, whatever its nature, often leads to a great sense of personal loss in those affected. A good helping relationship will allow the service user to explore the loss and adapt to it more effectively. The primary purpose here is to try and facilitate a grief response following a major and significant personal loss. Grieving is a very natural process; experiencing grief is part of being human.

The death of a loved person is perhaps the most striking loss that most will experience. When caring for a person who has experienced such a loss it may be helpful to use the assessment framework outlined in the article by Cook and Dworkin (1992). They recommend that the nurse collect factual data about a person's particular situation, their social context and coping styles as well as more subtle aspects of the interaction such as nonverbal behaviour and the nurse's personal reactions to the service user's story.

Some aspects of the nature of the relationship between people following a primary loss (wife, husband, child, lover, friend or colleague) will often emerge and need to be explored fully over time, along with the secondary losses that may have occurred. The secondary losses might involve changes in a service user's social standing and friendships, changed relationships with children and so on. Other secondary losses might include changing

roles and responsibilities, financial security, family structures and companionship (Payne et al., 1999). Within the framework of attachment theory, Bowlby (1980) argued that the stronger the attachment to the lost person (spouse, parent or child), the greater the intensity of distress for the service user.

People may have different coping styles following a great loss in their lives. Some may not talk to anyone about their loss for some time. They may experience strong feelings of depression, anger, resentment and low self-worth and may have thoughts of suicide. Others may not express the pain and grief from the loss openly but suppress these feelings over time to avoid being seen as 'wounded', 'abandoned' or a 'failure' in relationships. It is important to be able to express the pain and anger that follows a significant personal loss. Accepting the loss is one of the key tasks in mourning (Worden, 2001) and this acceptance then enables the service user to work on the pain of grief and make adaptive adjustments (Payne et al., 1999).

Some elements of the physical impact of the loss can emerge: lack of sleep, poor eating pattern and associated weight loss. In addition, the influence of religion, spirituality and available support systems will be important elements in determining how an individual copes. These would also form important facets of any good assessment.

Personal loss comes in many forms – loss of a spouse, a child, a parent, a pregnancy or a companion animal – and the significance of these losses can spark a crisis in people's lives. Children and adolescents experience losses too (parents, grandparents, sisters, brothers or friends) and may need even more creative support to help them express their pain and distress.

A sad story can induce sadness and stimulate reflection about the ways people sometimes treat each other and how lonely it must be to face a crisis and its aftermath (a marriage separation, domestic violence, sexual abuse, suicide in the family). This reaction is something that the nurse should discuss with a supervisor, mentor or preceptor.

Being there for the service user

It is important to spend time with the service user and allow them to tell their story. At this time strong feelings may be evoked and this is often one of the most testing times for a nurse: not knowing what to say or do. Being there and listening attentively is of great value. It is important not to try and rescue the service user from the pain or distress that is being described. Try to be a 'companion' and 'walk alongside the service user' in a 'meaningful relationship' (Geldard, 1998). This approach will help to ensure that the pace of the session is appropriate and unrushed. Many important emotional reactions can be unpacked and may need to be revisited later on. It is important for the service user to remain in the driving seat and for the nurse to follow them.

Allowing the service user to express emotional pain

It is usually helpful to allow the service user the time and space to work with their feelings if they raise them in the session. Sometimes just being silent will signal to the service user to pick up the threads again and expand on these in their own way and in their own time. It is important to try to avoid 'normalizing' the feelings a service user expresses, while acknowledging and validating their feelings. It will be helpful to reflect the service user's feelings, to build empathy at several points during the session (e.g. You felt 'abandoned', 'worthless', 'in great pain'). These help to acknowledge the strong feelings that the service user is experiencing or has felt in the past (see Chs 22 and 23 for further discussion of communication skills).

Being sensitive to cultural considerations in death and dying

There are some important cultural differences with respect to death and dying that a nurse must be aware of when helping service users and their families. These differences shape the way people view the world: 'From an anthropological perspective, members of a society view the world in a similar way because they share the same culture; people differ in how they view the world because their cultures differ' (Robbins, 1997, p. 4). In commenting on the attitudes to death and dying that are prevalent in Western societies, Kübler-Ross (1981) argued that people in Western societies tend to spend a great deal of time denying the reality of death, as seen in the euphemisms employed to describe a dead person. This is not so in other societies, where death is accepted as part of the cycle of life.

Regardless of the cultural setting and experiences, each person's grief is individual and each person will react differently to bereavement. People need to retain their individuality in a professional helping setting to ensure that they grieve in their own appropriate way (McKissock, 1992). Nevertheless, Worden (2001) argues that despite cultural differences, and individual reactions to death and dying, a common theme is the wish to regain the lost person and the belief that the dead person will be met again in some form of afterlife.

Acknowledging the meaning of death and dying in different cultures

The meaning assigned to events and experiences shapes people's view of the world and tells them how to react to death and dying in culturally expected ways. In some groups, death marks the passage from one world to another, while for others death is an ending or part of a cycle of birth, death and rebirth (Robbins, 1997). For example, the Kwakiutl of British Columbia believe that a dead person's soul leaves the body and enters the body of a salmon. The soul is later released and is free to enter the body of another person when the salmon is caught and eaten.

Robbins (1997) describes a number of cultural differences to indicate how some societies fear the dead, while others revere them. The traditional Chinese household may construct shrines to family ancestors whose advice is sought when important family decisions are faced. The dead become part of the world of the living. This is common in many Japanese and other Asian families (Johnson, 1987). In contrast, in Southern Italy, useful objects such as coins are placed near the dead person to discourage them from returning to disturb the living.

Culture provides a social context for the actions of survivors. Public outpourings of grief and mourning may characterize grieving and lead to culturally expected behaviours. In other cultures such overt displays of emotions may be seen as embarrassing. The Dani of New Guinea expect a close female relative of the deceased to sacrifice part of a finger, while Southern European widows were expected to shave their heads. In traditional times, when North American Apaches died, their shelters and homes were burned down; in traditional India, widows were cremated at their husbands' funerals (Robbins, 1997).

These culturally appropriate beliefs and behaviours are in stark contrast to what is expected at a funeral the UK, Australia or the USA, where 'survivors of the deceased are expected to restrain their grief almost as if it were a contagious disease' (Robbins, 1997, p. 6). This is especially so for men in Western society, who have been socialized to believe that open expressions of emotion are unacceptable. In contrast to this expectation, a death in a Jewish community is considered to be a public loss and is shared with the community. The family of the deceased person becomes the focus of community attention and the community shares responsibility for the burial and the care of the bereaved family.

Some cultures accept death as a natural and inevitable process, while others perceive it to be caused by some form of sorcery that must be met with acts of vengeance. Sometimes these culturally appropriate beliefs and behaviours elicit a sense of disbelief in someone from another culture and may even lead a health professional with a Western orientation and training to conclude that the bereaved person is 'mentally ill'. For example, the Chewa of Malawi in Africa believe that illness and death are the result of sorcery and that there is a link between sorcery and social tension. If people disagree on important issues they may practise sorcery against each other (Robbins, 1997). If the relative of a deceased person were to make claims of this nature to their Western GP, they might be referred to a psychiatrist for antipsychotic treatment.

Although death is universal, people's responses to death can be shaped by culture (DeSpelder and Strickland, 1992). For example, the type of death can be problematic and perceived differently. In many cultures, suicide is one of the most difficult things for survivors to accept; yet, in Japan, suicide may be seen as an honourable way to die (Moos, 1995). Understanding some of the cultural perspectives that exist can help counsellors and nurses to be more open in their attitudes to service users from different cultures. Cultural reactions to death and dying are extremely diverse and multifaceted. Accepting and understanding this diversity can lead to a nonjudgemental attitude and genuine helping for the service user.

Not to be aware of some of the deeply rooted cultural customs surrounding a particular death may give the impression that the nurse of a bereaved service user is not genuinely concerned about the service user, and this could cause further distress. An attitude of flexibility and sensitivity is vitally important (Sherr, 1989). This attitude is also sensible, as the nurse cannot possibly know everything about every religious group. In addition, the diversity is further complicated by the way individual service users may respond to a death in a particular case (Sherr, 1989). The nurse must be *prepared*: seeing others in despair may trigger despair in the nurse too.

Finally, it is important to remember, especially in a multicultural country like the UK, that many people identify strongly with their traditional cultural background at times of crisis, much more so than at other times in their lives (Cook and Dworkin, 1992). This may be a source of structure and emotional strength for them but it may also elicit personal conflicts and feelings of guilt about neglecting the values or religious practices that were so important at an earlier age. It may be difficult for those around them to accept this change (see also Ch. 6).

Acknowledging difficulties

Professional nurses need to acknowledge their difficulty in understanding other people's perspectives on life crisis, loss, death and dying, especially if those perspectives are far removed from their own core values. A nurse who develops a better awareness of the impact of culture is in a much better position to make a thorough assessment of the service user experiencing bereavement and other types of loss. The assessment should include a description of the cultural beliefs and experiences of the service user and how they responded to any similar losses in the past. It should clarify how the loss and other secondary losses will affect the service user's life. It is important that the nurse or helper does not transfer their own cultural beliefs and values back onto the service users and their families (Sherr, 1989).

The nurse who has a good understanding of the service user's cultural background is in a much better position to decide whether the grieving is normal or abnormal. Worden (2001, p. 34) noted that if counsellors are to make accurate predictions about how a person will grieve, they need to know 'something about the social, ethnic and religious background of the survivor'. For example, if a service user has been socialized not to speak ill of the dead, they may be unable to express the anger they feel towards a deceased relative, and the counsellor will have to work with the service user to help them to arrive at and express a 'balanced' perspective.

People from other (non-Western) cultures may be less likely to seek out professional help for fear of 'losing face' in their own community. Even if they do, they may be less trusting of the helper because their culture has taught them not to rely on outsiders. In contrast, a helper who is close to the service user culturally may be perceived as a threat to confidentiality and this may have a negative impact on the process, making it difficult to establish a trusting relationship in which the service user feels comfortable disclosing personal information (d'Ardenne and Mahtani, 1989).

It is important also to note that the relationship aspects of the process will remain crucial whatever cultural factors come into play. Horvath (1995, p. 12) described a meta-analysis that explored the relationship between the quality of the alliance the therapist has with their service user and the outcome of therapy, over a 15 year period. He noted that the quality of the alliance was a 'robust predictor of therapy outcome'. Nurses who expand their counselling role will need to ensure that relationships with their service users have an appropriate affective/emotional bond. This may be harder to establish and maintain when caring for someone with a different cultural background.

Finally, the nurse who is committed to his or her service users may then feel overwhelmed and emotionally exhausted by despairing service users and families in crisis. As a result, the nurse will not be able to help service users effectively and the nurse's own health will suffer. To guard against this, the nurse will need to work with colleagues who can provide some form of supervision and debriefing so that suitable boundaries between the nurse and those seeking help are established. This will also help the nurse to achieve greater clarity in the helping process and ensure that the service user's issues are being addressed.

Exploring opportunities for advanced training

Dealing with crisis requires great skill, and nursing interventions can be enhanced with advanced training. Some of the theoretical frameworks developed in other areas, notably psychology and counselling, are very well suited to the nursing practice context (see, for example, Barker, 2003; Watkins, 2001). Some approaches that offer great scope in this area are the person-centred approach to counselling following Carl Rogers (Merry, 2000), the gestalt approach developed by Frederick Perls (Ellis and Leary-Joyce, 2000) and the narrative approach espoused by Michael White (Payne, 2000).

155

The use of suitable theoretical approaches provides a framework for providing comfort to the service user (and their family) and addressing the intense feelings associated with a crisis. They will also help the service user to clarify events and preferred options in their life, and to identify the primary resources and sources of support available to them. In short, they will help the service user to be the author of their own life and to strive to live in the way that they prefer. Nursing interventions that are underpinned by appropriate counselling and therapy theory can be of great help to the service user as they strive to adapt effectively to a crisis in their life.

A PERSONAL NARRATIVE

In my weekly practice as a psychologist I regularly see people who are dealing with significant personal distress and losses in their lives. These losses take many forms: fractured or changing relationships leading to unfulfilled lives, loss of unrealized potential through the onset of a serious mental illness, loss of identity through sexual or psychological abuse, loss of career opportunities or loss of a partner or child through unexpected death. Although I see distressed people most weeks, I rarely feel burdened by the work.

This work teaches me to have a new appreciation of life and the gifts it provides. I often find clients' stories of how they dealt with loss inspiring and filled with hope and sometimes humour.

This helps me to avoid making judgements about people generally, to view the world with 'softer' eyes and to have a greater appreciation of people. It helps me to be influential and helpful but to also be acutely aware of the fact that it is the clients who do the work and make changes in their lives, not me. There are of course occasions when my relationship with a client does not work, and I do find this hard. I find it helpful to talk about the positive and negative aspects of this work with supportive colleagues, to continue to develop myself professionally through study and therapy workshops, and to go to the gym every week.

CRITICAL THINKING CHALLENGE 9.3

Careen (42 years old) is a qualified architect and partner in a busy city office. She is an attractive woman with an intermittent history of bipolar disorder and has been happily married to James for 20 years. They have two daughters: Siobhán (17) and Oonagh (15). It is clear that the family love Careen very much and when she has been ill they have coped admirably. On this occasion, Careen has had to be admitted to hospital because she has not been sleeping and her behaviour has become more erratic and unpredictable: driving recklessly and putting people at risk, threatening to kill a shop assistant when he responded rudely to her, turning up for work at 3.30 in the morning with no clothes on and being sexually provocative with strangers. The level of disinhibition she displayed was such that she was assessed by the crisis team as being a risk to herself and others and was admitted to the acute mental health unit on a short-term basis.

David is a registered mental health nurse of some years' experience. He is very conscientious and has a very good rapport with service users, their families and other healthcare professionals. He is currently studying for a Master's degree and is in charge of the unit on night duty. When doing his rounds of the unit at 5.30 a.m. he found Careen having unprotected sex with Nick in her room. Nick has a long history of mild depression, alcohol and intravenous drug misuse.

- ◆ What should David do to care for Careen and her family in the coming weeks?
- ◆ Who should be informed about the incident? What guidelines could David use to structure his choices and decisions?

CONCLUSION

Dealing with crisis is a normal part of life for everyone. Nurses, however, will be exposed to crisis and its aftermath on a regular basis, no matter what area of nursing they specialize in. Nursing exposes its practitioners to the pain and suffering that unfolds daily in other people's lives. It does so in an intense way and sometimes over a very short and compressed period of time. This level of exposure will elicit attendant emotional reactions and upset in the nurse and others. Nurses also have to learn to cope with the stressful events in their own lives that emerge from time to time. These can interfere with the nurse's ability to help others, so it is important to make sure they are dealt with in order to limit their impact on work-related issues.

Learning to cope with crisis and respond positively through enhanced self-awareness, the development of specialist counselling skills and increased cultural sensitivity will not only help the nurse to function more effectively at work, but will also help the nurse to stay healthy. To conclude, it is important to remember that people do survive even the most harrowing of experiences and existences. It might help to do further reading in the area, such as the most remarkable account of survival found in Dave Pelzer's *My Story*, which is three books in one describing his journey of survival from the most horrifying abuse by his mother who was dependent on alcohol (Pelzer, 2002). These stories are inspiring reading for any health professional.

EXERCISES FOR CLASS ENGAGEMENT

When written in Chinese the word 'crisis' is composed of two characters. One represents danger and the other represents opportunity.

John F Kennedy

You gain strength, courage and confidence by every experience in which you really stop to look fear in the face. You are able to say to yourself, 'I lived through this horror. I can take the next thing that comes along.' You must do the thing you think you cannot do.

Eleanor Roosevelt

- Take a pencil and a sheet of paper. Write a short summary of a particular crisis in your life. Describe the event or time and recall how you felt and how you responded to it. See if you can name the people who were most helpful. What did they do or say that helped you to get through? What particular skills, competencies or personal qualities did you find in yourself that helped you to get through this crisis period? How has the experience enhanced your coping skills since then?

- Share this story with your group, and together consider how your experiences might help or hinder your ability to help people in crisis.

- Seán and Conor were brought up in a small, staunchly Catholic and conservative town where everyone went to Mass on Sunday and most families knew each other well. They had known since their early teens that they were both gay but had not disclosed this to family members or teachers. Feeling greatly burdened and out of step with the community, they decided to speak to the Parish priest and told him about their sexual orientation. The priest chased them out of his house and told them that they would both 'roast in Hell'. Seán and Conor stopped going to Mass and soon after left the town for city life, returning only for occasional visits to their families.

  - How might this reaction to their disclosure have affected the lives of Seán and Conor?
  - Consider how you might respond if a close friend or relative made this type of disclosure to you.

- Briefly describe a few changes and losses, other than the death of someone close to you, that you have experienced in the past few years.

  - With your group, discuss some of the ways in which each type of loss is similar to and yet different from the other. List commonalities and unique aspects of each loss.
  - See if you can identify any secondary losses.

- Two cars were being driven fast and in opposite directions along a winding country lane. It was late summertime, and the hedgerows on either side of the lane were lush and high. It was impossible to see around any of the corners.

- Both drivers, because of the heat of the day, had their windows wound down, and their minds were focused on the road ahead and their destination. And, as it happened, the driver of one of the cars was a man and the other was a woman.

- They approached the final bend at speed, and they only just managed to see each other in time. They slammed on their brakes and just managed to slide past each other without scraping the paintwork.

- As they did so, the woman turned to the man, and through the open window she shouted, 'Pig!'

- Quick as a flash the man replied, 'Cow!'

- He accelerated around the corner ... and crashed into a pig.

  - Can you think of a time when you assumed something to be the case and found out later that you were wrong? How did you cope with that?

- What kinds of assumptions might you make when caring for someone from a different cultural background to yours? Or that they might make about you? What difficulties might arise as a result? How could such issues be managed effectively by nurses and other healthcare workers? Share your findings with your group.

- Deirdre (46) was a nurse and single parent of two identical twins, Gavin and Tim. She worked in casualty for many years on night duty alongside a very good team of staff. There was a really good supportive atmosphere in the unit and they were collectively a very competent emergency team. On the night of their twenty-first birthday Gavin and Tim went out partying and borrowed Deirdre's car while she was working.

- At 2 a.m. three ambulances arrived at the casualty following a high-speed collision on the freeway. A number of people were killed and others were seriously injured. As the accident and emergency department staff helped to unload the ambulances, Deirdre saw the bodies of her two sons in the back of one of the ambulances, and fainted.

- Write down your responses to the following questions and then share these in the larger group setting:

  - What emotions would be elicited in Deirdre and her colleagues by this shocking trauma?
  - How do you think you would have felt if you were one of Deirdre's colleagues that night?
  - How could the team help Deirdre to deal with these events initially and in the following weeks?
  - What particular resources or activities might prove helpful for Deirdre and the team in the healing process?
  - How could the staff deal with the 'awkward' feelings they experience around Deirdre when she returns to work several weeks later?
  - What would you like to take with you from this story that might help you in your future clinical work? Why are these important to you? What do they suggest about the type of nursing professional you aspire to be?

Source: Rabbi Lionel Blue, on 'Thought for the Day', BBC Radio 4, Today Programme. Cited in: Owen, 2001.

REFERENCES

Aguilera, D.C., 1998. Crisis Intervention. Theory and Methodology, eighth ed. Mosby, St Louis.

Audit Commission, 1993. What Seems to be the Matter: Communication Between Hospitals and Patients. HMSO, London, (National Health Service Report 12).

Barker, P. (Ed.), 2003. Psychiatric and Mental Health Nursing: The Craft of Caring Arnold, London.

Bowlby, J., 1980. Attachment and Loss. Volume 3, Loss—Sadness and Depression. Hogarth Press, London.

Caltabiano, M.L., Byrne, D., Martin, P.R., et al., 2002. Health Psychology: Biopsychosocial Interactions. John Wiley & Sons, Australia.

Carnelley, K., Bolger, N., Wortman, C., et al., 2006. The time course of grief reactions to spousal loss: evidence from a national probability sample. J. Pers. Soc. Psychol. 91 (3), 476–492.

Cook, A.S., Dworkin, D.S., 1992. Helping the Bereaved: Therapeutic Interventions for Children, Adolescents and Adults. Basic Books, New York.

Cuvelier, M., 2002. The mentally ill are six to seven times more likely to be murdered. Psychol. Today May/June:23.

d'Ardenne, P., Mahtani, A., 1989. Transcultural Counselling in Action. Sage, London.

DeSpelder, L.A., Strickland, A.L., 1992. The Last Dance: Encountering Death and Dying. Mayfield, Mountainview, CA.

Doyle, M., 1999. Organizational responses to crisis and risk: issues and implications for mental health nurses. In: Ryan, T. (Ed.), Managing Crisis and Risk in Mental Health Nursing. Stanley Thornes, Cheltenham, pp. 40–56.

Ellis, M., Leary-Joyce, J., 2000. Gestalt therapy. In: Feltham, C., Horton, I. (Eds.), Handbook of Counselling and Psychotherapy. Sage, London, pp. 337–342.

Furman, L., 2007. Grief is a brutal but empowering teacher: a

social worker's reflections on the importance of spiritual assessment and support during the bereavement process. Illness, Crisis Loss 15 (2), 99–112.

Geldard, D., 1998. Basic Counselling Skills, third ed. Prentice Hall, Sydney.

Gillies, J., Neimeyer, R., 2006. Loss, grief and the search for significance: toward a model of meaning reconstruction in bereavement. J. Constr. Psychol. 19 (1), 31–65.

Hedtke, L., Winslade, J., 2004. Remembering Lives: Conversations with Dying and the Bereaved. Baywood, New York.

Helman, C.G., 1990. Culture, Health and Illness. An Introduction for Health Professionals. Butterworth-Heinemann, London.

Hembree, E., Foa, E., 2003. Interventions for trauma-related emotional disturbances in adult victims of crime. J. Trauma. Stress 16 (2), 187–199.

Hogman, G., Meier, R., 1995. One in Ten: a Report by the National Schizophrenia Fellowship into Suicide and Unnatural Deaths involving People with Schizophrenia. National Schizophrenia Fellowship, London.

Holahan, C.J., Moos, R.H., Schaefer, J.A., 1996. Coping, stress resistance and growth: conceptualizing adaptive functioning. In: Zeiderner, M., Endler, N.S. (Eds.), Handbook of Coping. Theory, Research and Applications. John Wiley & Sons, New York.

Holmes, T.H., Rahe, R.H., 1967. The social readjustment rating scale. J. Psychosom. Res. 11 (2), 213–218.

Horvath, A.O., 1995. The therapeutic relationship: from transference to alliance. Session: Psychother. Pract. 1 (1), 7–17.

Jalland, P., 1997. Death in the Victorian Family. Oxford University Press, Oxford.

Johnson, K., 1998. Trauma in the Lives of Children. Crisis and Stress Management Techniques for Counsellors, Teachers and Other

Professionals. Hunter House, Alameda, CA.

Johnson, S.E., 1987. After a Child Dies: Counselling Bereaved Families. Springer, New York.

Kinnear, P., Graycar, A., 1991. Abuse of Older People: Crime or Family Dynamics. Trends and Issues in Crime and Criminal Justice 113. Australian Institute of Criminology, Canberra.

Kübler-Ross, E., 1981. On Death and Dying. Macmillan, New York.

Levine, M., Perkins, D.V., 1997. Principles of Community Psychology. Perspectives and Applications, second ed. Oxford University Press, New York.

Lively, S., Friedrich, R.M., Buckwalter, K.C., 1995. Sibling perception of schizophrenia: impact on relationships, roles, and health. Issues Ment. Health Nurs. 16 (3), 225–238.

Lorion, R.P., Parron, D.L., 1985. Countering the countertransference: a strategy for treating the untreatable. In: Pedersen, P. (Ed.), Handbook of Cross Cultural Counselling and Therapy. Greenwood Press, Westport.

McKissock, M., 1992. Coping with Grief, revised ed. ABC Books, Sydney.

Mann, J., 2002. A current perspective of suicide and attempted suicide. Ann. Intern. Med. 136 (4), 302–311.

Mann, J., Apter, A., Bertolote, J., et al., 2005. Clinician's corner. Suicide prevention strategies: a systematic review. J. Am. Med. Assoc. 294 (16), 2064–2074.

Merry, T., 2000. Person-centred counselling and therapy. In: Feltham, C., Horton, I. (Eds.), Handbook of Counselling and Psychotherapy. Sage, London, pp. 348–352.

Moos, N., 1995. An integrative model of grief. Death Stud. 19 (4), 337–364.

Moos, R.H., Schaefer, J.A., 1986. Life transitions and crises: a conceptual overview. In: Moos, R.H. (Ed.), Coping with Life Crisis: An

Integrated Approach. Plenum, New York, pp. 3–28.

Morrison, P., Gaskill, D., Meehan, T., et al., 2000. The use of the Liverpool University neuroleptic side-effect rating scale (LUNSERS) in clinical practice. Aust. N. Z. J. Ment. Health Nurs. 9, 166–176.

Office for National Statistics 2011. Suicide rates in the United Kingdom, 2000–2009. <http://www.statistics.gov.uk/statbase/Product.asp?vlnk=13618>.

Owen, N., 2001. The Magic of Metaphor. Crown House Publishing, Carmarthen.

Parry, G., 1990. Coping with Crises. British Psychological Society in Association with Routledge, London.

Payne, M., 2000. Narrative Therapy. An Introduction for Counsellors. Sage, London.

Payne, S., Horn, S., Relf, M., 1999. Loss and Bereavement. Open University Press, Oxford.

Pelzer, D., 2002. My Story. Orion, London.

Pilgrim, D., Rogers, A., 2003. Mental disorder and violence: an empirical picture in context. J. Ment. Health 12 (1), 7–18.

Robbins, R.H., 1997. Cultural Anthropology. A Problem-Based Approach, second ed. FE Peacock, Itasca, IL.

Rodger, M., Sherwood, P., O'Connor, M., et al., 2006/2007. Living beyond the unanticipated sudden death of a partner: a phenomenological study. OMEGA, J. Death Dying 54 (2), 107–133.

Schulberg, H., Bruce, M., Lee, P., et al., 2004. Psychiatry and primary care. Preventing suicide in primary care patients: the primary care physician's role. Gen. Hosp. Psychiatry 26 (5), 337–345.

Schwartz, S., 2000. Abnormal Psychology. A Discovery Approach, Mayfield, CA.

Scileppa, J.A., Teed, E.L., Torres, R.D., 2000. Community Psychology. A Common Sense Approach to Mental Health. Prentice Hall, NJ.

Sharkey, S., 1999a. Crisis and risks associated with schizophrenia. In: Ryan, T. (Ed.), Managing Crisis and Risk in Mental Health Nursing. Stanley Thornes, Cheltenham, pp. 59–74.

Sharkey, S., 1999b. Crisis risks associated with depression. In: Ryan, T. (Ed.), Managing Crisis and Risk in Mental Health Nursing. Stanley Thornes, Cheltenham, pp. 90–104.

Sherr, L., 1989. Death, Dying and Bereavement. Blackwell, Oxford.

Shrank, W., Kutner, J., Richardson, T., et al., 2005. Focus group findings about the influence of culture on communication preferences in end-of-life care. J. Gen. Intern. Med. 20, 703–709.

Slaikeu, K.A., 1990. Crisis Intervention. A Handbook for Practice and Research, second ed. Allyn & Bacon, Boston.

Van der Veer, G., 1998. Counselling and Therapy with Refugees and Victims of Trauma: Psychological Problems of Victims of War, Torture and Repression, second ed. John Wiley & Sons, Chichester.

Watkins, P., 2001. Mental Health Nursing. The Art of Professional Care. Butterworth-Heinemann, Oxford.

Wheeler, I., 2001. Parental bereavement: the crisis of meaning. Death Stud. 25 (1), 51–66.

Worden, J.W., 2001. Grief Counselling and Grief Therapy. A Guide for the Mental Health Practitioner, third ed. Springer, New York.

Wright, B., 1993. Caring in Crisis. A Handbook of Intervention Skills, second ed. Churchill Livingstone, Edinburgh.

Zadravec, T., Grad, O., Sočăn, G., 2006. Expert and lay explanations of suicidal behaviour: comparison of the general population's, suicide attempters', general practitioners' and psychiatrists' views. Int. J. Soc. Psychiatry 52 (6), 535–551.

Zink, T., Jacobson Jr., C., Regan, S., et al., 2004. Hidden victims: the healthcare needs and experiences of older women in abusive relationships. J. Womens Health 13 (8), 898–908.

Chapter | 10 |

Assessment and diagnosis

Jan Barling

CHAPTER CONTENTS

DOI: http://dx.doi.org/10.1016/B978-0-7020-4493-9.00010-X

CHAPTER POINTS

- Assessment and diagnosis are critical in ongoing care delivery for people with a mental disorder.
- Comprehensive biopsychosocial assessment requires specific interviewing skills.
- A biopsychosocial model of assessment gathers information based on psychiatric, physical, spiritual and cultural data.
- Risk assessment is essential in triage assessment.
- A range of measures are available to determine service user status and outcome.
- The ICD-10 and DSM-IV TR are current classification systems used in mental health.
- The use of classification systems for the diagnosis of mental disorders has raised cultural, social and professional issues.

KEY TERMS

- biopsychosocial comprehensive assessment
- classification of mental disorders
- diagnosis of mental disorders
- DSM-IV TR
- ICD-10
- mental health outcome measures
- mental status examination
- physical assessment
- risk and triage assessment
- spiritual and cultural assessment

LEARNING OUTCOMES

The material in this chapter will assist you to:

- explain the rationale for assessment, diagnosis and classification of mental disorders,
- understand current diagnostic and classification systems in mental health,
- develop an understanding of triage assessment,
- identify essential interviewing skills required for the assessment process,
- identify information required to conduct a comprehensive biopsychosocial assessment,
- describe the mental status examination,
- explain risk assessment,
- gain knowledge of observations, tests and procedures required to complete a comprehensive physical assessment,
- identify appropriate outcome measures for use in mental health services.

INTRODUCTION

The cornerstone of mental health nursing is an accurate and thorough biopsychosocial, spiritual and cultural assessment. The initial assessment determines whether the person has a mental health problem, what the problem is, what the most suitable treatment may be and if there are any concurrent social or health problems that may also need attention or treatment. Therefore, a comprehensive assessment is essential in determining the service user diagnosis and developing an appropriate treatment plan.

This chapter introduces the skills and knowledge that will assist you in performing a comprehensive and accurate biopsychosocial assessment and in developing a plan of care in collaboration with the service user. This individual plan of care will determine future treatment interventions that will contribute to the service user achieving their determined goals. This chapter also introduces the diagnostic classification systems used in mental health services.

CLASSIFICATION SYSTEMS

The nineteenth century saw the establishment of asylums for the treatment of people suffering from a mental disorder. This period corresponded with the beginnings of scientific methodology and the classification of mental disorders through experimentation and observation.

Emil Kraepelin developed the first comprehensive classification system in the late nineetheenth century. Kraepelin classified all mental disorders known at the time into 13 categories. He grouped the disorders according to common aetiology and descriptive categories based on symptom similarities. The descriptive diagnostic classification systems that are used today are based on the one devised by Kraepelin (Schwartz, 2000).

Classification systems provide a functional, standardized and validated means of grouping objects or phenomena (Weir and Oei, 1996). A mental health professional classifies mental disorders according to patterns of behaviour, thought and emotion. Research has led to the development of a universal system of classifying mental disorders: the *Diagnostic and Statistical Manual of Mental Disorders*, 4th edition (text revision) (DSM-IV TR) (American Psychiatric Association, 2000) and the *International Statistical Classification of Diseases and Related Health Problems* (ICD-10) (World Health Organization, 1992).

An understanding of classification systems enables mental health nurses to communicate effectively and professionally with other health disciplines, to participate collaboratively in service user care, to contribute to clinical research, and to organize and use data in clinical problem-solving and in choosing effective interventions (Clinton and Nelson, 1996).

ASSESSMENT

Assessment is the first step in the diagnosis of mental disorders. A mental health assessment 'is a complex intellectual activity that includes formulating hypotheses about a person, deciding what data are necessary to confirm or disconfirm these hypotheses, gathering the required data, interpreting them and finally drawing conclusions' (Schwartz, 2000, p. 96). Mental health assessment occurs in conjunction with a full clinical assessment: 'clinical assessment is the systematic evaluation and measurement of psychological, biological, and social factors in an individual presenting with a possible psychological disorder' (Barlow and Durand, 2005, p. 69).

A broader definition of assessment is:

gathering, classifying, categorising, analysing and documenting patient information about health status. It starts with the process of establishing a therapeutic alliance between the patient and/or client and the mental health worker and forms the basis of care planning. The process of assessment should be approached with empathy and compassion to support the development of trust between the patient and/or client and the mental health worker.

(New South Wales Health, 2001, p. 21)

Performing thorough, accurate and ongoing assessment is a major part of the role of the mental health nurse. Assessment is a complicated process, as the diagnosis arrived at from assessment determines the treatment for the person presenting with a mental health problem. A thorough assessment gives the opportunity to gauge service user strengths as well as needs.

Assessment rarely involves one function. We might assess people to find out who they are, to describe and measure specific problems of living or to describe their assets and personal and social resources (Barker, 2003a). A comprehensive assessment involves all of these. Through assessment it is hoped that we gain some understanding of meaning and human significance of the person's problem (Barker, 2003a)

Assessment can be formal or informal. A formal assessment has an organized interview plan and uses tools such as checklists, questionnaires and rating scales to obtain relevant information to assist with the assessment interview. An informal assessment has less structure and questions are asked that the interviewer believes are relevant at the time. Barker (2003a) states that the formal interview has advantages over the informal interview as the

tools and structured interview plan means that people are assessed in more or less the same way. He states that our biases, opinions and other 'value judgements' are less likely to influence the interview, as can occur in an informal assessment. The choice of formal or informal assessment methods is determined by the person in care and the standardized assessment protocols that the mental health services have adopted.

Assessment methods

The aim of assessment is simple but the process is complex. We aim to answer the question 'What is really going on here, and how will this help us work out what we need to do, by way of a caring response?' (Barker, 2003b, p. 66). Information about people can be collected in two ways: by the person themselves or by other people who have observed the person's behaviour, such as family and carers or the person's treating team. What we need to know about the person will determine how we gather the information. If we need to know how a person thinks or feels, or their values and beliefs, we need to ask the person. If we need to know what other people think, feel or believe about the person, we need to ask those other people. If we need to know how a person might behave in certain circumstances, we ask the person to observe or reflect on their behaviour, or we ask someone to observe the behaviour, or both (Barker, 2003b). Understanding the lived experience of service users and carers is essential to assessment. Information essential for understanding the lived experience includes the service user's or carer's way of interpreting or understanding what is happening to him or her, in addition to knowledge about the person's life, including how previous aspirations and plans, personal and social resources and circumstances are affected by what is happening (Fossey, 2007). Leggatt (2007) states that family members and significant others should be engaged with the treating staff as early as possible because they have in-depth information about the development of the symptoms and also knowledge of the social and emotional environments that may contribute to the symptoms. The family and significant others can also provide information about the person's interests, abilities and personality characteristics.

Barker (2003b) has identified four major assessment methods:

* diaries and personal records,
* questionnaires and rating scales,
* direct observation,
* interviewing.

Diaries and personal records

This involves asking the person to keep a log or diary of thoughts, feelings and behaviours they experience during the day. The person needs to be aware of what information that would assist the treating team (Barker, 2003b).

Questionnaires and rating scales

Questionnaires and rating scales are designed to provide specific information on some aspect of a person's functioning. Questionnaires can be completed by the person or as part of the interview process. Some questionnaires require only a yes/no answer to gain a score on the specific aspect of a person's functioning. With rating scales the person is asked to rate the severity of the problem, or their performance, or to indicate the extent to which they agree or disagree with a certain statement. Rating scales can assess patterns of behaviour and measures beliefs, values and attitudes. All rating scales end with a numerical score. The score will reflect the extent to which some emotions are felt, some behaviours performed, some thoughts experienced or some beliefs held (Barker, 2003b).

Direct observation

Direct observation can be carried out by the person, members of the treating team or members of the person's family. Self-monitoring is an extension of keeping a diary or log, where the person is helped to identify specific targets so some kind of measure can be taken over time. The targets are usually specific behaviours, thoughts and feelings. The person usually monitors the duration (how long the behaviour lasts) or frequency of a specific pattern of behaviour (how often the person engages in the behaviour). In some cases the person may be asked to record how long it takes to complete a certain task. Self-monitoring is not easy for the person, as they are required to monitor their behaviour all day long. Appropriate assessment targets and simple observational methods are important in order for the person to remain engaged in the process of self-monitoring (Barker, 2003b). Barker advises that creative personalized ways of self-monitoring are important in ensuring that the person engages in this process.

Staff monitoring is assessment based on staff observation, such as how the person presented on interview, how they behaved during interview and during the course of inpatient assessment, and how they behaved during a family meeting or in a group. The observations are focused on what is visible or audible to the professional. This objective information needs to be augmented with information drawn from other sources, such as the person, family members and significant others, and other therapists and team members, in order to answer the question, 'What is really going on here?' (Barker, 2003b).

Interviewing

An interview is the process of asking questions of a person to gather the information required for an assessment. The interview is usually semistructured and the person is asked exploratory questions on various topics. Other questions arise out of the person's answers. The interview is orderly without being regimented and provides the latitude to follow different paths without losing the flow of the interview (Barker, 2003b).

The assessment process is the first step in developing a therapeutic nurse–service user relationship. The therapeutic relationship 'represents a time-bound alliance between the nurse and service user which is consciously entered into' (Carson, 2000, p. 202). This relationship depends on communication skills, the most important being *empathy* and *presencing*.

> *Empathy represents a mutual interpersonal process in which the nurse is able to capture the inner struggle of the patient, bring together different aspects of the patient's situation in a meaningful way, and communicate that understanding in a way that is understood as truth by the patient.*
>
> (Zderad 1969, cited in Carson, 2000, p. 217)

Egan has expressed empathy in the following stylized formula:

> *You feel … (name the correct emotion expressed by the client) … because or when … (here indicate the correct experiences and behaviours that give rise to the feelings).*
>
> (Egan, 1998, p. 84)

This formula allows the service user to feel heard and understood. Presencing has been defined as 'attempting to be nonjudgemental and nondefensive while creating a conducive environment for an open constructive conversation and allowing the experience of the client to affect you' (Glass, 2003, p. 55). Glass also states (p. 55) that 'presencing concerns a head and heart shift; it involves suppressing your own concerns and moving from your own space/happenings to the client's space/happening'. As such, presencing involves 'being in the moment' with the service user and giving your undivided attention. This skill has also been referred to as *immediacy* (refer to Ch. 22).

Chapter 22 addresses the communication skills that are needed to achieve empathy and immediacy when interviewing a service user. The following issues also need to be considered:

- Location of the interview: where possible the nurse should interview the service user in a location where the service user's dignity, privacy and comfort are respected. A quiet, private setting where service user and nurse can interact at eye level provides the structure for the formation of a therapeutic alliance.

- Service user's developmental stage: major crises that occur in life are often related to the transition required through each stage. For example, is a young mother's depression related to the transition from 'independent' career woman to 'dependent' mother? Is the 16-year-old's antisocial behaviour related to the transitional period of childhood to adolescence? A developmental perspective can assist the nurse in understanding the service user's perspective (refer to Ch. 8).
- Apprehension in the service user: most people presenting for assessment are fearful or confused about symptoms they have experienced. They may also be embarrassed about the stigma surrounding mental illness. In addition, some believe that professionals working in mental health can 'read' people's minds or at least have remarkable powers of insight into the individual. Some inexperienced nurses are apprehensive about communicating with people with a mental disorder. Being aware of the service user's apprehension may facilitate understanding of the problem.
- General questions first, then specific: the nurse should take a broad, holistic approach at the beginning of the interview. The first 3–10 min should be the most open-ended of the interview. Using open-ended questions will help the service user to begin to feel respected and listened to, and be more willing to focus on specific issues. The nurse's responses during the initial assessment phase should be focused on building rapport, and should consist of empathic silences, repeating the service user's last words, identifying the service user's affect ('That must have made you very sad') and requesting clarification.
  - As the nurse begins to develop an overall picture of the service user, questions become more specific and direct: 'Tell me more about this depression, Mr Jones'.
  - As the assessment interview progresses, the nurse should ask more focused questions: 'How long have you been feeling that life is hopeless?', 'How many kilos have you lost in the past month?' At this stage of the interview the nurse is trying to collect information related to when the symptoms appeared, whether they have been getting better or worse, what the symptoms are like, how severe they are and their relation to other symptoms. Collecting this information enables the nurse to formulate a diagnosis related to diagnostic criteria for specific mental disorders.
  - Finally, the nurse should focus on closed questions; that is, questions with a yes or no answer: 'Have you ever had blackouts?', 'Have you found yourself thinking that everyone is against you?'

The development of interviewing skills will ensure that the nurse and the service user can enter into a therapeutic relationship where problems are identified and a plan of care is established.

The craft of interviewing

Barker (2003c) speaks of the *craft* of interviewing. People know who they are through their stories. Barker (2003a) talks of the background of human identity: the stories that people are born into and become part of, through the telling of their story. The story involves more than the events a person experiences; the background stories are important as they frame the developing script of the story of the person here and now. Therefore, in an assessment interview it is important to ask, 'Who is this person?'. In this way you cannot divorce the person from all the stories that shaped the person's life story (Barker, 2003a). Barker (2003a) emphasizes the importance of knowing *why* we do an interview. He believes our motto should be 'to seek first to understand' (p. 65). To begin to understand, we are required to examine the situation with the person and enquire into their experience of what is happening. Then we need to understand why we have chosen one approach over another. But most importantly we need to understand how little we know about the person we are interviewing, and seek to understand through our interview something of value about the person and their experience (Barker, 2003a).

No assessment can be expected to succeed without basically sound interview techniques (Meadows, 2007c). Inadequate assessment will result in inadequate care (Barker, 2003a). The goal of interviewing is to collect as much relevant information as possible by the shortest route, and in this the questions and how they are asked are of importance (Barker, 2003c).

An interview can be an uncomfortable experience for the person and may promote anxiety. People may disguise their anxiety through hesitant answers, short replies or apparent striving to please. Appropriate questioning can reduce this. An important question that should be asked at the beginning is: 'Do you want to ask anything before we begin?' Other simple questions such as 'What have you brought along with you today?' or 'What brings you here?' give the person a chance to influence the direction of the interview and foster a sense of partnership (Barker, 2003c).

Meadows (2007c) provides the following strategies for encouraging a person to share their feelings later in the interview, after neutral information about them (such as age, address and occupation) has been collected.

- Put down your pen.
- Adopt a posture that has some echo of the service user's, providing an obvious physical expression of empathy and perhaps telling you something about what it feels like to adopt his or her posture.

- Allow a few moments of nonthreatening eye contact, and a few short moments of silence, including silencing of your own internal mental chatter.
- Note your impression of the interaction and your empathic sense of how the service user feels, as well as how you feel.
- Follow up this nonverbal initiative with a gentle but direct 'How are you?': this may yield more information in a minute than an hour spent in ways that are less likely to convey to the service user the impression of being an empathic and concerned fellow human being (Meadows, 2007c, p. 286).

Interviewers need to be nonjudgemental: in some situations people may make statements that are disturbing, such as admissions concerning suicide intent, sexual practices, past misdeeds that have inspired guilt or material considered bizarre or delusional. An expression of surprise, astonishment, reproach or even stunned silence will stifle any further admission or self-examination (Barker, 2003c).

The concept of *resistance* is used to explain difficulties with the interview process. Barker (2003c) believes that, to prevent resistance developing, we should see the interview from the person's perspective. He provides the following solutions for obstacles which may occur during the interview.

- Failure to respond: the person does not give the information asked for in the interview. This could be the result of a poorly phrased question, so try presenting the question in a different way.
- Difficulty answering the question: the person may answer but be unsatisfied with their reply. Offer some words of encouragement and provide discrete feedback to help the person find the words they need to explain the situation.
- Refusal to answer: try rephrasing the question, or nudging the person gently. Or respect the person's wishes and leave this issue for another time and place. Always let the person know why you have postponed the question.
- Going off on a tangent: one question can produce a number of answers, some relevant, some less so. The interviewer must decide whether to respond to some of these tangents or stick to the core question. Turning the decision over to the person as to whether they wish to discuss these tangents empowers the person's decision-making. It is important to gauge the flow of the conversation carefully (Barker, 2003c, pp. 81–82). Other issues related to the interview include the interview setting and safety.

CRITICAL THINKING CHALLENGE 10.1

Horsfall et al. (2000) suggest the following exercise to sensitize you to the words used in practice and their associated meaning for distancing or labelling a service user. This exercise can be conducted alone or with other mental health professionals in the clinical setting.

- In a notebook or on a piece of paper, write down all the key words you hear used by mental health professionals in describing the communication or actions of service users.

After you have generated an extensive list, which could take several days to compile, do the following.

- Count the frequency of each word on any given day.
- Look up the dictionary definition of each word. Does the dictionary definition of the word match the meaning intended by the mental health professional who used it?
- Think about how you might determine whether there is a discrepancy between the dictionary definition and the word as used by the mental health professional.
- Evaluate the usefulness of each word as it is expressed. How does it open up or close off understanding of the person?
- Decide whether there are any words that should be eliminated or replaced with terms that would more accurately depict observations.

Source: Horsfall et al. (2000), p. 87.

The interview setting

Sometimes a key determinant of how the assessment will be conducted is *where* it occurs (Meadows, 2007b). A person can be interviewed in their bedroom on the ward, the sitting room at home, a consulting room off the ward or an interview room at the clinic (Barker, 2003c). Meadows (2007b) states that the place in which a person is interviewed influences the power relationship of the interview and the actions that might follow. For example, in a family home, the assessor has been invited into the home, which gives control to the family members there. A difficulty with this is that the interviewer may be influenced by the dominant member of the family and it may be difficult for other members of the family to express their views.

People diagnosed with a mental health problem may live in poor-quality accommodation, such as a 'bedsit'. Often this accommodation has limited support structures and is a problematic environment in a practical sense. As such, the person's living skills may be modified and well attuned in order to survive in this type of accommodation.

A functional assessment of the person's living skills will need to take this into consideration. In contrast, mental health facilities provide high levels of support and basic needs, so a person's functional level may not be rated as high because the institution is providing for the person. In addition, privacy may be limited during the interview. People living on the street have very little privacy and their social networks are often broken. The person needs high levels of coping skills in order to survive in such an environment. If a person is creating a public disturbance, the mental health worker may feel pressured to label the person as 'mentally ill', as this provides resolution of the problem. Assessment may be made difficult by the inability to secure privacy, pressure on time and other uncontrolled interventions by members of the public. Responsibilities may be unclear and negotiations about these responsibilities to other groups, such as the police, may be difficult and complex (Meadows, 2007b).

Primary care settings provide similar features to public places. General practice clinics provide mental health services, but given the nature of the setting they can be problematic, as the setting and time constraints may limit assessments. If mental health workers are required to conduct assessments in such settings they need to be aware of their status as guests. It is often helpful to have an understanding of the dynamics of the particular practice, including the reactions of the administrative and reception staff. Medical care facilities include hospitals, accident and emergency departments and inpatient settings. The power relationship is skewed towards the mental health worker as the service user is in less familiar and possibly threatening territory. Finally, assessment may be conducted at the police station, remand centre or prison. Such settings have their own particular rules and hierarchies. Awareness of the legal context in which the interview is being conducted is important in understanding the person's situation. The mental health worker needs to establish the purpose of the interview and the limitations of the assessment interview within this legal context (Meadows, 2007b).

Safety

Most people with mental health problems present no risk of violence. On most occasions where violence does occur, the violence has been anticipated. Sensible precautions minimize the risk to the mental health worker when interviewing service users.

Meadows (2007b) provides key points for mental health workers to follow, to ensure their safety.

- Be aware of the need to anticipate violence, and do not ignore the presence of weapons, threats, cues that the person is angry or a history of violent behaviour.
- Be prepared to involve the police: for instance, in disarming an armed person.

- In an assessment situation, be mindful of the availability of escape routes.
- Avoid being alone with a person unless you are confident that the risk of violence is low.
- Listen to your intuitive and emotional responses to the situation, and be open to acting on them. Be prepared to escape from a situation in which you feel threatened, or call for help.
- Be clear about the limits of tolerable and acceptable behaviour in the assessment context. For instance, be prepared to insist that the person being assessed is not armed. Be prepared to terminate the interview, possibly abruptly, on the grounds of concern for your safety.
- On occasions, it may be important to acknowledge the existence of violent impulses that the service user may have, but not necessarily be frightened of them. However, do not confuse this with bravado or machismo.
- Successful restraint requires enough (often at least five) properly trained people.
- Avoid presenting as threatening to the person being assessed. People who are experiencing paranoia are often violent because they are frightened.
- Administering sedative drugs, particularly intramuscularly and intravenously, in a setting without full medical support has been associated with fatalities and is to be avoided (Meadows, 2007b, p. 287).

In addition to these key points, the following strategies can help provide a safe assessment setting in the event that the mental health worker feels threatened.

- Multiple exit routes with outward-opening doors can prevent the mental health worker being trapped in a room.
- Spaces without movable furniture which can be used to blockade doors are preferred.
- Potential weapons should be considered and removed.
- The mental health worker carries a concealed personal alarm system.
- Arrangements are made to provide backup staff if there is potential for violence during an interview (Meadows, 2007b, p. 288).

BIOPSYCHOSOCIAL MODEL OF ASSESSMENT

A biopsychosocial assessment involves a comprehensive assessment of all aspects of the service user's problem – biological, psychological, sociological, developmental, spiritual and cultural – with information derived from interviews with the service user and their family, or others as appropriate. Concerns need to be addressed regarding how they may have led to the illness developing and how they may be maintaining the problem behaviour for the service user (Onyett, 1998).

Assessment is completed with all service users, regardless of the setting. The forms used and details sought may vary, but the principal information gathered is similar. Broadly speaking, the information gathered in an assessment interview provides the framework for a comprehensive biopsychosocial assessment of the service user's current presentation to mental health services.

When assessing a person for the first time, information needs to be gathered to answer the following questions.

- Does the person have a mental health problem? If so, what is the problem?
- What is the most suitable treatment for the individual?
- Can the team provide appropriate treatment? If not, to whom can the individual be referred?
- If the individual is accepted for treatment, are there concurrent social or health problems that need urgent attention before psychiatric treatment commences?
- What effect might the intervention have on the individual's health status? (adapted from Treatment Protocol Project, 2004, p. 8)

Other issues to consider include:

- access: how will you best be able to gain access to this person?
- engagement: are there factors which may make it difficult for you to engage with the person?
- rapport: how best might you build a therapeutic alliance with this person?
- location: is the location of the assessment conducive to good communication? Do you have adequate support in case of problems?
- local protocols: are you aware of local policies and protocols governing suicide assessment and management?
- local resources: are you aware of local resources that could be used to manage a person's risk?
- existing information: have you checked for any existing information available about this person?

Mental health assessment

The purpose of the mental health assessment is to develop an understanding of the person presenting for help. It involves taking a basic psychiatric history and a mental status assessment. The following information is required in conducting a comprehensive psychiatric assessment:

- identifying information,
- reason for referral,
- presenting problem and/or precipitating factors,
- previous mental health history/medical history/drug history,
- developmental/psychosocial/relationship history,
- risk factors,
- assessment of strengths,
- assessment of mental health status.

Identifying key information

Identifying information includes name, age, sex, present address, telephone number, languages spoken, general practitioner, marital status, occupation and next of kin. Some forms will require additional information about children, education level attained and family of origin, for example.

Example

Mary Jones is 32 years old, married with four children, lives at 22 Brown Street and her telephone number is 8888 888. She speaks English and is working part time in an estate agent's office. Her regular GP, Max Smith, is aware of her coming to the mental health clinic today.

Reason for referral

This should include:

- who has asked for the service user to be seen and why,
- the nature of the problem,
- events that led to this presentation,
- any recent suicide attempts,
- any recent episodes of self-harm.

Example

Mary presented to a community mental health clinic with her husband. She was referred by her GP, who was concerned about Mary's deteriorating mental state over the past 3 months and requested a mental health assessment. There have been no recent suicide attempts or episodes of self-harm.

Presenting problem

Obtain a brief description of the principal complaint and the time frame in the service user's own words. Listening to the service user facilitates the development of a therapeutic alliance.

You will need to obtain the following information:

- specific symptoms that are present and their duration,
- time relationships between the onset or exacerbation of symptoms and the presence of social stressors/ physical illness,
- any disturbance in mood, appetite, sexual drive or sleep,
- any treatments given by other doctors or specialists for this problem,
- the individual's response to treatment.

The following narratives provide examples of how the mental health nurse can maximize the quality of information obtained.

First, determine the service user's perception of the situation.

Example

Nurse: Mary, Dr Smith asked me to see you today because he is concerned about some of the things you have been saying and doing. Can you tell me what you think has been going on?

Mary: I have been feeling really confused and upset for the last few months and just not right.

Nurse: What are some of the things that may be making you feel just not right?

Mary: I don't seem to be able to cope with everyday living and lately I have been hearing voices, which are really upsetting me.

Nurse: How are the voices upsetting you?

Mary: They are in my head all the time and they keep telling me to kill myself. It's horrible.

Second, get an overview of the precipitating factors/ events. Ensure that the chronology of the events and the emergence of the symptoms is clear. The context of the presenting problem is also important. Box 10.1 details the social and environmental precipitating events that may have triggered the episode or be maintaining the behaviour.

Example

Nurse: How long have you been feeling 'not right'?

Mary: It seemed to happen soon after Jenny was born. At first, I would cry all the time and couldn't manage any of the housework. It was really difficult trying to look after Jenny and the other kids. Sometimes I would go to bed because I just didn't want to face the day. I thought there was something really wrong, because I wasn't sleeping or eating and I kept getting headaches, muscle aches and pains and an upset stomach. I have been seeing Dr Smith a lot, hoping he could fix me up.

Nurse: When was Jenny born?

Mary: June the 18th. She will be 3 months old tomorrow.

Nurse: You said you told Dr Smith about the voices this morning. Have the voices been bothering you ever since you felt not right, after Jenny was born?

Mary: No, the voices only started about a month ago, but they are getting worse and I don't know what to do. It feels like I'm going mad.

> ### Box 10.1 **Precipitating environmental and social problems**
>
> - Problems with primary support: death of family member, health problems in family, disruption of family by separation, divorce or estrangement, removal from home, remarriage of parents, sexual or physical abuse, parental over-protection, neglect of child, inadequate discipline, discord with siblings, birth of siblings. Note: suspected child abuse is 'everybody's business' and must be reported.
> - Problems related to social environment: death of family member, inadequate social support, living alone, difficulty with acculturation, discrimination, adjustment to life-cycle transition, care of animals if admission required.
> - Educational problems: literacy, academic problems, discord with teachers and classmates, inadequate school environment.
> - Occupational problems: unemployment, threat of job loss, stressful work schedule, difficult work conditions, job dissatisfaction, job change, discord with boss or coworkers.
> - Economic problems: extreme poverty, inadequate finances, insufficient welfare support.
> - Problems with access to healthcare: inadequate healthcare services, transportation to healthcare facilities unavailable, inadequate health insurance.
> - Problems related to interaction with the legal system: arrest, incarceration, litigation, victim of crime.
> - Other psychosocial and environmental problems: exposure to disasters, war, other hostilities, discord with nonfamily caregivers such as counsellor, social worker or physician, unavailability of social service agencies.

The nurse would have to ask more open-ended questions to determine whether any other social or environmental problems may have precipitated or be contributing to the problem.

Mental health history

Information required includes the number of admissions to mental health inpatient units, the number of episodes of self-harm, attempted suicide or occasions of assault, and an indication of any mental health treatments received. This information is usually obtained from the service user, previous clinical notes, a letter from the doctor or history provided by relatives or friends.

Example

Nurse: Mary, what you are experiencing must be pretty scary. Has this ever happened before?

Mary: No, this is the first time I have ever felt like I have been going mad and the voices really frighten me.

Nurse: What about after the other three kids were born. How did you feel then?

Mary: I had no problem at all. Everyone has always said how together I am. That's why this is really freaking me out.

Medical history

Information includes major medical and surgical history. If relevant, the service user's consent should be sought to obtain a detailed medical history from the treating doctor.

Example

Nurse: Have you ever been in hospital for an operation or a medical complaint?

Mary: No, I was just in hospital for the birth of the kids. The last one was pretty tiring and hard.

Nurse: Did you have any medical problems after the birth?

Mary: No, I just have long births and lots of pain.

Nurse: Do you have any physical problems for which the doctor is treating you?

Mary: No, apart from the last 3 months with the headaches and stomach aches.

Nurse: To help us obtain a better picture of your health, will you give us your consent to obtain information from your doctor if we need to?

Drug history

Gather information related to the current medications the person is taking. This includes prescription and nonprescription medication, including complementary medication.

Other important information includes:

- the medication regimen,
- all prescribed and nonprescribed medications, including natural remedies,
- an indication of dosage, frequency and prescriber,
- when drugs were last used,
- any adherence problems with taking the medication,
- whether the service user has ever had any adverse reactions to any drugs,
- whether the service user is allergic to any drugs.

Example

Nurse: Are you taking any medication that the doctor has prescribed for you?

Mary: Not that I can remember.

Nurse: So, you are not taking any medication to help with things that have been happening in the last three months?

Mary: Just over the last month I have been taking Valium to help me sleep at night.

Nurse: Can you remember how much?

Mary: Yes, 5 mg.

Nurse: How often do you take it?

Mary: Every night.

Nurse: Can you think of any other medications the doctor has prescribed?

In some services, specific assessment charts are provided in order to obtain detailed information on drug and alcohol intake.

Psychosocial/relationship history

This outlines circumstances that are significant for understanding current issues, and covers many aspects of the individual's life, such as relationships, family background, work or school history and, possibly, developmental stages.

Obtain information about:

- infancy (especially important if the presenting service user is a child),
- childhood and adolescence,
- work history,
- marital history,
- relationships with others,
- children,
- illegal activities.

Example

Mary is the middle of three children, both siblings being males. Her parents are alive, retired and living 100 miles away. Mary remembers that her parents' relationship was tense (when she was young) but seemed to improve as she and her brothers grew older. She believes her relationship with John, her husband (of 10 years), is 'okay' and that with four children and her job there is no time for arguments. The children are aged 8 years, 6 years, 5 years and 3 months, and Mary says she enjoys the company of the older children. She enjoys her part-time work, 12 h per week, although it has been more difficult since her youngest child was born.

Determining risk factors

Several risk factors need to be assessed for each service user:

- harm to others,
- harm to self,
- suicide,
- absconding,
- vulnerability to exploitation or abuse (sexual),
- vulnerability to exploitation or abuse (violence).

Assessment of the above risk factors is documented in the triage section of this chapter.

Example

Nurse: *You mentioned that the voices were frightening and that they were telling you to kill yourself. How do they do this?*

Mary: *They tell me to do certain things like jump in front of a train. It's awful.*

Nurse: *Are the voices so strong that you think you might try and harm yourself?*

Mary: *No, I am managing to stay in control, but it is a constant battle.*

Nurse: *How do you stay in control?*

Mary: *I just think of what it would do to the family. But at times I think I would be better off dead.*

Nurse: *So you have no plan to harm yourself?*

Mary: *No, I have never thought about how I would kill myself. I'm just concerned about the voices.*

Nurse: *Do the voices say anything else?*

Mary: *Sometimes they tell me to take Jenny with me as she would be better off dead. They say things like, 'Take the baby and go and stand on the road'.*

Assessment of strengths

There is little within any of the formal assessment tools that assesses the strengths of the service user. In Mary's case, noting that she has financial or family support can be seen as a positive feature in this regard.

Examples of strengths and resources include:

- intelligence,
- education,
- support systems,
- religious and spiritual beliefs,
- motivation,
- physical health.

Rapp (1996) and Rapp and Goscha (2006) have developed a conceptual framework with a set of principles and methods which assess the strengths of individuals and their communities. The focus on strengths and opportunities rather than pathology creates opportunity for growth. The strengths identified in this conceptual framework include the individual's interests, aspirations, skills, competencies and talents (Rapp, 1996). The focus on communities in this framework views the community as an oasis of resources. The community is seen to provide opportunities, people who care and support, facilities and natural resources.

Essential for implementation of the strengths model is a strength assessment, which involves gathering information about personal and environmental strengths across six domains:

- independent living,
- vocational and educational,
- socialization and leisure,
- health,
- financial and legal,
- transportation.

Collaborative assessment of strengths

Adees (2003, in Meadows et al., 2007) suggests that strengths may go unrecognized or become devalued in the context of negative life experience. Therefore a strengths assessment should be a collaborative process of discovering and developing a person's self-awareness of strengths. Keen and Keen (2003) believe that collaborative assessment results in the promotion of users' views, choices and responsibility in care and treatment programmes. Stuart and Laraia (2005, p. 198) define *collaboration* as 'Decision making, problem-solving, goal-setting and assumptions of responsibility by people who work together co-operatively and with open communication'. The three key ingredients of collaboration are:

- active and assertive contributions from each person,
- receptivity and respect for each person's contribution,
- negotiations that build on the contributions of each person to form a new way of conceptualizing the problem (Stuart and Laraia, 2005, p. 198).

Keen and Keen (2003) consider that a collaborative assessment process enables the nurse to discover the person's abilities, needs and aspirations, so the service is able to respond helpfully. Solution-focused therapy and narrative therapy have been identified as forms of collaborative therapy which can uncover a person's strengths. Hoyt (2000, cited in Keen and Keen, 2003) summarizes the approaches that tend to uncover the strengths of a person, as opposed to traditional psychiatric approaches.

- Possibility versus certainty: traditional approaches seek to discover the truth quickly and to do something effective about it. If the truth cannot be discovered, temporary hypotheses are formulated to explain the phenomena under investigation. These hypotheses often become part of professional quasiscientific certainties. These quasiscientific certainties can influence professional thinking and professionals can become convinced of their reality and approachability. In contrast, collaborative assessment believes that these hypotheses or quasiscientific certainties are discussed with the service user and are abandoned or reformulated if the service user does not agree with them. This requires an assessment approach of fascinated curiosity and the identification of possibilities.

- Egalitarian versus expert: mental health professionals can believe that their clinical knowledge, technical skills and therapeutic skills provide them with life-changing expertise. Service users can be potentially disempowered by such professional pride and assumed expertise. But having knowledge about the human condition does not provide absolute authority about the human condition or intuitive comprehension of the person being assessed. Service users prefer the sense of partnership developed from feeling understood and equal. This is best achieved by a collaborative conversation between equals.

- Competency versus pathology: traditional mental health assessment procedures tend to explicitly or subliminally explore aspects of pathology. Collaborative assessment is solution-focused and strength-based. The primary focus is to establish what skills or abilities the person has. The collaborative assessor, even when confronted with extremely disturbed behaviour, believes that the person has disguised, hidden or temporarily displaced competence and seeks to uncover it. Collaborative assessment requires that both person and assessor have a role in the development of new understanding and coping methods.

- Systemic versus unilateral thinking: systemic thinking involves assessment of a broader perspective rather than focusing on individual pathology. It involves exploring interactions occurring in the person's family and understanding political, social, cultural and economic stressors of the individual. In families, a systematic view of the problem requires a circular, reciprocal understanding of the problem and its maintenance, which highlights the fact that the action of each person influences the other person, whose behaviour in turn influences them. Unilateral thinking, on the other hand, provides a linear description of a person's behaviour which supposes that one person's behaviour influences how another person thinks, acts and feels, and that this person does not in turn influence how the other thinks, acts or feels; in other words, the person is the problem, not the system in which the person lives. The systemic view also requires that the assessor take into account the influence of broader society on a person's thoughts, behaviour and feelings. Societal and world events can create sadness, anxiety and different behaviour in some people. In summary, systemic thinking involves not overestimating the individual's disposition as a cause of the problem or underestimating situational and environmental factors which could be related to the problem.

Mental status examination

The mental status examination (MSE) is a semistructured interview used mainly as a screening tool to assess a person's current neurological and psychological status along several components. The exam involves observations as well as an interview.

Example

Mary presents as neatly dressed with make-up applied and hair combed. She does not make eye contact and sits with her hands clenched in her lap. She speaks quietly, using full sentences. Mary states that she feels depressed, and her affect is flat. She states that she feels suicidal and reports auditory hallucinations. Mary is orientated to time and place and says that it is 'not normal' to hear voices. She is prepared to have treatment and appreciates the reassurance of safety.

Nurse: *It sounds like you have been having a rough time of it since Jenny was born. What are some of the things that have been bothering you?*

Mary: *I don't seem to be able to enjoy things anymore…. It is a real struggle for me to get out of bed in the morning and day-to-day chores are very difficult…. I feel very sad and I cry all the time…. It is so bad that I sometimes feel life is not worth living.*

Nurse: *You sound depressed and unhappy…. You mentioned that you sometimes think life is not worth living. Have you ever thought of harming yourself?*

Mary: *Sometimes I think about killing myself but I manage to talk myself out of it. I know I would never do anything as drastic as that but I feel so low sometimes that I think about it a lot.*

Nurse: *Do you know why you are here today?*

Mary: *Yes, Dr Smith referred me to the community mental health centre because he was worried about the voices I have been hearing for the last month.*

Nurse: *Are you worried about the voices as well?*

Mary: *Yes. I know this is not normal and they are starting to frighten me.*

Nurse: *You mentioned thinking about killing yourself and that the voices are telling you to kill yourself and maybe Jenny. Do you believe the voices are powerful enough to convince you to run in front of a train or to take Jenny out on the road?*

Mary: *They are very scary, and I am frightened that they may take control. That is why I really need help.*

Nurse: *It concerns me that you are frightened by the voices which are telling you to kill yourself and that you sometimes think about killing yourself. I think we may need to put a plan of action in place that ensures that you and Jenny are safe. Is that okay with you?*

Mary: *Yes, anything so I can start feeling normal again.*

Nurse: *Would you be willing to see the psychiatrist and see where to go from there, maybe start some medications?*

Mary: *Yes, if it will stop the voices and start making me feel better, I'll do anything.*

Overview

Following is an overview of the MSE followed by a discussion of relevant observations for each component (Treatment Protocol Project, 2004, pp. 10–19).

Overview of MSE:

- appearance and behaviour:
  - appearance,
  - attitude to situation and examiner,
  - motor behaviour;
- speech:
  - rate,
  - volume,
  - quantity of information;
- mood and affect:
  - mood (e.g. depressed, euphoric, suspicious),
  - affect (e.g. restricted, flattened, inappropriate);
- form of thought:
  - amount of thought and rate of production,
  - continuity of ideas,
  - disturbance of language or meaning;
- content of thought:
  - delusions,
  - suicidal thoughts,
  - other;
- perception:
  - hallucinations,
  - other perceptual disturbances (derealization, depersonalization, heightened/dulled perception);
- sensorium and cognition:
  - level of consciousness,
  - memory: immediate, recent, remote,
  - orientation: time, place, person,
  - concentration: serial 7 s,
  - abstract thinking;
- insight:
  - extent of individual's awareness of the problem.

Appearance and behaviour

The aim of this section is to observe and describe the manner and appearance of the individual at the time of assessment.

- Describe the individual's physical appearance (grooming, hygiene, clothing (including shoes), nails, build, tattoos and other significant features).
- What is the individual's reaction to the present situation and the examiner (hostile, friendly, withdrawn, guarded, cooperative, uncommunicative, seductive)?
- Describe the individual's motor behaviour (psychomotor retarded, restless, repetitive behaviours, hyperactive, tremor, hand-wringing, bizarre) (include description).

Speech

The physical aspects of speech can be described in terms of rate, volume and quantity of information (slow, rapid, monotonous, loud, quiet, slurred, whispered). Some particular characteristics of speech you might consider are:

- mutism: total absence of speech,
- poverty of speech: replies to questions are brief and monosyllabic,
- pressure of speech: speech is extremely rapid, difficult to interrupt, loud and hard to understand.

Mood and affect

- *Mood* describes internal feeling or emotion, which often influences behaviour and the individual's perception of the world. *Affect* refers to the external emotional response. Both aspects can provide useful diagnostic information.
- Describe the individual's mood (depressed, euphoric, labile (alternating between extremes), suspicious, fearful, hostile, anxious, irritable, self-contemptuous).
- Describe the individual's affect. Note whether the emotional response is appropriate, given the subject matter being discussed. Some terms you may need to be familiar with are:
  - normal: expected variations in facial expression, voice, gestures and movements that are congruent with the context or topic of discussion,
  - restricted: decreased intensity and range of emotional expression,
  - blunted: severe decrease in intensity and range of emotional expression,
  - flat: almost complete or complete absence of emotional expression with accompanying expressionless face and monotonous voice.

Form of thought

This is assessed according to:

- amount of thought and its rate of production (poverty of ideas, flight of ideas, slow or hesitant thinking, vague);

- continuity of ideas (the logical order or flow of ideas). Individuals may or may not be able to stick to the topic of conversation. They may digress into irrelevant conversation, completely lose their train of thought, or talk 'around' the topic;
- disturbance in language (the use of words that do not exist or conversations that do not make sense). Some important terms that indicate disturbance in form of thought are listed in the glossary.

Thought content

Assessment is of delusions, suicidal thoughts and others.

Delusions are beliefs that are firmly held despite objective and contradictory evidence and despite the fact that other members of the culture do not share the same beliefs. There are numerous types of delusions, some of which tend to be associated with different disorders. For example, common delusions which are associated with schizophrenia include the following.

- Delusions of persecution: where a person believes that they are being deliberately wronged, conspired against, or harmed by another person/agency.
- Delusions of reference: the belief that events or other people's actions or words refer specifically to the individual and have a special meaning for the individual.
- Delusions of control, influence or passivity: the belief that one's feelings, impulses, thoughts or actions are not one's own. The person believes they have no will of their own and are controlled by an external force (other than God or fate).

Other delusions, which may be found in schizophrenia but also other disorders, include the following.

- Religious delusions: where the individual believes they have a special link with a religious figure (such as God). This excludes intense religious or cultural beliefs.
- Nihilistic delusions: are often associated with depressive episodes. The individual believes that the self or part of the self does not exist, or is dead, or that others or the world do not exist.
- Grandiose delusions: which refer to the exaggerated belief in one's importance, power, knowledge or identity. Often associated with manic episodes or schizophrenia.
- Fantastic delusions: the belief that the individual has had a remarkable adventure or experience. Often associated with manic episodes.

Suicidal thoughts will be dealt with in more detail when examining the assessment of risk factors in the context of a comprehensive biopsychosocial assessment.

Other types of thought content include obsessions, compulsions, antisocial urges, phobias, intentions, hypochondriacal symptoms and preoccupations (perhaps with physical illness).

Perception

Assess for hallucinations. A *hallucination* is a false sensory perception in which the individual sees, hears smells and senses or tastes something that other people do not. The hallucination occurs in the absence of appropriate external stimulus. Hallucinations are not necessarily associated with a psychotic disturbance and can occur when falling asleep (hypnogogic hallucinations), when waking up (hypnopompic hallucinations) or in the course of an intense religious experience. The type of hallucination and the content should be described. Some types of hallucination and perceptual disorder are described in Box 10.2.

Box 10.2 **Types of hallucination and other perceptual disorder**

- Auditory hallucinations: may be nonverbal (tapping, humming, music, laughing) or verbal (conversation, accusatory; often associated with depression). An auditory hallucination is probably the most common type of hallucination.
- Visual hallucinations: being able to see objects, people or images that others cannot see. Most commonly occurs in organic mental disorders.
- Olfactory hallucination: smelling things that do not exist. Most commonly occurs in organic mental disorders.
- Gustatory hallucinations: relate to a sense of taste. Most commonly occurs in organic mental disorders.
- Tactile hallucination: the false perception of touch or surface sensation, such as from an amputated (phantom) limb, or crawling sensations on or under the skin.
- Somatic hallucinations: the false perception that things are occurring in or to the body.

Other perceptual disturbances include the following.

- Derealization: the external world appears different and unfamiliar. The individual feels distanced from the world and things may seem colourless and dead. Derealization may be associated with extreme anxiety, stress, fatigue and affective disorder, or with hyperventilation, which is a symptom of panic disorder.
- Depersonalization: the perception of the self seems different or unfamiliar. The individual may feel unreal, or that their body is somehow distorted, or may have a sense of perceiving themselves from a distance. In its severe form the individual may actually feel as if they are dead. May be associated with extreme anxiety, stress or fatigue.
- Heightened perception: perceptions are extremely vivid. For example, sounds are unnaturally loud, clear or intense, colours are more brilliant or beautiful, and details of the environment tend to stand out in an interesting way.
- Dulled perception: perceptions are experienced as dark, uninteresting and flat. For example, tastes are blunted, colours muddied or dirtied, and sounds are impure or ugly. Excludes the individual lacking interest in things.

Sensorium and cognition

Assessment is of the following aspects.

- Level of consciousness: impairment of consciousness usually indicates organic brain disease.
- Memory: the three main areas of memory are: immediate, recent (the nurse may ask the service user to remember three random words and ask them to repeat the words immediately, and then at 5- and 15-min intervals) and remote (events from years ago). The clinician often obtains most of the information about the individual's memory through responses to other questions during the course of the interview.
- Orientation: obvious disturbances in orientation usually indicate organic brain disease. The commonly used categories for assessment of orientation are time, place and person. Impairments usually develop in this order and, if treatable, usually clear in the reverse order.
- Concentration: concentration may be assessed by asking the individual to subtract serial 7s from 100. This task is only necessary if you suspect that there is some degree of impairment. Performance anxiety, mood disturbance, an alteration of consciousness or a lack of education may interfere with this task.
- Abstract thought: abstract thinking involves the ability to:
  - deal with concepts,
  - extract common characteristics from groups or objects,
  - juggle more than one idea at a time,
  - interpret information.

Abstract thinking may be assessed by asking the individual to interpret the meaning of common proverbs (e.g. a bird in the hand is worth two in the bush). Care needs to be taken when using proverbs with different cultural groups. A lack of abstract thinking is often associated with organic brain disease or thought disorder.

The Mini-Mental State Examination (MMSE) is the most commonly used instrument for screening cognitive function. The examination is useful for assessing cognitive impairment such as dementia or head injury. The MMSE provides measures of orientation, registration (immediate memory), short-term memory (but not long-term memory), as well as language functioning (Folstein et al., 1975).

Insight

Insight refers to the individual's awareness of his or her situation or illness. There are varying degrees of insight. For example, an individual may be aware of the problem but may believe that someone else is to blame for it. Alternatively, the individual may deny that a problem exists. The assessment of insight has clinical significance, because lack of insight generally means that it will be difficult to encourage the individual to accept treatment.

CRITICAL THINKING CHALLENGE 10.2

It is important to be comfortable with the mental state exam because it is the cornerstone of mental healthcare. It provides the basis for collecting information in order to diagnose and treat an individual presenting to the service.

- If you have the opportunity, conduct a mental state exam and obtain a service user history of a person presenting to a service (alternatively, use a case study/ role play from this book).
- What were some of the difficulties you encountered with conducting the interview?
- Do you know of alternative concepts that may be useful in conducting a service user interview?

Reflect on these concepts and strategies.

- How do they contradict the norms and sanctions related to conducting a service user interview?
- What do you perceive would be the consequences for the service user and yourself in using these concepts in practice?

Physical assessment

No biopsychosocial assessment is complete without an examination of the service user's physical status. When attempting a physical assessment, the factors described below should be addressed.

Present and past health status

Check:

- availability of recent medical evaluations and test results,
- past hospitalizations and operations,
- cardiac problems including cerebrovascular accidents, myocardial infarctions and childhood illnesses,
- respiratory problems,
- neurological problems, head injuries, seizure episodes or the experience of loss of consciousness,
- endocrine disorders, in particular unstable diabetes or thyroid or adrenal dysfunction,
- immune disorders, particularly HIV and autoimmune disorders,
- use of, exposure to, abuse of or dependence on substances, including alcohol, tobacco, prescription and illegal drugs (adapted from Boyd, 2005).

Physical examination

Some people presenting with what appears to be a mental health problem may actually have an underlying physical problem or a physical problem which may be contributing to the mental health problem. For this reason it is essential that any person presenting for a psychiatric assessment also has a thorough assessment of all systems of the body. A medical doctor conducts this systems review. Nurses augment this systems review with a nursing physical assessment.

Physical functions

An assessment of the person's physical functions provides a baseline for the nurse to implement nursing intervention. The following functions are assessed and documented:

- elimination: the service user's daily urinary and bowel habits. This information acts as a baseline in order to assess changes in habits as a result of medication,
- activity and exercise: the service user's daily level of activity and exercise is assessed to ensure that the service user maintains or increases their fitness level as a form of nursing intervention,
- sleep: changes in sleep patterns can affect a person's emotions or may be symptoms of a mental disorder such as depression, anxiety or mania,

- appetite and nutrition: changes may reflect depression, anxiety, possible eating disorders and problems with body image,
- hydration: as for appetite,
- sexuality: it is important to assess changes in sexual activity and comfort with one's own sexuality. Questions should be asked in a matter-of-fact, nonjudgemental manner,
- self-care: a service user's ability to care for self or carry out activities of daily living may be indicative of their mental state (adapted from Boyd, 2005).

Laboratory results

Laboratory tests are required to screen for physical problems that may influence the diagnosis of a mental disorder. These tests are ordered by the medical officer. A few investigations, such as a full blood count and general biomedical indices (renal, liver function, electrolytes and thyroid function) are almost universally indicated. Table 10.1 lists the laboratory tests and their relevance to mental disorders.

Table 10.1 Haematological tests related to psychiatric disorders

Test	Possible results	Possible cause or meaning
Full blood count (FBC)		
Leucocyte count (WBC)	Leucopenia (decrease in leucocytes)	May be produced by: phenothiazines, clozapine, carbamazepine
	Agranulocytosis (decrease in the number of granulocytic leucocytes)	Lithium causes a benign mild-to-moderate increase
	Leucocytosis (increase in leucocyte count above normal limits)	Neuroleptic malignant syndrome (NMS) also associated with an increase
WBC differential	'Shift to the left' from segmented neutrophils to band forms	Shift often suggests bacterial infections
		Has been reported in about 40% of cases of NMS
Red blood cell count (RBC)	Polycythaemia (increased RBCs)	Primary form: caused by several disease states
		Secondary form: compensation for decreased oxygenation, such as chronic pulmonary disease
		Blood is more viscous, and the service user should not become dehydrated
	Anaemia (decreased RBCs)	Related to some form of anaemia which requires further investigation
Haematocrit (Hct)	Increase	May be due to dehydration
	Decrease (related to anaemia)	May be associated with a wide range of mental health changes including asthenia, depression and psychosis
		20% of women of childbearing age have iron deficiency anaemia
Haemoglobin (Hb)	Decrease	Another indicator of anaemia
Erythrocyte indices: red cell distribution width (RDW)	Elevated RDW	Suggests a combined anaemia related to chronic alcoholism, resulting from vitamin B_{12}, folate and iron deficiencies

(continued)

Table 10.1 Continued

Test	Possible results	Possible cause or meaning
Other haematological measures		
Vitamin B$_{12}$	Deficiency	Neuropsychiatric symptoms such as psychosis, paranoia, fatigue, agitation, marked personality change, dementia and delirium may develop
		Oral contraceptives decrease B$_{12}$
Folate	Deficiency	Alcohol, phenytoin, oral contraceptives and oestrogens may be responsible
Platelet count	Thrombocytopenia: decrease	Psychiatric medications such as carbamazepine, phenothiazines, clozapine or other nonpsychiatric medications
		Several medical conditions
Serum electrolytes		
Sodium	Hyponatraemia: low serum sodium	Significant mental state changes may ensue
		Associated with: Addison's disease, syndrome of inappropriate secretion of antidiuretic hormone (SIADH), polydipsia (water intoxication) and carbamazepine use
Potassium	Hypokalaemia: low serum potassium	Produces weakness, fatigue, electrocardiogram changes, paralytic ileus and muscle paresis
		Associated with: bulimia, psychogenic vomiting, use and abuse of diuretics and laxative abuse
		Can be life-threatening
Chloride	Increase Decrease	Increases to compensate for lower bicarbonate Associated with: bingeing/purging behaviour and repeated vomiting
Bicarbonate	Increase Decrease	Associated with bingeing and purging, excessive use of laxatives, psychogenic vomiting
		May develop in some service users with hyperventilation syndrome and panic disorder
Renal function tests		
Blood urea nitrogen (BUN)	Increase	Cause may be dehydration
		Associated with mental status changes, lethargy and delirium
		Toxicity of medications cleared by the kidney (such as lithium) may increase
Serum creatinine	Increase	Does not usually become elevated until 50% of the nephrons in the kidney are damaged
Serum enzymes		
Amylase	Increase	Associated with bingeing/purging behaviour in eating disorders
Alanine aminotransferase (ALT)	ALT>AST	Common in acute forms of viral and drug-induced hepatic dysfunction
Aspartate aminotransferase (AST)	Increase	Use of sodium valproate

(continued)

Table 10.1 Continued

Test	Possible results	Possible cause or meaning
	AST>ALT	Severe elevations in chronic forms of liver disease and in some myocardial infarctions
Creatine phosphokinase (CPK)	Increase	Muscle tissue injury
		Neuroleptic malignant syndrome
		Repeated intramuscular injections, e.g. depot antipsychotics
Thyroid function		
Serum triiodothyronine (T3)	Decrease	Hypothyroidism
		Individuals with depression may convert less T4 to T3
		Lithium and sodium valproate may suppress thyroid function
Serum thyroxine (T4)	Increase	Hyperthyroidism, T3 toxicosis, may produce mood changes, anxiety and symptoms of mania
Thyroid-stimulating hormone (TSH)	Increase Decrease	Hyperthyroidism as a cause, symptoms as in increase of T3
		Hypothyroidism: symptoms similar to depression, except for cold intolerance, dry skin, hair loss and bradycardia
		Lithium may also cause increase
		Considered nondiagnostic: may be hyperthyroidism, pituitary hypothyroidism

Source: Reprinted from Boyd M, Psychiatric Nursing, 3e, 2005, with permission from Lippincott, Williams and Wilkins, http://www.lww.com.

Spiritual assessment

The spiritual dimension is often overlooked in assessment. It is important because it provides a deeper understanding of the service user, their social setting and the possible origins of the problem. Carson proposes that 'the presence and intensity of faith in God, degree of religious commitment, and sense of purpose and meaning along with basic life values, strongly affect the service user's potential for recovery' (Carson, 2000, p. 253).

Elkins et al. (1998) identify the following characteristics of spirituality:

- provides a transcendental dimension, possibly but not necessarily experienced as a personal god,
- acts as a source of meaning in life, filling an existential vacuum,
- creates a sense of mission or vocation and of the sacredness of life,
- enables experiences of awe, reverence and wonder,
- promotes an awareness and acceptance of the tragic as part of life,
- frequently challenges material values,
- usually promotes altruism and idealism,
- may change all aspects of being and living,
- may be experienced without formal religion.

Spirituality is often neglected in the understanding of mental health problems. Meadows (2007a) believes that service users may be hesitant to talk about their spiritual experiences as they believe that the experience will be interpreted by the clinician as abnormal or 'crazy'. Even if the clinician accepts the reality of the service user's experience, team and organizational factors may hinder further discussion. It is important to realize that each individual has their own unique spiritual interpretation of the universe and, as such, none of us can claim to understand the correct spiritual nature of things (Post et al., cited in Meadows, 2007). It is therefore important not to overlook the spiritual dimension of an assessment. To facilitate this form of assessment, it is important to create a setting in which the person feels safe to talk about the spiritual dimension of their being. Table 10.2 lists questions that may be of benefit in conducting a spiritual assessment.

Cultural assessment

Cultural assessment is a complex issue. Given the diversity of cultures in the UK it would be impossible for the mental health nurse to understand all cultures. Despite this, mental health nurses need to engage the service user and the

Table 10.2 Questions to use in spiritual and philosophical assessment

Concept of God	Is religion or God important to you? If so can you describe how? Do you use prayer in your life? If so, does prayer benefit you in any way? Do you believe that God or a deity is involved in your personal life? If so how? What is your God or deity like?
Sources of strength and hope	Who are your support people? Who is the most important person in your life? Are people available to you when you are in need? Who or what provides you with strength and hope?
Religious practices	Is your religious faith helpful to you? Are any religious practices meaningful to you? Has your mental health problem affected your religious practices? Are any religious books or symbols helpful to you?
Meaning and purpose	What gives your life meaning and purpose? What makes you get up out of bed every morning and do what you have to do? Do you feel that your life makes a difference? If so in what ways? In what ways has your mental health problem had an impact on your meaning and purpose?

Source: Reprinted from Carson V, 2000, Mental Health Nursing: the Nurse–Patient Journey, 2nd edn. W B Saunders, Sydney, with permission from Elsevier.

family so that appropriate care can be given. Adoption and application of the underlying principles of cultural safety (see Ch. 6) by nurses will enable appropriate assessment.

Attitudes that interfere with appropriate assessment include the following.

- Ethnocentrism: the belief that one's own world view, based on the values and norms of our culture, is superior to those of others and is the only valid world view (Frisch and Frisch, 2006, p. 106).
- Stereotyping: the failure to identify individual variations and differences within cultural groups. It results in the expectation that all individuals within a certain cultural group will have the same values, beliefs, customs and behaviours. Individuals within that cultural group are labelled according to the stereotype (Frisch and Frisch, 2006, p. 107).
- Cultural blindness: an attempt to treat all people fairly by ignoring differences within a culture and acting as though the differences do not exist. Such cultural blindness can be seen as insensitivity just as much as stereotyping and ethnocentrism (Frisch and Frisch, 2006, p. 107).

Being aware of these attitudes in ourselves and others is the first step in developing awareness of our values and how they affect practice.

Failure to communicate effectively with service users can cause delays in diagnosis and treatment, and can have tragic results (Crisp and Taylor, 2005). Crisp and Taylor (2001, p. 132) identify some barriers to communication, of which nurses and other healthcare workers should be aware:

- the formal use of one national language (such as English),
- institutional racism and prejudice,
- racist and prejudicial attitudes of both nurses and service users towards each other,
- ethnocentrism and stereotyping,
- cultural differences,
- differences in class and education between service users and nurses,
- different experiences,
- different perceptions of health and illness,
- unfamiliar healthcare systems,
- different expectations of healthcare,
- culture shock.

Box 10.3 highlights the communication skills that may assist when communicating with people from different cultural backgrounds.

Narayan (2003) has developed a cultural assessment checklist that may assist nurses during the first interview to develop a rapport with the service user and an understanding of the service user's culture (see Table 10.3).

TRIAGE ASSESSMENT

A triage assessment refers to the decision-making process that occurs when alternatives for acute care are being considered. The factors that influence the decisions made need to be based on a holistic system of care. A thorough biopsychosocial approach, where all relevant aspects of the person's symptoms and current situation are considered, is most appropriate. The principle of any triage system is for the right person to be directed to the right place at the right time for the right reasons.

A triage assessment is completed at a face-to-face presentation at an accident and emergency department or mental health acute-care service. Key questions that need to be asked at the presentation of the service user are as follows.

- Is this an acute medical or surgical rather than mental health emergency?
- Is this service user at acute risk for assaulting staff or other service users?
- Is the service user at acute risk of serious harm to self?
- Should the service user be able to leave if he or she wishes to?
- Does the service user need to be seen immediately or can he or she safely wait a while?
- Does the service user need to be seen at all? (Treatment Protocol Project, 2003, p. 40)

Box 10.3 Communicating with people from different ethnic backgrounds

- Speak slowly, audibly and distinctly, and use terminology that service users from other cultures can understand.
- Use simple words and avoid jargon.
- Listen as much as you speak; do not interrupt, because this can be seen as rude.
- Allow extra time to communicate with someone whose language is not your own. Trying to understand each other may take extra effort and time.
- Respect silence; do not fill every gap in the conversation.
- When you experience frustration or sense conflict or misunderstanding in a cross-cultural situation, stop and ask yourself whether the conflict is due to cultural differences. Try to see a common basis or understanding.
- Adapt your style to the demands of the situation. Speak the service user's language.
- Do not make judgements about people based on their accent or language fluency.
- Be open and sensitive about how you give feedback.
- Know who in the family is the appointed head or decision-maker.
- Understand the 'hot buttons' that can lead to conflict.
- Avoid using slang.
- Do not use racial or ethnic epithets.
- Avoid verbal and nonverbal behaviour that does not meet accepted cultural norms, including definite pronouncements about a culture that is not your own.
- Ask the service user if he or she uses herbs and what the expected benefits are.
- Learn to identify culturally relevant rituals.
- Stress the service user's strengths and demonstrate respect and caring.

Source: Reprinted from Carson V, 2000, Mental Health Nursing: the Nurse–Patient Journey, 2nd edn. W B Saunders, Sydney, with permission from Elsevier.

Table 10.3 Cultural assessment checklist

Degree of acculturation	
Language and communication	How strictly does the service user adhere to the beliefs and values of their culture of origin in comparison to internalization of new cultural norms?
	What language is the service user most comfortable speaking and reading?
	Does the service user require an interpreter?
Nonverbal patterns of communication	
Eye contact	Is eye contact considered polite or rude?
Tone of voice	Is special meaning attached to loud or whispered conversations?
Personal space	Is personal space wider or closer than in your culture?
Facial expressions, gestures	What is the meaning behind certain facial expressions and hand/body gestures?
Touch	When, where and by whom can a service user be touched?
Etiquette and social customs	
Typical greeting	How would you like to be greeted/addressed by our staff?
Social customs before business	What behaviour is expected of guests? Taking off shoes, accepting food and drink?
Direct or indirect communication	Is it polite to engage in small talk before getting down to business?
Patterns	Should discussion be direct and forthright or subtle and indirect?

(continued)

Table 10.3 Continued

Service user's explanation of the problem	
Diagnosis	What do you call this problem? How would you describe this problem?
Onset	When and how did the problem begin? Why then?
Cause	What caused the problem? Why do you think you developed this problem and not someone else? What might other people think is wrong with you?
Course	What are the chief problems this condition has caused you?
Prognosis	What do you fear most about the problem? How serious is the problem? Do you think it is curable?
Treatment	How have you treated the problem so far? What have you done to feel better?
	Who in your family/community/religious group can help you? Are you consulting other healers?
Nutrition assessment	
Pattern of meals	What is eaten? When are meals eaten? Perform a 2-day diet recall. Could this pattern interfere with the plan of care?
Sick food	What foods are thought to promote health? What foods are considered good for sick people?
Food intolerance and taboos	Is there potential for food/drug interactions with traditional foods?
	Are there religious food prescriptions and restrictions?
Pain assessment	
Cultural patterns of coping with pain	Does the service user tend to be stoic or expressive when in pain?
What does pain mean to the service user?	What is the worst pain you have ever had? How did you cope with it?
Service user's perception of severe pain	How well did the treatment work?
Appropriate treatments	What is the service user's attitude towards taking pain medication?
Medication assessment	
Service user's perception of Western medication	Is the service user's attitude towards Western medication valuing or distrusting?
Possible pharmacogenetic variation	Could there be a genetic variation in the way the service user responds to medication?
	Are there traditional remedies, such as herbs, teas or ointments that the service user uses?
	In past experiences with the healthcare system, what has the service user found helpful? Offensive? Confusing?
Psychosocial assessment	
Family structure Family resources	Who do you consider family? What impact does the mental health problem have on your family?
	Who is the head of the family? With whom should we discuss your care? Is there someone who helps you make decisions?
Community resources	Who helps when you are sick? How do they help you? How would you like them to help you?
	What health/support services are available through the service user's cultural community?

Source: Adapted from Narayan M, 2003, Cultural Assessment and Care Planning, Home Healthcare Nurse, with permission from Lippincott, Williams and Wilkins, http://www.lww.com.

A Crisis Triage Rating Scale (CTRS) (Bengelsdorf et al., 1984) has been developed to screen emergency mental health service users rapidly. The scale evaluates service users according to three factors. A descriptive statement accompanies each score.

- Dangerousness (1 = most dangerous to self or others, 5 = least dangerous).
- Support system (1 = poor or absent, 5 = excellent).
- Motivation and cooperation (1 = least likely to cooperate, 5 = most likely).

This scale is useful in predicting whether hospitalization is required. The three scores are added to give a minimum of 3 and a maximum of 15. A score of less than or equal to 9 indicates a need for hospitalization; above 9 indicates that another form of intervention is required (Bengelsdorf et al., 1984). A critical appraisal of the service user's risk status is essential in triage. Risk status is rated on a four-point scale from low to extreme, and is assessed in four domains:

- harm to others,
- harm to self,
- suicide,
- absconding.

Risk of harm to others

Persons rated as low on the scale would present with no indication of violence or aggression prior to assessment, while service users who rated at the extreme end of the scale would be engaging in aggressive behaviours such as verbal abuse and physical aggression. They may be openly threatening harm and have access to weapons. Behaviours related to the moderate and high risk of harm to others would include a previous history of violence, poor impulse control, being in a delusional state, the content of the delusions, evidence of substance abuse and/or withdrawal, and body language consistent with potential aggression, such as fist clenching, pacing, restlessness, agitation and disruptive behaviour.

Risk of harm to self

Persons rated low on the scale would have had no indication of self-harm prior to assessment, while those rated as extreme would be engaging in self-harm or self-mutilating activities. Some service users may be engaging in self-harming activities as a result of command hallucinations (auditory hallucinations that tell the person to perform acts that they do not want to), or acting on delusional beliefs that involve self-harm activities. Behaviours equating to moderate- and high-risk status include a history of previous self-harm behaviour, intrusive thought of self-harm behaviour, attempting to

reduce stress by such behaviours as picking and pinching skin or pulling hair, seeking instruments to induce self-harm and having a delusional belief system that involves self-harm.

Risk of suicide

Persons assessed as low suicide risk would present with no indication of suicide prior to assessment, while those rated as extreme are intent on committing suicide, with access to the means and a well-developed plan. The person has limited social support or has disengaged from social supports. The person has no future orientation and may have experienced a recent loss. Those assessed as moderate may have some suicidal thoughts with no plan or intent, while those people deemed to be at high risk may have intrusive thoughts of suicide that are difficult to be distracted from. They may feel hopeless and helpless and lack the problem-solving ability to change the situation. The person may be thinking about how they will commit suicide, including where to obtain the means. The person may be disengaging from social supports and have a past history of suicide attempts.

The chapter on crisis and loss (Ch. 9) provides a more in-depth assessment of self-harm and suicide.

Risk of absconding

Assessing for a person's risk of absconding is related to the person's ability or willingness to accept treatment. The person deemed to be at moderate risk of absconding has ambivalence about being in hospital or continuing their relationship with community services. Staff find themselves regularly encouraging the person to stay in treatment. Those at high risk have had a previous history of absconding and express their reluctance to stay in the healthcare facility or to continue to live in the present community.

The information obtained from the assessment of the service user's risk status and the service user's CTRS score results in the service user being assigned to one of five categories. The categories represent how urgently the service user needs to be assessed by a mental health professional. Table 10.4 provides an example of the categories and management guidelines.

Vulnerability to exploitation or abuse

Some people living with a mental disorder are vulnerable to exploitation or abuse through sex or violence. It is therefore important that in any triage assessment the person's vulnerability to exploitation and abuse be recorded and protective measures put in place to avoid

Table 10.4 Triage guidelines

Description	Observation/treatment acuity	Typical presentation	General principles of management
1. Immediate life-threatening illness Immediate danger to self or others	Immediate intervention (life-threatening: immediate)	Cardiorespiratory arrest Actively violent, aggressive behaviour Actively self-destructive behaviour Possession of weapon	Continuous visual surveillance Provide safe environment for service user and others Ensure adequate personnel to provide restraint/detention Consult mental health specialist
2. Probable danger to self or others Severe behavioural disturbance	Constant observation (emergency: within 10 min)	Extreme agitation/restlessness Aggressive Confused/unable to cooperate Threat of self-harm Threat of harm to others May have police escort	Continuous visual surveillance Provide safe environment for service user and others Ensure adequate personnel to provide restraint/detention Consult mental health specialist
3. Possible danger to self or others Service user is very distressed or psychotic Service user is experiencing a situational crisis and is very disturbed	Close observation (urgent: within 30 min) Confusion/withdrawn	Presence of psychotic symptoms Presence of affective disturbance Suicidal ideation Agitation/restlessness Bizarre/disorganized/intrusive behaviour	Consult mental health specialist Re-triage if evidence of increasing behavioural disturbance (restlessness, intrusiveness, increasing distress)
4. Service user has a longstanding, semi-urgent mental disorder/problem Moderate distress	Periodic observation (semi-urgent: within 60 min)	No agitation/restlessness Irritability without aggression Cooperative Gives coherent history Symptoms of anxiety or depression without suicidal ideation	Re-triage if evidence of increasing behavioural disturbance (restlessness, intrusiveness, increasing distress)
5. Service user has a longstanding, nonacute mental disorder/problem No danger to self or others No acute distress No behavioural disturbance	General observation (nonurgent: within 120 min)	Cooperative, communicative Compliant with instructions Request for medication Financial/social/accommodation/relationship problems	Referral to mental health specialist/team Mobilize or establish support network Known service user

Source: Reprinted from the Commonwealth Department of Health and Ageing Emergency Triage Education Kit, used by permission of the Australian Government.

such exploitation. The nurse will need to be extremely diligent if the person presents with any of the following indicators:

- extensive documented past history of sexual abuse,
- unawareness of social boundaries regarding dress or personal space,
- frequent and intense thoughts or discussion of sexual activity from which the individual is unable to be distracted,
- no recognition of, and continued contact with, an individual demonstrating predatory behaviour.

People vulnerable to exploitation by violence or abuse may present with the following characteristics:

- past history of violent relationships,
- evidence of hostile/dependent or passive personality traits,
- increasingly intrusive behaviour,
- some or limited recognition of a violent relationship/environment,
- limited ability to express their needs within this relationship,
- evidence of significant substance use.

A person who is at extreme risk has expressed a desire to return to the violent relationship/environment with no recognition of personal control of the situation. In a mental health facility, a person's care level is determined by the risk assessment. The risk assessment in the community determines the interventions that will be required to ensure a person's safety and the safety of others.

MENTAL HEALTH ASSESSMENT AND OUTCOME MEASURES

Traditionally, most mental health professionals have used their clinical judgement to determine change. Assessment and outcome measures are often associated with rigorous research and are not a part of everyday practice. However, clinical judgement is not always accurate, as the clinician may under- or over-rate treatment effectiveness, may concentrate on only one of the problems, such as symptoms, and not observe other problems such as social functioning. The use of outcome measures that are standardized in their content and scoring procedures can provide an accurate assessment of presenting problems and a measure of change (Andrews et al., 1994). The measurement of outcomes can:

- allow the individual to monitor his or her progress,
- allow the clinician to monitor the individual's progress,
- allow the clinician to monitor his or her performance as a clinician,
- help with decision-making regarding which treatments are effective and should be supported, and which treatments are less effective and in need of review (Treatment Protocol Project, 2003, p. 20).

What to measure?

The following areas may be considered when measuring service user outcomes:

- measure of symptoms,
- measure of functioning,
- measure of quality of life,
- measure of burden,
- measure of satisfaction with the service,
- multidimensional measures.

Stedman et al. (1997) identified six outcome measures that were considered appropriate for use as routine outcome measures for service users and service provision. The six selected measures are:

1. Behaviour and Symptom Identification Scale (BASIS-32) (Eisen et al., 1994),
2. Mental Health Inventory (MHI) (Davies et al., 1988; Veit and Ware, 1983),
3. Medical Outcomes Study Short Form 36 (SF-36) (Ware and Sherbourne, 1992; Ware et al., 1993),
4. Health of the Nation Outcome Scales (HoNOS) (Wing et al., 1996),
5. Life Skills Profile (LSP) (Parker et al., 1991; Rosen et al., 1989),
6. Role Functioning Scale (RFS) (Goodman et al., 1993; McPheeters, 1984; Newman, 1980).

Measures that are used for assessment of a particular mental disorder are discussed in the chapter related to that disorder.

Methods of administering service user outcome measures

Outcomes can be measured by having:

- the service user complete a questionnaire,
- the carer or clinician complete a questionnaire about the service user,
- the clinician interview the service user in a structured or unstructured fashion,
- the clinician or carer make a rating of the service user's level of functioning on the basis of information already available to them from their interaction with the person (Andrews et al., 1994).

The Health of the Nation Outcome Scales (HoNOS)

The Health of the Nation Outcome Scales (HoNOS) were designed as a brief, easily administered tool for routine clinical use to gather information about key areas of mental health and social functioning, specifically for service monitoring and outcome measurement. The HoNOS comprise 12 scales, each measuring a type of problem that service users of mental health services may present with. The scales are:

1. overactive, aggressive, disruptive or agitated behaviour,
2. nonaccidental self-injury,
3. problem drinking or drug taking,
4. cognitive problems,
5. physical illness or disability problems,
6. problems associated with hallucinations and delusions,
7. problems with depressed mood,
8. other mental and behavioural problems,
9. problems with relationships,
10. problems with activities of daily living,
11. problems with living conditions,
12. problems with occupation and activities.

The HoNOS have advantages over a number of other symptom and functioning inventories in that they are not diagnostically specific and so have practical applicability across a range of service user groups and mental health settings. HoNOS also have potential usefulness for service monitoring (Stein, 1999).

The HoNOS are not a structured clinical interview; the information is gathered through the comprehensive assessment process used in routine practice.

CLASSIFICATION OF MENTAL DISORDERS

The American Psychiatric Association (APA) classifies mental disorders as conditions that can be:

... conceptualized as a clinically significant behavioral or psychological syndrome or pattern that occurs in an individual and that is associated with present distress (a painful symptom) or disability (impairment in one or more important areas of functioning) or with significantly increased risk of suffering death, pain, disability, or an important loss of freedom. In addition, this syndrome or pattern must not be merely the expectable and culturally sanctioned response to a particular event, for example the death of a loved one ... Neither deviant behavior (e.g. political, religious, or sexual) nor conflicts that are primarily between the individual and society are mental disorders unless the deviance or conflict is a symptom or dysfunction of an individual as described above.

(American Psychiatric Association, 2000, p. xxiii)

At present the DSM-IV TR and the ICD-10 provide the foundation for psychiatric classification, formulation and diagnosis in mainstream mental health services. Each of the categories is accompanied by a description of the disorder in question. A diagnosis is formulated by comparing the behaviour of the service user with the descriptions of the disorder. The service user is diagnosed according to the description that fits best.

ICD-10: *International Classification of Diseases*

The ICD-10 provides broad categories that may be used by any clinician but especially those who do not feel comfortable in providing a clinical diagnosis. The ICD-10 mental health manual lists 458 types of mental disorder, of which some are discrete disorders and others subtypes of major psychiatric disorders. The ICD-10 consists of a comprehensive listing of clinical diagnoses, each associated with a unique numerical code. Similar disorders are linked together so that similar codes apply to closely related conditions. The ICD codes can be evaluated by computer and closely related diagnostic categories can

be clustered together for statistical analysis. The ICD is sometimes referred to as the F scale, as this letter is the prefix for the numbering of the disorders.

ICD-10 diagnostic categories

Categories are as follows:

*   F00–F09 organic, including symptomatic, mental disorders: types of dementia and delirium,
*   F10–F19 mental and behavioural disorders due to psychoactive substance use: alcohol and other substance use, and associated disorder,
*   F20–F29 schizophrenia, schizotypal and delusional disorders: types of schizophrenia and disorders with similar symptoms,
*   F30–F39 mood disorders: types of depression, mania and mixtures of these,
*   F40–F48 neurotic, stress-related and somatoform disorders: types of phobias (fears), anxiety problems and maladaptive reactions to stress, such as physical complaint or psychological attempts to escape,
*   F50–F59 behavioural syndromes associated with physiological disturbance and physical factors: disorders of natural functions such as eating, sleep and sexual dysfunction, not caused by an organic cause or disease,
*   F60–F69 disorders of adult personality and behaviour: distortions of personality, impulse control disorders, sexual identity and preference problems,
*   F70–F89 mental retardation and disorders of psychological development: degrees of learning disability, difficulties with language and scholastic skills, pervasive developmental disorders (e.g. autism),
*   F90–F98 behavioural and emotional disorders with onset usually occurring in childhood and adolescence: behavioural disturbances, problems with early relationships and social functioning, and tic disorders, stammering and bed wetting/soiling.

The ICD lists the names of the clinical condition – for example, 'mild depressive episode' – without further definition of the diagnostic label. Therefore the ICD can be used to label a diagnosis but is less useful for describing clinical symptoms. The benefit of the ICD is its strength in the coding of diagnosis, which can provide statistical analysis of the major diagnostic groups that are presenting to a service. The coding system also lends itself to larger epidemiological studies.

DSM-IV TR: *Diagnostic and Statistical Manual*

The main DSM-IV TR diagnostic categories, and a brief description of each, are as follows:

*   disorders usually first diagnosed in infancy: these range from pervasive disorders that affect every aspect of life to minor ones, such as elimination,

- childhood and adolescence disorders: the common bond is the age at first diagnosis,
- mental retardation and learning disorders: disorders of intellectual functioning and communication,
- delirium, dementia, amnestic and other cognitive disorders with presumed neurological causes (brain damage, brain disease): mainly disorders of memory and cognitive function,
- eating disorders: undereating and overeating,
- mental disorders due to illness: includes emotional and cognitive effects of physical and general medical conditions,
- substance-related disorders: alcohol and drug (prescription and illicit) problems,
- schizophrenia and other psychotic disorders: disorders marked by lack of contact with reality and disturbed thought processes,
- mood disorders: includes depression, extreme elation and mood alteration,
- anxiety disorders: a mixed group of fear- and dread-related conditions,
- somatoform disorders: disorders with physical complaints,
- factitious disorders: intentional faking of physical illness,
- dissociative disorders: loss of memory and personal identity,
- sexual- and gender-identity disorders: problems with sexual functioning and gender identity,
- sleep disorders: sleep difficulties with various causes,
- impulse-control disorders not elsewhere classified: a mixed group of disorders including shoplifting, fire setting, gambling and others,
- adjustment disorders: reaction to life circumstances (death, divorce and parenthood),
- personality disorders: disorders of 'character' such as antisocial, dependent and histrionic personality disorders,
- other conditions that may be the focus of clinical attention: a wide variety of problems that may require clinical intervention (academic, occupational, intellectual) (adapted from Schwartz, 2000, p. 123).

Multiaxial classification

In formulating a diagnosis from the DSM-IV TR, the mental health practitioner assesses the service user across five axes. The purpose of these is to gather information from five different domains, which helps the clinician plan treatment and predict outcome. The multiaxial system provides the framework for organizing and communicating clinical information, for capturing the complexity of clinical situations and for describing the differences in people presenting with the same diagnosis. It also acts as a guide for a comprehensive assessment by focusing on different domains that may have been overlooked if the focus had been on a single presenting problem (American Psychiatric Association, 2000).

- Axis I contains a person's primary clinical diagnosis.
- Axis II is used to describe any existing personality disorder. This ensures that the mental health practitioner does not ignore long-term patterns of behaviour that may influence the primary diagnosis.
- Axis III describes nonpsychiatric medical conditions that may play a role in the person's treatment and diagnosis.
- Axis IV indicates a person's psychosocial and environmental issues that may influence the diagnosis, treatment or functioning of the service user.
- Axis V assesses a person's overall level of functioning. This assessment is usually made using the Global Assessment of Functioning Scale. This scale describes psychological, social and occupational functioning. The lowest score describes people who are having difficulty with everyday living, with marked behavioural problems, difficulty with relationships, lack of social networks and limited employment opportunities. The highest score describes people who are employed, have intact and healthy relationships, a developed social network and no behavioural problems. Ratings can be made on current or past level of functioning. The scale can be used to assess the person's level of functioning on admission to the service and to track the progress of the person through treatment interventions (American Psychiatric Association, 2000).

CRITICAL THINKING CHALLENGE 10.3

Interview a service user in your care to identify areas of strength in the service user. How does the recognition of strength influence your final treatment plan?

Does the multiaxial assessment system in the DSM-IV TR provide a comprehensive assessment of factors that may be contributing to a person's mental disorder? Can you think of any factors that may have been excluded?

What would you see as being problematic if a universal classification system were not used?

CONCLUSION

This chapter has given an overview of the assessment process initiated when a person presents to the mental health system and other areas such as accident and emergency departments. The view of the service user is of paramount importance. If nurses understand the meaning that the service user assigns to the situation, development of an integrated, collaborative care plan is likely to occur. The diagnosis and assessment of mental disorders requires advanced interview skills, and nurses are required to develop their interpersonal skills to ensure that the person is comfortable with the nurse. These advanced interpersonal and interviewing skills result in the person trusting the nurse, and accurate and relevant assessment information being obtained. This then ensures that the person is provided with the best care and treatment for their situation.

EXERCISES FOR CLASS ENGAGEMENT

David is a 17-year-old student studying for his A levels. Five months ago his mother noticed that he was spending more time in his room and little time with friends. In recent weeks he has started listening to loud music with lyrics associated with violence and suicide. When his mother asked him about this he stated that there was nothing wrong, that he just needed time on his own and that this is the music that most of his friends are listening to. His room is always dark, with the blinds drawn, and dirty clothes, magazines, books and stale food over the floor and bed. He rarely showers and has been wearing the same clothes for the past 2 weeks. On Friday night when he was called to dinner, he yelled, 'Get out of my head! If you don't leave me alone you'll be sorry!' Later that night David's parents were woken by David yelling and punching the wall and screaming, 'I can't take it any more!' His father has called the after-hours crisis team for an assessment interview.

Have three members of the class role play David.

- In the first role play, David has a substance use disorder.
- In the second role play, David has a depressive disorder.
- In the third role play, David has a psychotic disorder.

Ensure that other members of the class are unaware of the disorder David is role playing.

- Have other members of the class conduct an assessment interview with David.

- Those not involved in the role play should form a fishbowl around those in the role play.
- Have the students forming the fishbowl observe:
  - the nonverbal and verbal behaviour of David and the assessor,
  - appropriate nursing skills for an assessment interview,
  - questions that assist in the formulation of the diagnosis.
- At the end of the interview, have those in the role play give feedback to the group on what they thought went well and what they thought didn't go well.

There are many issues associated with assessment and diagnosis of mental disorders. Divide the class into three. Each group should discuss one of the following issues:

- social issues,
- professional issues,
- issues related to diagnosis and classification.

Each group should then report back to the rest of the class.

If you are interested in the pros and cons of the DSM-IV TR you might want to visit the following website, which provides arguments for and against labelling and classifying human behaviour as it relates to the DSM-IV TR: http://www.apa.org.

REFERENCES

American Psychiatric Association, 2000. Diagnostic and Statistical Manual of Mental Disorders, fourth ed., text rev, international version. American Psychiatric Association, Washington DC.

Andrews, G., Peters, L., Teeson, M., 1994. The Measurement of Consumer Outcome in Mental Health: A Report to the National Mental Health Information Strategy Committee. Clinical Research Unit For Anxiety Disorders, Sydney.

Barker, P., 2003a. Assessment—the foundation of practice. In: Barker, P. (Ed.), Psychiatric and Mental Health Nursing: The Craft of Caring. Arnold, London.

Barker, P., 2003b. Assessment methods. In: Barker, P. (Ed.), Psychiatric and Mental Health Nursing: The Craft of Caring. Arnold, London.

Barker, P., 2003c. Interviewing as craft. In: Barker, P. (Ed.), Psychiatric and Mental Health Nursing: The Craft of Caring. Arnold, London.

Barlow, D., Durand, 2005. Abnormal Psychology: An Integrative Approach. Thomson Learning, Melbourne.

Bengelsdorf, H., Levy, L., Emerson, R., et al., 1984. A crisis triage rating scale: brief dispositional assessment of patients at risk of hospitalisation. J. Nerv. Ment. Dis. 172 (7), 424–430.

Boyd, M., 2005. Psychiatric Nursing: Contemporary Practice, third ed. Lippincott, New York.

Carson, V., 2000. Mental Health Nursing: The Nurse–Patient Journey, second ed. W B Saunders, Sydney.

Clinton, M., Nelson, S., 1996. Mental Health and Nursing Practice. Prentice Hall, Sydney.

Crisp, J., Taylor, C. (Eds.), 2001. Potter and Perry's Fundamentals of Nursing. Elsevier, Sydney.

Crisp, J., Taylor, C. (Eds.), 2005. Potter and Perry's Fundamentals of Nursing, second ed. Elsevier, Sydney.

Davies, A., Sherbourne, C., Peterson, J., et al., 1988. Scoring Manual: Adult Health Status and Patient Satisfaction Measure Used in RAND's Health Insurance Experiment. RAND Corporation, Santa Monica.

Egan, G., 1998. The Skilled Helper: A Problem-Management Approach to Helping, sixth ed. Brooks/Cole, Melbourne.

Eisen, S., Dill, D., Grob, M., 1994. Reliability and validity of a brief patient report instrument for psychiatric outcome evaluation. Hosp. Commun. Psychiatry 45 (3), 242–247.

Elkins, D., Hedstorm, L., Hughes, L., et al., 1998. Towards a humanistic-phenomenological spirituality. In: Meadows, G., Singh, B., Grigg, M. (Eds.), 2007. Mental Health in Australia: Collaborative Community Practice. Oxford University Press, Melbourne.

Folstein, M., Folstein, S., McHugh, P., 1975. Mini mental state: a practical guide for grading the cognitive state of patients for the clinician. J. Psychiatr. Res. 12 (3), 189–198.

Fossey, E., 2007. Understanding the lived experience of carers and consumers. In: Meadow, G., Singh, B., Grigg, M. (Eds.), Mental Health in Australia: Collaborative Community Practice. Oxford University Press, Melbourne.

Frisch, N., Frisch, L., 2006. Psychiatric Mental Health Nursing, third ed. Delmar, Melbourne.

Glass, N., 2003. Interpersonal Relating: Study Guide. School of Nursing and Health Care Practices, Southern Cross University, Lismore, New South Wales.

Goodman, S., Sewell, D., Cooley, E., et al., 1993. Assessing levels of adaptive functioning: the role functioning scale. Commun. Ment. Health J. 29 (2), 119–131.

Horsfall, J., Stuhlmiller, C., Champ, S., 2000. Interpersonal Nursing for Mental Health. McLennan & Petty, Sydney.

Keen, T., Keen, J., 2003. Developing collaborative assessment. In: Barker, P. (Ed.), Psychiatric and Mental Health Nursing: The Craft of Caring. Arnold, London.

Leggatt, M., 2007. Carer's perspective on assessment consumers. In: Meadow, G., Singh, B., Grigg, M. (Eds.), Mental Health in Australia: Collaborative Community Practice. Oxford University Press, Melbourne.

McPheeters, H., 1984. State wide mental health outcome evaluation: a perspective of two southern states. Commun. Ment. Health J. 20 (1), 44–55.

Meadows, G., 2007a. The importance of spirituality. In: Meadows, G., Singh, B., Grigg, M. (Eds.), Mental Health in Australia: Collaborative Community Practice. Oxford University Press, Melbourne.

Meadows, G., 2007b. Assessment in context. In: Meadows, G., Singh, B., Grigg, M. (Eds.), Mental Health in Australia: Collaborative Community Practice. Oxford University Press, Melbourne.

Meadows, G., 2007c. Mindfulness in assessment. In: Meadows, G., Singh, B., Grigg, M. (Eds.), Mental Health in Australia: Collaborative Community Practice. Oxford University Press, Melbourne.

Meadows, G., Singh, B., Grigg, M. (Eds.), 2007. Mental Health in Australia: Collaborative Community Practice. Oxford University Press, Melbourne.

Narayan, M.C., 2003. Cultural assessment checklist. Home Health Care Nurse 21 (9), 611–618.

New South Wales Health, 2001. NSW Mental Health Outcome and Assessment Training (MH-OAT) Facilitator's Manual. NSW Health, Sydney.

Newman, F., 1980. Strengths, uses and problems of global scales as an evaluation instrument. Eval. Program Plann. 3 (4), 257–268.

Onyett, S., 1998. Case Management in Mental Health. Chapman & Hall, London.

Parker, G., Rosen, A., Emdur, N., et al., 1991. The life skills profile: psychometric properties of a measure assessing function and disability in schizophrenia. Acta Psychiatricia Scand. 83 (2), 145–152.

Rapp, C., 1996. Theory, principles and methods of the strengths model of case management. In: Bergman, H., Harris, M. (Eds.), Case Management for Mentally Ill Patients: Theory and Practice. Harwood, Sydney.

Rapp, C., Goscha, R., 2006. The Strengths Model: Case Management of People with Psychiatric Disabilities. Oxford University Press, New York.

Rosen, A., Hadzi-Pavlovic, D., Parker, G., 1989. The life skills profile: a measure assessing function and disability. Schizophr. Bull. 15 (2), 325–337.

Schwartz, S., 2000. Abnormal Psychology: A Discovery Approach. Mayfield, London.

Stedman, T., Yellowlees, P., Mellsop, G., et al., 1997. Measuring Consumer Outcomes in Mental Health. Department of Health and Family Services, Canberra.

Stein, G., 1999. Usefulness of the health of the nation outcome scales. Br. J. Psychiatry 174 (5), 375–377.

Stuart, G., Laraia, M., 2005. Principles and Practice of Psychiatric Nursing, eighth ed. Elsevier, Sydney.

Treatment Protocol Project, 2003. Acute Inpatient Psychiatric Care: A Source Book, second ed. World Health Organization Collaborating Centre for Evidence in Mental Health Policy, Sydney.

Treatment Protocol Project, 2004., fourth ed. Management of Mental Disorders, vol. 1. World Health Organization, Collaborating Centre for Evidence in Mental Health Policy, Sydney.

Veit, C., Ware, J., 1983. The structure of psychological distress and wellbeing in general populations. J. Clin. Consult. Psychiatry 51 (5), 730–745.

Ware, J., Sherbourne, C., 1992. The MOS 36-item short-form health survey (SF 36): 1. Conceptual framework and item selection. Med. Care 30 (6), 473–481.

Ware, J., Snow, K., Kosinski, M., et al., 1993. SF-36 Health Survey Manual and Interpretation Guide. The Health Institute, New England, Boston, MA.

Weir, D., Oei, T., 1996. Mental disorder: conceptual framework, classification and assessment. In: Clinton, M., Nelson, S. (Eds.), Mental Health and Nursing Practice. Prentice Hall, Sydney.

Wing, J., Curtis, R., Beevor, A., 1996. Health of the Nation Outcome Scales: Report on Research. Royal College of Psychiatrists, London.

World Health Organization, 1992. ICD-10: International Statistical Classification of Diseases and Related Health Problems, tenth rev. World Health Organization, Geneva.

Part | 3 |

Understanding mental health problems

Chapter | 11 |

Learning disabilities

Charles Harmon, Philip B. Petrie, and Kay Mafuba

CHAPTER POINTS

- Definitions and systems of classification exist for learning disabilities.
- Learning disability and other nurses need to liaise effectively with health and social care services for people with learning disabilities.
- People with a learning disability can fail to receive assessment and treatment services.
- Nurses are involved with the acute nursing assessment and management of individuals with a dual diagnosis of learning disability and mental disorder.
- Assessment and communication issues need to be considered.
- Pitfalls in the assessment process need to be negotiated.
- Continuous care for people with dual diagnosis needs to be facilitated.
- Discharge planning and the Care Programme Approach (CPA) plans are significant nursing responsibilities.

KEY TERMS

- assessment and treatment services
- best interests
- Care Programme Approach (CPA)
- carer
- challenging behaviour
- continuity of care
- dual diagnosis
- health action plan
- health facilitation
- learning disability

DOI: http://dx.doi.org/10.1016/B978-0-7020-4493-9.00011-1

- learning disability services
- mental capacity assessment
- normalization
- nursing assessment
- nursing management
- social inclusion
- stakeholders
- support
- support worker

LEARNING OUTCOMES

The material in this chapter will assist you to:

- analyse factors that contribute to difficulties in the diagnosis and management of people with a dual diagnosis (i.e. people with a learning disability who also have a mental disorder),
- discuss the definitions and features of learning disability according to the ICD-10, DSM-IV TR and the American Association on Mental Retardation,
- outline reasons why the term 'learning disability' is preferred in the UK context,
- outline the service philosophy pertinent to services for people with a learning disability,
- discuss the factors that contribute to a thorough mental health nursing assessment for individuals with a dual diagnosis,
- discuss the nursing care and management appropriate for individuals with a dual diagnosis who have acute care requirements due to mental health problems,
- discuss the nursing strategies relevant to ensuring continuity of care for people with a dual diagnosis in the first month after their discharge from the care of an assessment and treatment service.

INTRODUCTION

This chapter provides information on the nursing care and management of service users who have a dual diagnosis – that is, a diagnosis of a mental disorder comorbid with a learning disability – in the context of assessment and treatment service provision. To assist readers who have little first-hand experience with people with a learning disability, a number of case studies are included. Essentially, good-quality nursing care for service users with a learning disability is the same type of care offered to any other member of the community, with some important differences, as follows.

- It might be necessary for the nurse to modify the way in which she or he communicates with the service user,

in order to accommodate a level of understanding appropriate to the service user's disability.
- A modification of the assessment process may provide the nurse with information vital to the management of the service user.
- The process of forming a therapeutic relationship with the service user will be greatly enhanced by promoting a cooperative relationship between the relevant mental health professionals and the service user's usual carers and/or service providers.
- The service user should be supported upon discharge from assessment and treatment services via the design and implementation of a Care Programme Approach (CPA) plan.

THE LANGUAGE OF LEARNING DISABILITY SERVICES

In order to fully appreciate the subject of learning disability and mental disorder, it is necessary to learn some of the language used by learning disability professionals (see also the list of key terms at the beginning of this chapter). Much of the literature, particularly regarding definition of terms and the prevalence of dual diagnosis, has been written by British or American authors, and guidance is provided here on understanding the varied terminology used in these sources and applying the information in a UK context.

Terminology

The term *dual diagnosis* is most often used by mental health professionals in reference to service users who have a diagnosis of mental disorder as well as a substance abuse problem. (This form of 'dual diagnosis' is addressed in Ch. 19.) There is, however, another form of dual diagnosis that provides a label for people diagnosed with a mental disorder who have a comorbid learning disability. Dual disability in this chapter refers to the latter definition.

Many terms have been used to describe people who in some way represent a departure from the usual. Labels such as 'feebleminded' and 'mentally subnormal' have been used in the past to describe people with a learning disability but these terms have, thankfully, been superseded. Indeed, terms such as 'idiot', 'imbecile' and 'moron' were also once used by the scientific community to describe people with a learning disability but these terms are no longer in everyday professional use, because of the way in which their meaning has altered over time. Internationally, the terms *intellectual disability, learning disability, mental retardation* and *intellectual handicap* remain in use, depending on the country or jurisdiction. In the

UK, however, the descriptor *learning disability* is preferred by service users and health and social care professionals, mainly because it is felt that terms such as 'mental retardation' are stigmatizing.

In the UK there are three distinct approaches to defining learning disability. These are *scientific/international*, *social* and *legal*. The scientific/international approach uses the terms 'mental retardation' and 'intellectual disability'. The *International Classification of Diseases* (ICD-10) refers to 'a condition of arrested or incomplete development of the mind' with significant impairment of intellectual functioning and 'reduced level of intellectual functioning resulting in dimished ability to adapt to the daily demands of the normal social environment' (World Health Organization, 1992, pp. 226 & 227). The *social approach* uses predominantly two terms: 'learning disability' or 'learning difficulty'. In this approach the focus is on an individual's social functioning assessment and the main tools used are Adaptive Behaviour Scales (ABS). The legal approach is enshrined in the Mental Health Act 1983, amended 2007. The Act uses the term 'mental impairment' which refers to 'incomplete development of mind' and 'impairment in social functioning' (intelligence quotient (IQ) 55–69). It also refers to 'severe mental impairment', which refers to 'severe impairment of intelligence' and 'social functioning' (IQ >54) (Mental Health Act 1983, amended 2007). The term 'mental impairment' was replaced with 'learning disability' in the 2007 amendments to the 1983 Mental Health Act. However, the 2007 Act made only very minor amendments to provisions in the 1983 Act relevant to people with dual diagnosis.

Systems of classification

The term intellectual disability is defined in the *Diagnostic and Statistical Manual of Mental Disorders*, fourth edition (DSM-IV TR) as:

> *... significantly subaverage general intellectual functioning ... accompanied by significant limitations in adaptive functioning in at least two of the following skill areas: communication, self-care, home living, social/interpersonal skills, use of community resources, self-direction, functional academic skills, work, leisure, health, and safety ... occur[ring] before age 18 years.*

(American Psychiatric Association, 2000, p. 41)

Subaverage intellectual functioning is defined as below an intelligence quotient (IQ) of 70 and is principally subdivided into four levels of increasing severity, from mild (IQ range 50–55 to 70), moderate (IQ range 35–40 to 50–55), severe (IQ range 20–25 to 35–40) to profound (IQ below 20–25). According to this system of classification, of the 2–3% of the general population who

might be diagnosed with learning disability, about 85% are thought to belong to the mild category, 10% in the moderate category and approximately 5% in either the severe or the profound categories (American Psychiatric Association, 2000, pp. 42–44). In a similar vein, the ICD-10 (World Health Organization, 1992) employs a system of categorization that emphasizes IQ.

The American Association on Learning Disability (2002, p. 39) defines intellectual disability as 'a disability characterized by significant limitations both in intellectual functioning and in adaptive behaviour as expressed in conceptual, social, and practical adaptive skills ... [that] ... originates before age 18'. This definition is similar to the DSM-IV TR definition because it maintains that learning disability occurs below a threshold IQ score of around 70. However, it differs from the DSM-IV TR definition in that it emphasizes levels of functioning based on adaptive behaviour rather than IQ. Furthermore, according to the American Association on Learning Disability, the individual is assessed according to their support requirements and categorized according to 'the intensity of needed supports'; that is, intermittent, limited, extensive or pervasive (American Association on Learning Disability, 2002, p. 152).

The ICD-10 Classification of Mental and Behavioural Disorders clinical descriptions and diagnostic guidelines define mental retardation as 'a condition of arrested or incomplete development of the mind, which is especially characterized by impairment of skills manifested during the developmental period, which contribute to the overall level of intelligence, i.e. cognitive, language, motor, and social abilities' (World Health Organization, 1992, p. 226). There are four broad categories: mild mental retardation (IQ 50–69), moderate mental retardation (IQ 35–49), severe mental retardation (IQ 20–34) and profound mental retardation (IQ >20).

Although there is no such thing as the 'typical' person with a learning disability, the following stories are nevertheless intended to give you a general idea of the characteristics of individuals who might fit into the American Association on Learning Disability intensity-of-support categories.

- Ruth has a moderate learning disability. She is 20 years old and lives in a rented flat in a manner much like the rest of the community. Ruth used to attend a supported employment scheme but has recently taken up employment in a local supermarket, having learned the necessary vocational skills at an evening college. She lives a fairly independent life with the support of her family but receives two visits each week from her social services department, who assist her in planning meals and budgeting. Ruth has limited numeracy skills but she can competently manage money transactions and perform everyday mathematical calculations. She reads slowly and hesitantly but can read an article in her local paper with few difficulties.

- Barry is 25 years old and has a mild learning disability. He lived at home with his parents until he was 20 but now shares a supported housing scheme with two other men. Barry works in a supported employment scheme but occasionally works on weekends as a labourer with his uncle's landscape-gardening business. Although he makes friends easily and is well known at his local community soccer club, Barry has difficulty budgeting and using his money wisely. He also has a history of trouble with the police because he has occasionally got into fights following drinking sessions. Consequently Barry receives 5 h of contact per week with a disability worker who assists him in learning financial management skills and in conducting himself responsibly when socializing.

- Jan is a 40-year-old woman who has a severe learning disability. She has a hearing impairment and regularly takes medication for her epilepsy. After the death of her parents when she was 12 Jan was institutionalized in a large, state-owned residential facility, where she lived with 30 other individuals in a dormitory-style unit. At age 25 she was placed in a home in the community with four other people with similar support needs. The home is staffed by residential support workers and the service users attend a local day centre where they are provided with opportunities to participate in community activities and improve their living skills. Jan has a limited spoken vocabulary but with the assistance of a hearing aid can understand much of what is said to her. She can read important words like her own name, 'hot' and 'danger', but cannot read a newspaper or the captions in a television programme. She can perform many tasks associated with self-care and personal hygiene, and assists in the preparation of meals and other domestic chores around the house.

- Petra is a 10-year-old girl who has a profound learning disability. Apart from her learning disability, she has cerebral palsy (a disorder that limits her ability to move and coordinate her limbs) and epilepsy. These disabilities greatly limit her developmental opportunities and her independence. Petra lives at home with her parents and attends a school that caters for her specific needs. She has great difficulty speaking, because of her cerebral palsy, but can indicate her needs using sounds and gestures that her parents understand and with the aid of a 'pointer board', which she uses to point to symbols to indicate a range of things from concrete needs (such as food or drink) to emotions (such as happy). Petra also has a computer device that has a keyboard featuring the symbols on her pointer board and the capacity to electronically 'speak' for her. Petra is unable to walk independently but has a 'walker', a complex mechanical device that assists in mobilization, and a motorized wheelchair. Petra's parents hope that she can one day lead an independent life away from her family home just like any other young adult.

CAUSES OF LEARNING DISABILITY AND ASSOCIATED DISORDERS

Learning disability may result from impediments to intellectual development and/or neurological damage caused by factors that include:

- heredity (e.g. genetic causes such as Down's syndrome and fragile-X syndrome),
- alterations in embryonic development (e.g. foetal alcohol syndrome),
- familial and environmental influences (including deprivation of learning/developmental opportunities due to an unstimulating home environment),
- autistic-spectrum disorders (e.g. autistic disorder),
- pregnancy and perinatal problems (including hypoxia or viral infections),
- general medical conditions after birth (including infections and traumas) (American Psychiatric Association, 2000, p. 45).

The best known are genetic causes such as Down's syndrome, which occurs in approximately one in 700–1000 births (Dykens et al., 2000, p. 61). According to Dykens et al. (2000, p. 5), however, only about 50% of people with a learning disability have known 'organic' causes for their condition, with an estimated one-third of all cases being due to genetic abnormalities. This statistic is indicative of the problem of disabilities as an under-explored field for researchers, but this situation may well change, given the prominence of the Human Genome Project and the wealth of data it has generated.

Learning disability may also be accompanied by other types of impairment such as hearing impairments, visual impairments and epilepsy (Gilbert et al., 1998). In addition, people with a learning disability often lack the ability to make healthy lifestyle choices and are especially prone to developing preventable medical disorders in adulthood (e.g. cardiovascular diseases, nutritional disorders and endocrine disorders), including mental health problems (Barr et al., 1999).

SERVICES FOR PEOPLE WITH A LEARNING DISABILITY

In the UK, most people with a dual diagnosis live in the community in a variety of services (Mansell, 2007). A significant proportion of people with learning disabilities live with their families or informal carers. Of this group of people living at home there is access to short-break or respite services. However, it is important to note that there are significant geographical variations in the provision of these respite services.

Following closure of most of the NHS's long-stay institutions most people with dual diagnosis were resettled into ordinary group homes in the community. Most group homes that specialize in supporting people with dual diagnosis are run either privately or by the voluntary sector. These services vary in size and research has shown that some of them are too large and therefore unable to provide person-centred care for people with dual diagnosis. Criticisms focus on the inability of such services to facilitate meaningful community access for people with dual diagnosis. Another critisism of this model of service provision is that some of these services are too far from the families of their residents. There is also a significant variation in the quality of these services (Mansell, 2007). In addition to staff group residential homes, although not new, there has been a recent shift towards supported-living schemes. This follows developments in recognition of housing rights, direct payments and individual budgets.

Studies have shown that for people with learning disabilities to live successfully in the community there is need for adequate provision of occupational and leisure opportunities. A study in Northern Ireland by McConkey (2004) highlighted the importance of day opportunities for people with learning disabilities. For people with dual diagnosis and associated behavioural challenges, traditional day centres have always provided limited opportunities, and the government's agenda to modernize day care provision provides new opportunities for people with dual diagnosis. Recent innovative approaches have focused on further education, vocational training, supported employment and self-advocacy provisions. For people with dual diagnosis these developments seem to offer new opportunities.

For people with dual diagnosis living in the community, specialist community learning disability services are vital for successful community living. Traditionally, community teams for people with learning disabilities support people with learning disabilities living in the community. Recently these teams were based in social services departments. Generally these teams comprise learning disability nursing, psychology, psychiatry, social work, physiotherapy and occupational therapy. Recently multidisciplinary 'specialist crisis intervention teams' have been developed to focus on supporting people with dual diagnosis who are at risk of admission to hospital. Child and adolescent mental health services for children with dual diagnosis have also been developed in some areas.

A small proportion of people with dual diagnosis still live in long-stay hospitals. Although the NHS has closed down most of its long-stay campuses, there are new, privately run campus-style hospitals. The closure of long-stay institutions and the recent development of individualized budgets and direct payments is designed to ensure that most people with a learning disability live in their own homes or with their family carers. Although these developments are to be welcomed for people with dual diagnosis there are concerns regarding carers' experience or knowledge of working with people with learning disabilities who have a mental disorder. These factors can create difficulties for the person with a dual diagnosis in that their acute and/or long-term mental health needs might not be met effectively.

Service philosophy in learning disability services

The principles of normalization, first fully articulated by Wolfensberger (1972), have been a philosophical driving force behind the creation and design of services for people with a learning disability. This set of principles accounts, to some degree, for the various changes in the services of people with learning disabilities in the UK over the past few decades. More recently, O'Brien's model (1987) has provided direction with respect to the normalization of services. O'Brien identifies measures to ensure that people with a learning disability have:

- an increased physical presence in the community,
- choice in how they live their lives,
- the opportunity to acquire and develop skills that promote independent living,
- respect as citizens,
- the opportunity to participate in the community (O'Brien, 1987, p. 182).

This model emphasizes a humanist perspective in which citizens with a learning disability are given the same rights and opportunities as any other citizens, even if they need the support of appropriate services. Importantly, proponents of this model advocate the use of generic services (that is, services that any citizen would use, such as public transport, private banking services or general hospitals), rather than specialist disability-based services, in the quest for integration between the disabled and nondisabled populations.

PREVALENCE OF DUAL DIAGNOSIS

Prevalence studies generally indicate higher rates of mental disorder among the learning disabled population than among the general population (Benson, 1985; Borthwick-Duffy, 1994; Jacobson, 1990; Taylor et al., 2004). Some authors have theorized that people with a learning disability have a higher probability of developing mental health problems than the general population because their deficits with respect to communication, processing skills, cognitive functioning and social skills cause them to be more vulnerable to stress (Reiss, 1994; Sovner, 1996). Gilbert et al. (1998) noted that learning disability may be accompanied by other types of impairment that have been associated with mental health problems in the general population, such as hearing impairments, visual impairments and epilepsy, and that socioeconomic factors such as unemployment and poverty may also contribute to higher rates of mental disorders in this group.

A study of people with learning disabilities living in community settings in Wales (Deb et al., 2001) found that some 4.4% of the sample ($n=90$) met ICD-10 criteria for schizophrenia, 2.2% for depressive disorder, 2.2% for generalized anxiety disorder, 4.4% for phobic disorder and 1% for delusional disorder. According to Deb et al.:

> ... the overall rate of functional psychiatric illness (point prevalence) was similar to that found in the general community (16%). However rates of schizophrenic illness and phobic disorder were significantly higher in the study cohort compared with those in the general population (0.4% and 1.1% respectively).
>
> (Deb et al., 2001, p. 495)

Studies that estimate the prevalence of dual diagnosis in other countries like Australia and New Zealand are small in number. In a Queensland study, Edwards and Lennox (2002) estimated that between 7.4 and 20.2% of service users using services for people with a learning disability ($n=7196$) also had a diagnosis of a mental disorder. The validity of this study was, however,

compromised to some extent by the failure of 33% of the surveyed agencies to provide data to the researchers. A more exhaustive study of the prevalence of dual diagnosis in Australia came from White et al. (2005), who conducted a secondary analysis of the data from the national Disability, Ageing and Careers Survey 1998. The authors concluded that 1.3% of the sampled intellectually disabled population had a psychotic disorder, 8% had a diagnosis of a depressive disorder and 14% had a diagnosis of an anxiety disorder (White et al., 2005, p. 398).

FALLING THROUGH THE CRACKS

McIntyre et al. (2002) reported on the negative impact of mental ill health upon individuals with a learning disability and their families. Because of a range of difficulties, however, people in the intellectually disabled population who also have a mental disorder remain undiagnosed, are often ignored or do not have equitable access to assessment and treatment services (Chaplin, 2004; Fletcher and Poindexter, 1996; VanderSchie-Bezyak, 2003).

Part of the problem appears to be that carers and professionals tend to lack the skills required to meet the additional mental health needs of these people (Coyle, 2000). Equally, however, health professionals lack skills in dealing with this population (McConkey and Truesdale, 2000; Naylor and Clifton, 1994) and many may even be unwilling to treat them (McConkey and Truesdale, 2000, p. 159). Given these problems, much can go wrong in the care of people with dual diagnosis, as the case studies of Roy and John illustrate.

CASE STUDY: ROY

Roy had his first admission to a long-stay mental health facility for people with learning disabilities at the age of 15 and by age 20 he was a permanent inpatient with a diagnosis of moderate mental impairment and bipolar disorder. After considerable trial and error, his mental health problems were successfully treated with the assistance of the mood stabilizer lithium carbonate and the 'typical' antipsychotic medication, chlorpromazine. By the age of 20 Roy was living in Mimosa Lodge, a large rehabilitation unit run by the local NHS trust, where he was supported by learning disability nurses and psychiatrists.

At the age of 50 Roy moved from the rehabilitation unit to a group home run by a local charity. He appeared to settle in well and was regarded as a bit of a joker, always attempting to cuddle the female staff. However, very little documentation accompanied him to the new service and there was a minimum of information regarding the history and management of his mental disorder. Without records there was nothing to indicate when he had commenced

antipsychotic medication, or why the treatment was started. The staff presumed that his medication had been initiated to manage challenging behaviours that were no longer in evidence. There were also concerns that Roy's shuffling gait and sleep difficulties were medication-related and so his new GP halved the quantity of chlorpromazine.

Roy's sleep pattern deteriorated rapidly, his speech and movements became accelerated, he became more insistent on cuddling both male and female staff and these physical contacts became more overtly sexual. Pre-existing behaviour-management techniques (such as identifying and avoiding triggers for Roy's behaviour, ignoring Roy's inappropriate behaviour, redirecting him to more appropriate tasks and asking him to spend time in the garden when he was otherwise unmanageable) became ineffective and Roy began to initiate low-level physical assaults upon staff. Additional staff were needed to support Roy at night and the overall support structure started to fracture. After 6 weeks nurses from the local community team for people with learning disabilities arranged for Roy's admission to an assessment and treatment unit where he spent 8 weeks being stabilized on a regimen of lithium carbonate and the 'atypical' antipsychotic medication, quetiapine. Nursing care

consisted of the standard practices for a person diagnosed with bipolar disorder.

Following this bout of acute illness Roy was able to return to the group home, where he has been able to resume his usual lifestyle.

CASE STUDY: JOHN

John is a 20-year-old man who has a moderate learning disability. He uses little verbal communication but understands much of what is said to him and augments his limited speech with gestures and hand signs similar to those used by some people with severe hearing impairments. He can perform most self-care activities but is unable to read and write, except for a few words including his own name.

John was 17 when his mother died, and this event marked the occurrence of challenging behaviours including sudden displays of aggression directed towards others as well as himself. Because his father could not cope with these behaviours John was subsequently moved from his family home to a residential home for people with a learning disability. John displayed a range of problem behaviours including high-level verbal and physical assaults, theft from staff and other residents, lying, monopolization of staff time and self-abusive behaviours such as pulling his own hair out and picking the scabs off cuts and abrasions. The house manager sought a full physical examination because blood had been noted in the toilet bowl after John had used it. John became angry and abusive when he was asked about it, but investigations found no physiological cause for the blood in the toilet.

In his assessment, the psychologist identified a grief reaction to the loss of John's mother and 'attention seeking' as the primary cause of his difficult behaviours. A range of behaviour-support strategies were subsequently designed and implemented by nurses, including educative programmes designed to provide him with more independence in leisure skills, and outings and other activities that John enjoyed. Enjoyable activities were

approved on the proviso that he had not stolen property or displayed aggression towards others, and John was distracted and redirected to other activities if he engaged in inappropriate behaviours (see Ch. 23 for behaviour therapy and other therapeutic nursing interventions).

Nevertheless, over the next 6 months the behavioural programmes appeared to be having little impact and John's behaviour continued to deteriorate. At the request of the house staff, John was seen by the mental health team but was uncommunicative and, although staff provided written and verbal information to the assessing psychiatrist describing John's behaviours and their possible motivation, it was determined that John did not have a mental disorder.

John's behaviours continued to be highly problematic and 10 months after his placement at the residential home he was taken by ambulance to the local hospital for the emergency surgical removal of a length of fencing wire that was lodged in his urethra. The surgeon noted that there was evidence of repeated trauma to the urethra and the neck of the bladder and that it was probable that these were self-inflicted injuries that had been sustained over a number of months (see Ch. 22 for self-harm, and Ch. 9 for grief and bereavement). Concerns about the extent and apparent duration of the self-injurious behaviours resulted in a request by the surgeon for an assessment of John by the hospital's mental health liaison nurse. Further assessment by a psychiatrist resulted in John receiving a provisional diagnosis of major depression. Community learning disability nurses were subsequently engaged to assist residential home staff with his ongoing management.

Comments on Roy and John's case studies

It is clear that the outcomes in both cases could have been catastrophic, particularly if either Roy or John had sustained more serious permanent injury. In Roy's case, changing his antipsychotic medication (chlorpromazine) dose had unfortunate consequences that could have been avoided if adequate documentation had accompanied him in his move from one service to the next. Such documentation would have advised the new service of Roy's long-term mental health diagnosis and alerted personnel to the need to consult a specialist psychiatrist rather than

the GP when seeking a review of his antipsychotic medication. Similarly, the management of his behaviour immediately after the halving of his chlorpromazine dose was not informed by standard mental health management practices and, indeed, learning disability professionals were not engaged until his behaviour had reached crisis point.

In John's case relevant professionals were consulted at an appropriate time but he did not receive appropriate management until his depression was severe and he had engaged in potentially serious self-harm activities. What was required in both instances was effective communication between disability assessment and treatment services, accompanied by a thorough mental health assessment of the service users and the creation of a management plan understood and implemented not only by assessment and treatment services but also carers in the service users' home settings (see acute assessment and management, on the following pages).

CRITICAL THINKING CHALLENGE 11.1

How might the nurse obtain an adequate history regarding Roy's mental health problems?

What information should nurses obtain from Roy's carers in order to ensure a thorough assessment of his mental health status?

How likely is it that Roy had had previous episodes of mental distress during his stay at Mimosa Lodge?

CRITICAL THINKING CHALLENGE 11.2

Analyse possible factors that may have contributed to the delays in treatment for John's mental disorder.

How might the nurse establish communication with John, given his limited vocabulary?

ACUTE ASSESSMENT

Acute assessment here refers to assessment of an individual with a diagnosis of a mental disorder comorbid with a learning disability.

Just like the rest of the community, people with a learning disability can display a range of unusual or disturbed behaviours in response to adversity. Unlike most of the community, however, people with a learning disability often have difficulty communicating the reasons for their maladaptive behaviour, which might range from stereotypical (or repetitive) behaviours (such as hand flapping or body rocking), to 'acting out' behaviours (such as displays of yelling and violent body movements), self-injurious behaviours (such as scratching at their skin or old wounds) or aggression towards others.

Sovner (1996) proposed that people with a learning disability might develop disturbed behaviours as part of their usual behavioural repertoire because they had limited developmental opportunities and/or inappropriate learning situations when they were young. Equally, however, disturbed behaviours may develop as a response to the pain and discomfort of general medical conditions or the distress associated with mental health disorders. The mental health assessment of service users with a learning disability can thus become something of an art when one is faced with the task of ascertaining the origins of behaviour and its meaning in relation to the service user's mental health problem.

Assessment and communication issues

A further difficulty for the nurse is that service users with a learning disability often have limited capacity for conversation because of their primary disability or because of concurrent disabilities such as hearing impairment. In addition, service users with higher support needs may experience problems in generalizing (or transferring) communication skills from familiar environments, such as their home, to less familiar environments, such as assessment and treatment units. Another common problem is that the service user may become shy or confused and, as a consequence, use regressed or echolalic speech (repeating what has been said), as in this example.

Nurse: **How are you today, Robyn? You look a bit sad.**

Robyn: **A bit sad.**

The service user may also tend to answer 'Yes' to questions in order to please the interviewer or because they have interpreted questions literally:

Nurse: **Do you hear voices, Robyn?**

Robyn: **Yes, I hear voices all the time.**

Employing the assistance of carers, family members and significant others to assist with the communication process is most advisable, particularly if the service user has a significant communication impairment (for example, is semi- or nonverbal) and uses augmentative forms of communication such as sign language (signing), pointer boards (also known as communications or symbol boards) or computer devices.

Further information on augmentative and alternative communication is beyond the scope of this chapter but is available in the literature (Abudarham and Hurd, 2002; Cascella, 2005; Cockerill and Carroll-Few, 2001; Linfoot, 1994; von Tetzchner and Grove, 2003). In addition, a useful website on sign language is http://www.britishsignlanguage.com/. Note that sign languages may vary from one country to the next, just as with spoken languages. Having said this, British, Australian and New Zealand hand signs are similar, but US signs are often quite different.

Coombs and Martin (2002) have shown that mental health clinicians typically obtain information during the assessment and review processes either directly from the service user or from their own observations of the individual, rather than using other sources of information such as the service user's family or usual carers. However, Silka and Hauser (1997) assert that, in the case of service users with a learning disability, it is necessary to gather information from all possible sources to obtain a full clinical picture, especially if the service user has significant communications deficits and cannot participate in an assessment process that relies on their ability to respond verbally to questions.

In all instances the approach to obtaining information about a service user should be calm and non-threatening, using concrete, open-ended questions and avoiding jargon, complex technical terms or abstract questions (Hamer, 1998). For service users with a learning disability, the nurse will need to use skills in both observation and communication, verbal and nonverbal, in carrying out the assessment. If the service user's usual carers are willing to participate in this process it is helpful to interview them to obtain information about the service user's usual behaviour patterns (Moss and Lee, 2001). It is also important to ask the carer how the service user's presenting behaviour is a departure from the usual. This information may help to identify the 'typical' signs that indicate mental disorder as well as 'atypical' signs, which are behaviours peculiar to the service user following the onset of the mental disorder, including stereotypical (or repetitive) behaviours, 'acting out' behaviours and self-abusive behaviours (Ross and Oliver, 2002).

Other data pertinent to the assessment process should include information that may assist in developing the service user's history, including information from other service providers such as their GP, social workers and psychologists. In particular, a medication history should be established.

NURSE'S STORY: COMMUNICATING

Using augmentative forms of communication can be a difficult task for the novice but basic communication can be achieved quite quickly with the aid of motivation and some basic education. I had the pleasure of supervising a group of nursing students at a clinical placement that was a residential school for children and adolescents with autistic spectrum disorders. Very few of the children had speech that could be understood by the nursing students and so we commenced the process of teaching the students to communicate via communication boards, which display symbols that can be used to indicate meaning. Needless to say, the students were daunted by the task ahead of them, particularly when they entered the classrooms and were confronted by children seated at desks decorated with symbols and enthusiastically gesturing to them to come over and 'have a chat'.

I'd tried to plan for this experience by giving the students some prior reading and a brief demonstration of the use of communication boards. Essentially, however, the classroom teachers and I had contrived the learning environment so that the children would teach the students how to communicate via this medium. This was very exciting for me as I watched the students struggle with the new information and the pressure exerted on them

by their eager 'teachers'. Within about 10 min, however, you could see progress being made. One nursing student yelled: 'She went to the movies with her mum, in her mum's car, and saw a movie with a handsome actor: Tom Cruise!' The child smiled proudly. When the nursing student guessed the title of the movie the young child was absolutely delighted. The two had struck up a rapport and communication flowed much more quickly from this point.

Charles Harmon, RN

One of the first questions asked during the initial assessment should be whether the service user has recently undergone a full medical examination. A deterioration in skills or behaviour can be due to an undiagnosed physical complaint or exacerbation of an existing one. Barr (1998) has asserted that physical illness in this group of people is often not detected and that many conditions are diagnosed too late, making treatment less effective. *Healthcare for All* (Michael, 2008) noted that there is significant evidence suggesting that people with learning disabilities experience high levels of suffering because of untreated, but treatable, ill health. For people with dual diagnosis, a Disability Rights Commission (2006) report identified diagnostic overshadowing as a significant factor contributory to the high incidence of untreated mental and physical ill health.

Enhancing the assessment process

Where possible, standard assessment formats such as the mental status examination and self-harm and/or risk assessment should be used in the assessment of all mental health service users (see Ch. 10 for mental status examination, Ch. 22 for self-harm and Ch. 23 for risk assessment).

There are other tools available, however, to assist with the assessment of service users with learning disabilities when the standard tools are considered ineffective because of the service user's limitations in cognition and communication. Five such instruments are described below.

- The Psychiatric Assessment Schedule for Adults with Developmental Disabilities (PAS-ADD) is a diagnostic tool suitable for the nurse or other mental health professional adept at clinical interviewing (Moss et al., 1993).
- The Mini Psychiatric Assessment Schedule for Adults with Developmental Disabilities (Mini PAS-ADD) is a relatively more accessible tool for most nursing staff, although specific training is required for its effective use. Essentially, the Mini PAS-ADD consists of a life-events checklist as well as a four-point scale upon which clinicians may 'rate' the service user's symptoms of depression, anxiety, expansive mood, obsessive–compulsive disorder, psychosis and autism (Prosser et al., 1998).

• In addition to the above, Hamer (1998) recommends the use of the JOMAAC assessment tool (see Box 11.1), in which the adult service user is assessed according to observations of their judgement, orientation, memory, affect, attitude and cognition. The main advantage of this form of ongoing assessment is that the nurse can draw some conclusions about the service user's current mental status based on direct observation, with minimal reliance on the service user providing dialogue.

Box 11.1 JOMAAC assessment at a glance

Judgement

• Perception of events or stimuli
• Appropriateness of appearance, such as grooming, touching and language
• Interpretation of vulnerable situations (observations such as hitting a bigger, stronger service user)
• Aggression towards self
• Aggression towards others
• Aggression towards property
• Suicidal gestures
• Responses to recent significant life events
• No behavioural improvement despite consistent, high-quality behavioural programming
• Awareness of surroundings
• Awareness of internal stimuli
• Awareness of name, location and reason for hospitalization
• Impaired level of consciousness

Orientation

• Awareness of surroundings
• Awareness of internal stimuli
• Awareness of name, location and reason for hospitalization
• Impaired level of consciousness

Memory

• Recent memory tests (What did you have for breakfast? What activity did you just do?)
• Ability to repeat what was said
• Remote memory tests (the name of community caregiver)

Affect

• Acting-out behaviour
• Emotional status (laughing, crying, flat, constricted)
• Verbalization of fear
• Withdrawal behaviour

• Reluctance to perform a learned skill
• Reluctance to be with familiar people
• Multiple complaints, somatization
• Reluctance to be in familiar surroundings
• Response to known upcoming event
• Response to current or near-current event
• Temper tantrum
• Change in activity level
• Facial expression, tone
• Aggression
• Hand or body gestures
• Appropriateness of emotional state
• Range of emotional state
• Sleep disturbance
• Changes in eating patterns
• Decreased concentration
• Loss of interest
• Statements regarding self-worth, suicide, hurting self or others
• Changes in person's behaviour or mood that occurs in all settings, versus just some settings
• Hypersexuality

Attitude

• Uncooperative
• Sarcastic
• Perplexed
• Hostile
• Apprehensive
• Unfeeling

Cognition

• Ability to keep thoughts focused
• Speech patterns (echolalic, mutism, intonation, pressure, rate, deterioration)
• Displays beliefs that are obviously false
• Gestured hallucinations
• Voiced hallucinations
• Poor interpersonal relationships
• Decreased ability to perform activities of daily living (feeding, dressing, toileting)
• Poor eye contact
• Bizarre rituals
• Emotional dissociation (including mood variability and impulsiveness)
• Catatonia
• Paranoid behaviour

Source: Reprinted from Hamer, BA, (1998) Assessing mental status in persons with mental retardation. *Journal of Psychosocial Nursing and Mental Health Services*, 36(5), 27–31, with permission from SLACK Incorporated.

- For the assessment of children and adolescents with a learning disability, the Developmental Behaviour Checklist (DBC) (Einfeld and Tonge, 1995) is a comprehensive 96-item carer-completed screening checklist that allows carers (including nurses) to rate the severity of a child's behavioural and emotional problems. This checklist has been modified to produce a version known as the Developmental Behaviour Checklist for Adults (DBC-A; Mohr et al., 2005). Both versions of the DBC facilitate a cut-off score that indicates the level of disturbance, which may be further investigated by an expert mental health clinician.

Other pitfalls in the assessment process

There are other difficulties that may occur from the perspective of the nurse who is assessing a service user with a dual diagnosis.

- The service user may display uncharacteristically impoverished or regressed social and communication skills, which might mask the signs of a mental health disorder.
- The service user may give unreliable or inappropriate responses to questions asked by clinicians at the time of assessment due to their lack of understanding of the abstract terms and concepts used in the assessment process (Hamer, 1998).
- Ross and Oliver (2002) asserted that the presence of atypical signs in response to mental disorder, such as the challenging behaviours exhibited by John and the stereotypical (or repetitive) behaviours exhibited by Margaret (in the next case study), may add another potentially confusing dimension to the assessment process.
- A related impediment is diagnostic overshadowing (Reiss et al., 1982), in which important indicators of mental disorder are simply attributed to the service user's learning disability rather than being interpreted as signs of mental disorder; that is, the service user's behaviour is overshadowed by their diagnosis of a learning disability (see the case study of Margaret for an example).

ACUTE NURSING CARE

The key to caring for service users who have a mental disorder comorbid with a learning disability lies in establishing effective communication with them, their carers and/or their families, combined with a thorough assessment.

There is ample evidence that service users with a dual diagnosis can benefit from a range of physical interventions, such as pharmacological treatments (Coughlan, 2000;

Jenkins, 2000) and electroconvulsive therapy (Ruedrich and Alamir, 1999), in much the same way as other members of the community who experience mental health problems (see Ch. 23 for a range of therapeutic interventions).

CASE STUDY: MARGARET

Margaret is a 35-year-old woman who normally lives with her mother and who has mild learning disability. Margaret has a small vocabulary but is able to understand much of what is said to her. She can perform self-help tasks and has developed competencies in occupational, leisure and social skills. Diagnostic overshadowing played a large part in the delay between the onset of severe symptoms and diagnosis for this service user.

The police brought Margaret into the accident and emergency department late one Sunday after local residents reported that she had been lying on the road outside a shopping centre. Margaret was very distressed and crying, and when asked why she lay on the road replied: 'You will get run over lying on the road and go to heaven, sorry Mr Policeman'. She was able to give her name, phone number and address to the attending nurse and a subsequent phone call found that Margaret lived at home with her mother and had gone to the local shops for bread. The accident and emergency department staff decided that Margaret could go home to the care of her mother as there was no history of mental disorder and she was able to say where she lived. Lying on the road was dismissed as 'behaviour' due to her learning disability. This proved to be *diagnostic overshadowing*.

Two days later, Margaret's mother Jean telephoned the assessment and treatment service staff to say that a local shopkeeper had brought Margaret home after he had found her lying on the road. Jean was told that someone from the mental health team would visit in the next couple of days, but this was not regarded as high priority, as the behaviour was seen as part of Margaret's learning disability. The following afternoon, community nurses visited and questioned Margaret, who became tearful and repeated: 'I'll get run over and go to heaven'. Jean told the staff that she had heard Margaret crying at night and that she had been awake early in the morning and needed to be told to shower. This was unlike Margaret but Jean said that she had been sad since her grandmother died 3 months previously and seemed to lack motivation.

On their way back to the office the nurses called in to the local shops and discovered that Margaret had been lying on the road intermittently for the past 4 weeks. At first she would get up as soon as someone called out to her but over the past 2 weeks she would cry: 'No I'll get run over and go to heaven'. The staff, recognizing her behaviour as suicidal, arranged for Margaret to be admitted to the assessment and treatment unit as a detained patient (i.e. she was deprived of her right to discharge herself from hospital on the grounds that there was a reasonable risk that she would harm herself). Margaret's subsequent nursing care is described below.

Collins (1999) points out that psychotherapy for service users with a dual diagnosis was often not used based on the belief that the person's intellectual capacity and limited communications repertoire rendered them ineligible. There is now evidence that a range of 'talking therapies' such as psychodynamic, behavioural and cognitive therapies are effective for those with functional language skills, albeit in an abridged form (Brown and Marshall, 2006; Dagnan, 2007; McKee, 2001; Raghavan, 1998; Romana, 2003). Similarly, Raghavan (1998) has commented on the reported efficacy of various relaxation techniques used to manage anxiety states for service users with a dual diagnosis. The nursing interventions described in Chapter 23 can be employed in much the same way as they are for the remainder of the population, with the addition of more comprehensive discharge planning.

The case study of Margaret (above) provides an example of the acute nursing care that would be provided for the dual diagnosis service user following their admission to an inpatient unit.

In Margaret's case, nursing and medical staff found that she was uncommunicative upon admission to the assessment and treatment unit and that she sat gently rocking and averting her gaze from staff. Fortunately, the staff were able to engage Jean (Margaret's mother) in the process of taking a history and for some of the assessment process. After medical staff had performed a physical examination of Margaret it was decided to take her to her bedroom and continue the assessment process once she had familiarized herself with her new environment. In the interim, a nurse was able to commence brief conversations with Margaret using gentle open-ended questions. Margaret was subsequently asked to unpack her suitcase and engage in self-care activities independently.

CRITICAL THINKING CHALLENGE 11.3

List the ethical considerations that should be taken into account when nursing Margaret in an acute-care setting. Discuss how each of these problems might be addressed.

Margaret lived at home and in such cases it is important to work with the family to gain their trust, to ensure the optimal outcome for the service user, and to obtain a reliable history of the service user's mental and physical status. Over the course of the next hour, the nurse was able to ascertain from Jean that Margaret was uncharacteristically withdrawn and that her movements were much slower than usual. Jean also revealed that Margaret's concentration had deteriorated in recent weeks, and Margaret was able to add that she felt terrible and that she didn't 'want to live anymore'. Apart from these typical signs of clinical depression (see the diagnostic criteria in Ch. 15), staff noted that Margaret's rocking had continued and that she made low, barely audible noises. Jean confirmed that rocking and moaning were atypical signs of Margaret's depression as they were not normally part of her behavioural repertoire.

Having gained the confidence of the new patient, the nurse was able to interview Margaret alone and, after some encouragement, found that she had retained her plan to kill herself by lying down in the middle of a road and being run over by a car. She did not have any other plans for her own death but repeated that what she really wanted was to die and go to heaven to see her grandmother. Eventually the nurse was able to complete the initial assessments for Margaret, including mental status assessment and a risk assessment, and was able to write admission notes that described her signs and symptoms including the atypical signs of depression. Margaret was subsequently placed on half-hourly general observations with four-hourly observations using the JOMAAC tool as a format for further assessment of mental status. Although primary nursing was not a part of the unit's policy on patient care, Margaret was allocated a single nurse for each subsequent morning and afternoon 'shift' on the first 2 days of her admission to facilitate communications and to assist in the process of ongoing assessment. Despite these arrangements, Margaret remained largely uncommunicative and chose to speak only with a few of the staff.

Apart from the interventions outlined above, the management of Margaret's depression was much like that afforded to other patients (see Ch. 15). While she was being stabilized on an antidepressant (in this case venlafaxine) Margaret was offered grief counselling (see Ch. 9) to help her to cope with the loss of her grandmother. Although Margaret was quick to understand that she needed to take her medication with her morning and evening meals until her doctor said to stop, she was unable to grasp education given to her by staff about the physiology of her depressive disorder and the need to be vigilant regarding the symptoms of relapse. She also had a very limited understanding of the way in which her medication was helping her.

At the suggestion from Margaret's mother, and with Margaret's permission, it was decided to devise a mental health support plan (see Figure 11.1) in order to disseminate information about Margaret's management strategies to her carers when she had been discharged. The plan featured possible relapse signs (such as social withdrawal and 'rocking') and management strategies should Margaret again decide to harm herself (such as removing Margaret from harmful circumstances, clarifying Margaret's intentions and contacting the community learning disability team if Jean required assistance).

MENTAL HEALTH SUPPORT PLAN

Name: Ms Sophie Jones   **Date commenced:**
Date of birth: 04/07/88   **Written by:** Norma Cloonan (Nurse Consultant)

Rationale and aims

This plan is designed to give Sophie's parents and support service personnel guidance in how best to support her in managing her mental health problems, including preventative strategies for minimizing the occurrence of acute psychotic symptoms and reactive strategies when her symptoms are acute and difficult for her to self-manage.

Sophie has experienced symptoms of an acute psychotic episode with an associated functional disability, and has a moderate learning disability. She lives at home with her parents and works in a factor assembling electronic components. There is no known family history of mental disorder, and Sophie's condition, while it is unclear when it began, only became a problem for her and her family about 4 months ago. After a period of inpatient assessment and stabilizing of her condition she was discharged back into the community with the Community Mental Health Team continuing to monitor her progress.

This Mental Health Support Plan has been developed through consultation with Sophie and the people in her support network and will be reviewed at least three-monthly.

The aim of the Mental Health Support Plan is to support Sophie to maintain her lifestyle in the community, including her living arrangements and her employment, through preventative treatments and strategies and through early response and intervention should her mental health problems re-occur.

Signs and symptoms

When Sophie is experiencing acute symptoms of psychosis she may exhibit the following signs.

- Sophie may sit and talk to herself, perhaps looking at one place near her as she speaks (note that her speech may be conversational, as if she is talking to and listening to another person).

- Sophie may refuse to change her clothes, as she may believe that her mother has been putting 'bad things' in her clothing.

- She may talk repetitively about her mother and father being 'bad'.

- She may be suspicious of other people, particularly if they are known friends of her parents.

- She may become easily distracted, perhaps not listening to speakers or simply ignoring them, or she may need questions to be repeated several times before she answers them.

- Sophie may isolate herself in her bedroom, perhaps coming out only for meals.

- She may become aggressive towards her family or towards herself (striking the side of her head with the palm of her hand).

Triggers: things that contribute to the emergence of Sophie's symptoms

The following situations and events have been identified as having possible influence on triggering an exacerbation of her psychosis.

These are listed to draw your attention to ensuring that they are avoided where possible.

1. **Missed medication and medication non-adherence** – Sophie has been observed spitting her medication out when she thinks no one is looking.

2. **Alcohol consumption** – while she does not seek out alcohol, it has been noticed that even light beer on a special occasion has a negative effect on her mental state.

3. **Lack of sleep** – Sophie has been more withdrawn and guarded when she has not had adequate sleep.

4. **Stress** – extra pressure at work, other people pressuring her, being 'picked on', etc.

Figure 11.1 Example of a mental health support plan .

Prevention strategies

The following strategies are to be implemented in the effort to prevent further acute episodes of psychosis experienced by Sophie.

1. **Supervise her taking medication** – make sure she has a drink with her medication and that she takes it before a meal. Keep an eye open for discarded medication and report any incidents of medication non-adherence to her community mental health nurse.

2. The community mental health nurse is to **monitor Sophie's progress** by meeting with her weekly and responding to calls from the family or employer as required.

3. Sophie is to be seen by her Responsible Clinician **once every three (3) months** for a medication review. The community mental health nurse will make and attend each appointment.

4. Sophie's parents and workplace supervisors are to **report immediately any of the above signs or symptoms** of psychosis to the community mental health nurse on the appropriate form, which can be completed and faxed as required.

Responding to a crisis

Sophie may require more assessment and support when she experiences symptoms of psychosis than can be offered by those in her community support network. The following procedures are to be followed if the signs and symptoms of psychosis (or any other behaviours of concern) are observed.

1. **Give her one dose of her PRN medication (as required)** – Sophie has PRN medication in a rosette box which she has at home and takes to work with her. She may go to sleep within 20 min, although when she is very poorly the medication may appear to have little effect.

2. **Contact the community mental health nurse** (during business hours phone: 07555 555 999) or **the community mental health team** after hours (phone: 5551 9993) and inform them of Sophie's condition.

3. **Follow instructions** – a decision about how to manage the situation will be made after consultation with the mental health team.

4. **If she is to be taken to the local hospital for admission**, this will be done by the mental health team or the police. Make sure you pack a bag for her and send any records or notes that may assist the mental health team in assessing her condition and reviewing her treatment.

Note: If Sophie is admitted to the local hospital, this plan must be reviewed before discharge.

Signatures of agreement to this plan

Author's signature: ____Norma Cloonan_____   Date: _____23rd January 2012_____

Signatures of

Name: FRED SMITH_____   Signature: ____Fred Smith____ Date: 23/1/12_____

Name: SALLY JONES_____   Signature: ____Sally Jones____ Date: 23/1/12_____

Name: SOPHIE JONES_____   Signature: ____SOPHIE_____ Date: 23/1/12_____

Name: Dr PETER BLOGGS_____   Signature: ____P. Bloggs_____ Date: 23/1/12_____

Name: MARGARET MEAD_____   Signature: ____Marg Mead____ Date: 23/1/12_____

Plan review date:

Note: This sample mental health support plan (MHSP) has been designed to demonstrate the presentation of information for this textbook chapter. The information in this sample has been kept to a minimum and is not to be considered a clinical model for the management of any individual client who has a diagnosed psychotic disorder.

Figure 11.1 (Continued)

FACILITATING CONTINUOUS CARE

According to Yamada et al. (2000) the achievement of lasting positive outcomes for service users with a dual diagnosis and the avoidance of unnecessary hospitalizations due to acute relapse of mental disorder are highly dependent on the commitment of staff to the discharge planning process. The following discussion about the long-term, ongoing care of service users with a dual diagnosis recognizes that these service users typically access a range of services for their ongoing or continuous care and support (Accordino et al., 2001; Barlow, 1999; Silka and Hauser, 1997). It is also important to recognize that those individuals living with their family or in their own home typically have contact with a range of statutory and other services and that those service users who live in supported living schemes frequently maintain a high level of contact with and support from their family members. In addition, the role of the family, apart from providing typical family relationships, is often to fulfill the role of substitute decision-maker or advocate.

Understanding disability support services

Although it is difficult to outline all the salient features of learning disability services, one common component of these services that is vital to this discussion is the process of individual planning. Individual plans, also known by a variety of other names such as individual care plans, individual programme plans and person-centred plans, are considered the core documents that guide service providers in planning for and delivering a service that endeavours to meet the individual needs and aspirations of each service user. The plan is usually developed on initial entry to the service, monitored regularly and reviewed at least annually. The development of the plan typically involves assessment of the service user and consultation with other stakeholders, with prioritized goals forming the key performance indicators for the service.

Person-centred plans, while varying in the scope of outcomes targeted, are based on the needs of the service user, and may also guide the service user's support network in assisting them to attain a preferred lifestyle and living environment. Person-centred plans may include an array of behaviour intervention and support plans (Whitworth et al., 1999), including:

- ecological interventions: changing the service user's environment to help them to achieve a quality of life while minimizing toxic stimuli,
- positive skill-development programmes: teaching the service user diverse skills such as social or leisure skills,

- focused interventions: using behaviourist approaches based on reinforcement of positive behaviours and the non-reinforcement of inappropriate behaviours,
- reactive strategies: plans aimed at minimizing harm when the service user exhibits inappropriate behaviours (LaVigna et al., 1989).

In disability services, holistic support is attained through the development of documented individual (multi-elemental) support plans, which can direct support services in assisting the service user to achieve some level of personal success, self-esteem and quality of life (Fletcher and Poindexter, 1996).

Another feature of many learning disability services that should be discussed is the professional background of the people they employ. There is often a misconception among health professionals that all learning disability services, particularly those providing residential accommodation and care management services, are equipped to fully care for, manage and treat people with a dual diagnosis. This is often far from reality. Many organizations that support people with learning disabilities do not specifically employ staff with nursing backgrounds but traditionally draw their staff from the fields of social care, or any number of unrelated and various employment backgrounds (Holt et al., 2000). Where a service user requires a specialist service for addressing their specific needs (e.g. health needs), the role of social care staff is to assist the service user to access appropriate generic community health services (that is, the services used by any member of the community).

When a service user with a dual diagnosis is discharged back into the care of a community care provider, the nurse needs to have a clear understanding of the service, its service features, the skills of the staff and the function it is funded to provide. This understanding should minimize confusion or misunderstandings in the implementation of management programmes and ensure that the service user does not get caught in any voids created by interagency disputes over roles and responsibilities. Of course this level of understanding must be afforded to the family and carers of the service user living at home, as they may or may not have the skills, knowledge and experience required to effectively support the individual through the treatment process (Pridding et al., 2007; Spiller and Hardy, 2004).

Discharge planning

The purpose of discharge planning is, ideally, to return the service user to his or her prior environment or another suitable community-based setting. Effective discharge planning should commence at the time of the service user's initial presentation to the assessment and treatment service and should include elements such as a schedule for outpatient follow-up and the provision of any other additional services as required (Silka and Hauser, 1997).

In facilitating the discharge planning process the nurse should first identify the service user's support network and establish effective communication with the relevant personnel. The two services should then work together to facilitate the inclusion of the discharge plan in the service user's person-centred plan in the CPA plan, an important phase of which is identifying the roles and responsibilities of each of the members of the service user's multidisciplinary team, as well as resources required. The plan should be documented (including monitoring and review phases) in a functional format that all personnel can follow and implement. Information about the service user's mental disorder and its care, treatment and management should then be supplied as necessary to the service user, their family, carers, support staff and/or advocacy personnel.

Silka and Hauser (1997) recommend that, before discharge, a conference be held between all members of the support network to ensure that the relevant responsibilities and processes of support are articulated, negotiated, agreed to, understood and documented, including: steps to be taken to avoid future inpatient stays, further tests or assessments, any appropriate additional referrals for further support, and criteria and processes for responding to critical incidents.

Information sharing

Holt et al. (2000) suggest that the ability of service users, family members, carers and others to respond quickly and early to an episode of acute illness is diminished if they have little insight into or training about mental disorder and how it affects the service user. Family members, carers and support workers who are educated in the issues of dual diagnosis, or who are supported in identifying and accessing information resources, are more likely to provide effective support to the service user and work more effectively with (other) service professionals. Additionally, the inclusion of psychoeducational strategies (such as providing information about the signs, like poor sleep patterns or agitation, indicating that the person may become acutely unwell, or the effects, side effects and protocols for administration of neuroleptic medications) in the service user's treatment plan has been demonstrated to have positive results in treatment compliance and the overall wellbeing of the service user (Coyle, 2000; Pekkala and Merinder, 2002).

Person-centred plans

Service providers, as part of the individual planning process, are now developing a broad array of specific healthcare plans to ensure that the medical and health needs of the service user are planned, implemented and monitored by appropriate health professionals. Specific to the discussion here are Health Action Plans (HAP) and the CPA.

A HAP 'details the actions needed to maintain and improve the health of an individual' with a learning disability, and outlines all the help needed for meeting the health needs (Department of Health, 2002). The role of the learning disability nurse as a health facilitator is important in facilitating access to appropriate services and professionals for people with dual diagnosis. HAP and health facilitation are central to improving and maintaining the health of people with learning disabilities (Department of Health, 2008). This chapter deals with the mental health needs of people with learning disabilities and therefore more focus is on the CPA.

An example of a CPA plan that relates to the case study of Sophie is shown in Figure 11.1. Often developed by nurses and the multidisciplinary team who work with the service user while they are in the assessment and treatment unit, the CPA is a requirement for people detained under the Mental Health Act 1983, amended 2007. The CPA provides staff, carers, families and individuals with clearly documented guidelines that can be used for a number of purposes, including:

- providing a forum for the inclusion of significant others in the development, implementation and review of the service user's treatment,
- ensuring that prescribed treatments are provided as directed by the approved clinician and/or other related health professionals,
- the clear documentation of strategies, routines and programmes,
- ensuring that early intervention strategies are identified (including understanding the early signs of acute illness and the appropriate use of medications), thus minimizing the need for acute admissions.

CASE STUDY: SOPHIE

Sophie is a 19-year-old woman with a moderate learning disability who normally lives at home with her family. She was admitted under Section 3 of the Mental Health Act 1983, amended 2007, after she was provisionally diagnosed with a first-episode psychotic disorder.

The community learning disability team had obtained a history of Sophie's recent mental status changes from Sophie's parents and initially communicated with her with the assistance of her brother, whom she trusted. During her initial assessment Sophie explained that she was afraid of her parents and that she believed them to be evil. She indicated that she had 'voices' in her head but was unable to communicate what these voices were telling her. Her parents added that, in the months before her admission,

Sophie had been reluctant to shower, spent a lot of time in her room and could be heard talking to herself. When asked if anything was wrong, she became evasive, stating that she was just singing to herself. Sophie became more withdrawn and disorganized in her behaviour, eventually becoming aggressive when approached by her parents. Her personal hygiene deteriorated, she refused to change her clothes and remained in her room, coming out only for meals. Staff noted that, apart from her aggression, Sophie displayed 'atypical' signs such as making strange noises and hitting the side of her head when she became stressed.

In the weeks after her admission, staff used the JOMAAC tool to assess Sophie's progress until some of the nursing staff managed to build up a rapport with her. She continued to take her prescribed antipsychotic medication (risperidone) and otherwise received the nursing care afforded to a person with a psychotic disorder (see Ch. 14). As Sophie's condition stabilized in the protective environment of the assessment and treatment unit, the named nurse commenced discharge planning including the preparation of a CPA plan.

In order to ensure that an effective CPA is devised it is the responsibility of the named nurse to provide input during the planning process, either through attending CPA meetings or by providing information as required. It should also be recognized that the CPA is an appropriate clinical tool for families and other nonprofessional or unpaid carers to ensure that treatment goals are achievable in the less formal environment of the family home and also to assist carers in their preparation for crises that may arise from exacerbation of their family member's mental health problems.

Assessment and treatment services for people with dual diagnosis

At the time of writing, policy and practices in respect of dual diagnosis are undergoing significant change following changes to the NHS and recent changes to mental health policy and legislation. There are some excellent examples of innovative practice, but there are significant variations between the four countries and within each of the countries.

In the UK people with dual diagnosis can be treated in hospital informally or they can be detained to receive assessment and or treatment. In England and Wales this is done under the Mental Health Act 1983, amended 2007. In Scotland the similar provisions are through the Mental Health (Scotland) Act 1984 and Mental Health (Care and Treatment)(Scotland) Act 2003. In Northern Ireland people with dual diagnosis receive assessment and treatment services under the provisions of the Mental Health Act (Northern Ireland Order) 1986.

In England and Wales assessment and treatment services for people with dual diagnosis are provided by the NHS and private hospitals. The Mental Health Act Commission has been collecting relevant data since 2005 (Emerson et al. 2010). For example, in 2009 there were 3501 (2487 NHS and 1014 independent) adult patients in England (Care Quality Commission 2009). It is, however, important to point out that there is geographical variation in the provision of these services across England and Wales. Following recent reorganization of the NHS many of these assessment and treatment services have been integrated with mental health services.

NURSE'S STORY: LIVING WITH A RELATIVE WITH DUAL DIAGNOSIS

As a community nurse working for disability services I often met people who were distressed because they lived with a relative with a dual diagnosis. Byron's family was just one example. Byron was 26 years old and had a learning disability, along with some challenging behaviours (including screaming, punching walls and sometimes destroying furniture) which had developed since the onset of his psychotic disorder 4 years previously. His parents, both aged in their mid-sixties, were the only people who could engage with Byron as he was very slow to accept and trust any new people in his life. At the time of my professional involvement with them, however, they were deeply upset with their son's behaviour and confused about what they could do to take control of their lives.

It can be very difficult to maintain the required professional focus when confronted with a crisis such as this. While empathic understanding is important, it is equally important to stay objective. I have learned that, in order to help, it is important for me in my role as a nurse to recognize that the problem at hand is not my personal problem but that I have much to offer in empowering families to take control of their situation. I left that first visit filled with a deep sense of sadness for these people, but also with a tinge of excitement because I could see a future of hope. I wanted to get back to this family quickly, to understand what was happening and to assist in making things right.

The main focus of my involvement with the family was not just about addressing the more obvious problems. My role was more about helping the family to cope and stay engaged with their son. Working in partnership with Byron's parents I was able to help them devise some strategies that would enable them to take turns in caring for their son and, when they were not doing so, to participate in relaxation and other therapies aimed at minimizing the amount of stress in their lives.

I also assured Byron's parents that there were others in their situation and was able to encourage their communication with a support group for families living with dual diagnosis. In addition, I was able to bring health professionals to the table who could offer interventions that enabled more effective management of Byron's symptoms and his eventual reintegration back into a community-based activities programme.

While Byron came to accept me as one of his carers, this initial engagement with his parents was the key to facilitating care. I maintained contact with Byron's family for some months after this initial contact and was delighted that his parents achieved a happy medium between caring for their son and meeting their own needs. I still see Byron and his family from time to time, and take great pride in the fact that I played a small part in helping them to reestablish control of their lives. As a nurse it is tempting to try and take control of other people's problems but, for me, the biggest reward is seeing people develop to a point where I am no longer needed.

Philip Petrie, RN

MENTAL CAPACITY

Research studies have long highlighted abuse and safeguarding issues for people with learning disabilities and how this contributes to mental ill health (Cooke and Sinason, 1998). *Death by Indifference* (Mencap, 2007) and the Six Lives report (Parliamentary and Health Service Ombudsman and Social Services Ombudsman, 2009) highlighted the vulnerability of people with learning disabilities. The Care Quality Commission's (2011) report following media reports of ill treatment of people with dual diagnosis at the Winterbourne View private hospital in Bristol further highlights the importance of safeguarding and acting in the best interests of people with learning disabilities.

Central to safeguarding people with learning disabilities is the Safeguarding of Vulnerable Adults (SOVA) scheme and the Mental Capacity Act 2005 (see Ch. 4). The SOVA scheme is beyond the scope of this chapter but further information is available at http://www.isa.home-office.gov.uk/.

The Mental Capacity Act 2005 is underpinned by five key principles, which are:

1. the presumption of capacity,
2. support for individuals to make their own decisions,
3. unwise decisions: individuals deemed to be making unwise decisions not to be assumed to lack capacity,

4. best interests: an act taken or decision made to be in the best interest of the individual,
5. least-restrictive options: actions and decisions made for or on behalf of a person with a learning disability to be least restrictive of human rights and freedom.

The Mental Capacity Act 2005 presumes that adults (people aged 18 and above in the UK) have capacity to make their own decisions about their care and treatment unless proven otherwise. The Act aims to protect people with learning disabilities and others with cognitive conditions. It provides guidelines and processes about how to make appropriate decisions in particular situations. For people with dual diagnosis one of the positive changes is the need for assessment for lack of capacity. Mental capacity assessment is decision- and time-specific, meaning that assumptions about incapacity can no longer be made by simply referring to an individual learning disability or dual diagnosis.

Under the Mental Capacity Act 2005, nurses, carers and other professionals are required to make decisions or act in the best interests of individuals in their care who lack capacity. Central to acting in the best interests of individuals is the provision of a nonexhaustive checklist of considerations any decision-maker needs to go through to ensure they are acting in the best interest of the individual. Another key provision is the right of carers and relatives to be consulted about an individual's best interests. The creation of the Independent Mental Capacity Advocacy (IMCA) under the Act make it a statutory requirement for NHS and local authority organizations to involve an IMCA when making major decisions involving individuals with learning disabilities who have no others to advocate on their behalf. The role of the IMCA supersedes the role of generic advocacy services.

CASE STUDY: MENTAL CAPACITY

Martin is a 40-year-old man with a dual diagnosis of mild learning disability and schizophrenia. Martin used to work in a sheltered employment scheme for people with learning disabilities before the onset of schizophrenia when he was 30 years old. He was admitted to an assessment and treatment unit for people with dual diagnosis where he stayed for 6 years before he was discharged into a residential home which specializes in working with people with dual diagnosis.

Martin has an uncontrollable appetite for fast foods and since he moved into the residential home he has gained weight and is now considered to be clinically obese. The residential home with the support of a local NHS dietician have tried to support Martin to adopt a healthier diet but without success. This has resulted in Martin neglecting himself and in the deterioration of behaviour towards staff and other residents if he is denied access to the foods he likes. Martin has also recently started on occasions to refuse to take medication for symptoms of schizophrenia.

He has been recently diagnosed with Type 2 diabetes following admission to hospital with a chest infection. Martin has no known relatives and the staff in the residential home have asked the GP to consider referring Martin for gastric bypass surgery.

CRITICAL THINKING CHALLENGE 11.4

Consider and discuss how staff in the residential home can demonstrate that they are acting in Martin's best interests.

Does Martin have capacity to make a decision for himself with regard to interventions about his obesity?

CONCLUSION

Providing nursing care for service users with a dual diagnosis is a challenging task that requires nurses to alter their practice to accommodate the specific needs of the service user and also to liaise with carers and other stakeholders. The nurse must also anticipate that not all health professionals can work effectively with this service user group, sometimes because of a lack of specific skills and knowledge and sometimes because of personal prejudices. With the improvement of services and the greater availability of information, however, it is anticipated that future nurses will be better informed about this important issue and that they may be better prepared and motivated to address the specific needs of service users with a dual diagnosis.

EXERCISES FOR CLASS ENGAGEMENT

Prepare a list of derogatory terms you have heard used to describe people with a learning disability. Prepare a list of nondiscriminatory terms used to describe people with this form of disability. Compare your lists with those of your group members. Which is the longest list? What are the reasons for this discrepancy?

How do individual group members feel about working with people who have a learning disability? Identify the impediments to providing care for these people.

What factors might interfere with the achievement of a positive outcome for the service user with dual diagnosis within assessment and treatment services and within disability services? Outline strategies to overcome these barriers.

ACKNOWLEDGEMENTS

The authors wish to acknowledge Mr Philip Petrie (Deputy CEO, The Centre BHCCA) for the mental health support plan format in Figure 11.1. We also acknowledge our colleagues Ms Norma Cloonan and Mr Irvin Savage for their contributions.

The authors would also like to acknowledge Dr Carolyn Mohr, Department of Psychological Medicine, Faculty of Medicine, Nursing & Health Sciences, Monash University, and Ms Chris Taua, Principle Lecturer in the School of Nursing at Christchurch Polytechnic Institute of Technology, for their helpful suggestions in the writing of this chapter.

DISCLAIMER

REFERENCES

Abudarham, S., Hurd, A. (Eds.), 2002. Management of Communication Needs in People with Learning Disability. Whurr, London.

Accordino, M.P., Porter, D.F., Morse, T., 2001. Deinstitutionalization of persons with severe mental illness: context and consequences. J. Rehabil. 67 (2), 16–21.

American Association on Learning Disability, 2002. Learning Disability: Definition, Classification and Systems of Supports, tenth ed. American Association on Learning Disability, Washington DC.

American Psychiatric Association, 2000. Diagnostic and Statistical Manual of Mental Disorders, fourth ed., text rev. American Psychiatric Association, Washington DC.

Barlow, C., 1999. Issues in the management of service users with the dual diagnosis of learning disability and mental illness. J. Disabil. Nurs. Health Soc. Care 3 (3), 159–162.

Barr, O., 1998. Responding to the health needs of people with learning disabilities. In: Thompson, T., Mathias, P. (Eds.), Standards and Learning Disability, second ed. Baillière-Tindall, London.

Barr, O., Gilgun, J., Kane, T., et al., 1999. Health screening for people with learning disabilities by a community learning disability nursing service in Northern Ireland. J. Adv. Nurs. 29 (6), 1482–1491.

Benson, B.A., 1985. Behaviour disorders and learning disability: associations with age, sex and level of functioning in an outpatient clinic sample. Appl. Res. Learn. Disabil. 6, 79–85.

Borthwick-Duffy, S.A., 1994. Epidemiology and prevalence of psychopathology in people with learning disability. J. Consult. Clin. Psychol. 62 (1), 17–27.

Brown, M., Marshall, K., 2006. Cognitive behaviour therapy and people with learning disabilities: implications for developing nursing practice. J. Psychiatr. Ment. Health Nurs. 13 (2), 234–241.

Care Quality Commission, 2010. Count Me In 2009. Care Quality Commission, London.

Cascella, P.W., 2005. Expressive communication strengths of adults with severe to profound learning disabilities as reported by group home staff. Commun. Disord. Q. 26 (3), 156–163.

Chaplin, R., 2004. General psychiatric services for adults with learning disability and mental illness. J. Learn. Disabil. Res. 48 (1), 1–10.

Cockerill, H., Carroll-Few, L. (Eds.), 2001. Communication Without Speech: Practical Augmentative and Alternative Communication. MacKeith, London.

Collins, S., 1999. Treatment and other therapeutic interventions: psychological approaches. Tizard Learn. Disabil. Rev. 4 (2), 20–27.

Cooke, L.B., Sinason, V., 1998. Abuse of people with learning disabilities and other vulnerable adults. Adv. Psychiatr. Treat. 4, 119–125.

Coombs, T., Martin, C., 2002. Information and risk assessment: what do nurses think is important? Paper presented to the Conference of the Australian and New Zealand College of Nurses, Sydney, 15–18 October.

Coughlan, B.J., 2000. Psychopharmacology in the treatment of people with learning disabilities: a review. Ment. Health Care 3 (9), 304–307.

Coyle, D., 2000. Meeting the needs of people with learning disabilities and mental health problems: a review. Ment. Health Care 3 (12), 408–411.

Dagnan, D., 2007. Psychosocial interventions for people with learning disabilities. In: Bouras, N., Holt, G. (Eds.), Psychiatric and Behavioural Disorders in Intellectual and Developmental Disabilities. Cambridge University Press, Cambridge.

Deb, S., Thomas, M., Bright, C., 2001. Mental disorder in adults with learning disability. 1: prevalence of functional psychiatric illness among a community-based population aged between 16 and 64 years. J. Learn. Disabil. Res. 45 (6), 495–505.

Department of Health, 2002. Action for Health – Health Action Planning and Health Facilitation, Good Practice on Implementation for Learning Disability Partnership Boards. TSO, London.

Department of Health, 2008. Valuing People Now – A New Three-Year Strateguy for People with Learning Disabilities. Department of Health, London.

Disability Rights Commission, 2006. Equal Treatment: Closing the Gap – A Formal Investigation into Physical Health Inequalities Experienced by People with Learning Disabilities and/or Mental Health Problems. Disability Rights Commission, Stratford upon Avon.

Dykens, E.M., Hodapp, R.M., Finucane, B.M., 2000. Genetics and Learning Disability: A New Look at Behaviour Interventions. Paul Brookes, Baltimore.

Edwards, N., Lennox, N., 2002. Dual Diagnosis Project. University of Queensland, Brisbane.

Einfeld, S.L., Tonge, B.J., 1995. The developmental behaviour checklist: the development and validation of an instrument to assess behavioural and emotional disturbance in children and adolescents with learning disability. 1: rationale and methods. J. Autism. Dev. Disord. 25 (2), 81–104.

Emerson, E., 2010. People with Learning Disabilities in England 2010. Department of Health, London.

Fletcher, R.J., Poindexter, A.R., 1996. Current trends in mental health care for persons with learning disability. J. Rehabil. 63 (1), 23–26.

Gilbert, T., Todd, M., Jackson, N., 1998. People with learning disabilities who also have mental health problems: practice issues and directions for learning disability nursing. J. Adv. Nurs. 27, 1151–1157.

Hamer, B.A., 1998. Assessing mental status in persons with learning disability. J. Psychosoc. Nurs. 36 (5), 27–31.

Holt, G., Costello, H., Oliver, B., 2000. Training direct care staff about the mental health needs and related issues of people with developmental disabilities. Ment. Health Aspects. Dev. Disabil. 3 (4), 132–139.

Jacobson, J.W., 1990. Do some mental disorders occur less frequently among persons with learning disability? Am. J. Learn. Disabil. 94 (6), 596–602.

Jenkins, R., 2000. Use of psychotropic medication in people with learning disability. Learn. Disabil. Nurs. 9 (13), 844–850.

LaVigna, G.W., Willis, T.J., Donnellan, A.M., 1989. The role of positive programming in behavioral treatment In: Cipani, E. (Ed.), The Treatment of Severe Behavior Disorders: Behavior Analysis Approaches, vol 12. Monographs of the American Association on Learning Disability, pp. 59–83.

Linfoot, K. (Ed.), 1994. Communication Strategies for People with Developmental Disabilities: Issues from Theory to Practice McLennan & Petty, Sydney.

McConkey, R., 2004. Pressures, Possibilities and Proposals: Northern Ireland Review of Day Services for People with Learning Disabilities. EHSSB, Belfast.

McConkey, R., Truesdale, M., 2000. Reactions of nurses and therapists in mainstream health services to contact with people who have learning disabilities. J. Adv. Nurs. 32 (1), 158–163.

McIntyre, L.L., Blacher, J., Baker, B.L., 2002. Behaviour/mental health problems in young adults with learning disability: the impact on families. J. Learn. Disabil. Res. 46 (3), 239–249.

McKee, R., 2001. Therapeutic interventions in the support of people with learning disabilities who present mental health problems. Assignment: Ongoing Work of Health Care Students 7 (3), 4–8.

Mansell, J., 2007. Services for People with Learning Disabilities and Challenging Behaviour or Mental Needs, rev. ed. Department of Health, London.

Mencap, 2007. Death by Indifference. Following up the Treat me Right Report. Mencap, London.

Michael, J., 2008. Healthcare for all – report of the independent inquiry into access to healthcare for people with learning disabilities. <http://www.dh.gov.uk/prod_consum_dh/groups/dh_digitalassets/@dh/@en/documents/digitalasset/dh_106126.pdf>.

Mohr, C., Tonge, B.J., Einfeld, S.L., 2005. The development of a new measure for the assessment of psychopathology in adults with learning disability. J. Learn. Disabil. Res. 49 (7), 469–480.

Moss, S., Lee, P., 2001. Mental health. In: Thompson, J., Pickering, S. (Eds.), Meeting the Health Needs of People who have a Learning Disability. Baillière Tindall, London.

Moss, S.C., Patel, P., Prosser, H., et al., 1993. Psychiatric morbidity in older people with moderate and severe learning disability (learning disability). Part 1: development and reliability of the patient interview (the PAS-ADD). Br. J. Psychiatry. 163, 471–480.

Naylor, V., Clifton, M., 1994. People with learning disabilities: meeting complex needs. Health Soc. Care 1 (6), 343–353.

O'Brien, J., 1987. A guide to lifestyle planning: using the activities catalogue to integrate services and natural support systems. In: Wilcox, B., Belamy, G.T. (Eds.), A Comprehensive Guide to the Activities Catalogue. Paul H Brooks, Baltimore.

Parliamentary and Health Service Ombudsman and Social Services Ombudsman, 2009. Six Lives: The Provision of Public Services to People with Learning Disabilities. TSO, London.

Pekkala, E., Merinder, L., 2002. Psychoeducation for Schizophrenia. The Cochrane Library, Oxford.

Pridding, A., Watkins, D., Happell, B., 2007. Mental health nursing roles and functions in acute inpatient units: caring for people with learning disability and mental health problems—a literature review. Int. J. Psychiatr. Nurs. Res. 12 (2), 1459–1470.

Prosser, H., Moss, S., Costello, H., et al., 1998. Reliability and validity of the Mini-PAS-ADD for assessing psychiatric disorders in adults with learning disability. J. Learn. Disabil. Res. 42, 264–272.

Raghavan, R., 1998. Anxiety disorders in people with learning disabilities: a review of literature. J. Learn. Disabil. Nur. Health Soc. Care 2 (1), 3–9.

Reiss, S., 1994. Handbook of Challenging Behaviour: Mental Health Aspects of Learning Disability. IDS, Columbia.

Reiss, S., Levitan, G.W., Szyszko, J., 1982. Emotional disturbance and learning disability: diagnostic overshadowing. Am. J. Ment. Defic. 86 (6), 567–574.

Romana, M.S., 2003. Cognitive-behaviour therapy: treating individuals with dual diagnosis. J. Psychosoc. Nurs. 41 (12), 31–35.

Ross, E., Oliver, C., 2002. The relationship between levels of mood, interest and pleasure and 'challenging behaviour' in adults with severe and profound learning disability. J. Learn. Disabil. Res. 46 (3), 191–197.

Ruedrich, S.L., Alamir, S., 1999. Electroconvulsive therapy for persons with developmental disabilities: review, case report and recommendations. Health Aspects. Dev. Disabil. 2 (3), 83–91.

Silka, V.R., Hauser, M.J., 1997. Psychiatric assessment of the person with learning disability. Psychiatr. Ann. 27 (3), 162–169.

Sovner, R., 1996. Six models of behaviour from a psychiatric perspective. Habilitative Ment. Health Care Newsl. 15 (3), 51–54.

Spiller, M.J., Hardy, S., 2004. Developing a guide to mental health for families and carers of people with learning disability. Learn. Disabil. Pract. 7 (8), 28–31.

Taylor, J.L., Hatton, C., Dixon, L., et al., 2004. Screening for psychiatric symptoms: PASS-ADD checklist norms for adults with learning disabilities. J. Learn. Disabil. Res. 48 (1), 37–41.

VanderSchie-Bezyak, J.L., 2003. Service problems and solutions for individuals with learning disability and mental illness. J. Rehabil. 69 (1), 53–58.

von Tetzchner, S., Grove, N., 2003. Augmentative and Alternative Communication and Developmental Issues. Whurr, London.

White, P., Chant, D., Edwards, N., et al., 2005. Prevalence of learning disability and comorbid mental illness in an Australian community sample. Aust. N. Z. J. Psychiatry 39 (5), 395–400.

Whitworth, D., Harris, P., Jones, R., 1999. Staff culture and the management of challenging behaviours in people with learning disabilities. Ment. Health Care 2 (11), 376–379.

Wolfensberger, W., 1972. Normalization: the Principle of Normalization in Human Services. National Institute on Learning Disability, Toronto.

World Health Organization, 1992. ICD-10: International Statistical Classification of Diseases and Related Health Problems, tenth rev. World Health Organization, Geneva.

Yamada, M.M., Korman, M., Hughes, C.W., 2000. Predicting rehospitalisation of persons with severe mental illness. J. Rehabil. 66 (2), 32–39.

USEFUL WEBSITES

British Sign Language: <http://www.britishsignlanguage.com/>.

Department of Health, Learning Disabilities. <http://www.dh.gov.uk/en/SocialCare/Learningdisabilities/index.htm>.

Department of Health, Valuing people now. <http://www.valuing-peoplenow.dh.gov.uk/>.

Learning Disability Observatory. <http://www.improvinghealthand-dlives.org.uk/>.

Monash University Lifespan Project, investigating the mental health of people with learning disability across the lifespan. <http://www.med.monash.edu.au/spppm/research/devpsych/lifespan.html>.

PAS-ADD, assessment tool and associated information. <http://www.pasadd.co.uk/>.

Chapter | 12 |

Working with children and young people

Mike Groome, Kristin Henderson, and Jem Masters

CHAPTER POINTS

- The prevalence of emotional problems in the earlier years of life ranges from 10 to 20% within developed countries.

- Mental health problems cannot be seen as operating in isolation from other aspects of young people's lives.
- A child or adolescent experiencing behavioural or emotional problems may be indicative of problems within the family.
- Working with children and adolescents can be challenging but very fulfilling.
- It is essential to clarify the young person's perception of the problem and their goals for 'treatment', as well as that of the parents.
- 'Engagement' is the establishment of a therapeutic alliance, or rapport, to achieve desired outcomes and goals. This occurs from the initial interview. Understanding young people's language and communicating effectively is integral to engaging with them and vital to the success of their ongoing treatment.
- Children and young people may differ in their form of presentation when compared to adults with similar disorders.
- Nurses involved in the care of children and adolescents admitted to mental health facilities often have to deal with legal issues relating to duty of care, child protection and mental health legislation.
- Service user and carer participation is increasingly important when working with families.

KEY TERMS

- child and adolescent mental health nursing
- cross-cultural issues
- engagement
- externalizing problems
- Gillick competence
- internalizing problems

DOI: http://dx.doi.org/10.1016/B978-0-7020-4493-9.00012-3

- medication adherence
- psychoeducation
- resocialization
- service user and carer participation (advocacy)

LEARNING OUTCOMES

The material in this chapter will assist you to:
- develop an introductory understanding and overview of childhood and adolescent mental health problems and disorders,
- gain awareness of the extent of childhood and adolescent mental health problems and disorders,
- gain an awareness of the range of services provided to children and adolescents,
- explore the role of the nurse in working with children and adolescents with mental health needs and their families.

INTRODUCTION

As in everyday life children and adolescents cannot simply be considered little adults, so within the field of mental health and ill health there are differences between early life and adulthood. This chapter introduces the field of child and adolescent mental health nursing. It explores the role of the nurse and then, using case studies from clinical practice, gives some examples of disorders experienced by children and adolescents and interventions that nurses can use to help them.

Although some disorders are shared across generations, they may differ in their form of presentation at different developmental stages. For example, children suffering from symptoms of depression may be more agitated or have a variety of somatic symptoms, whereas some depressed adolescents might be antisocial, aggressive, withdrawn or involved in substance use (Thompson and Mathias, 2000). Some problems common to adults may start in childhood or be influenced by events that occurred early in life. Some problems may resolve with neurological development or emotional maturity, or with a stable, supportive environment. Likewise, with effective intervention and treatment there may be other comorbid health problems from which the young person may be able to achieve a complete recovery.

Over the past decade, discoveries in neurological research have reinforced the idea that the human brain is quite 'plastic' and that some areas are influenced during development by the environment, including such factors as the level of stress or anxiety a young person experiences. There is also greater awareness of the interaction between genetic endowment and the surrounding world.

These developments are helping to provide new understanding of how individual children cope with emotional difficulties and gain control over their lives. They have also reinforced the effectiveness of a wide range of therapeutic interventions (Hoagwood and Serene, 2002).

An important factor in considering the effect of any kind of health problem, whether physical or mental, on young people is the disruption it may bring to every aspect of development and education. Although in adulthood our lives can be dramatically changed through ill health, we have usually completed the basic developmental tasks of life and have finished the foundations of education. For the child or adolescent, however, various problems may develop simply due to the interruption caused by health problems. Bowlby and Robertson (cited in Walker et al., 2004) illustrated the effects on young children of being separated from their family during hospitalization and hospitals now have liberal attitudes to parents and siblings being able to maximize contact with the sick child. In addition, mental health professionals, including mental health nurses, are also able to offer expert opinion and support for children and young people and their families when dealing with severe or prolonged physical illness.

If one takes the view that there are critical periods in life when particular development tasks can be achieved, it is possible that these problems may have a long-term effect on people's lives (Brannon and Feist, 2000; see also Ch. 8). For example, 'mental health problems in children are associated with educational failure, family disruption, disability, offending and antisocial behaviour, placing demands on social services, schools and the youth justice system. Untreated mental health problems create distress not only in the children and young people, but also for their families and carers, continuing into adult life and affecting the next generation' (Department of Health, 2004, p. 6).

It is important therefore that services be developed and extended to more young people and that issues of equitable access to services are pursued vigorously.

DIAGNOSIS IN CHILD AND ADOLESCENT MENTAL HEALTHCARE

The American Psychiatric Association, in its *Diagnostic and Statistical Manual of Mental Disorders*, fourth edition (DSM-IV TR; American Psychiatric Association, 2000) lists the disorders usually first diagnosed in infancy, childhood or adolescence (see below). The major categories within child and adolescent services are listed, with some examples of specific diagnoses. The list below is not exhaustive; for complete descriptions, refer to the DSM-IV TR:

- learning disorders;
- motor skills disorder;
- communication disorders:
  - stuttering;

- pervasive developmental disorders:
  - autistic disorder,
  - Rett's disorder,
  - Asperger's disorder;
- attention-deficit and disruptive behaviour disorders:
  - attention-deficit/hyperactivity disorder,
  - conduct disorder,
  - oppositional defiant disorder;
- tic disorders:
  - Tourette's disorder,
  - chronic motor or vocal tic disorder;
- elimination disorders:
  - encopresis,
  - enuresis.

Because some disorders are not unique to this stage of life, they are not included in the DSM-IV TR list. Depressive disorders are an example, although depression is becoming increasingly common in children and adolescents (Sawyer et al., 2000).

The diagnostic categories listed above are internationally recognized mental health problems can also be assessed using the child behaviour checklist (see Box 12.1). As you can see, this checklist places stronger emphasis on behaviour and problems than categories of disorders. Problems are categorized into two general and eight specific areas, as shown. Viewing problems within such a framework helps us to understand young people as having issues related to predominant personality traits, developmental factors or incidents and influences within their family and wider social environment.

By contrast, static diagnostic systems can tend to lose the fluid, changing and reorganizing nature of young people's experience as they progress towards adulthood, and may also run the risk of encouraging a focus on one 'problem' in isolation (Hoagwood and Serene, 2002). For this reason, this chapter describes mental health problems in the context in which symptoms are observed, rather than in relation to categorical diagnostic criteria.

INCIDENCE

Writers in various Western countries have often expressed concern about the prevalence of emotional problems in the earlier years of life. In countries surveyed the incidence ranges from 10 to 20%. The World Health Organization has predicted that these figures will double by 2020, making emotional problems one of the more common causes of illness and disability in children (World Health Organization, 2001). In the UK, approximately 10% of children and young people aged between 5 and 16 years have a clinically diagnosed mental disorder. Of these, 4% have an emotional disorder (such as anxiety or depression), 6% have a conduct disorder while 2% have a hyperkinetic disorder. Some children (2%) have more than

---

Box 12.1 Child behaviour checklist

General areas

Internalizing problems: inhibited or over-controlled behaviours, such as anxiety or depression.
Externalizing problems: antisocial or under-controlled behaviours, such as delinquency or aggression.

Specific areas

Somatic complaints: recurring physical problems that have no known cause or cannot be medically verified. These may include headaches, or a tendency to develop signs and symptoms of a medical disorder.
Delinquent behaviour: behaviour where rules set by parents and/or communities are broken, such as property damage, theft of cars and other items.
Attention problems: concentration difficulties and an inability to sit still, including school performance problems.
Aggressive behaviour: bullying, teasing, fighting and temper tantrums.
Social problems: where individuals have impairment of their relationships with peers.
Withdrawal: where the individual is specifically inhibited by shyness and being socially isolated.
Anxious/depressed behaviour: a range of feelings of loneliness, sadness, feeling unloved, a sense of worthlessness, anxiety and generalized fears.
Thought disorders: or what might be seen as bizarre behaviour or thinking.

Reprinted from Sawyer MG, Arney FM, Baghurst PA, et al, 2000, Promoting the mental health and wellbeing of children and young people. Discussion paper: key principles and directions. Used by permission of the Australian Government.

---

one type of mental health problem (Office of National Statistics, 2005). Approximately 45 000 young people with a severe mental health disorder and 1.1 million children and young people under 18 may require care from specialist services (Department of Health, 2004).

However, although problems that are externalized are more noticeable and may therefore demand and receive more attention, introversion and depression may go undetected because the child is often well behaved and sometimes what may be considered 'too good' by family members or 'overly compliant' by professionals.

MENTAL HEALTH PROBLEMS IN CONTEXT

Mental health problems can affect many other aspects of young people's lives and therefore the problems must be seen in context. The more significant the mental health problem an individual has, the greater the possibility of problems in other areas of their lives. Furthermore, parents and other family members may often see these problems as affecting their own lifestyles and activities. Not enough is known about the long-term outlook for these young people, but it is important for professionals to see young people in the context of their everyday experience. Help may be needed across a broad range of life issues: with family functioning, social skills or school problems, for example. While the mental health problem may have caused these difficulties, it is equally important to consider that the life issue may have been the cause or an aggravating factor in the disorder (Sawyer et al., 2000). A balanced view is required, so that causal factors are not attributed to one area without adequately observing what is happening in other aspects of the young person's life. It may be that the child or adolescent is acting as a 'barometer' for problems existing in the family: the young person may be presenting with symptoms that reflect problems in the family or between parents. This may not be recognized initially and may only be revealed after some time. That is why an important aspect of assessment of children and adolescents includes an evaluation of the family's functioning and coping skills.

SERVICES AVAILABLE TO CHILDREN AND YOUNG PEOPLE

It is believed that one in five young people suffering from mental health problems throughout the Western world will receive the expert help they need (National Institute of Mental Health, 2002). In most Western countries, specialized services are usually called child and adolescent mental health services (CAMHS). Previously known as child guidance clinics, the services have expanded their scope considerably, offering a range of specialist assessment and treatment options. However, the provision of specialist child and adolescent mental health services across the UK is patchy with wide local and regional variations (Department of Health, 2008). CAMHS services include primary care (so-called Tier 1 services), specialist mental health workers in primary care (Tier 2), specialist, multiprofessional services for child and adolescents with complex, severe mental health needs (Tier 3) and day units and specialist outpatient and inpatient units (Tier 4) (Department of Health, 2004).

Emphasis has also been placed in recent years on early intervention and mental health promotion with young people and there have been developments of specific interventions, such as tackling bullying and increasing awareness of mental health issues (Department of Health, 2001, 2004). Early Intervention in Psychosis Services (EIPS) were established in 2001 for people aged between 14 and 35 with a first presentation of psychotic symptoms and/or during the first 3 years of psychotic disorder (Department of Health, 2001). The services were designed to:

- 'reduce the stigma associated with psychosis and improve professional and lay awareness of the symptoms of psychosis and the need for early assessment,
- reduce the length of time young people remain undiagnosed and untreated,
- develop meaningful engagement, provide evidence-based interventions and promote recovery during the early phase of illness,
- increase stability in the lives of service users, facilitate development and provide opportunities for personal fulfilment,
- provide a user-centred service, i.e. a seamless service available for those from age 14 to 35 that effectively integrates child, adolescent and adult mental health services and works in partnership with primary care, education, social services, youth and other services,
- at the end of the treatment period, ensure that the care is transferred thoughtfully and effectively' (Department of Health, 2001, pp. 43–44).

The current number of young people each year aged 15–35 who experience a first episode of psychosis is estimated at 6900 in England (London School of Economics Personal Social Services Research Unit, 2011). Recently the Coalition Government has broadened out the debate concerning early intervention in its *Early Intervention: The Next Steps* report (Cabinet Office, 2011). It states: 'Early Intervention enables every baby, child and young person to acquire the social and emotional foundations upon which our success as human beings depends' (Cabinet Office, 2011, p. 3). As such, the report emphasizes the importance of promoting physical and mental wellbeing among children and young people as well as building and supporting their social and emotional capabilities.

For adolescents in particular, simply providing a traditional outpatient or inpatient service may not be enough. Many teenagers worry about what others would think if they asked for help. Even more say they prefer to take care of their own problems, as they struggle with their sense of identity and relationships with adults. Unlike children, because of the adolescent's striving for increasing autonomy, a family approach may not be useful. A variety of unhealthy or 'at-risk' behaviours may be present. Half of adolescents with mental health problems also smoke or drink and a third report binge drinking. There is also a close link between mental health problems and suicidal behaviour or thinking (Sawyer et al., 2000). Many health services and programmes tend to focus on single issues, such as drugs and alcohol, or medical treatment, with insufficient attention paid to comorbidity (Andrews et al., 1999). There is a need for more collaboration and more funding for generalized adolescent health services and outreach programmes.

The treatment provided also varies from service to service, depending on the major problems presenting locally, age range, treatment philosophy, theoretical models, expertise available and the living circumstances of the young person and their family. Interventions may include behaviour therapy, cognitive behavioural therapy, couples therapy, parenting programmes, play therapy, psychodynamic individual or group work, socialization and social skills programmes, systems-based family therapy or individual therapy for a parent. Sometimes approaches are combined to achieve better outcomes. For example, a child may benefit from behaviour therapy to help them deal with problematic behaviour, but the family may also require assistance to enable them to develop positive styles of functioning together. As with adult services, nurses have a range of roles, often developing expertise in various modes of therapy.

CRITICAL THINKING CHALLENGE 12.1

Why do GPs, paediatricians and schools have such a vital role in early detection of mental health problems in children and young people?
  What interventions might GPs, paediatricians and schools provide?

THE NURSING ROLE

Working with children and adolescents can be challenging but fulfilling and rewarding. As children and adolescents are still developing as individuals, an intervention in their young lives can often make a dramatic difference for the rest of their life. Early intervention is often more effective than managing difficulties that have extended into adulthood. With adequate care and a supportive environment, young people can grow stronger emotionally, psychologically and physically. Working with a child and adolescent mental health team provides the opportunity to use a wide range of clinical treatment strategies and therapies. A multidisciplinary team approach is frequently used. Nurses often play a significant role in various aspects of care, including that of therapist. It is usually expected that a nurse wishing to enter this field will have some years of experience as a mental health nurse and further education, thus possessing a solid grounding in theory and clinical practice.

Raphael (2000) has pointed out the need for child and adolescent mental health services to recruit health professionals with a high level of knowledge and skills. The following list of core knowledge and traits regarded as fundamental for all professionals working in child and adolescent mental health services has been generated

from unpublished research by Limerick (1999, cited in Limerick and Baldwin, 2000):

- child development theories,
- theories that support child and adolescent mental health practice,
- initial interview skills,
- therapeutic interventions,
- evaluating skills,
- professional management skills,
- communication skills,
- professional development skills,
- practitioner qualities including trust, confidence and support.

Possessing these attributes, mental health nurses can become a significant resource for their service users. However, to be able to intervene effectively with service users the nurse needs to master the art of engaging with children and young people, both as individuals and in the context of their families.

CRITICAL THINKING CHALLENGE 12.2

Have a brainstorming session, either individually or in a group: list all the skills that a child and adolescent mental health nurse would require. Subdivide these into skills that you think may be specific to either a community mental health nurse or a mental health nurse working in an inpatient setting.

ENGAGING WITH CHILDREN AND YOUNG PEOPLE

One of the most useful skills the mental health nurse can acquire and refine is the ability to engage service users and establish rapport. Engagement between nurses, young people and their families is fundamental to developing a relationship based on trust. A relationship founded on trust will foster a willingness to work together towards change. Faber and Mazlish (2005) identify the outcome that the beginning mental health nurse working with young people should aspire to as essentially mastering communicating so that children and teenagers will listen, but also being so good at listening that the young person is more likely to communicate.

Mental health nurses working with children and adolescents also need to develop and refine the skill of discreet observation of the young person's mood and behaviour, and their interactions with their peers, family, friends and others. Observation of these factors, considered in the broader psychosocial context, will enable the nurse to achieve a comprehensive assessment of the factors contributing to the current difficulties experienced by the young person and their family.

Ongoing discussion with parents (carers) should clarify the understanding of which specific factors may be contributing to current problems. With a more specific diagnosis, the nurse and family may then begin the process of exploring solutions (planning). Any solutions agreed upon with the family are best implemented with the family's support and commitment, thus maximizing the probability of positive change. Constant monitoring (evaluation) of behavioural interventions and responses by family members is essential to ensure that the mental health team, the young person and their family continue to share a common understanding about the management of the problem and a commitment to recovery.

The participation of young people and their family in mental healthcare should not be confined solely to therapeutic outcome. Organizations have much to learn from service users about planning environments that are sensitive to the needs of young people. 'Family-friendly' environments also need to include processes that are responsive to the specific needs of younger people, particularly those who are experiencing significant emotional or mental health difficulties.

Engagement of young people and families across cultural contexts is key to accurate diagnosis and comprehensive treatment planning. There are implications for the way in which mental health professionals approach the assessment of their service users and families in multicultural countries. The nurse's understanding of specific cultural practices and beliefs held by service users is imperative to developing trust. Asking for information in a way that recognizes cultural norms will promote the service user's confidence in the care provided (see Ch. 5 and Ch. 6). Service users are more likely to provide accurate information if they believe that the nurse understands their cultural needs and has genuine respect and commitment to a recovery plan that is culturally sound.

Children

As outlined above, a myriad of factors contribute to and affect the mental health of young people. Familial or genetic predisposition to mental disorders, the presence of a coexisting medical or neurological problem, developmental problems or growing up in a chaotic or deprived environment are just a few of the considerations of which the mental health nurse should be mindful when beginning assessments of young people and their families. Furthermore, these factors will also affect the direction taken with goal planning and nursing interventions. It should be remembered that the nursing care plan is in fact a recovery plan for the young person and family; therefore the goals must be achievable and the strategies must be practical when implemented by the child and family (with nursing support). If the plan is based on

what the nurse can achieve rather than what the family can realistically accomplish, then the medium- to long-term success for recovery may be severely impaired and continuity of care lost. A case study and exploration of the issues discussed thus far will illustrate some key concepts.

CASE STUDY: ADAM

A mother contacts the community child and adolescent mental health service, unsure whether it is appropriate to seek help regarding her 9-year-old son, Adam, who she describes as 'becoming increasingly anxious and who has developed a fixation with tidiness', so much so that it is causing disruption in the family. The family consists of two female siblings, aged 11 and 7, and a father who is an accomplished musician who frequently travels for extended periods performing nationally and internationally. The mental health nurse receiving the call assures the mother that her concerns warrant a further assessment by a member of the mental health team, as her child appears to be highly anxious. He is unable to relax and appears to be developing maladaptive behaviours (excessive tidying). Furthermore, his anxiety is having an adverse effect on his relationship with his siblings. The nurse gathers more specific information by phone and explains to the mother that this referral will be discussed at the next team meeting and that she will receive a call within a week regarding an appointment for her, her husband and their son, for further assessment.

Discussion of case study: Adam

Within the first minutes of the mother's description of her son's problem, the mental health nurse was able to discern a role for the mental health team in assisting this family. The mother was assured that her concerns were well founded. The nurse spent a little more time gathering only the information necessary to discuss the case (assessment) with the team so that a plan for a further face-to-face interview could be made. Thus the mother feels reassured by the prospect of an appointment (implementation). A therapeutic alliance has been initiated between the family and the mental health service.

This early process reflects the beginning of the nurse's role in engaging the family in the therapeutic alliance and emphasizes how important each team member's role is in promoting a positive impression on the family (even before meeting them personally). The impression the family gains from an initial phone call can colour their perception of further interactions with the mental health team. Furthermore, the feeling of confidence in the mental health nurse and other team members will likely have an impact on the confidence of the child and siblings. This is important, as all family members will be involved in the child's recovery.

CRITICAL THINKING CHALLENGE 12.3

Imagine you are contacting a health service about worries and concerns you have for a member of your family. What nursing attributes and skills would you find reassuring during the first phone contact?

The foundation and building of a therapeutic relationship with the young person and the family will usually begin at the time of the initial phone call or face-to-face interview. This interview can be difficult for the young person, who may not perceive that there is a problem and therefore may not fully understand why they are attending an assessment at the mental health service. The skilled mental health nurse will use this opportunity to establish the young person's understanding of their need for an appointment. If the young person seems unsure (or unwilling to concede), they can often be encouraged to describe some difficulties which are occurring at home that they think may have led to their needing this appointment.

It is essential to clarify the child or young person's perception of the problem and their goals for treatment, as well as those of the parents. The nurse's role is to facilitate expression of the difficulties and to make explicit the goal that the service user and family have regarding recovery. This is necessary so that all parties (child, family and mental health team) can agree on the treatment plan.

Another case study will illustrate these key issues. While a diagnosis such as attention-deficit hyperactivity disorder might possibly be indicated in this situation, the case illustrates that it is important to concentrate on the presenting problems and any associated difficulties, rather than giving priority to diagnostic classification. Involvement in diagnostic controversies can potentially misdirect the focus of care from the individual needs of the child and family.

CASE STUDY: TIM

Tim is a 6-year-old boy who is attending his first appointment at a community child and adolescent mental health service, accompanied by his parents. He is the oldest of three children and has a young brother and baby sister. His parents report an escalation in Tim's behaviour just before he turned 3: 'It's like he never grew out of the "terrible twos". He just kept on going at a hundred miles an hour,' reported his mother. Tim's father concurred: 'The more limits I set, the worse he gets'. Tim's reply when asked if he knew why he was there was simply: 'I've been naughty'.

Discussion of case study: Tim

The skilled mental health nurse will attempt to clarify these comments using objective language and will eventually identify some very specific behaviours that the parents regard as priorities for change. The nurse will attempt to match the parents' goals with those of their son.

The nurse's response to Tim's perception that he has been 'naughty' might be: 'Naughty, what does that mean?' The aim for the nurse is to guide Tim to use specific words to tag specific behaviours, and if these match those identified by his parents, a simple goal may be developed to achieve an outcome that is satisfying to both parties. Tim's descriptions of how he sees 'the problem' may also assist the nurse to establish more accurately what the problem might be. Consider this further exchange between Tim and the nurse.

Nurse: 'Naughty', what does that mean?

Tim: When I run away or squeal.

Nurse: So you run away?

Tim: My brother … he's 3 … he runs away too…. When he runs away from Mummy, she chases him.

Nurse: And does your brother squeal?

Tim: No, but when my baby sister squeals, Daddy helps Mummy play with her.

This exchange demonstrates how, through active listening, the nurse has gathered some very specific information about the family dynamics that provides a possible explanation for some of Tim's behaviour. It could be that he is mimicking the behaviours of his younger siblings to receive the same attention from his parents that he perceives his brother and sister receive when they run away or squeal.

Encounters with children and adolescents and their families as illustrated in these case studies demonstrate how the nurse and other team members can engage young people in ongoing treatment, and how treatment will be influenced by further findings. The initiation of a sound therapeutic alliance with the child and family is an achievement, although the alliance also requires nurturing.

Generally, a therapeutic alliance is accomplished when respect is paramount in the nurse–service user relationship. Like adults, young people respond most positively to being treated with genuine respect. Young people feel respected when they are listened to and given opportunities to make choices and contribute to solving problems. As Faber and Mazlish (2005) identify, making choices gives the child valuable practice in making decisions; opportunities for problem-solving give them courage to follow things through independently. A commitment by the mental health nurse to facilitating choice and promoting problem-solving opportunities for young people will be further enhanced by a belief in the humanistic idea that all behaviour has meaning. If we as mental health nurses explore the meaning behind the behaviours we observe, we can plan appropriate strategies to modify behaviour and promote positive change.

In the UK child and adolescent mental health services work with many young people who present in acute emotional distress. Some will internalize their distress and may become withdrawn and depressed. Others may externalize their emotional pain. When this occurs the child will demonstrate altered behaviours, which may include rigid thinking, compulsive patterns of behaviour, agitation, impulsivity and, in severe cases, aggression. If the nurse has established a therapeutic alliance with the child, the shared trust and respect will provide a foundation for choice-giving and problem-solving. An example from practice will best illustrate this concept.

CASE STUDY: FIONA

Fiona is 12 years old and is attending the child and adolescent mental health service for the first time, accompanied by her mother, with whom she lives. Her younger brother has lived with her father since their parents separated 3 years ago. Fiona's mother is extremely concerned about a gradual change in Fiona's mood over the past 2 years. She has reportedly become angry and unpredictable, a dramatic change from the quiet but confident child she used to be. Her mother describes instances where Fiona has impulsively run from home and engaged in risky behaviours such as riding her bike recklessly on their busy street. When met by members of the mental health team, Fiona is at first passive, refusing eye contact, seeming to ignore the conversation between her mother and the nurse and refusing to respond when spoken to directly. Several times during the conversation, however, Fiona interrupts with a hostile comment, countering information provided by her mother.

Discussion of case study: Fiona

Skills required

In the case study of Fiona, even though Fiona is refusing to be involved in the initial assessment her behaviours and her brief interjections are a valuable source of assessment information. The nurse will document Fiona's behaviours and her comments. In context, this will reflect some family dynamics and give some indication of how Fiona currently feels about her life. The challenge for the nurse will be to initially engage Fiona in a shared interest of hers that is nonemotional and therefore less threatening.

Rather than attempting to engage Fiona too early, the nurse wisely chooses to wait for an opportunity. This does not arise until the very end of the initial interview,

when the nurse announces that the assessment is almost complete. 'About time,' Fiona grumbles, 'I just want to get in the car and listen to my new CD'. The nurse grasps this opportunity:

Nurse: *Ah, a new CD ... which group?*

Fiona: *No one you'd know.*

Nurse: *Try me.*

To Fiona's surprise, the nurse has recently bought the same CD and although Fiona feigns horror that an adult would even know the band, she cannot completely disguise her admiration.

Nurse: *See you in a fortnight then?*

Fiona: *If I'm not too busy with my music.*

Fiona's choice of words ('If I'm not too busy ...') indicates that she is trying to sound uninterested while still leaving her options open.

Approach taken and outcome achieved

Troubled children and adolescents are not always easily engaged. Often the factors contributing to their need for mental health support have affected their ability to trust others; in many cases they have felt let down by adults. The nurse who recognizes this will allow time for the young person to engage, initially on his or her own terms, so the fragile therapeutic alliance can gradually strengthen. Fiona's hostility was ignored; the nurse chose instead to preserve Fiona's fragile sense of dignity. Respecting Fiona's ability to make sound decisions, the nurse did not assume that she would be returning in a fortnight, but rather posed it as a question; this approach was aimed at reassuring Fiona that she had a choice. Her choice to return in a fortnight would demonstrate her courage in recognizing that a problem exists, and her willingness to explore some supports.

NURSE'S STORY: REFLECTION

As an experienced mental health nurse, I'd regarded myself as a spontaneous, reflective clinician, confident that my responses to and interactions with patients were at all times respectful, helpful and kind. I was taken by surprise then, when I began working with young people in an inpatient mental health setting, that I now felt hesitant and doubtful about how to respond. What was appropriate? What would be a better response? My confidence and spontaneity had given way to feeling stilted and unsure ... until a defining moment, when I realized that opening my senses to cues from others, taking time to (literally) look in the mirror, could deepen my understanding of how others see themselves. This is my story…

With his bath finished and his pyjamas on, 8-year-old Cobey and I stand in front of the full-length mirror looking straight at ourselves, occasionally glancing across at each other's reflection, then back to our own. As we look into the mirror, I wonder what we each see.

I see myself: casually dressed, complete and unchanging … and looking a wee bit tired! I suspect that Cobey, like me, sees an image of himself; but I can only speculate on what self-image that might be…

I kneel down beside Cobey to try and observe his reflection as he might be seeing it. There is a small crack in the glass near where Cobey is standing. The mirror has been damaged, but because of the safety component of the glass it has not shattered but simply absorbed the knock, leaving three fractures darting out from the one stress point. As I had anticipated, Cobey's image is disjointed, and the symbolic implications momentarily tug at me.

'What do you see?' I ask him quietly.

No answer. There he is, looking into a broken mirror, observing a fragmented self: lots of small pieces, together, but not quite. He moves bodily up and down and sideways, all the time trying to piece together his reflection in a harmonious union. But it is not to be: whichever position he views himself from, he is in several pieces, a fragmented whole.

'I'm in pieces … nothing fits together properly,' he eventually says, giggling. Then for a few more minutes he moves about, trying to find where he might place himself so that the pieces of him do come together as they should. In a short while, in frustration, he curses the mirror and leaves the room. I stand stunned. Cobey's complex and distressing childhood history symbolically laid bare before the mirror. So much about us both reflected in this brief encounter.

Kristin Henderson

CRITICAL THINKING CHALLENGE 12.4

In the case study of Fiona, what might the outcomes have been if the nurse had persisted in asking Fiona questions early in the interview?

What assumptions could be made regarding Fiona's need to interrupt while her mother and the nurse were speaking?

Adolescents

When adolescents and their family (carers) present to a healthcare facility, there is an expectation by family and carers that treatment will achieve the desired outcomes, in terms of the physical, emotional and mental state of the young person. However, it is possible that these outcomes may not be achieved, because of many situational factors. One such factor may be the young person's lack of willingness to be part of the referral, assessment and treatment process due to their not recognizing or acknowledging that they have a significant problem. Mental health nurses providing mental healthcare for adolescents need to acknowledge that possible influencing factors such as poor insight, resistance to treatment or challenging of authority may be part of normal adolescent behaviour.

Mental health nurses should attempt to form a relationship with the young person through engagement and foster a sense of purpose with the treatment plan for the adolescent. Engagement is the process of forming a relationship based on interactions where there is an ongoing conversation or acknowledgment of a partnership. Green and Jacobs (1998) write that engagement is the establishment of a therapeutic alliance to achieve the desired outcomes and goals of the perceived processes in which people enter into a relationship. Therefore an important element of engagement is building a rapport, which encompasses not only the formal aspects of mental healthcare such as completing a diagnostic interview, but also the social interactions and nonverbal communication that occur. Sharman (1997) states that nonverbal forms of communication may be more significant than verbal interactions when interviewing and engaging young people with mental health problems.

For mental health professionals, language is the key to open communication and creation of an environment that can augment engagement. Adolescents may use language and jargon that differs according to their age group or subculture, especially when it comes to 'street lingo'. Adolescents may have a culture that at times seems alien to their parents, caregivers and health professionals. Adolescents and their peer groups may use words and phrases that have a significantly different meaning than that to which adults may be accustomed: for example, 'sick' or 'gross' may mean 'good'. Healthcare professionals who work with adolescents may need to clarify with the young person what they actually mean by their phrases or words, if the professional does not understand them. This may be particularly relevant when discussing illicit drugs and the street names used for marijuana, amphetamines and hallucinogens.

Understanding language and communicating effectively is integral to engaging with young people and vital to the success of their ongoing treatment. We stated earlier that this chapter will not deal with specific classified conditions, but rather, the principles of nursing care relating to groupings of disorders. The following section explores the principles of mental health nursing that promote engagement with adolescents with challenging behaviours arising from psychosis, depressive symptoms and social–emotional issues. Examples of practice situations will highlight some appropriate responses to consider.

CRITICAL THINKING CHALLENGE 12.5

As a small-group exercise, discuss some strategies that nurses can use to foster engagement with an adolescent who is sullen and guarded.

Psychosis and behaviour issues

Psychotic symptoms can be a common reason for adolescents being admitted to child and adolescent mental health inpatient unit. Inpatient care is often suggested, in order to ensure safety, to stabilize the condition and to introduce appropriate medication and therapy in promoting ongoing psychological security. The symptoms associated with psychosis can be frightening for young people. It can often be a difficult time for parents, when their child is disturbed by hallucinations and delusions and is lacking insight into their current mental or emotional state. Nurses working with adolescents need to understand and practise basic concepts of engagement to optimize outcomes of providing care for the adolescent and their family.

To engage the adolescent in a therapeutic relationship that will promote treatment and ultimately result in regaining wellness, nurses need to encourage and allow the adolescent to develop trust. Trust is difficult for a young person to develop, especially if they are attending an appointment begrudgingly or have been hospitalized against their will. To promote a therapeutic relationship that supports trust it is essential to be honest and consistent in any approach to treatment. Adolescents can appear to be more guarded or sensitive than adults with similar disorders. For example, an adolescent may have difficulty in complying with medications. This might be for a variety of reasons, including a fear of being sedated, possible drug sensitivity, potential to develop adverse side effects from prescribed medications or, if delusional, perhaps even the suspicion of being poisoned. Adverse side effects of some antipsychotic medications may result in weight gain. Adolescents may dislike this. Young people may experience muscle spasm or rigidity as another adverse effect of antipsychotic medication. Some medications may require regular blood tests. This can be a frightening experience and some may consider it as frightening as the symptoms of the psychosis. Because of these considerations, adherence with medication can be difficult and a confusing issue for the adolescent.

Mental health nurses are pivotal in providing information and psychoeducational programmes aimed at promoting wellness, and in providing an opportunity for the young person to gain insight into their health and condition. Throughout the nurse's contact with young people, opportunities to provide psychoeducation in regard to a service user's mental health status and their treatment are vital. Early recovery can be facilitated by psychoeducation. This may include discussing issues of causation and the likely medium- to long-term outcomes of their care and treatment.

CASE STUDY: DAVID

A 15-year-old boy, David, has been referred to the Early Intervention Service. He is experiencing a psychotic episode as a result of smoking marijuana for several months. He has been hearing auditory hallucinations (voices telling him he is useless and a nuisance to be around). In the past 6 months there has been a decline in David's academic performance and he has been isolating himself from his friends and family. Within the past 2 months he has been verbally and physically abusive towards his parents and siblings.

Discussion of case study: David

The presentation (to Early Intervention Services) of a young person like David, experiencing their first episode of psychosis, is not uncommon. In considering David's care, the nurse's first priority is to ensure that David is physically safe and that those around him also feel safe. When a person's thinking is altered by psychotic phenomena, they may act irrationally as a consequence of feeling fearful and insecure. This may include aggressive behaviour. It is important that the nurse appears confident and takes a role in calming the current situation by offering reassurance and firm guidance with statements such as, 'David, what you are experiencing must be frightening. We will help you'. Short, clear statements made firmly but quietly and with genuine empathy will be reassuring for David and his family. It is important that it is made clear that, whatever David says or does, he has been heard. At this stage, the nurse should avoid disputing the service user's irrational thoughts. Rather, David should be encouraged to verbalize his confusion and distress. This may assist in diffusing his agitation and may lead to his feeling calmer, thereby reducing the risk of him becoming aggressive. Aggression is often a response to feeling frightened, threatened or overwhelmed.

Another important priority is involving the family as early as possible, providing them with much-needed support, so that they can, in turn, provide support to David. The family can also be helpful in providing an accurate history of family health. This will assist in establishing any familial predispositions to mental disorder and the nature of onset. This information may help the mental health worker to establish the likely severity and prognosis for the diagnosed disorder and organize an individualized treatment plan that will have a higher probability of a positive outcome. Recovery from mental health problems demands a high level of support from family, friends and staff. The best prognosis and quality of life are achieved when all work collaboratively.

Working with adolescents with psychosis is extremely challenging. However, if the nurse follows the aforementioned guidelines in attempting to engage them, the ability to support the service user and family through the difficult times will prove ultimately rewarding. Once safety has been established and the service user and family have begun to engage with staff, the medium- to long-term relief of symptoms and psychoeducation can ensue.

Other care and treatment modes could include hospitalization, resocialization through group therapy and individual goal setting that focuses on peer support and reestablishing a social network. Individual goal planning, peer support and group therapy can each promote socially adaptive and acceptable behaviour. Adolescence is a period of personal development involving challenging authority and pushing against the norms of society. The 'normal' adolescent behaviours should not be stifled through treatment but recognized and supported, so that David can return to his peer group and family with minimal residual effects of the psychotic episode. One aspect of hospitalization that can have negative longer-term effects is the labelling of the condition suffered by David. Nurses should remember that one episode of psychosis might not justify labelling David with 'schizophrenia'.

Depression and suicide

Although the number of successful suicides of young people is decreasing (Office of National Statistics, 2011), depression and risk of suicide is a major problem in the community. The psychological and physical trauma associated with young people who have attempted suicide may be difficult for mental health nurses to come to terms with. The young person should be reassured that their safety is the treatment team's priority, while at the same time providing support to the family. Youth suicide and attempts at self-harm may challenge mental health nurses and family members to consider their own mortality and the question of why people attempt suicide. It is important that mental health nurses develop skills that enable them to feel comfortable addressing these issues directly with the service user and family.

Engagement

Adolescents who are experiencing symptoms of depression or who are suicidal can be extremely difficult due to their tendency to socially withdrawn and isolative behaviour or due to cognitive impairment. Nurses are able to engage adolescents through social interactions, groups and individual therapy. It is often the nurse who spends long hours with the young person and is present with them as their mood shifts throughout the day who may be alerted to a subtle increase in risk to the young person's emotional or physical safety. The nurse's ability to reassure the young person of his or her availability as needed helps the young person feel free to discuss issues with the nurse when the time seems most right for them.

An issue that can be confusing for nurses is the fact that at times adolescents who are clinically depressed may present with aggressive traits or behaviours. Some adolescents are not able to communicate their emotions verbally. As a result, their only means of expressing distress may be through verbal or physical aggression, towards themselves or others. Engagement of these young people may be aided by involvement in physical activities, sport or music and the arts. Sharing the young person's physical space and activities may help in forging a therapeutic alliance. The use of diversional activities can enable the mental health nurse to further engage the young person and further develop the therapeutic relationship. Establishing a confidante may be the turning point in the young person's care and treatment.

CASE STUDY: JULIE

Julie is a 14-year-old who, over the past year, has become increasingly withdrawn from her peer group. She was previously an A-grade student in a school with a good reputation, but over the past 4 months her school grades have dropped noticeably and she is not completing her homework. She no longer has an interest in playing netball or attending her athletics club. Julie's mother states that Julie has been aggressive towards her and has been harming herself by cutting her wrists with any sharp object available. Julie was commenced on antidepressant medication by her GP 6 weeks prior to admission but there has been minimal change in her mental state.

Discussion of case study: Julie

In the case study Julie requires intensive therapy, which may include cognitive behavioural therapy, family therapy, individual psychotherapy and a review of her medication. Psychosocial issues also need to be considered during Julie's treatment. This may include exploring school issues, and whether Julie has been physically, emotionally or sexually abused or has experienced significant losses that have contributed to her depression.

In assisting young people like Julie, the mental health nurse will need to establish rapport and maintain engagement. It will be important to gain the service user's confidence from the initial meeting, as there will be many sensitive issues to address. Adolescents seeking help from adults will not always commit time for a therapeutic relationship to grow, if they doubt in any way the sincerity of the person in whom they are confiding.

In some instances, the action of inflicting harm upon oneself can provide a sense of relief from severe emotional distress and psychic pain. It is therefore essential that the nurse recognizes this possibility and, while working with the young person, makes every effort to ensure that they feel respected and not judged on the behaviour that has led to them seeking help. Medical care, such as attention to a wound, should be addressed discreetly and professionally (National Institute for Health and Clinical Excellence, 2004).

The key aspect of providing care for the young person is establishing their current level of safety and working with them on how this can best be achieved. It will be helpful to ensure that the young person has adequate support networks, so they can strengthen these connections with a view to obtaining help in more adaptive ways in the future.

CRITICAL THINKING CHALLENGE 12.6

List the potential barriers to establishing a therapeutic alliance with Julie.

WORKING WITH FAMILIES

Ideally, nurses working with children and adolescents should incorporate all members of the family in their care. A major component of child and adolescent mental health nursing is the involvement of the family in assessment, treatment, discharge and follow-up. Working with young people and families may include family therapy. It is acknowledged that family therapy is discussed within the context of mental health therapeutic interventions (see Ch. 23). It is important, however, to consider family therapy within the context of child and adolescent mental health.

Family therapy has been constantly evolving since its conception in the middle of the twentieth century. Traditionally, family therapy has focused on the identified problems with the child or adolescent and how the family has dealt with these issues. In recent times there has been a shift in focus towards family-centred mental health nursing, which includes family-based assessments and treatments and attention to the whole family rather than focusing on the identified young service user.

Benner Carson (2000, pp. 343–349) states that family therapy works within the following concepts.

- Problems in families are best understood and treated from a circular rather than a linear perspective.
- Families experiencing problems need to discover their own problem-solving abilities.
- Family members' ability to change depends upon their ability to alter their perception of the problem.
- A family understanding a problem does not itself lead to change.

- A therapeutic context for change must be created for families.
- Problems or symptoms may serve a positive family function.
- More positive outcomes will be achieved if problems are treated by seeing the family as an interacting system.

From these key aspects of family involvement nurses can formulate their own methods of working with families to best suit their clinical environment. Nurses can use various frameworks derived from family therapy. The approach may be structured, systemic, brief, solution-focused or narrative. Nurses involved in such work require ongoing clinical supervision and support in order to ensure that optimal relationships are maintained and that the family achieves their desired outcomes.

CONFIDENTIALITY

An important issue for young people is being able to understand how the information shared during interactions with team members is documented and knowing who has access to these records. It is important to them that confidentiality be maintained. However, when there are risk factors involved the young person must know that nurses and their colleagues are bound to impart information that has a direct effect on their safety or the safety of others.

Interviews with adolescents should not be restricted to the formality of interview rooms. As long as safety can be assured, some adolescents may prefer to be interviewed in a more public place, such as a courtyard. Flexibility (and not a small dose of ingenuity) is the key to providing a quality service that will encourage young people in crisis to return.

MEDICATION ADHERENCE

As stated previously, medication adherence is a major issue for adolescents, regardless of their condition. Many young people do not want to be different from their peer group. This may include not wanting to be seen as different by needing tablets. The rationale for taking medication should be explained and adverse effects discussed, together with how to reduce the complications of medication therapy. Problem-solving with the young person about ways to discreetly include the taking of prescribed medication in their daily lifestyle pattern will be of benefit. The risk of taking nonprescribed medications should be highlighted. This can be achieved by maximizing therapeutic interventions. In adolescent mental health, engagement through developing rapport and trust are key elements to achieving change. Without these elements, minimal change can be achieved.

The case studies in this chapter have sought to reinforce the importance of engagement. Demonstrating empathy and performing with absolute sincerity are important factors in caring for children and adolescents. It is important that young people feel that they are the priority for the nurse at this particular time.

A further important consideration for nurses working with children and adolescents is legal issues related to the treatment of young people who have mental health problems.

LEGAL ISSUES

Nurses involved in the care of young people admitted to mental health services often have to deal with legal issues relating to duty of care, child protection and mental health legislation.

Children and younger adolescents must have their parents' or guardian's consent to seek treatment for any form of medical intervention, including mental health assessments and treatment. Young people can give their own consent to receive medical or nursing treatment, as long as their parents are aware and the health professionals believe that the young person is competent to give consent. The ability for young people to consent to medical treatment or seek medical consultations is referred to as *Gillick competence* (Gillick v. West Norfolk and Wisbech Area Health Authority (1986) 1 AC 112). Medical and nursing staff may question whether the young person is 'Gillick competent' or has the cognitive ability to make an informed judgement to give their own consent for treatment. The legal precedent is the case where a parent took the local health authority to court after one of her children received treatment from a GP without her consent. This case has had a major impact on the provision of paediatric healthcare and is cited across legal and healthcare systems in the Western world as a basis for establishing how consent is obtained from young people. In mental health, as with general healthcare, consent could be challenged by parents and doctors; however, to ensure the safety and wellbeing of young people, mental health legislation provides strong guidelines and rights of appeal. Mental health nurses who treat young people should be aware that it is unethical and legally unsafe to engage a young person in treatment without informing their parent(s). Healthcare services and inpatient units tend to have specific protocols and policies to address this issue.

The legal process by which young people can be admitted to mental healthcare services is similar to that for adult service users. This ensures that legal processes and due process are followed in regard to human rights, issues of liberty and the protection of the rights of others. It is always preferable that young people are admitted voluntarily. If the safety of an adolescent is at risk and they are unable to consent to voluntary treatment, the Mental Health Act can be enacted. Younger people are usually regarded as voluntary if their parents have provided consent. The other main legal issues that need to be observed in child and adolescent mental health are child protection and statutory orders in regard to custody.

CONCLUSION

This chapter has highlighted skills that nurses require when working for the first time with children and adolescents in the mental health field. It has focused primarily on engagement: establishing a therapeutic relationship and forging a therapeutic alliance. The authors believe that nurses must first master strategies for engaging young people and their families before more advanced skills in mental health nursing can be consolidated effectively. Engaging young people and families early and initiating a therapeutic relationship will enhance the quality of assessment information provided by the service users. Furthermore, a sense of trust among parties will promote commitment to a shared treatment plan created in partnership among the young person, their parents or carers and the mental health team.

EXERCISES FOR CLASS ENGAGEMENT

Contact your nearest child and adolescent mental health service and request information on the services available to children and young people. Share this information with your group.

◆ Are these services proactive and responsive?
◆ Does the service actively promote early intervention?

Contact a nurse working in a community setting and another from an inpatient unit, and ask them to speak to your group about their roles. Note any differences between the mental health nursing of young people in the community and that of young people in an inpatient setting.

In small groups, nominate one person to act as a mental health nurse and another to play the role of a sullen, guarded adolescent. Remaining group members are to observe and document the difficulties presented in establishing rapport.

Contact a child and adolescent mental health service and arrange to speak with a person who has experience with depressed or suicidal youth. Then clarify your responses to Critical thinking challenge 12.2.

Read http://www.education.gov.uk/munroreview/downloads/8875_DfE_Munro_Report_TAGGED.pdf and summarize key points in establishing an effective child protection system. Share your findings.

REFERENCES

American Psychiatric Association, 2000. Diagnostic and Statistical Manual of Mental Disorders, 4th ed., text rev. American Psychiatric Association, Washington DC.

Andrews, G., Hall, W., Teeson, M., et al., 1999. The Mental Health of Australians. Mental Health Branch, Commonwealth Department of Health and Aged Care, Canberra.

Benner Carson, V. (Ed.), 2000. Mental Health Nursing: The Nurse–Patient Journey, 2nd ed. W B Saunders, Philadelphia.

Brannon, L., Feist, J., 2000. Health Psychology. Wadsworth, Belmont.

Cabinet Office, 2011. Early intervention: next steps. <http://www.dwp.gov.uk/docs/early-intervention-next-steps.pdf>.

Department of Health, 2001. Mental health policy implementation guide. <http://www.dh.gov.uk/prod_consum_dh/groups/dh_digitalassets/@dh/@en/documents/digitalasset/dh_4058960.pdf>.

Department of Health, 2004. The Mental Health and Psychological Well-Being of Children and Young People. Department of Health, London.

Department of Health, 2008. Children and young people in mind: the final report of the National CAMHS Review. <http://www.dh.gov.uk/en/Publicationsandstatistics/Publications/PublicationsPolicyAndGuidance/DH_090399>.

Faber, A., Mazlish, E., 2005. How to Talk so Kids will Listen and Listen so Kids will Talk. Avon, New York.

Green, J., Jacobs, B., 1998. Inpatient Child Psychiatry. Routledge, London.

Hoagwood, K., Serene, O.S., 2002. The NIMH blueprint for change report. Research priorities in child and adolescent mental health 41(7), 760–767.

Limerick, M., Baldwin, L., 2000. Nursing in outpatient child and adolescent mental health. Nurs. Stand. 15 (13–15), 43–45.

London School of Economics Personal Social Services Research Unit, 2011. Economic case. <http://www.iris-initiative.org.uk/silo/files/mental-health-promotion-and-prevention-the-economic-case.pdf>.

National Institute for Health and Clinical Excellence, 2004. Self-harm: the short-term physical and psychological management and secondary prevention of self-harm in primary and secondary care. <http://www.nice.org.uk/nicemedia/pdf/CG016NICEguideline.pdf>.

National Institute of Mental Health, 2002. Brief notes on the mental health of children and adolescents. <http://www.slideshare.net/dennis43/brief-notes-on-the-mental-health-of-children-and-adolescents>.

Office of National Statistics, 2005. Mental health of children and young people in Great Britain, 2004. <http://www.statistics.gov.uk/downloads/theme_health/summaryreport.pdf>.

Office of National Statistics, 2011. Suicide rates in the United Kingdom, 2000–2009. <http://www.statistics.gov.uk/pdfdir/sui0111.pdf>.

Raphael B., 2000. Promoting the mental health and wellbeing of children and young people. Discussion paper: key principles and directions. Australian Government, Canberra. <http://www.health.gov.au/internet/wcms/Publishing.nsf/Content/48F5C63B02F2CE07CA2572450013F488/$File/promdisc.pdf>.

Sawyer, M.G., Arney, F.M., Baghurst, P.A., et al., 2000. Child and Adolescent Component of the National Survey of Mental Health and Well-Being. Mental Health and Special Programs Branch, Commonwealth Department of Health and Aged Care, Canberra.

Sharman, W., 1997. Children and Adolescents with Mental Health Problems. Baillière Tindall, London.

Thompson, T., Mathias, P., 2000. Lyttle's Mental Health and Disorder, 3rd ed. Baillière Tindall, London.

Walker, J., Payne, S., Smith, P., et al., 2004. Psychology for Nurses and the Caring Professions, 2nd ed. Open University Press, Maidenhead.

World Health Organization, 2001. Fact sheet no. 265, December 2001. <http://www.who.int/whr/2001/media_centre/en/whr01_fact_sheet1_en.pdf>.

Chapter | **13** |

Mental disorders of older age

Wendy Moyle

CHAPTER POINTS

- The UK population is ageing and it is older people that nurses will most likely be providing care for in the future.
- Most older people are healthy and do not require health and social support.
- Staff attitudes are important in influencing the delivery of care to older people.
- Nursing care and treatment of mental health problems in older people should include listening to the individual, encouraging an active and healthy lifestyle, and cultivating an interactive therapeutic nurse–service user relationship.
- In assessing an older person the nurse should avoid making ageist assumptions, such as assuming that dementia is the cause of changes in behaviour and activity.
- Mental health nursing staff should not assume that deterioration in function is a normal part of ageing.
- Mental health disorders in older age include depression, anxiety, delirium, dementia and schizophrenia. The most common disorder is depression.

- ageing
- ageism
- assessment
- delirium
- dementia
- depression
- mental disorders

LEARNING OUTCOMES

The material in this chapter will assist you to:

- demonstrate an understanding of the common mental disorders that occur in older adults,
- explore management of the following mental disorders in older people: depression, anxiety disorders, suicide, substance misuse, delirium, dementia and schizophrenia,
- explore strategies to promote mental health in older people,
- reflect on your own and others' attitudes towards older people.

INTRODUCTION

The UK is an ageing society. It is imperative that nurses understand and can work with older people, as they are likely to be the population that nurses will increasingly be required to provide healthcare for in the future. This chapter provides an overview of mental health problems that are common in the older adult population, and explores the issues and principles underlying their assessment and treatment, including a number of general strategies to promote mental health. In addition, some negative attitudes towards older people are discussed, along with the implications of these negative attitudes for attempts to enhance the quality of care for older people.

DEMOGRAPHY OF AGEING IN THE UK

Over the last quarter of a century there has been an increase of 1.7 million people aged 65 and over (Office for National Statistics, 2010). In 1984, people aged 65 and over formed 15% of the population, rising to 16% in 2009. It is projected that by 2034 23% of the population will be aged 65 and over (Office for National Statistics, 2010). In particular, those people aged 85 years and over have the fastest population increase: from 660 000 people in 1984 to 1.4 million in 2009.

By 2034 it is estimated that 3.5 million people will be aged 85 and over: 5% of the total UK population. Consequently, the median age of the UK population has increased from 35 years in 1984 to 39 years in 2009 and this is projected to increase to 42 years by 2034. It also appears that the gender gap has narrowed, with the median age of the female UK population in 2009 being 40 years and the median UK male population age standing at 38 years (Office for National Statistics, 2010).

Although older people may not necessarily be dependent on others, ageing brings with it an increase in certain disease processes. Mental health problems are not, however, a normal occurrence of ageing, although the risk of developing mental disorders does increase with age. In particular, risk factors for depression, such as loss and grief, social isolation, medical illness and disability and being a caregiver, are more common in older age (Murray et al., 2006). The predicted increase in the older population is therefore expected to multiply the numbers of adults with diagnosed mental disorders (Bartels and Smyer, 2002).

It is difficult to have a firm sense of how many older people have a mental health problem as prevalence figures vary considerably according to the populations surveyed and the methodologies used (Lawlor and Radic, 1994). In addition, there are also a number of negative stereotypical perceptions of age and older people that may inhibit the diagnosis and treatment of physical illness and mental distress. In 1969 Butler coined the term 'ageism' to define the systematic stereotyping of and discrimination against people because they are old (cited in Butler, 1975). We have come to realize that ageism can apply to any age group, not just older people. Thus, ageism has more recently been defined as discrimination against people on the grounds of their age alone, as a consequence of which stereotypical assumptions are made about how people are viewed throughout life (Behrens, 1998).

Unfortunately, health professionals are not immune to ageist attitudes (Karlin et al., 2005; Moyle, 2003). Over the past decade a number of studies have investigated how healthcare professionals feel about caring for older people. Nursing students' attitudes to older people have frequently been found to be negative (Martell, 1999; Robinson and Cubit, 2005; Stevens and Crouch, 1992). Ageist views may in turn also affect the prevalence rates of mental health in the older population through misdiagnosis or an unwillingness to diagnose individuals because they are seen as 'old'.

Older people living alone are 3.3 times more likely to be diagnosed with depression than those residing in a household with others (Schulman et al., 2002). It is important, however, not to stereotype older people as being unwell, and to remember that not all older adults require hospital services and assistance.

ASSESSMENT OF OLDER PEOPLE

All staff working with older people should begin by learning about the normal process of ageing. The world is full of active and healthy older people and most older people do not require additional health and social support.

The main reasons for assessing older people are:

- to obtain a baseline assessment of function: this can assist in avoiding unrealistic goals,
- to demonstrate positive changes to service users and to gather evidence for relatives, nurses and other health professionals,
- to ascertain the presence and, if present, the extent of cognitive decline,
- for selection purposes (e.g. in research), to ensure that groups of people are of similar levels,
- to evaluate a new approach, treatment programme or service,
- for legal purposes (e.g. complications following a head injury),
- to assist diagnosis and prognosis.

Most of the time nurses are involved with obtaining a baseline assessment of function and assisting with diagnosis and prognosis. The most common cognitive screening instrument is the Mini-Mental State Examination (MMSE; Folstein et al., 1975). The use of observation skills and a brief assessment of the service user's cognitive functioning through the use of the MMSE provide valuable baseline data on which to base subsequent observations and care (see Ch. 10). The severity of cognitive impairment is frequently defined by MMSE scores, which may give an indication of dementia (NICE, 2011a):

- mild Alzheimer's disease: MMSE score of 21–26,
- moderate Alzheimer's disease: MMSE score of 10–20,
- moderately severe Alzheimer's disease: MMSE score of 10–14,
- severe Alzheimer's disease: MMSE score of less than 10.

There are, of course, many reasons why someone may present with a cognitive impairment and whereas MMSE scores may give an indication of dementia it is not a definitive diagnostic tool. It is vital, therefore, that a full assesment is undertaken to exclude other health issues, such as physical health problems, depression or delirium (see below). Investigations should include:

- routine haematology,
- biochemistry tests (including electrolytes, calcium, glucose, and renal and liver function),
- thyroid function tests,
- serum vitamin B_{12} and folate levels (NICE, 2011b).

Structural neuroimaging should be used in the assessment of people with suspected dementia and, in general, magnetic resonance imaging (MRI) is recommended to assist with early diagnosis and detect vascular changes (NICE, 2011b). A review of a person's medication should also be undertaken in order to identify and minimize use of drugs, including over-the-counter products, which may have an impact cognitive functioning (NICE, 2011b).

When making a diagnosis of mental health problems, cultural concepts related to physical and mental wellbeing must be considered. However, common tools, such as the MMSE (Folstein et al., 1975) are of particular concern as they do not take into consideration an individual's educational attainment, language or culture. Such considerations must be taken into account when any mental health assessment is undertaken.

Ageism in assessment

Although there are many safe ways to investigate the reasons behind a change in behaviour and ability, conclusions are often drawn too quickly. It is too easy to assume, because a 70-year-old person fails to recognize familiar faces, and rambles and behaves strangely, that a dementing condition is the cause. There could be any number of reasons for this behaviour, from delirium to depression, and therefore it is important that nurses spend time with the service user and their spouse or carers, to ensure a thorough and accurate assessment and to reduce the influence of ageist staff attitudes.

NURSE'S STORY: DOLORES

I was working in accident and emergency when Dolores was brought into the department in an unkempt and confused state. She was initially assumed by staff to be suffering from a dementing syndrome such as Alzheimer's disease, as she was 'aged', incoherent and lay chanting on the stretcher.

On examination Dolores was found to be wearing several layers of clothing, each soiled with excrement. While one nurse undressed Dolores, another asked her husband Jack for information about her condition, how long she had been in this state and whether there was any underlying condition or medication that may have contributed to the situation. Jack indicated that his wife had been coherent, with clarity of thought, up until the previous week. She had not recently had an operation or ingested any medication or substance that might have caused a chemical-induced delirium.

The nurses were alerted to the possibility of a toxic delirium as Jack informed them that Dolores had a large chest wound and that she had not been receiving medical care. Under the many layers of clothing Dolores was found to have a fungating breast cancer. Early in her illness she had asked her elderly husband to nurse her at home and to promise that he would never take her to see a doctor.

As her illness progressed she would not allow Jack to undress her, and as she became cold and soiled he placed new clothing over her existing clothing.

Dolores did not have Alzheimer's disease. She was suffering from delirium as a result of a chemical imbalance due to her physical deterioration. Unfortunately, her condition deteriorated quickly and she survived only another 5 h in hospital.

Nursing staff were distressed by the sight of Dolores in her many layers of wet and dirty clothing, and some staff felt that Jack had not cared for or about her. They assumed that a caring husband would have taken her for medical treatment earlier. But this assumption was incorrect: a neighbour and another relative spoke of Jack's devotion to Dolores and his desire to carry out her every wish, even if it meant caring for her without medical and nursing assistance. It was during a debriefing, at the end of the day, that several staff came to recognize that despite their knowledge and education they had all too quickly jumped to an incorrect diagnosis because on initial observation Dolores was seen as being elderly and confused. It was timely to initiate continuing education sessions in the department to concentrate on such issues.

CRITICAL THINKING CHALLENGE 13.1

Reflect upon the nurse's story about Dolores. Consider why the conclusion of dementia was so readily presumed and how you might ensure, when assessing older service users, that this does not happen in practice.

MENTAL HEALTH PROBLEMS IN THE OLDER POPULATION

Although a number of conditions – such as depression, anxiety disorders, suicide, substance misuse, delirium, dementia and schizophrenia – fall within the context of mental health problems in old age, they do not occur because of ageing. It is predicted, however, that the incidence of such disorders may continue to increase as the population ages (Nadler-Moodie and Gold, 2005). Each of these disorders is explored in the following sections.

Depression

One of the most common mental health problems of old age is depression (Djernes, 2006, Schulman et al., 2002). Depression in older adults has often been found to be associated with vascular brain changes (Snowdon, 2001).

Presentation

The presentation of depression (see Ch. 15) in older age is often less obvious than in younger people as older people will often focus attention on their physical symptoms and are less likely to acknowledge feeling depressed (Snowdon, 2001). Although they may exhibit the cardinal features of depression, such as lowered mood and loss of interest (American Psychiatric Association, 2000), older people will often attribute these feelings to their physical condition rather than to a psychological state.

It is important to interview a spouse or carer as both a corroboration of the service user's history and to substantiate a professional assessment, as well as to gather additional information to assist in the assessment. A spouse or carer will commonly report changes that the individual has not recognized, such as social withdrawal, irritability, avoiding family and friends, poor hygiene and memory change. Losses such as status, income and bereavement can contribute to feelings of dejection (see Ch. 9).

Diagnosing depression in an older population is compounded by the difficulty of differentiating it clinically from dementia and delirium (explored later in this chapter). Depression and dementia may both present with psychomotor slowing, apathy, impaired memory, fatigue, sleep disturbance and poor concentration.

Prevalence

There are varying accounts of the prevalence of depression among people over the age of 65. One in four older people living in the community have symptoms of depression, and the risk increases with age: 40% of people aged 85 years and over may be affected (National Mental Health Development Unit, 2011). Forty per cent of people who live in care homes may be depressed (National Mental Health Development Unit, 2011). Variance in prevalence rates also results from epidemiologists generally only recording cases of major depression and dysthymia. They commonly have not included individuals with minor depression, which is common in old age as a result of a depression arising from functional decline and medical symptoms. Individuals with minor depression may have significant depressive symptoms but not fulfill all the *Diagnostic and Statistical Manual of Mental Disorders*, 4th edn (DSM-IV TR), criteria for major depression or dysthymia (see Ch. 15 for diagnostic criteria). Prevalence rates for depression are approximately 50% higher in women than in men (Bagley et al., 2000).

Aetiology

There is a common perception that older people become depressed as a part of the normal ageing process. This is not so, but older people are vulnerable to experiencing a depressive episode because of age-related biochemical changes and psychological factors. Depression is frequently associated with many common medical conditions found in later life such as stroke, cancer, myocardial infarction, diabetes, rheumatoid arthritis and Parkinson's disease (Snowdon, 2001). Psychological risk factors are bereavement, medications and losses related to physical illness, financial security, accommodation and independence (Bruce, 2002; Norman and Redfern, 1997; Snowdon, 2001). Furthermore, older adults who are institutionalized face a number of changes to their normal routine as they often struggle to adjust to living in an environment with lots of people, noise, rituals and habits that seem strange to them. Such factors may make them vulnerable to mental ill health (Manion and Rantz, 1995). See Chapter 8 for more information about mental health across the lifespan.

Assessment

It is essential that nurses are involved in the assessment of older service users and their psychosocial situations to assist in an early intervention nursing care plan. Assessment and management requires collaboration between health professionals who are skilled and educated in the care and management of older people with mental health problems (Moyle and Evans, 2007). It can be very difficult, especially with older service users, to distinguish between depression and dementia because both conditions share common features such as poor concentration, low mood and social isolation. To make this distinction even more difficult, depression often coexists with dementia. Furthermore, the diagnosis may be hindered where the person also has a physical illness which leads health professionals to believe that the person's depressive symptoms are understandable given their physical status. Undiagnosed and untreated depression places the person at risk of mental suffering, poor physical health, social isolation and suicide.

A depression screening instrument such as the Geriatric Depression Scale (GDS; Yesavage et al., 1983; see Table 13.1) may assist in making the diagnosis, referral for treatment and in providing a baseline assessment against which to measure the effect of treatments. The GDS consists of 30 questions that focus on the individual's thoughts and feelings of depression experienced over the previous week. Unlike other screening instruments the GDS avoids asking questions about physical symptoms, as this generation of people traditionally tends to concentrate on physical symptoms and avoid discussing emotional symptoms. They may also regard the presence of depressive symptoms as a part of their ageing process and neither ask for nor expect help with such symptoms. Where a differential diagnosis cannot be made, psychiatric consultation and/or a trial of antidepressant therapy may be warranted. While cognitive deficits are common in both dementia and depression in older people, they will normally resolve with recovery from depression.

Table 13.1 Geriatric depression scale (GDS)

1. Are you basically satisfied with your life?
2. Have you dropped many of your activities and interests?
3. Do you feel that your life is empty?
4. Do you often get bored?
5. Are you hopeful about the future?
6. Are you bothered by thoughts you can't get out of your head?
7. Are you in good spirits most of the time?
8. Are you afraid that something bad is going to happen to you?
9. Do you feel happy most of the time?
10. Do you often feel helpless?
11. Do you often get restless and fidgety?
12. Do you prefer to stay at home, rather than going out and doing new things?
13. Do you frequently worry about the future?
14. Do you feel you have more problems with memory than most?
15. Do you think it is wonderful to be alive now?
16. Do you often feel downhearted and blue?
17. Do you feel pretty worthless the way you are now?
18. Do you worry a lot about the past?
19. Do you find life very exciting?
20. Is it hard for you to get started on new projects?
21. Do you feel full of energy?
22. Do you feel that your situation is hopeless?
23. Do you think that most people are better off than you are?
24. Do you frequently get upset over little things?
25. Do you frequently feel like crying?
26. Do you have trouble concentrating?
27. Do you enjoy getting up in the morning?
28. Do you prefer to avoid social gatherings?
29. Is it easy for you to make decisions?
30. Is your mind as clear as it used to be?

Scoring for the scale

Score one point for each of the answers given below:

1	no	11	yes	21	no
2	yes	12	yes	22	yes
3	yes	13	yes	23	yes
4	yes	14	yes	24	yes
5	no	15	no	25	yes
6	yes	16	yes	26	yes
7	no	17	yes	27	no
8	yes	18	yes	28	yes
9	no	19	no	29	no
10	yes	20	yes	30	no

Cut-off

Normal: 0–9

Mild depressive: 10–19

Severe depressive: 20–30

The GDS is a public domain scale developed through US Government funding. Information about the scale can be found at http://www.stanford.edu/~yesavage/GDS.html.

The possibility of a depressive episode should be considered in older people if they develop cognitive impairment or anxiety. To assist with the diagnosis of depression in an older person, keep in mind the following when caring for older individuals.

- Check for the presence of depressive symptoms using a screening instrument for this age group, such as the GDS (see Table 13.1).
- Individuals can suffer from depression, a physical disorder and/or dementia, all at the same time.
- Do not assume that symptoms can be easily related to the individual's life circumstances or their age.

Nursing care of people diagnosed with depression

Most depressive disorders in older adults respond to treatment (Snowdon, 2001). However, in older service users diagnosed with severe depression associated with dementia, the prognosis is poor.

Psychotherapeutic support

The most effective treatment for depression is early intervention. Nurses are in a unique and important position within the healthcare team as they have more contact with service users in hospital and community settings, which makes the early recognition of depressive symptoms and early intervention possible. Nurses are invaluable in giving psychotherapeutic support to enable service users to talk about their feelings. Psychosocial therapies such as cognitive therapy (CT), cognitive behavioural therapy (CBT), interpersonal therapy, group therapy and counselling are useful, especially when the depressive episode is loss-related. Cognitive therapy and CBT identify distorted or illogical thinking processes and maladaptive patterns of behaviours and then attempt to replace them with more reality-based thinking and adaptive behaviours (Beck et al., 1979). Interpersonal therapy identifies and modifies interpersonal problems resulting from grief, role disputes and transitions, or interpersonal deficits (see Ch. 23 for more information about these treatment modes).

Pharmacotherapy and electroconvulsive therapy

Pharmacotherapy (e.g. antidepressants, antipsychotics) and electroconvulsive therapy (ECT) may be prescribed and used alone or in conjunction with the psychosocial therapies (see Chs 23 and 24). Although depression may be greatly improved with pharmacotherapy it is imperative that older service users are monitored for medication side effects that can have adverse effects on their cardiac condition. For example, tricyclic antidepressants and monoamine oxidase inhibitors (MAOIs) are known to affect cardiac conduction, rate, contractility and rhythm and may also cause orthostatic hypotension (Slordal and Spigset, 2006). Therefore, monitoring of physical functioning should be incorporated into the nurse's daily routine, and results that deviate from the person's baseline results must be reported. In recent years, selective serotonin-reuptake inhibitors (SSRIs) have been prescribed, as they are known to have fewer cardiac side effects. However, there is always an increased risk of drug interactions when service users are prescribed multiple medications, and older service users who have been associated with the healthcare sector are highly likely to be on a number of medications. It is also important to establish whether service users are using complementary and alternative medications, as some of these (e.g. St John's wort) can cause potentially fatal reactions when taken with antidepressant medication. Ginseng and St John's wort, for example, may cause potentiation of MAOI activity, adverse effects and hypertensive crisis (Holt and Kouzi, 2002). Furthermore, fever, sweating and dizziness can occur as a result of an interaction between SSRIs and St John's Wort (Holt and Kouzi, 2002).

The case study of Linda provides an example of how a depressive episode affects an individual and their family. It also demonstrates the importance of an individualized nursing care plan that focuses not only on the condition but also on preparation for discharge, future rehabilitation and prevention.

CASE STUDY: LINDA

Linda is a 67-year-old married woman. She has spent all her married life helping her husband run a small business in a country town. She has adult children living in the country who she sees frequently. Linda's family brought her to see her GP, although Linda had not wanted to come as she stated she was too tired to go out of the house. Linda's family reported to the GP that she had recently lost interest in everything that she had once enjoyed, such as visiting her grandchildren and entertaining friends and family at home. She had taken to staying in bed until late, not showering and refusing to take part in family activities. Linda was eating very little and had lost a significant amount of weight, and she appeared severely emaciated, her clothes appearing to be several sizes too large for her. Limited communication and retarded motor functioning made communication with Linda difficult.

The GP made an urgent referral to a psychiatrist, who admitted Linda to a mental health facility where she was diagnosed with major depression with severe psychomotor retardation. She had had an admission 13 years previously for the same diagnosis. She was prescribed antidepressants and commenced a course of ECT, as ECT had proved helpful in her previous admission.

The nursing care plan for Linda included spending time with her to establish rapport and trust, and allowing Linda time to respond (this was imperative because of Linda's severe psychomotor retardation). Nurses used CBT to assist Linda to talk about her feelings and helped her to identify distorted or illogical thinking processes, such as her fear that the family business would not be sustainable. CBT helped Linda to replace these illogical ideas with reality-based thoughts and assisted her with new coping strategies. Linda responded well to the treatment and was discharged after 6 weeks into the care of a GP and a community mental health nurse. The long-term plan was for Linda to stay on antidepressants, to undertake regular consultation with her healthcare team and for Linda or her family to report if she again started to feel anxious and depressed, as early intervention was important in keeping Linda well and out of hospital.

CRITICAL THINKING CHALLENGE 13.2

Reflect on the case study of Linda and determine the priorities for Linda's care in the acute stages of her diagnosed disorder and upon admission to hospital. How would the priorities change prior to discharge, so that recovery and the prevention of future episodes of depression can be addressed?

Anxiety disorders

Anxiety disorders (see Ch. 17) and alcohol abuse and dependence (see Ch. 19) are often comorbid with depression in late life (Devanand, 2002). Symptoms of anxiety are commonly associated with major depression, and in older depressed adults there is considerable variability in the severity of the disorder (Flint and Rifat, 1997a). The most common anxiety disorders associated with depression in older adults are generalized anxiety disorder and phobias (Devanand, 2002). Although treatment for depression may reduce anxiety, this is not always the case, with anxiety symptoms persisting despite the resolution of other depressive symptoms (Flint and Rifat, 1997b). Comorbid anxiety disorder with major depression lowers the rate of service user recovery and is also associated with a higher rate of suicide (Coryell et al., 1992).

Suicide

The older service user should be assessed to determine whether they are suicidal at the time of assessment for depression. The risk of successful suicide in the older population is very real and should never be discounted as a possibility. Any talk of suicide by an older individual should be taken seriously and reported to a medical practitioner or specialist services if the service user is in the community, or to senior nursing staff and specialist services if the service user is hospitalized. Never assume because a service user is an older person and hospitalized, or in a nursing home, that they are not capable of hoarding medications to use in a suicide attempt. If the service user offers information about their intended suicide, identifying how, when and by what means the level of risk can be assessed (see Ch. 23 for risk assessment). Personality, physical illness and recent bereavement are known contributing factors to suicide in older people not suffering from diagnosed mental disorders at time of death (Harwood et al., 2006).

Prevalence

Older adults tend to use more violent methods in their suicide attempts and this generally accounts for their high success rates (Snowdon, 1997). In 2009 the overall UK suicide rate was 17.5 per 100 000 for men and 5.2 per 100 000 women (Office for National Statistics, 2011). However, the male suicide rate was lowest amongst those males aged 75 and over at 13.6 per 100 000. Likewise, the female suicide rate for women aged 75 and over was 4.7 per 100 000 (Office for National Statistics, 2011).

Substance misuse

Substance misuse involving illicit drugs is rare in older adults, but dependence on prescription medications such as benzodiazepines is not uncommon (Blixen et al., 1997), as a high proportion of older people experience sleep disturbances for which they seek medication. However, substance misuse in older service users is reported to be under-recognized, under-reported and under-treated (Sivaraman et al., 2011; Weintraub et al., 2002). In the 2009/2010 British Crime Survey, for example, people aged over 59 years were not asked about substance misuse (Sivaraman et al., 2011).

People who abuse alcohol are likely to suffer from significant symptoms of depression (Devanand, 2002). We also know that alcohol and drug misuse are associated with a variety of medical problems and high rates of medical treatment (Moos et al., 1994; Weintraub et al., 2002) and that undiagnosed substance use in older service users may lead to serious withdrawal syndromes during hospitalization (Foy et al., 1997).

Christensen et al. (2006) report the higher rates of alcohol use among older people who experience chronic pain. They recommend that pain assessments are undertaken alongside alcohol screening in older people. It is imperative therefore that nurses assess service users for substance misuse during their preliminary assessment, especially when older service users are admitted for surgery. Rather than asking if a service user drinks alcohol, ask them, 'How much alcohol do you drink per day?'. If they state 'not much' or 'I only drink socially', ask the service user to tell you exactly how much alcohol this involves. From personal experience, older service users could relate that they don't drink 'much', but consider that six bottles of beer and two whiskies a day constitutes being a social drinker! (See also Ch. 19.)

Delirium

Delirium may be defined as 'a disturbance of consciousness … manifested by a reduced clarity of awareness of environment [in which the] ability to focus, sustain, or shift attention is impaired' (American Psychiatric Association, 2000, p. 136). Delirium is a syndrome that constitutes a characteristic pattern of signs and symptoms and can be caused by anything that rapidly damages the brain. The condition is very common in older people, especially those people in hospital or a nursing home. Delirium is also associated with high rates of morbidity.

Differentiating between delirium and dementia can be more difficult in older people (see Table 13.2). Delirium develops over a period of hours to days and tends to fluctuate during the course of a given day. Dementia, on the other hand, is progressive and presents as a gradual failure of brain functioning. The exact nature of the pathophysiology of delirium is unknown. Both cortical and brainstem functions are impaired in delirium, the cortex mediating cognitive function and the brainstem wakefulness. Delirium is ruled out if a dementing syndrome accounts for the disturbance in consciousness. However, it is not unusual for delirium to coincide in people with dementia as a result of a medical condition. In this case the person may present with additional symptoms of short duration that are above and beyond that which can be accounted for by the dementia.

There are few data on the time course of delirium in older service users, possibly because it is often missed unless family or nursing staff are in constant contact with the individual. Most service users have a prodromal stage lasting from a few hours to a day or so. This refers to a change in the person's habitual behaviour and cognitive functioning (sleep disturbance, restlessness and irritability, general malaise and anxiety).

Table 13.2 Comparison of dementia, delirium and depression

	Dementia	Delirium	Depression
Onset	Chronic	Rapid onset, usually hours or days	Often abrupt and may coincide with life events such as death of a loved one
Course	Slow, progressive cognitive failure; symptoms may be worse in evening (sundowning)	Short, diurnal fluctuations in symptoms	Diurnal fluctuations, worse in morning
Duration	Months to years	Hours to days	6 weeks to years
Signs and symptoms	Conscious	Clouding of consciousness	Conscious
	Sleep disturbance is not usually a feature but the sleep–wake cycle may be set at the wrong time frame	Sleep disturbance	Sleep–wake disturbance
	Behaviour tends to be worse in the evening	Fluctuations noted during the course of the day	Selective disorientation
	Aimless wandering or searching	Restless and uneasy	May appear to be 'slowed up'
	Hallucinations are rare	Visual hallucinations that are usually disturbing	Delusions and hallucinations are rare
	Mood may be flattened or labile	Emotional lability and distress	Sad, with feelings of hopelessness and helplessness

It is important to establish early recognition of delirium because if the disease or damage that is causing it can be treated, the confusion will resolve. A midstream urine test should always be carried out if delirium is suspected (NICE, 2011b). Among older service users there may be a tendency for nursing staff to pass off behavioural changes as part of ageing and they may therefore avoid carrying out a thorough assessment. This may result in no treatment or inappropriate treatment being given, whereas if the delirium is related to biochemical changes due to an infection, for example, this could be resolved by a course of antibiotics.

Risk factors

Being older places individuals at risk of delirium. There are also a number of other risk factors that predispose older people to delirium:

- pre-existing brain damage,
- pre-existing dementia,
- sensory impairment.

Additional risk factors are:

- infections, especially urinary tract or chest,
- cardiac failure and other major heart conditions,
- respiratory failure resulting in raised carbon dioxide levels,
- kidney failure resulting in raised levels of protein and urea,
- constipation (although the reason for this has not been established),
- medications,
- drug withdrawal, including alcohol (delirium tremens, DTs).

Prior to an older person undergoing surgery it is important that the nurse assesses the service user to ensure that any changes in behaviour following surgery can be detected and early intervention given. There are two established risk factors for older people undergoing surgery: previous alcohol or drug abuse, and prolonged operating time under a general anaesthetic.

Schizophrenia

Although usually apparent before age 45 years, schizophrenia may be of late onset (Palmer et al., 2002). There is evidence that about 20% of older adults diagnosed with schizophrenia develop symptoms in middle age, known as 'late-onset schizophrenia' (Harris and Jeste, 1988). Service users diagnosed with psychotic disorders have been shown to have a high prevalence of aggressive behaviour (Bowie et al., 2001), which makes the nursing care of these service users challenging.

Antipsychotic medications are generally effective in managing psychotic symptoms, but they are not a cure for this disorder. In recent times, nonpharmaceutical support through therapies such as CBT and social skills training has proved useful to older service users with schizophrenia (Granholm et al., 2002; McQuaid et al., 2000). Although further research is required, nurses may be able to assist older service users diagnosed with schizophrenia using these therapeutic interventions.

The move to reduce the number of long-stay psychiatric facilities has resulted in a greater number of older service users diagnosed with schizophrenia being discharged to nursing homes and other care settings. It is therefore important for nurses working in long-term care to understand this condition and how the service user might react to the transition.

The case study of Lorraine demonstrates the difficulties for care staff when they have limited mental health education and resources to assist the service user, staff and other residents with the transition.

CASE STUDY: LORRAINE

Lorraine is a 76-year-old woman who was recently admitted to a new residential care facility. She has a diagnosis of paranoid schizophrenia and medical diagnoses including diabetes mellitus and ischaemic heart disease. She has had a number of long-term admissions to mental health facilities and has required community support whenever she is out of hospital. Her medical and mental health problems have made it difficult for Lorraine to self-care and she was considered to be at risk if left in the community. She was happy to be admitted to the nursing home, as she felt unsafe in her unit.

Lorraine proved to be a challenge for the nursing home staff, who were not used to having a resident with a diagnosis of schizophrenia. Staff identified that Lorraine lacked insight and that she provoked staff and other residents with inappropriate comments and verbal outbursts. She wanted constant staff attention and if she did not receive this she screamed and demanded attention. Her screaming made staff and residents very uncomfortable, as she would not stop until a staff member paid attention to her and spent time either walking or talking with her. Staff complained that they did not have the time that Lorraine demanded they spend with her. After a week in the facility Lorraine refused to get out of bed, crouching under the bed clothes and stating that no one liked her and that she wanted to go home, where she had friends.

Staff complained that Lorraine was manipulative and they asked not to be her nurse. They openly expressed their dislike of Lorraine, and there were occasions where it appeared that they were either deliberately avoiding her or provoking her as a form of punishment. This resulted in Lorraine's withdrawing from staff and other residents.

Following an assessment of the situation by the care manager, a mental health assessment team was asked to assess Lorraine and to suggest strategies to manage her behaviour. The mental health team suggested the following strategies:

- Provide Lorraine with firm guidance on behaviours which are appropriate to the social setting.
- Reassure her that her needs would be met as soon as possible.
- Acknowledge socially appropriate behaviour.
- Ask her to refrain from making inappropriate comments to other residents
- Use distracting techniques such as walking, music and art.

A staff education programme was commenced with a focus on mental health disorders such as schizophrenia, conflict resolution, CBT and needs-centred care. As staff began to respond more favourably to Lorraine, she also responded more appropriately and there were fewer episodes of inappropriate behaviour.

CRITICAL THINKING CHALLENGE 13.3

Reflect on the case study of Lorraine. Explore in more detail how you would plan, implement and evaluate Lorraine's care. Finally, describe strategies that could be used to help staff adjust to Lorraine's challenging behaviours.

Dementia

Dementia is a neurodegenerative illness which is incurable, characterized by loss of memory, language impairment, disorientation, changes in personality, difficulties with activities of daily living including self-neglect, symptoms of mental disorder (such as apathy, depression or psychosis) and behaviour that is out of character (such as aggression, sleep disturbance or disinhibited sexual behaviour, although the latter is not typically the presenting feature of dementia) (NICE, 2011b).

Published in 2009, the Department of Health's national dementia strategy, *Living Well with Dementia* (Department of Health, 2009), identified dementia as a national priority. It set out three key steps to improve the quality of life for people with dementia and their family and carers:

1. ensure better knowledge about dementia and reduce stigma,
2. ensure early diagnosis, support and treatment for people with dementia,
3. develop services to better meet changing needs (Department of Health, 2009).

The strategy recognized that there remains much ignorance in the UK society about dementia and seeks to raise awareness, inform and educate people about these disorders. It also recognized that many people with dementia do not always get a clinical diagnosis, especially in the early stages of the illness, and so there may be a delay in receiving timely care which could improve a person's quality of life during the initial stages of the disorder (Department of Health, 2009). The strategy has a key objective in encouraging people to seek help when they suspect they are experiencing early symptoms of dementia, and subsequently that they will experience an ease of access to services which can offer them appropriate support and treatment. There is also an emphasis on intermediate care, in assiting people to remain in their own homes for longer.

Prevalence

Dementia is not a normal part of life or ageing. However, the number of people with dementia is increasing in the UK as more people live longer and the prevalence of dementia increases exponentially with age. People in the early stage of dementia usually live in the community. People with higher levels of cognitive loss as a result of dementia are usually accommodated in residential care facilities. In the UK, between 36 and 53% of people who experience mild symptoms of dementia live in the community, while 35% of people with significant needs live at home supported by family and carers (British Psychological Society and Royal College of Psychiatrists, 2007). The overall cost of caring for people with dementia was estimated in 2009 to be £17 billion, rising to a predicted £50 billion in 2038 (Department of Health, 2009).

Dementia affects approximately 5% of people over the age of 65 in the UK, rising to 20% of people aged 80 and over. The estimated UK prevalence rates are 1.4 (males) and 1.5 (females) per 100 people aged 65 and over, rising to 19.6 (males) and 27.5 (females) amongst those aged 85 and over (British Psychological Society and Royal College of Psychiatrists, 2007). It is estimated that between 50 and 64% of people with Alzheimer's disease may have mild to moderately severe symptoms of dementia, while approximately half of people have moderately severe to severe symptoms (NICE, 2011a).

Aetiology

Alzheimer's disease is the commonest form of dementia, followed by vascular dementia (British Psychological Society and Royal College of Psychiatrists, 2007). Many of the remainder suffer from a mixed dementia. As well as Alzheimer's disease and vascular dementia there are other causes of dementia, such as Lewy body type, Parkinson's disease, frontal lobe dementia, physical or toxic damage, genetic disorders, infections, vitamin deficiencies and endocrine disorders. Many older adults with dementia exhibit significant depressive symptoms, and depression may be an early symptom of Alzheimer's disease (Mendez and Cummings, 2003).

Clinical features

The following features should be observed, monitored and treated where appropriate.

- Cognitive abnormalities:
  - memory impairment:
    - demonstrable evidence of impairment of both short- and long-term memory,
    - impairment in abstract thinking;
  - impaired judgement: inability to deduce the consequences of their actions or to make appropriate judgement on how to organize their lives;
  - impaired higher cortical function: aphasia (loss of ability to identify objects by their proper names), apraxia (inability to perform movements when asked), agnosia (difficulty in recognizing parts of one's own body), deficits in constructional ability (inability to assemble objects in their correct spatial relationship to each other);
  - personality change: exaggeration of previous character traits, or a complete change from the individual's former habitual 'state of being'.
- Non-cognitive abnormalities:
  - disorders of mood: depression, anxiety and, rarely, mania,
  - disorders of perception: hallucinations (visual or auditory), misidentifications,
  - delusions: seen in the earlier stages of disease as one requires relatively intact cognitive functioning for delusions.
- Disorders of behaviour:
  - wandering: movement without purpose, or semi-purposeful,
  - aggression: verbal or physical, generalized or focal,
  - inappropriate social or sexual behaviour,
  - restlessness: generalized, constant, purposeless movement.

The above features, and in particular the disorders of behaviour, often result in behavioural problems that are challenging for care staff to manage. An increase in behaviour problems occurring in the evening hours and beginning at a time near sunset has been termed 'sundowning' (Kim et al., 2005). Staff and relatives often report that the individual exhibits an increase in disorientation, restlessness and aggressive behaviour during the evening hours. This increase in disorientation has been attributed to diurnal variations in hormone and light, as well as to fatigue and a search for familiar surroundings in which to rest. However, in some individuals this pattern is reversed: they are more disoriented in the morning. There is also an argument that this could be a socially constructed syndrome created by people around the individual.

Although the cause of sundowning is not known, it is important to assess individuals to help guide the formulation of an individualized care plan. People with dementia are often highly responsive to the environment they find themselves in. Therefore, the environment needs to be made safe, and made familiar with objects that have meaning for the individual (e.g. family photographs). Unnecessary changes to routines should be avoided.

In the mid-1980s Dr Tom Kitwood and colleagues at the Bradford Dementia Group commenced work on a theory of caring for people with dementia that was underpinned by the need to rebalance the 'technical framing' of dementia and complement it with a philosophy that was constructed from 'person-hood' and 'person-centred values' (Kitwood, 1988; Kitwood and Bredin, 1992). Kitwood (1988) argued that dementia is not the problem; rather, it is our inability to accommodate the dementia sufferer's view of the world. Kitwood and Bredin (1992) suggested that this created a 'them and us' dialectic tension, which is sustained by the devalued status of someone who has dementia. Kitwood (1988) argued that the limitations of care environments produced what he termed a 'malignant social psychology'. As a means of addressing this, Kitwood and Bredin (1992) reconceptualized the dementing process along the following lines:

Dementia is viewed as the product of the following elements (P + B + H + NI + SP):

- P: personality, which includes coping styles and defences against anxiety,
- B: biography and responses to the vicissitudes of later life,
- H: health status, including acuity of the senses,
- NI: neurological impairment, separated into its location, type and intensity,
- SP: social psychology, which constitutes the fabric of everyday life.

Pharmacological treatment for dementia

The National Institute for Health and Clinical Excellence (NICE) recommend donepezil, galantamine and rivastigmine as treatment options for people with mild to moderate Alzheimer's disease (NICE, 2011a). These drugs are acetylcholinesterase (AChE) inhibitors which have been shown to improve cognitive function in 50–60% of people diagnosed with Alzheimer's disease (McGleenon et al., 1999). Another drug, memantine, has been recommended by NICE as a treatment option for people diagnosed with severe Alzheimer's disease, or for those who have not been able to tolerate AChE inhibitors (NICE, 2011a). Regular assessment of cognitive function is vital and the use of medication should only continue while it is having a positive effect on cognitive, global, functional or behavioural symptoms.

Concern has been expressed in the last few years about the overuse of medication, particularly antipsychotics, to 'control' behavioural and psychiatric symptoms of dementia (Committee on Safety of Medicines, 2004), with some 180 000 people with dementia being treated with antipsychotic medication in the UK every year (Banerjee, 2009). Whereas some people appear to derive some benefit from this treatment, there also appears to be an increased risk of adverse cerebrovascular events, such as strokes, with the atypical antipsychotics risperidone and olanzapine (Committee on Safety of Medicines, 2004) and implications for patient safety associated with sedation and drowsiness. Overall, it appears that the use of such medication for service users with dementia is limited in terms of its positive effects and has implications for patient safety (Banerjee, 2009).

Pharamacological treatments for specific mental health problems are discussed in the appropriate chapters.

Psychological interventions and therapies for dementia

There are many psychological interventions which can be used to improve the overall health and wellbeing of people with dementia. In the early stages of dementia CBT can assist the person to develop memory improvement strategies. The use of music can be an important form of sensory stimulation and 'reality orientation programmes' have been shown to have some, albeit slight, improvement in cognitive functioning (British Psychological Society and Royal College of Psychiatrists, 2007). Group work can help the person with dementia to mantain social contact and communication skills, and can include a focus on physical activity, reminiscence, arts and crafts. Nursing interventions which seek to support self-care can be an important strategy in assisting the person to maintain their independence. Environmental strategies, such as adapatations for people living at home and use of signposting and orientation aids in hospital and day centre settings and a focus on providing a safe and hygienic environment (including reminders about trip hazards, appropriate footwear and floor surfaces) can also be helpful in maintaining a person's mobility and safety, while reducing their distress (British Psychological Society and Royal College of Psychiatrists, 2007; NICE, 2011b). In later stages of dementia, emphasis may be placed on ensuring a relaxing environment to reduce agitation and distress, including hand massage and aromatherapy (British Psychological Society and Royal College of Psychiatrists, 2007).

When inpatient care is required for people with dementia, NICE recommends that care plans consider:

- 'consistent and stable staffing,
- retaining a familiar environment,
- minimizing relocations,
- flexibility to accommodate fluctuating abilities,
- assessment and care-planning advice regarding activities of daily living (ADL), and ADL skill training from an occupational therapist,
- assessment and care-planning advice about independent toileting skills: if incontinence occurs all possible causes should be assessed and relevant treatments tried before concluding that it is permanent,
- environmental modifications to aid independent functioning, including assistive technology, with advice from an occupational therapist and/or clinical psychologist,
- physical exercise, with assessment and advice from a physiotherapist when needed,
- support for people to go at their own pace and participate in activities they enjoy' (NICE, 2011b, pp. 28–29).

Equally important is the care of carers and families, including an assessment of their own health and social care needs, psychoeducational programmes aimed to increase their understanding of dementia, support and respite care, treatment for anxiety and depression where such problems have been identified, and peer support (British Psychological Society and Royal College of Psychiatrists, 2007). When a person has been diagnosed with dementia, NICE recommends that, unless the person objects, their family should be provided with the following information:

- the course and prognosis of the condition,
- treatments,
- local care and support services,
- support groups,
- sources of financial and legal advice, and advocacy,
- medicolegal issues, such as driving,
- local information sources, including libraries and voluntary organizations (NICE, 2011b).

Psychological intervention treatments for specific mental health problems are discussed in the appropriate chapters.

Comparing delirium, dementia and depression

It is important to differentiate between delirium and dementia so that early intervention for delirium can take place, and to distinguish whether features displayed by an individual are a result of dementia or depression. Any of these conditions may present with very similar features. Table 13.2 provides an overview of the different facets of these conditions. However, service users require adequate assessment in order to establish a diagnosis (see also Ch. 10).

NURSING CARE AND TREATMENT OF OLDER PEOPLE

Mental health initiatives for older people are often vague and unspecific or tend to concentrate on dementia to the exclusion of other mental disorders. There also appears to be a need for greater cohesion of services for older people. A number of nursing interventions have been identified as being of assistance to older people.

- It is important to listen to the individual in an active way, in particular to listen to the feelings and emotions behind the words.
- Encourage older people to participate in physical and social activities that invite them to focus on aspects of their life apart from ill health.
- Assist older people to understand disease processes, how to take medications and to maintain a physically and mentally active lifestyle.
- Help them to select coping strategies to assist them with any losses such as a decline in health or financial status or bereavement.
- If bereavement is a problem, help the person to work through the pain of grief and to adjust to an environment where the deceased is no longer available (see Chs 9 and 10).

These interventions are generalized, and so it is important to evaluate care processes regularly to ensure that the interventions are appropriate for the situation. It is also imperative that healthcare professionals consider the individual's culture, as decisions about care may be affected by cultural differences. For example, some cultural groups may not be willing to seek institutional care for family members as such services may appear to be culturally inappropriate for their needs.

THE NURSE–SERVICE USER RELATIONSHIP

An interactive therapeutic nurse–service user relationship, where the nurse brings a positive approach and attitude to the service user, and nurtures the therapeutic interaction between nurse and service user, will assist the service user's health and wellbeing (Beeber, 1998; Moyle, 1997, 2003). Indeed, 'helpfulness and friendliness are two characteristics that older people value in a nurse as well as warmth, cheerfulness, being decent and kind rather than giving care in a cold, surly, harsh, sharp or stern

manner' (Nursing and Midwifery Council, 2009, p. 17). Professional nursing care is based on a trusting relationship where values are respected as the nurse listens to service user's concerns, provides information and advice, relieves distress by encouraging the expression of emotion, improves service user morale through review of their capacities or satisfaction, and encourages the service user to practise self-help (Beeber, 1998; Evans, 2007). If the nurse–service user relationship develops well it can play a large part in sustaining the service user in the face of their emotional difficulties (see Ch. 2).

The nurse–service user relationship should remain professional. Identification of the nurse–service user relationship with emotion is viewed as being 'over-involved' and not therapeutic. Such an involved relationship may result in the service user being overly dependent on the nurse and losing their self-reliance. However, research findings (Moyle, 1997, 2003) have identified that the therapeutic relationship is a learned skill that does not come instinctively to nurses, and that attention to establishing a therapeutic nurse–service user relationship is required. Nurses will therefore benefit from an education process that both teaches them about the importance of such a relationship and encourages its development.

Maintaining health and function

Nurses can assist older service users in maintaining function by ensuring that service users have small, frequent meals, are well hydrated and maintain bowel function through a high-fibre diet, hydration and exercise. Service users should be encouraged to mobilize and be independent, and the nurse should ensure that they have undisturbed rest and relaxation. Other therapies that nurses may find therapeutic for older service users are hand and back massage, and pet therapy.

CASE STUDY: JOAN

Joan is an 83-year-old woman who has been widowed for 10 years. She lives with her son and daughter-in-law in a granny flat in a section of a large house. Joan has always been active both physically and mentally and has contributed to the running of the household, organizing meals and driving the grandchildren to school or extracurricular activities. Joan is prescribed medication for hypertension, which has been well controlled for the past 3 years.

While taking the youngest granddaughter shopping, Joan had a car accident, hitting a car as she pulled out of the shopping centre car park. Joan was taken to the local hospital accident and emergency department where she was diagnosed with whiplash, a fracture of the lumbar spine and concussion. She was admitted to a medical ward for a period of rest and recuperation. Following admission

Joan became agitated and complained that she felt 'locked up' and started calling out loudly for her son to take her home. She was also incontinent of urine. As this was now late at night and Joan's calling out was disturbing other service users, the nurse organized for Joan to be prescribed 5 mg of haloperidol PRN. This medication appeared to calm Joan, and she soon slept peacefully. Unfortunately, upon waking and in trying to get to the bathroom she fell and suffered a fractured femur of the left leg.

Joan was moved to the orthopaedic ward where she spent several weeks recuperating. During the time in the orthopaedic ward Joan appeared to become more confused and staff complained that she was uncooperative, particularly when bathing and eating. Joan was reluctant to eat the hospital food and was rapidly losing weight. Staff feared that Joan would fall again and nursed her either in bed with bed rails up or in a chair that she was unable to get out of. She was given sedation regularly to keep her settled. Joan had not undergone a mental health assessment during her hospital stay. The health professional focus was on whether her femur was 'mending'. Little consideration was given to a rehabilitation programme as staff had by this stage decided that Joan had been suffering from dementia and that she would require nursing home care. Joan's family did not accept this diagnosis and were concerned to see Joan in such a frail and confused state since her hospital admission. Joan's physical and mental status deteriorated while she was hospitalized until upon discharge she demonstrated a poor ability to self-care, poor mobility and low motivation and cooperation.

When Joan was admitted to the nursing home an assessment of the documentation that arrived with her brought into question whether she had been adequately assessed during her hospitalization. It also appeared that little attention had been paid to developing a rehabilitation plan. It seemed that staff had decided that Joan had a dementing syndrome and felt that there was no chance of her re-entering the community outside a nursing home. At the time of the nursing home admission Joan was given a diagnosis of depression, adjustment reaction and anxiety.

CONCLUSION

The outcome for Joan may have been different if an adequate assessment had been carried out throughout the time of her hospitalization and if a rehabilitation and discharge plan had been encouraged.

CRITICAL THINKING CHALLENGE 13.4

Reflect on the case study of Joan. Examine the care Joan was given and develop a nursing care plan that would allow for the setting of priorities for her rehabilitative process (see Ch. 1 for partnership, self-help, recovery, rehabilitation and service user issues).

STAFF ATTITUDES

Healthcare professionals as well as the public often have negative images of ageing (Moyle, 2003) as well as poor attitudes to and tolerance of mental health problems. It is this negative image of old age and mental health that may prevent the provision of a quality mental health service for older people. It is imperative that staff counter the belief that deterioration in cognitive functioning is a normal part of ageing. This requires a refocusing of attention from disease towards education that promotes older people as skilled and valued human beings. The challenging of poor practice, including negative attitudes and behaviour and the safeguarding of older people is, for the Nursing and Midwifery Council, an important aspect of the professional nursing care of the older person (Nursing and Midwifery Council, 2009). For the Nursing and Midwifery Council, 'The essence of nursing care for older people is about getting to know and value people as individuals through effective assessment, finding out how they want to be cared for from their perspective, and providing care which ensures that respect, dignity and fairness are maintained' (Nursing and Midwifery Council, 2009, p. 6).

Sadly, however, there is evidence of poor service offered by healthcare services and professionals to older people. For example, the term 'confusion' is often used by nurses to describe any number of service user behaviours from inattention to inappropriate vocalization, and the term lacks precision and clarity and may often be used towards uncooperative service users. The case study of Joan demonstrates how poor attitudes can influence both the assessment of and care planning for older service users. The case study also demonstrates the importance of mental health education for nurses working in all settings.

In February 2011, the Parliamentary and Health Service Ombudsman published its investigations into 10 cases of older people in the NHS who have suffered '… unnecessary pain, indignity and distress while in the care of the NHS. Poor care or badly managed medication contributed to their deteriorating health, as they were transformed from alert and able individuals to people who were dehydrated, malnourished or unable to communicate' (Parliamentary and Health Service Ombudsman, 2011, p. 7). Entitled *Care and Compassion?*, the report '… presents[s] a picture of NHS provision that is failing to respond to the needs of older people with care and compassion' (Parliamentary and Health Service Ombudsman, 2011, p. 6). The report, while harrowing and distressing, is required reading for any nurse, who should reflect on their own practice and the practice of others who provide care to vulnerable older people.

CONCLUSION

As people age they experience psychosocial factors such as bereavement and loss of physical and mental functioning. This may place older people at risk of mental disorders and in particular depressive episodes. However, mental disorders are not a normal part of ageing and service users require adequate assessment and diagnosis to ensure that their symptoms are not related to, for example, adverse effects of medications.

The diagnosis, care and treatment of mental disorders in older adults can be difficult. Furthermore, comorbid conditions and negative stereotypical ageist assumptions make treatment and diagnosis especially difficult. Although mental disorders are not a normal part of ageing, older people have a high success rate for suicide, and therefore it is imperative that they are assessed and treated effectively.

Nurses have an important role to play in the assessment, care and treatment of mental health problems amongst older people. Their skills in establishing a therapeutic nurse–service user relationship and in using psychotherapeutic support such as CBT and interpersonal therapy to assist the older service user to recognize distorted or illogical thinking processes and maladaptive patterns of behaviours resulting from grief, role disputes and transitions, or interpersonal deficits, can, along with pharmacotherapy, improve the older service user's quality of life. Although depression is the most prevalent diagnosed mental disorder among older people, it is also a treatable condition. The establishment of a nurse–service user relationship provides the opportunity for nursing staff to recognize the symptoms of depression and to suggest further assessment and treatment if required.

EXERCISES FOR CLASS ENGAGEMENT

Discuss the following with your group or class members.

- Document and discuss the differences between delirium and dementia in relation to time course, cause and clinical features.
- Identify the risk factors for delirium and discuss how you might assess for delirium.

- Why is it important to consider the diagnosis of delirium and dementia when care planning?
- Explore the reasons that it is difficult to differentiate depression clinically from dementia and delirium.
- How might the symptoms of depression affect the relatives and friends of the depressed older person?

REFERENCES

American Psychiatric Association, 2000. Diagnostic and Statistical Manual of Mental Disorders, fourth ed. text rev. American Psychiatric Association, Washington DC.

Bagley, H., Cordingley, L., Burns, A., et al., 2000. Recognition of depression by staff in nursing and residential homes. J. Adv. Nurs. 9 (3), 445–450.

Banerjee, S., 2009. The use of antipsychotic medication for people with dementia: time for action. <http://www.dh.gov.uk/prod_consum_dh/groups/dh_digitalassets/documents/digitalasset/dh_108302.pdf>.

Bartels, S.J., Smyer, M.A., 2002. Mental disorders of aging: an emerging public health crisis? Generations 26 (1), 14–20.

Beck, A.T., Rush, A.J., Shaw, B.F., et al., 1979. Cognitive Therapy

of Depression. Guilford Press, New York.

Beeber, L.S., 1998. Treating depression through the therapeutic nurse–client relationship. Nurs. Clin. North Am. 33 (1), 153–172.

Behrens, H., 1998. Ageism: real or imagined? Elder. Care 10 (2), 10–13.

Blixen, C.E., McDougall, G.J., Suen, L.J., 1997. Dual diagnosis of elders discharged from a psychiatric hospital. Int. J. Geriatr. Psychiatry 12 (3), 307–313.

Bowie, C.R., Moriarty, P.J., Harvey, P.D., et al., 2001. Aggression in elderly schizophrenia patients: a comparison of nursing home and state hospital residents. J. Neuropsychiatry Clin. Neurosci. 13 (3), 357–366.

British Psychological Society and Royal College of Psychiatrists, 2007. Dementia: the NICE–SCIE guideline

on supporting people with dementia and their carers in health and social care. <http://guidance.nice.org.uk/nicemedia/live/10998/30320/30320.pdf>.

Bruce, M.L., 2002. Psychosocial risk factors for depressive disorders in late life. Biol. Psychiatry 52, 175–184.

Butler, R., 1975. Why Survive? Being Old in America. Harper & Row, New York.

Christensen, H., Low, L., Anstey., K., 2006. Prevalence, risk factors and treatment for substance abuse in older adults. Curr. Opin. Psychiatry 19, 587–592.

Committee on Safety of Medicines, 2004. Atypical antipsychotic drugs and stroke. <http://www.mhra.gov.uk/home/groups/pl-p/documents/websiteresources/con019488.pdf>.

Coryell, W., Endicott, J., Winokur, G., 1992. Anxiety syndromes as epiphenomena of primary major depression: outcome and familial psychopathology. Am. J. Psychiatry 149 (1), 100–107.

Department of Health, 2009. Living well with dementia. <http://www.dh.gov.uk/prod_consum_dh/groups/dh_digitalassets/@dh/@en/documents/digitalasset/dh_094051.pdf>.

Devanand, D.P., 2002. Comorbid psychiatric disorders in late life depression. Biol. Psychiatry 52 (3), 236–242.

Djernes, J.K., 2006. Prevalence and predictors of depression in populations of elderly: a review. Acta Psychiatr. Scand. 113 (5), 372–387.

Evans, A.M., 2007. Transference in the nurse–patient relationship. J. Psychiatr. Ment. Health Nurs. 14, 189–195.

Flint, A.J., Rifat, S.L., 1997a. Anxious depression in elderly patients: response to antidepressant treatment. Am. J. Geriatr. Psychiatry 5 (2), 107–115.

Flint, A.J., Rifat, S.L., 1997b. Two-year outcome of elderly patients with anxious depression. Psychiatry Res. 66 (1), 23–31.

Folstein, M.F., Folstein, S.E., McHugh, P.R., 1975. Mini-Mental State: a practical method for grading the state of patients for the clinician. J. Psychiatr. Res. 12, 189–198.

Foy, A., Kay, J., Taylor, A., 1997. The course of alcohol withdrawal in a general hospital. Q. J. Med. 90 (4), 253–261.

Granholm, E., McQuaid, J.R., McClure, F.S., et al., 2002. A randomised controlled pilot study of cognitive behavioural social skills training for older patients with schizophrenia. Schizophr. Res. 53 (1/2), 167–169.

Harris, M., Jeste, D., 1988. Late-onset schizophrenia: an overview. Schizophr. Bull. 14 (1), 99–113.

Harwood, D., Hawton, K., Hope, T., et al., 2006. Suicide in older people without psychiatric disorder. Int. J. Geriatr. Psychiatry 21 (4), 363–367.

Holt, G.A., Kouzi, S., 2002. Herbs through the ages. In: Bright, M.A. (Ed.), Holistic Health and Healing. E A Davis, Philadelphia. pp. 135–160.

Karlin, N.J., Emick, J., Mehls, E.E., et al., 2005. Comparison of efficacy and age discrimination between psychology and nursing students. Gerontol. Geriatr. Educ. 26 (2), 81–96.

Kim, P., Louis, C., Muralee, S., et al., 2005. Sundowning syndrome in the older patient. Clin. Geriatr. 13 (4), 33–36.

Kitwood, T., 1988. The technical, the personal and the framing of dementia. Soc. Behav. 3, 161–180.

Kitwood, T., Bredin, M., 1992. Towards a theory of dementia care: personhood and well-being. Ageing Soc. 12, 269–287.

Lawlor, B., Radic, A., 1994. Prevalence of mental illness in an elderly community-dwelling population using Agecat. Ir. J. Psychol. Med. 11 (4), 157–159.

McGleenon, B., Dynan, K., Passmore, A., 1999. Acetylcholinesterase inhibitors in Alzheimer's disease. Br. J. Clin. Pharmacol. 48 (4), 471–480.

McQuaid, J.R., Granholm, E., McClure, F.S., et al., 2000. Development of an integrated cognitive-behavioural and social skills training intervention for older patients with schizophrenia. J. Psychother. Pract. Res. 9 (3), 149–156.

Manion, P.S., Rantz, M., 1995. Relocation stress syndrome: a comprehensive plan for long-term admissions. Geriatr. Nurs. 16 (3), 108–112.

Martell, R., 1999. Students shun elderly care despite enjoying placements. Nurs. Stand. 14 (8), 8.

Mendez, M., Cummings, J., 2003. Dementia: A Clinical Approach. Butterworth Heinemann, Philadelphia, pp. 477–502.

Moos, R.H., Mertens, J.R., Brennan, P.L., 1994. Rates and predictors of four-year readmission among late-middle aged and older substance abuse patients. J. Stud. Alcohol 55, 561–570.

Moyle, W., 1997. On being nurtured while depressed. Unpublished PhD thesis, Centre for Mental Health Nursing, QUT, Brisbane.

Moyle, W., 2003. Nurse–patient relationship: a dichotomy of expectations. Int. J. Ment. Health Nurs. 12 (2), 103–109.

Moyle, W., Evans, K., 2007. Models of mental health care for older adults: a review of the literature. Int. J. Older People Nurs. 2, 132–140.

Murray, J., Banerjee, S., Byng, R., et al., 2006. Primary care professionals' perceptions of depression in older people: a qualitative study. Soc. Sci. Med. 63 (5), 1363–1373.

NICE (National Institute for Health and Clinical Excellence), 2011a. Donepezil, galantamine, rivastigmine and memantine for the treatment of Alzheimer's disease. <http://guidance.nice.org.uk/TA217/Guidance/pdf/English>.

NICE (National Institute for Health and Clinical Excellence), 2011b. Dementia: supporting people with dementia and their carers in health and social care. <http://guidance.nice.org.uk/nicemedia/live/10998/30318/30318.pdf>.

Nadler-Moodie, M., Gold, J., 2005. A geropsychiatric unit without walls. Issues Ment. Health Nurs. 26, 101–114.

National Mental Health Development Unit, 2011. Management of depression in older people: why this is important in primary care. <http://www.nmhdu.org.uk/silo/files/management-of-depression-in-older-people.pdf>.

Norman, I., Redfern, S., 1997. Mental Health for Elderly People. Churchill Livingstone, New York.

Nursing and Midwifery Council, 2009. Guidance for the care of older people. <http://www.nmc-uk.org/Documents/Guidance/Guidance-for-the-care-of-older-people.pdf>.

Office for National Statistics, 2010. Ageing. <http://www.statistics.gov.uk/cci/nugget.asp?id = 949>.

Office for National Statistics, 2011. Suicide rates in the United Kingdom, 2000–2009. <http://www.statistics.gov.uk/pdfdir/sui0111.pdf>.

Palmer, B.W., Folsom, D., Bartels, S., et al., 2002. Psychotic disorders in late life: implications for treatment and future directions for clinical services. Generations 26 (1), 39–43.

Parliamentary and Health Service Ombudsman, 2011. Care and compassion? Report of the Health Service Ombudsman on ten investigations into NHS care of older people. <http://www.

ombudsman.org.uk/__data/assets/
pdf_file/0016/7216/Care-and-
Compassion-PHSO-0114web.pdf>.

Robinson, A., Cubit, K., 2005. Student
nurses' experiences of the body in
aged care. Contemp. Nurse 19 (1/2),
41–51.

Schulman, E., Gairola, G., Kuder,
L., et al., 2002. Depression and
associated characteristics among
community-based elderly people.
J. Allied Health 31 (3), 140–146.

Sivaraman, P., Wattis, J., Curran, S.,
2011. Substance misuse in the
elderly. Geriatr. Med. 41, 289–296.

Slordal, L., Spigset, O., 2006. Heart
failure induced by non-cardiac
drugs. Drug Saf. 29 (7), 567–586.

Snowdon, J., 1997. Suicide rates and
methods in different age groups.
Australian data and perceptions.
Int. J. Geriatr. Psychiatry 12 (2),
253–258.

Snowdon, J., 2001. Late-life depression:
what can be done? Aust. Prescr.
24 (3), 65–67.

Stevens, J., Crouch, M., 1992. Working
with the elderly: do student nurses
care for it? Australian J. Adv. Nurs.
9 (3), 12–17.

Weintraub, E., Weintraub, D., Dixon,
L., et al., 2002. Geriatric patients
on a substance abuse consultation
service. Am. J. Geriatr. Psychiatry
10 (3), 337–342.

Yesavage, J.A., Brink, T.L., Rose, T.L.,
1983. Development and validation
of a geriatric depression rating scale:
a preliminary report. J. Psychiatr.
Res. 17, 27.

Chapter | **14** |

Schizophrenic disorders

Murray Bardwell and Richard Taylor

CHAPTER CONTENTS

CHAPTER POINTS

- Schizophrenia is considered one of the most debilitating of the range of mental disorders prevalent in society.
- Schizophrenia as a mental disorder is poorly understood, although current and future research may shed greater light on its neuroanatomical causes.

DOI: http://dx.doi.org/10.1016/B978-0-7020-4493-9.00014-7

- Stress can be a trigger for those predisposed to mental health problems.
- Recognizing and understanding the impact of the prodromal phase of schizophrenia may enable better clinical outcomes for future management of this disorder.
- Treatment regimens that include behavioural and cognitive therapies combined with pharmacological therapies are likely to have better outcomes in the management of this disorder.
- The burden of the disorder and the associated stigma in schizophrenia make this one of the most socially debilitating conditions.
- Homelessness and schizophrenia are closely intertwined and prevalent in our society.

KEY TERMS

- affect
- agranulocytosis
- akathisia
- ambivalence
- apathy
- autism
- avolition
- blunted affect
- catatonia
- concrete thinking
- delusion
- dystonia
- echolalia
- echopraxia
- extrapyramidal adverse reactions
- hallucination
- ideas of reference
- incoherence
- loose associations
- neologism
- negative symptoms
- paranoia
- positive symptoms
- premorbid
- psychosis
- regression
- relapse
- schizophrenia
- tardive dyskinesia
- thought blocking
- thought disorder

LEARNING OUTCOMES

The material in this chapter will assist you to:
- define the term 'schizophrenia',
- discuss biological and environmental theories on the development of schizophrenia,
- distinguish the presentations of the prodromal, acute and chronic phases of schizophrenia,
- identify the major pharmacological strategies in the treatment of schizophrenia, their target symptoms and their major adverse effects,
- identify non-pharmacological strategies in the treatment of schizophrenia,
- distinguish the role of the nurse in the management of individuals diagnosed with schizophrenia,
- identify education strategies that may be employed in psychoeducation of the individual and family.

INTRODUCTION

Schizophrenia is one of the most debilitating and misunderstood of all mental health problems. Throughout history, schizophrenia has been feared, despised and misunderstood. People experiencing the effects of what we now know as schizophrenia have been burned at the stake as witches, imprisoned and held up for ridicule. Although our society no longer burns witches at the stake it could be argued that very little else has changed. It is still common in a society rich in health information for people to erroneously equate schizophrenia with split personality. Usually within this misunderstanding is the belief that behind the seemingly decent person known to have this disorder is an evil monster that ought to be feared (Schulze and Angermeyer, 2005). It is not uncommon for mental health professionals to be asked whether they think a person may have schizophrenia because they are agreeable one minute and hostile the next. The popular film industry occasionally features a character with schizophrenia, but such characterizations fail to accurately depict the manifestations of this disorder and its painful effects and more often than not perpetuate the common myths and stereotypes that surround this disorder. Children's television has been shown to convey negative images of those with mental disorder and has been implicated in the early socialization of children into the stereotyping of people with mental health problems (Wilson et al., 2000). The stigma that results becomes yet another burden that sufferers have to endure.

Gaining an understanding of schizophrenia can be a challenging and frightening experience. This chapter attempts to provide some insight into the condition and articulates the role of the nurse in helping the individual diagnosed with schizophrenia to reach their optimal level of health.

PREVALENCE

Schizophrenia is a disorder characterized by a major disturbance in thought, perception, cognition and psychosocial functioning and is one of the most severe mental disorders. Estimated prevalence rates vary widely between countries. The World Health Organization (WHO) estimates a worldwide prevalence rate of 0.7% or 7 per 1000 of the adult population. Schizophrenia is found in approximately 0.4% of the adult UK population (age 16–64; Office for National Statistics, 2001). In the USA the prevalence is thought to be 1.1% of the adult population (National Institute of Mental Health, 2009). The total societal cost of schizophrenia in England alone is estimated at £6.7 billion, including direct costs of treatment and indirect costs arising from, for example, unemployment, welfare payments and loss of productivity (British Psychological Society and Royal College of Psychiatrists, 2010).

Schizophrenia is not spread evenly throughout the population. Its onset tends to occur among those between the late teenage years and early adulthood (approximately 18–24 years of age). The diagnosed condition also tends to be more prevalent among the socially disadvantaged. The homeless population is one example where there are higher diagnosed rates of the condition (Caton, 1997). Caution needs to be observed in interpreting these social patterns. There is debate over whether the experience of the disorder results in a decline in the individual's social condition or whether the social disadvantage increases the likelihood of experiencing the disorder (Caton, 1997).

For many, especially the homeless and the destitute, access to much-needed healthcare remains a major issue. Of those who can access mental health services, many experience difficulties arising from the often serious and debilitating adverse reactions of medications required to manage their disorder. Adherence with treatment may be problematic and many choose to cease taking medication, which often results in a return to severe mental disorder and repeated admissions. This tragic pattern is commonly referred to in mental health contexts as revolving-door syndrome. There is room for optimism, however, brought about by greater emphasis on treatment of people living with schizophrenia in the community and on advances in pharmaceuticals. Schizophrenia should not be thought of as a single disorder or as a personality deficit. Schizophrenia is a complex syndrome with many varieties and symptoms that remains poorly understood by the community.

AETIOLOGY

Research has yet to determine the exact cause of schizophrenia. Researchers are increasingly turning to neurobiological explanations and away from psychodynamic explanations (Birtwistle and Baldwin, 1998; Sharma and Murray, 1993). Put simply, schizophrenia is more commonly viewed as a disorder of neurological functioning than a disorder of the mind. In all probability the cause of schizophrenia lies in a complex interaction between multiple combinations of genetic and environmental factors: for example, exposure to infection during gestation or birth (Brown, 2006; Venables et al., 2007), which may interfere with normal brain development and function. This complex interplay results in the constellation of behaviours collectively known as the 'schizophrenias' (Andreasen, 1999; Geddes and Lawrie, 1995; Levinson et al., 1998; Munk-Jorgensen and Ewald, 2001).

The fact that the brains of those diagnosed with schizophrenia differ from those without the disorder is now largely undisputed (Coffey, 1998; Cotter and Pariante, 2002). How or why these aberrations in brain biochemistry and anatomy affect the functioning of the brain remains a mystery, as does the reason that these abnormalities appear to remain dormant until late adolescence in most individuals (Cotter and Pariante, 2002).

Biological theories

The three most commonly discussed biological causative factors are brain anatomy, genetics and brain biochemistry. It would be erroneous to consider these three factors as mutually exclusive. Far more likely is the existence of a relationship between the three; for example, some as-yet-unidentified pattern of inheritance may predispose an individual to differences in anatomy or fluctuations in neurotransmitter biochemistry (Lewis and Murray, 1987, cited in Coffey, 1998).

Neuroanatomical abnormalities

Schizophrenia is often referred to as a neuropsychological disorder, which implies that the origins of the psychological disturbance lie in the neurological structure and function of the brain. Commonly, but not conclusively, modern imaging techniques reveal lower brain tissue volume and higher cerebrospinal volumes (Salokangas et al., 2002). Precisely how or why these changes occur is unknown. It is commonly thought that either genetics or environmental factors during gestation are responsible for the brain abnormalities, with the effects remaining dormant until adolescence. In contrast to this commonly held notion, some research suggests that the brain changes occur as a result of the disorder and may occur during or shortly after the first episode of psychosis (Lawrie et al., 2002). Clearly, a great deal more research between abnormal brain anatomy and schizophrenia is required. Both Farrison (2000) and Coffey (1998) cite a number of literature reviews that suggest that it is still too early to state conclusively that neuroanatomy is the causative factor in schizophrenia.

Genetic predisposition

As with neuroanatomical explanations, genetic explanations are far from conclusive. What seems most likely is that an individual's genetic make-up leaves them vulnerable to the development of the disorder to some degree. In other words, we inherit a certain level of risk for developing the disorder rather than inheriting the disorder itself. What seems apparent, however, is the pattern whereby the person who is most at risk of developing schizophrenia is the person who shares the most genes with a person with the disorder. That is, a person with a family member with schizophrenia is at higher risk of developing the disorder than a member of the general population.

The prevalence of schizophrenia in the UK is approximately 0.4%. This means that on average 4 in 1000 people are living with the symptoms of schizophrenia. It should be noted that this average figure has been shown to vary widely, depending on a range of environmental circumstances. A person is more likely to be diagnosed with schizophrenia, for example, if they grow up in an urban environment, belong to a lower socioeconomic group or were born in winter or spring (Haukka et al., 2001; Munk-Jorgensen and Ewald, 2001; Suvisaari et al., 2002; van Os, 2000). Nevertheless, symptoms of schizophrenia tend to be found in individuals who have relatives with schizophrenia. Individuals are far more likely to show symptoms of schizophrenia if one or more parents have the disorder (Birtwistle and Baldwin, 1998; Kety et al., 1994). This pattern is also found if an identical twin has been diagnosed with the disorder (Birtwistle and Baldwin, 1998; Kety et al., 1994) or if a fraternal twin or a nontwin sibling has a similar diagnosis (Birtwistle and Baldwin; 1998). The probabilities associated with the above patterns fail to follow any known pattern of inheritance. As a result it is suggested that a number of genes across a number of chromosomes could contribute to vulnerability to the disorder (US Department of Health and Human Services, 1999).

Biochemical theories

Biochemical theories share the belief that chemicals responsible for the transmission of nerve impulses across the synapse may be responsible for the development of schizophrenia. These chemicals are known as neurotransmitters. The most discussed theory on brain biochemistry involvement in schizophrenia relates to an abnormal amount or action of the neurotransmitter dopamine in the brain of the individual diagnosed with schizophrenia (Kapur and Seeman, 2001; Rivas-Vazquez, 2003). This theory is often referred to as the *dopamine hypothesis*, and it remains inconclusive despite the fact that it has been one of the most widely accepted theories for many years.

In very simple terms, the theory is a mix of known facts and hypotheses. The first of these facts is that antipsychotic medications such as chlorpromazine and thioridazine act by blocking some of the dopamine receptor sites in the brain and therefore the amount of effective dopamine is reduced (Birtwistle and Baldwin, 1998; Farrison, 2000; O'Connor, 1998). These medications also reduce symptoms such as hallucinations and paranoia.

A second fact is that certain substances, amphetamines in particular, increase the dopamine action and also mimic some of the symptoms of schizophrenia (Birtwistle and Baldwin, 1998). Where the theory is reduced to hypothesis and supposition is in the area of symptoms, such as lack of social interest (commonly referred to as negative symptoms). Until recently the antipsychotic medications such as those mentioned previously have had an effect on symptoms such as delusional thinking and hallucinations (commonly referred to as positive symptoms). It seems that dopamine excesses may only be responsible for part of the constellation of features in schizophrenia, namely the positive symptoms.

Similarly, negative symptoms are not produced by stimulants such as amphetamines, which are associated with dopamine excesses. In essence, dopamine-blocking agents are only effective in treating some aspects of the disorder. It is logical to assume therefore that the dopamine hypothesis only partially explains the symptoms commonly seen in schizophrenia.

It is recognized that serotonin, another commonly found neurotransmitter, may also be significant in the development of schizophrenia (Blin et al., 1996). A broad group of drugs collectively known as the atypical antipsychotics became increasingly popular in the early 1990s. Among this group are drugs such as clozapine, olanzapine and risperidone. These drugs block both serotonin and dopamine receptors and have been shown to be more effective in the treatment of many individuals suffering from schizophrenia and other schizophrenia-like psychoses. Whereas drugs such as the typical antipsychotic group almost exclusively target positive symptoms, the atypical antipsychotics are also effective against negative symptoms (Birtwistle and Baldwin, 1998). They are named 'atypical' because they contrast with the more conventional drugs such as chlorpromazine and thioridazine in their action and pharmacology.

The stress-diathesis model

The stress-diathesis model seeks to bring much of what is known about the cause of schizophrenia together into one model of understanding. The basic assumption behind the stress-diathesis model is that individuals are exposed to stressful events in the course of their lives and that these events may precipitate symptoms in some people who have a predisposition to mental health problems

(Zubin and Spring, 1977). Essential to this theory is the notion that some people are more vulnerable to mental disorder than others. In the case of schizophrenia this vulnerability may be related to genetics, environmental factors, aberrations in brain anatomy or biochemistry or, more likely, a combination of all these things (van Heeringen, 2000). Weisman (2005) expanded the understanding of the role of family as part of an individual's environment by examining the literature in this area. She asserts that a sufferer's family and home environment has the potential to affect the course of the disorder. More specifically, families that show high levels of expressed emotion, typified by excessive criticism, hostility or emotional over-involvement, do less well than families with patterns of relating that are not high in expressed emotion. The importance of this model and its more contemporary redevelopment, known as the stress-vulnerability-protective factors model, to clinical practice is the fact that it suggests a range of appropriate actions, from targeting vulnerable but as yet asymptomatic individuals through to symptom reduction by medication (Kopelowicz et al., 2003) and possibly family therapy and counselling (Weisman, 2005). Despite the fact that the stress-diathesis model of schizophrenia has merit, in that it integrates much of what is known, it still fails to bring us closer to a detailed understanding of schizophrenia (Hammen et al., 2000).

CRITICAL THINKING CHALLENGE 14.1

How might the stress-diathesis model explain the high rates of mental disorder among our society's homeless population?

DIAGNOSTIC CRITERIA

Diagnostic and statistical manual of mental disorders

The *Diagnostic and Statistical Manual of Mental Disorders* (4th edn, text revision), or DSM-IV TR (American Psychiatric Association, 2000), is a highly detailed listing of mental disorders and their corresponding diagnostic criteria. The benefit of the manual is that it allows clinicians to be consistent in their use of the term 'schizophrenia'. Because mental health problems have few, if any, laboratory tests or other diagnostic procedures that can either confirm or refute a diagnosis, the means available to make psychiatric diagnoses is through detailed history taking and skilled observation. The data gained from these processes are then measured against the diagnostic

criteria stated in the DSM-IV TR (American Psychiatric Association, 2000). In simple terms, the DSM-IV TR describes the clinical presentation that needs to exist for a diagnosis of schizophrenia to be made. This allows for common and consistent understandings in diagnosing the disorder of schizophrenia.

Although the term schizophrenia suggests a single disorder, schizophrenia is more accurately viewed as a constellation of conditions, with a number of common features along with differences that allow subtypes to be recognized. These features and differences are described by the DSM-IV TR (American Psychiatric Association, 2000) as follows.

A. Characteristic symptoms of schizophrenia

At least two of the following, which have been present during a period of 1 month:

1. delusions,
2. hallucinations,
3. disorganized (incoherent or erratic) speech patterns,
4. behavioural disturbance (catatonia or disorganization),
5. negative symptoms (blunting of affect or avolition).

If the delusions are considered bizarre, or if the hallucinations consist of a voice that makes a running commentary on the person's thoughts and actions, or if multiple voices are heard conversing with each other, then only one criterion from A is required.

B. Social/occupational dysfunction

Since the onset of symptoms there needs to be a noticeable impairment in the areas of work, relationships and self-care. If the onset occurs in childhood or adolescence, this impairment may be seen as a decline in academic performance as well as occupational and interpersonal relationships.

C. Duration

There needs to be evidence that the disturbance has existed for at least 6 months. Within this 6-month period the individual needs to display symptoms as listed in A.

D. Excluding other diagnoses

Other disorders such as mood disorders or schizoaffective disorder need to be excluded. The possibility that the individual may be affected by drugs or other general medical conditions needs to be excluded. If there is a history of autistic disorder or another pervasive developmental disorder, delusions and/or hallucinations need to also be present for at least a month (or less if treatment has been successful).

Schizophrenia subtypes

a. Paranoid type

This subtype is associated with a slightly later onset (twenties to thirties). Often there is no history of impairment in social or occupational functioning. Paranoid delusions and unfounded suspiciousness are dominant features, along with hallucinations and ideas of reference. The disorganization of behaviour and social functioning is often absent, as are affective disturbances. This subtype is one of the more common presentations of schizophrenia. The individual suffering from this disorder often performs quite well socially and occupationally. Often there is consistency between the hallucinatory material and the delusional thinking. For example, an individual may be suspicious of his or her neighbour. The individual may be experiencing hallucinatory voices that serve as a warning that he or she is in danger. Consistent with this hallucinatory material, the individual may believe that the neighbour is a spy. In addition to delusions of persecution, the individual may begin to feel that he or she has some special social or religious significance. These feelings then result in secondary delusions of a grandiose or religious nature.

It is understandable that if a person suffering from this subtype feels under threat with enough conviction they may resort to litigation or violence in order to defend themselves (American Psychiatric Association, 2000).

b. Catatonic type

Far less common than paranoid schizophrenia is the subtype of schizophrenia known as catatonia. The most obvious characteristic is severe and debilitating disorganization of motor behaviour. In general the condition comes in two forms. The first, where motor excitation is present, results in excessive and purposeless behaviour that is unrelated to the external environment. This form places the individual in danger of exhaustion, dehydration or injury from an impulsive act. The second form results in severe disturbance in voluntary motor behaviour, resulting in behaviours that include:

- negativism (resistance to instructions),
- mutism (where a person normally capable of speech is unable to do so),
- catalepsy (waxy flexibility),
- maintenance of rigid postures,
- echolalia (involuntary repetition of other people's verbalizations),
- echopraxia (involuntary repetition of other people's actions).

This form of catatonia can be so debilitating that it gives the individual an appearance of being unconscious. However, it has been found that the individual has a full awareness of the environment and often recalls events that occurred during this period of apparent unconsciousness (American Psychiatric Association, 2000).

c. Disorganized type

The disorganized type of schizophrenia is characterized by disinhibited, disorganized and regressive behaviour. The onset of the disorder is usually in the early twenties. The person's activities are described as purposeless and nonconstructive. Their affect is described as garrulous and inappropriate, marked by bouts of unstimulated laughter and grimacing. In lay terms, people experiencing this disorder are often described as 'silly' in their behaviour and appearance. The extreme levels of disorganized thought and behaviour make meaningful occupational activity, such as work or study, difficult or impossible.

In the disorganized type of schizophrenia the following criteria are met:

- disorganized speech,
- disorganized behaviour,
- flat or inappropriate affect, and the criteria for catatonic type are not met (American Psychiatric Association, 2000).

d. Undifferentiated type

In the undifferentiated type of schizophrenia, symptoms meet criterion A, and the criteria are not met for the paranoid, disorganized or catatonic type (American Psychiatric Association, 2000). This diagnosis is used where the symptoms do not have a strong pattern belonging to any one particular subtype of schizophrenia.

e. Residual type

Residual-type diagnosis is used when the symptoms are not of a sufficient intensity to be attributed to any other subtype. Emotional blunting, alogia, eccentric behaviour and illogical thinking mark the disorder. Positive symptoms of hallucinations and delusions are less prominent in this disorder and, if they do occur, they do not carry the same affectual disturbance.

The following criteria relate to the residual type:

- absence of prominent delusions, hallucinations, disorganized speech and grossly disorganized or catatonic behaviour,
- there is continuing evidence of the disturbance, as indicated by the presence of negative symptoms or two or more symptoms listed in criterion A for schizophrenia, present in an attenuated form (for example, odd beliefs, unusual perceptual experiences) (American Psychiatric Association, 2000).

HISTORICAL DEVELOPMENT IN UNDERSTANDING SCHIZOPHRENIA

Identifying and labelling the constellation of features now known as schizophrenia commenced in 1856 when Francois Morel used the term 'dementia praecox' (meaning precocious or early dementia) during the treatment of a young male experiencing the effects of mental disorder. The link that Morel, and later Emil Kraepelin (in 1902), made with their use of the word 'dementia' is interesting, as it is deliberate. By linking dementia with psychotic features, Kraepelin saw more than a causal link to his theory that the disorder was neurologically based, like forms of dementia, and also that the clinical pathway led to deterioration and chronicity, similar to dementia (Kaplan and Sadock, 2005). Collectively this view was far from optimistic and left minimal hope for the individual's recovery. What makes Kraepelin's theory interesting is the fact that contemporary research is beginning to demonstrate neurological links to the causation of schizophrenia (van Heeringen, 2000).

In comparison was the contribution made by Eugen Bleuler, as it was he who coined the term 'schizophrenia'. The term comes from two Greek words: schizo meaning 'split' and phrenia meaning 'mind'. The term refers to the disintegration and disjointedness of the personality and its associated functions such as mood display, speech and thought. Bleuler's approach diverges from Kraepelin's in a number of respects. Bleuler was more inclined to focus on the presentation of the disorder and classify it according to what could be observed, rather than the approach Kraepelin founded, which centred more on the course of the disorder. Bleuler was influenced strongly by the works of Sigmund Freud and consequently saw the disorder as a problem of mind and personality. Hence he saw it as a functional disorder rather than an organic one related to neurological dysfunction (Kaplan and Sadock, 2005). While Bleuler's work has contributed significantly to the understanding of the clinical picture of schizophrenia, the very name and the Greek meanings of the two words that make up this name have in many respects muddied the lay understanding of the disorder. Despite a great deal of media publicity and education, the common misunderstanding of the disorder is of split or multiple personality.

Although significantly divergent, the approaches of Kraepelin and Bleuler continue to contribute to the understanding of schizophrenia in contemporary society. Kraepelin's notion that the disorder has a biological basis continues to be researched and is most favoured as an explanation of causation even if not entirely proven or understood. His rather pessimistic outlook on the course of the disorder also remains valid for many individuals with schizophrenia despite major developments in the treatment of this disorder. Bleuler, on the other hand, simplified the identification of symptoms with his easily remembered 'four As':

- autism: the individual's tendency to retreat into an inner fantasy world, resulting in socially isolating or withdrawing behaviours and loss of contact with reality,
- ambivalence: the individual's tendency to hold conflicting views and feelings such as love and hate, rendering meaningful decision making difficult,
- affective disturbance: the individual's marked alteration in ability to express congruent emotions and affect,
- associative looseness: the individual's gross disturbance in ability to think logically and rationally and to decipher between related and unrelated thought processes (Kaplan and Sadock, 2005).

Bleuler was also associated with widening the diagnostic criteria, resulting in greater numbers of diagnoses. As a result more people were diagnosed and more people recovered, which may have given rise to greater levels of optimism (Healy et al., 2001).

CONTEMPORARY UNDERSTANDING OF SCHIZOPHRENIA

Prodromal phase

The initial markers of schizophrenia often develop in early adolescence. This development is poorly understood and even more difficult to identify. However, with hindsight, once the disorder has become severe enough to be diagnosed, prodromal features become identifiable and significant as the precursors of this disorder.

Although the prodromal features of schizophrenia are vague, nonspecific research has shown four central features relating to this period of the disorder. Davidson et al. (1999) identified deterioration from a previous level of functioning in the following areas:

- social functioning,
- organizational functioning,
- intellectual functioning,
- physical activity.

Acute phase

Schizophrenia has characteristic psychotic symptoms during the acute phase of the disorder which subside with treatment. The predominant presentation is a group of symptoms that alter the individual's perception of the world in such a way that it affects function in the context of society and environment. The person diagnosed with this disorder usually functions below a level previously achieved. Early manifestations may include poor or deteriorating school performance, poor social relations, decreased self-care and a failure to achieve expected milestones in childhood. In addition to the decline in social and occupational performance common to the prodromal phase of the disorder, the individual may present with all or some of the symptoms listed in Table 14.1.

Table 14.1 Commonly experienced symptoms: acute phase of schizophrenia	
Symptom	**Description**
Content of thought	
Delusion	Fixed belief that is inconsistent with one's social, cultural and religious beliefs which cannot be reasoned with by the use of logic Delusions that are multiple, bizarre and fragmented
Persecutory delusion	Belief that others are spying on them, spreading false rumours or planning to harm them
Ideas of reference	Belief that an insignificant or incidental object or event has special significance or meaning to that individual A common experience of ideas of reference is the perception that the newsreader on television is talking to the individual personally.
Thought disorder	
Thought insertion/ thought broadcasting	The feeling that one's thoughts are being read, or that people are taking the thoughts from one's head away or that one's feelings, impulses and actions are not their own but imposed by some external force
Loosening of associations	Ideas that fail to follow one another with a logical flow and sequence. This results in shifting from one subject to another, resulting in loss of significant meaning.
Incoherence	Verbal rambling in which recognition of any specific verbal content is impossible. May present with neologisms, clang associations and thought blocking.
Perceptual disturbances	
Auditory hallucinations	The hearing of voices that are coming from outside the person's head Voices may be familiar and usually comment on the person in a derogatory fashion. Voices that comment on the person's behaviour Voices that command a behaviour
Other hallucinations (less common)	Can involve any of the other senses
Affect	
Emotional blunting	Being 'flat' or inappropriate. Voice is a monotone, and the face is immobile.
Anhedonia	Loss of the feelings of pleasure previously associated with favoured activities
Incongruent affect	A mismatch between the person's thoughts and their emotional expression in a given situation. For example, a person may feel under great threat, but appear amused by the situation.
Psychomotor behaviours	
Catatonia	Some service users may become so withdrawn that they appear unconscious. It is believed that the person is so grossly involved in their delusional thinking and preoccupation that they are no longer capable of relating to external stimuli.

NURSE'S STORY: PRODROMAL

When I recall my school days, I think of a particular individual with whom I went to secondary school. At the time I would have described him as different rather than odd. He never fully engaged with others either individually or in a group and he certainly never initiated such engagement, yet when invited to participate in social activities he was quite capable of doing so. It seemed that despite engaging with others, as soon as he got the chance to return to a state of detachment from the larger social group, he took it. Although the term 'odd' would be too strong a word, his whole demeanour, including how he held himself, how he dressed and what occupied his time, seemed very distant from the rest of us. When I recall his schoolwork ability, nothing exceptional comes to mind.

Years later, as a psychiatric nurse, I was witness to his admission to the psychiatric facility in which I worked. He had been diagnosed with schizophrenia. When I recall my school days with him, I now understand the reasons he appeared strange and different. There was a very good chance that he had experienced prodromal features of schizophrenia during those days at school.

Chronic phase

Table 14.2 lists commonly experienced symptoms in the chronic phase. The more frequently occurring symptoms of schizophrenia can also be divided into two groups:

- Positive symptoms: thought processes, emotions and behaviours that appear as part of the onset and experience of the disorder. In other words,

Table 14.2 Commonly experienced symptoms: chronic phase of schizophrenia

Symptom	Description
Limited social engagement	The loss of drive toward developing and sustaining stimulating and rewarding social relationships. The person becomes reclusive.
Avolition	The loss of motivation resulting in impairment in goal-directed activity. This affects personal hygiene, attention to nutrition, occupation and work, and physical activity.
Alogia Poverty of ideas Poverty of speech	Tends to be limited in conversation and has a minimal number of topics or issues to think about or discuss. Tends to be short in response to questions, often favouring monosyllables.

Table 14.3 Positive and negative symptoms of schizophrenia

Positive symptoms	Negative symptoms
Hallucinations	Loss of energy (anergia)
Delusional thinking	Loss of drive (avolition)
Severe thought-process disturbance	Loss of living skills Blunted affect Loss of the experience of pleasure (anhedonia)

they are present in the person experiencing schizophrenia but absent in the person not experiencing the disorder.

- Negative symptoms: thought processes, emotions and behaviours that were present prior to the onset of the disorder but have since diminished or are absent following the onset of the disorder. In other words, they are present in the person without the disorder but absent or diminished in the person with the disorder. This is illustrated by examples in Table 14.3.

NONPSYCHOPHARMACOLOGICAL TREATMENT

Cognitive behavioural therapy

Cognitive behavioural therapy (CBT) interventions are ideally suited to the individual in the later stages of recovery or as maintenance when they are well. CBT should be delivered on a one-to-one basis over at least 16 planned sessions (NICE, 2009) with the aim of supporting people to:

- establish links between their thoughts, feelings or actions and their current or past symptoms and/or functioning,
- re-evaluate their perceptions, beliefs or reasoning related to the target symptoms,
- monitor their own thoughts, feelings or behaviours with respect to their symptoms or recurrence of symptoms,
- promote alternative ways of coping with the target symptoms,
- reduce distress,
- improve functioning (NICE, 2009, p. 12).

The underlying assumption behind CBT is that individuals can positively influence their symptoms by changing their behaviour and thinking. Moreover, the symptoms currently experienced are the result of habits in thinking and behaviour learned in the past and have a detrimental effect in the present (Turkington et al., 2002). The approach to therapy therefore is to unlearn the destructive ways of the past and replace them with more constructive approaches for the future.

CBT has no adverse effects, unlike antipsychotic medication, and has the potential to go on assisting the individual long after the symptoms subside and the therapy ceases (Tarrier et al. 1998, cited in Turkington et al., 2002). It can occur in highly systemized and comprehensive programmes, or it can occur at a very individual and informal level. The following are examples of how CBT may be used.

CBT interventions for hallucinations

Example: a person who hears frightening hallucinations while travelling on public transport may discover that listening to music through headphones and a portable music player can drown the voices out. In addition, the person can be encouraged to view the hallucinations as part of a disorder that can be managed and that these voices are harmless.

CBT interventions for delusional thinking

Service users experiencing delusional thinking can be encouraged to explore the content of these delusions. Delusional thinking may involve the belief that the neighbours are spying on the service user. The person may be encouraged to modify their thinking so that they view their neighbour's actions as being motivated by concern rather than malice. Getting to know and trust the neighbours may be a solution. It must be acknowledged that because of the nature of delusional thinking this approach may or may not be successful and in all likelihood will take a significant amount of time to be successful.

CBT interventions for stress and stigma

Many individuals diagnosed with schizophrenia live with the stigma associated with the disorder and as a result have poor self-esteem. CBT focuses on the person's strengths and abilities, which in turn improves self-esteem and goal achievement.

There has long been a belief that schizophrenia and psychosis along with other mental disorders may be a maladaptive and destructive response to poorly managed levels of stress (Kaplan and Sadock, 2005). This belief forms the basis of the stress-diathesis model of causation. CBT is effective in identifying stressors in an individual's life, ways of avoiding excessive stress and solutions to various unavoidable stressful situations.

RESEARCH BRIEF: CBT

In a British study a group of researchers studied the effects of CBT using a randomized trial involving over 400 service users divided into two groups. One group received CBT from suitably trained community mental health nurses in addition to their standard treatment. The other (control) group received their standard treatment. The findings of the study showed that CBT had the potential to increase the individual's level of insight and that this could be achieved safely and effectively.

Source: Turkington et al. (2002).

CRITICAL THINKING CHALLENGE 14.2

Why is CBT likely to be more successful in the late stages of recovery of schizophrenia than earlier in the treatment?

Supportive therapy

People who suffer from schizophrenia may experience additional impairments. These impairments relate largely to issues of everyday life, which the unaffected person seems to carry out with relative ease. Impairments arising from schizophrenia include impaired ability to perceive one's external social environment accurately, resulting in feelings of threat or peril, diminished ability to relate to others socially and to maintain relationships, poor self-esteem and failure to experience the range of normal emotions.

The role of supportive therapy in managing impairments arising from schizophrenia is considered just as important as treating the symptoms of the disorder and is central to any treatment regimen. The treatment approach in supportive therapy is based on the establishment of a therapeutic relationship that addresses individual needs. This reality-orientated approach enables the individual to explore aspects of their beliefs that are based in reality. Nursing interventions in supportive therapy for the management of schizophrenia are listed in Table 14.4. However, it must be pointed out that more research is needed to demonstrate the value of this approach to the service user's recovery (NICE, 2009).

Family intervention

Family intervention should be offered to families of people diagnosed with schizophrenia (NICE, 2009). (Families are considered those people who have a significant emotional connection to the service user, such as parents, siblings and partners.) There is strong evidence that family support and intervention can reduce replase rates, improve

Table 14.4 Nursing interventions

Service user's issue	Nursing management
Delusional thinking	Assess the risk the delusional thinking poses to self or others and take appropriate action to prevent such a threat, e.g. continuous close observation or use of *as-required* (PRN) antipsychotic medication. This action is designed to reduce the chances of the person acting on the delusional thinking.
	Attempt to understand the content of the delusional thinking. Delusional thinking often provides a clue to themes occurring in the person's thinking. It also acknowledges that the nurse believes the delusions are real to the service users. This conveys a concerned understanding and assists the development of trust.
	Don't reinforce delusional thinking by agreeing with the ideas presented and at the same time don't argue or attempt to prove their belief is false by using logic. Avoiding these approaches assists the service user in testing reality by using the nurse's system of beliefs as a reference point.
	Provide a quiet and peaceful environment if delusional thinking is increasing, and reduce or eliminate environmental factors that appear to be stimulating delusional thinking, e.g. television or radio.
Auditory hallucinations	Assess the extent and content of auditory hallucination.
	If the hallucinations are commanding certain actions, assess the degree to which these commands compel the person to act. Assess especially the impact of such commands on personal safety. Such hallucinations may pose threats to safety and require accurate assessment and immediate nursing intervention by way of *as-required* medication and close observation.
	Reassure the service user that hallucinations are a part of the disorder and cannot be heard by the nurse. This assists the service user to test reality.
	Identify with the service user activities that appear to stimulate hallucinations and devise ways of coping with such situations.
	Identify with the service user actions that reduce the impact of hallucinations, such as listening to music through headphones.
	Strategic use of as-required medication when hallucinations are most distressing.
Fear/anxiety/paranoia	Assess for the level of fear, anxiety or paranoia experienced.
	Reassure the service user that the environment is safe and that no harm will come to them.
	Be aware of your own behaviour and how it could be misinterpreted. Ensure that the nurse's approach is quietly confident, and mindful of the service user's need for an enlarged personal space.
	Don't touch the service user, as this could be interpreted as an attack.
	Don't whisper or laugh in the presence of the service user, as this may be misconstrued as being relevant to them.
	Strategic use of *as-required* medication when fear/anxiety/paranoia are escalating and distressing.
Disordered thinking	Assess the content and extent of disordered thinking.
	Assess the degree to which thought disorder affects the service user's activities of daily living.
	Speak using clear, unambiguous language as this facilitates clearer understanding.
	Assess the effectiveness of medications in the reduction of disordered thinking.
	Diversional activities may need to be tailored to the individual's ability, given the difficulties experienced as a result of disordered thought. Going for a walk may be more appropriate than a game of cards.
	Assess the impact that the level of environmental stimuli is having on the person's ability to think clearly, and modify the level of stimuli as needed.

(continued)

Table 14.4 Continued

Service user's issue	Nursing management
Lack of insight	Assess the service user's level of understanding of the disorder and the situation they are currently facing.
	Provide information about the disorder as appropriate given the service user's level of wellness.
	Reinforce the need to take antipsychotic medication according to medical instructions. One of the most common factors in nonadherence of medication regimens is lack of insight. This has a major impact on the person's prognosis.
Poor personal hygiene	Assess the service user's ability to meet their hygiene needs. Their current level of personal hygiene may be useful as an indicator.
	Assist the service user to meet their hygiene needs.
	Encourage/remind the service user to meet their hygiene needs to the best of their ability. Because service users have such difficulty in thinking clearly at times, personal hygiene is often neglected. In addition, a good level of personal hygiene would decrease the likelihood of the person experiencing harmful social rejection.
Inadequate nutritional intake	Assess hydration and nutritional status.
	Assess the degree to which poor nutritional intake is related to paranoid delusional thinking. Often service users have a fear that their food is poisoned or contaminated. This can be overcome by a number of nursing actions, which may include the service user assisting in the preparation of their food or using prepackaged tamper-proof food.

outcomes and treatment adherence among service users and reduce the burden of care (NICE, 2009). Support for families to cope with their relatives' mental health problem can include education, problem-solving techniques, methods of managing crises, reducing distress and improving communication. NICE (2009) suggest that family interventions should wherever possible:

- include the service user if practical,
- include at least 10 planned sessions over a period of 3 months to 1 year,
- take into account preference for single-family rather than multifamily interventions,
- take into account the relationship between the main carer and the service user,
- have a specific supportive, educational or treatment function,
- include negotiated problem-solving or crisis-management work.

PSYCHOPHARMACOLOGICAL INTERVENTION

A student studying mental health nursing or gaining clinical experience in specialist mental health facilities would find it hard to comprehend what it might have been like prior to the development of antipsychotic or neuroleptic drugs. In the era prior to the availability of effective drug treatments for people with mental disorders they were housed in large, harsh institutions offering little hope for recovery. It is even harder to imagine what life would have been like for individuals experiencing schizophrenia without any effective treatment. Yet this was the reality until the 1950s when the first of the antipsychotic medications were used in treatment of people with mental health problems.

In the 1950s a French surgeon, Henri Laborit, used the antihistamine drug chlorpromazine to reduce the amount of general anaesthesia required by his service users during surgery. He knew that complications following surgery were often a result of the anaesthetic agent. Chlorpromazine calmed the individual preoperatively, and so, when undergoing surgery, they required less anaesthesia and suffered fewer complications. It was reasoned that the calming effect of chlorpromazine might have application in the field of psychiatry, where there was a desperate need for effective drug treatments. Chlorpromazine was trialled successfully and the age of effective psychopharmacology was born (Keltner and Folks, 2005). Chlorpromazine, although rarely used these days, became the first of many drugs belonging to the phenothiazine group. The phenothiazines belong to a group of drugs collectively known as typical antipsychotics or conventional antipsychotics and include thioridazine, trifluoperazine and fluphenazine. Although not offering hopes of cure, they offered successful management of the symptoms of schizophrenia where this had previously been problematic. Although their use has been associated with problematic adverse reactions, the phenothiazines offered hope of successful management of the disorder and independent living.

In 1990 a new class of drugs emerged – the atypical antipsychotics – which promised less serious adverse effects than the phenothiazines and were more effective in treating psychotic disorders in both the early and residual stages (Muller et al., 2002). The superiority of these atypical antipsychotics in their therapeutic effect is subject to debate, however. What remains undisputed is their reduced adverse effects (Gardner et al., 2005). The first of these, clozapine, had been around since the 1960s but its habit of causing bone marrow suppression and resultant agranulocytosis, a blood disorder characterized by severe depletion of white blood cells, rendering the body almost defenceless against infection, ruled it out

as a drug with widespread practical application. Recent technology, however, has made monitoring and detection of blood dyscrasias more reliable. For many the benefits of this drug outweigh the risks, provided regular blood tests are undertaken. It now has its place as an intervention in treating schizophrenia and is especially effective in the treatment of negative symptoms of schizophrenia (Gardner et al., 2005; Oyewumi and Al-Semaan, 2000). Other drugs commonly referred to as atypical antipsychotics include risperidone, amisulpride, quetiapine and olanzapine.

CASE STUDY: JIM

Jim is a 20-year-old man with a recent history of unusual and disturbed behaviour. Jim's parents had become increasingly concerned about him to the point of contacting their GP, who in turn made the referral to the community mental health team.

RECENT HISTORY

Jim had spent his first semester at university and had lived at home for the past 2 months. At home his activities had been limited to lounging, listening to music, sleeping and eating from the refrigerator at night. He would then leave without tidying up after himself. This behaviour was unlike Jim, according to his parents. They stated that although quiet and pleasant in disposition normally, this considerate young man had undergone significant change in his personality in recent times.

However, it was a more significant behaviour witnessed by Jim's parents that gave rise to the referral. According to his parents, when Jim was spoken to about his behaviour he became defensive and verbally abusive. At one stage he threatened physical violence.

A community mental health nurse scheduled a meeting with Jim and his parents at his home.

ASSESSMENT INTERVIEW

A psychiatrist and a mental health nurse interviewed Jim. The assessment revealed a young man in quite a poor state of personal hygiene. His clothes were wrinkled as if he had been sleeping in them and a noticeable body odour was

present. Although cooperative throughout the interview, at times he appeared a little restless when questioned and often asked if he was legally compelled to answer the question. He appeared to be reassured that the questions were only to ascertain what sort of help would be required.

In conversation Jim appeared monosyllabic, with slowed speech that appeared to lack energy. His affect was flat and he admitted to having difficulty concentrating. He was asked if he had been hearing voices. To this he replied that he had and that they were making disparaging comments about him. When asked if he had an explanation for this, he replied that he hadn't but thought one of the voices was a female teacher from his school days. He then asked if the room was covered by video surveillance equipment, as he could feel its radiation. Further probing into his thought processes revealed experiences where Jim would walk past shop windows and see warning signs. An example he gave was of a female shop attendant wearing a red shirt.

As the level of risk appeared low and Jim was cooperative it was felt that twice-daily visits by the community mental health nurse were appropriate. The psychiatrist made a diagnosis of acute paranoid schizophrenia. Jim was commenced on:

- risperidone IM depot, 25 mg fortnightly,
- olanzapine 5 mg twice per day,
- procyclidine 5 mg *as required*.

(Refer to Ch. 24 for information about these medications.)

CRITICAL THINKING CHALLENGE 14.3

In Jim's case study, indicate the lifestyle changes Jim will need to undertake in order to return to a well state.

What advice would the family need in relation to their care of Jim?

What information would Jim need in relation to the commencement of his medication regimen?

Design a psychoeducation package that will assist Jim in understanding his mental health issue(s).

Goals of antipsychotic medication administration

The goals of antipsychotic drug administration are essentially twofold. The first is to control the symptoms of schizophrenia, particularly delusional thinking, bizarre behaviour, hallucinations, agitation and feelings of paranoia. While the typical antipsychotic medications are effective at combating these positive symptoms, they are less effective at targeting the negative symptoms such as emotional blunting, avolition, loss of energy and social withdrawal. In fact, these drugs can make such features

See also Box 14.1.

Box 14.1 Service users' education guidelines prior to commencement of antipsychotic medication

- It is important to take medication as prescribed.
- Inform service users of the likelihood of being on medication for a significant length of time.
- Antipsychotic medications commonly cause adverse reactions and these can be discussed with the mental health professional.
- Some medications cause sedation and fatigue, so great care must be taken when driving or operating heavy machinery.
- Medication will need to be reviewed if service user becomes pregnant.
- Medications interact with alcohol. Alcohol is best avoided when taking these medications.
- Do not mix illicit drugs (amphetamines, narcotics, etc.) with antipsychotics.
- If a dose is missed, wait until the next dose is due. Don't double up.
- Do not stop taking the medication simply because of feelings of good health. These medications are necessary to maintain good health. Not taking medication as prescribed creates the risk of relapse.
- Regular blood tests may be required if clozapine has been commenced.

Table 14.5 Adverse effects of antipsychotics

Peripheral nervous system effects	Dry mouth
	Headache
	Constipation
	Urinary hesitancy
	Photophobia
	Decreased lacrimation
	Sexual dysfunction (impotence, ejaculatory delay)
Central nervous system effects	Sedation
	Parkinsonian effects
	Akathisia
	Lowered seizure threshold
Severe adverse effects	Neuroleptic malignant syndrome
	Tardive dyskinesia
	Agranulocytosis
	Acute dystonic reaction (spasm)
Other effects	Photosensitivity
	Retinal deterioration
	Weight gain
	Hormonal interference (galactorrhoea, gynaecomastia, hypoglycaemia, hyperglycaemia)
	Anti-emetic effects

worse in some cases. In contrast, some of the atypical antipsychotics, clozapine in particular, are equally effective in combating both positive and negative symptoms (Gardner et al., 2005). The broader action of atypical antipsychotics has contributed to their use as the first choice in treatment. Achieving this goal would allow the individual to return to life much as it was prior to the onset of the disorder. See also Box 14.1.

The second goal is to prevent the relapse of the disorder. The period in which maintenance doses of medication will be required varies from individual to individual. The general guidelines suggest that for an individual who has experienced a single episode of psychosis, medication may be required for 1–2 years. For those who have experienced two or more severe episodes, a 5-year period of constant medication may be indicated (McGrath and Davies, 1999).

To continue taking medication that causes a wide range of unpleasant adverse reactions (see Table 14.5) long after the symptoms of the disorder have gone can take a large leap of faith. It is no surprise that many individuals fail to comply with taking their antipsychotic medication over the long term.

Adverse effects

An electrocardiogram (ECG) should be considered before a person commences antipsychotic medication, particularly if the person is at risk of cardiovascular disease (such as a diagnosis of high blood pressure or personal history of cardiovascular disease) or if the person is being admitted as an inpatient (NICE, 2009).

Weight gain

This is more likely to occur with clozapine and olanzapine but is also associated with chlorpromazine (Gardner et al., 2005).

Nursing interventions

Stress the importance of activity and exercise. Assess current dietary intake and suggest modifications if required.

Parkinsonian effects

These include a blank, mask-like expression, salivary drooling, noticeable tremor in the limbs, muscle rigidity, stiffness and a shuffling gait.

Nursing interventions

Reassure the service user that these adverse reactions subside with time (McCabe, 2002). Monitor for parkinsonian effects and administer anticholinergics as prescribed and as-required medication.

Akathisia

Akathisia is commonly referred to as restless leg syndrome. Those who experience it find it difficult to sit or sleep. Both activities are interrupted by the incessant urge to move the limb or to change positions.

Nursing interventions

Contact the physician, who may need to change the antipsychotic drug if adverse reactions cannot be tolerated. Anticholinergics may ameliorate adverse reactions.

Neuroleptic malignant syndrome

Neuroleptic malignant syndrome is the most serious and life-threatening adverse reaction to antipsychotic drugs. It generally develops in the first week or two following commencement of medication but has been known to occur at any time while the individual is taking the drug. It is usually associated with higher-potency typical antipsychotics such as haloperidol (Murty et al., 2002).

Symptoms are a combination of hyperthermia, severe motor rigidity and disturbances in levels of consciousness and cardiovascular functioning, blood pressure in particular and, more specifically, sweating, pyrexia, hypotension, tachycardia, stupor and muscular rigidity. It is a medical emergency with a mortality rate of 20–30%. Its overall incidence is unclear but is in all probability around 0.1–1% (Keltner and Folks, 2005). Treatment requires immediate cessation of the antipsychotic drug and referral to a physician.

Nursing interventions

If neuroleptic malignant syndrome is suspected, antipsychotics must be ceased immediately. Vigilance for the syndrome is essential, especially for those who are taking high-potency drugs such as haloperidol. Ensure effective levels of hydration are maintained. Should the syndrome develop, nursing care consists of monitoring and reduction of body temperature.

Tardive dyskinesia

Tardive dyskinesia literally means 'late-occurring movement disorder'. It is a devastating and possibly irreversible adverse reaction to long-term antipsychotic medication (Kane et al., 2002). The condition is associated particularly with high-potency drugs such as haloperidol. The effects can range in severity from mild to incapacitating and include uncontrollable coarse tremor, spasm-like movements of body, arms and legs, rolling of the tongue and smacking of the lips. It continues long after cessation of antipsychotics and is often made worse by the administration of antiparkinsonian drugs such as benzatropine.

Nursing interventions

Assess for involuntary movements and suspect tardive dyskinesia. Refer to physician for the possibility of lowering dosage. For long-term takers of antipsychotics, periodic tapering off of the dose is useful to assess the need for ongoing medication.

Acute dystonic reaction (spasm)

Muscle spasms are seen in the body trunk and the neck (opisthotonos and torticollis) and on occasion these spasms result in the eyes rolling up in a terrifying and uncontrollable fashion (oculogyric crisis). The most dangerous and life-threatening form occurs when the muscles surrounding the larynx spasm, resulting in airway occlusion. This is a medical emergency.

Nursing interventions

The development of this frightening and potentially fatal adverse effect warrants swift nursing intervention. Acute dystonic reactions respond swiftly to intravenous, intramuscular or oral (route depends on the level of acuity) administration of antiparkinsonian drugs such as benztropine (McCabe, 2002). This should be followed by careful observation. In the case of laryngeal spasm the service user may require airway support and oxygen therapy until it resolves.

Medication adherence

The reasons for nonadherence to medication regimens instituted in the care of people suffering from schizophrenia are abundant. Schizophrenia is a debilitating disorder that affects occupational, social and cognitive functions. Pharmaceuticals largely used to treat the disorder cause many adverse reactions, which add another layer of disability to be faced by the individual. Against such a backdrop, many individuals choose to be noncompliant. Some individuals diagnosed with schizophrenia do not have the insight to draw a relationship between the medications and the maintenance of a well status and often will cease taking their medications. Secondly, some individuals cannot understand the reasons for taking medication or the frequency with which they need to take it.

In some cases the clinicians have not provided the necessary education so that service users can be informed of medication regimens. Some clinicians treat service users in an authoritarian and paternalistic way, so genuine cooperation between clinician and service user is not maintained. Long-acting depot drugs allow an individual to receive just one injection every week or couple of weeks. One of these, long-acting resperidone, has been shown to be effective in reducing the severity of the disorder as well as fostering better compliance (Jarboe et al., 2005).

CRITICAL THINKING CHALLENGE 14.4

How can nurses encourage greater levels of adherence with antipsychotic medication among individuals diagnosed with schizophrenia?

LIVING WITH SCHIZOPHRENIA

Homelessness

Having a safe home that is conducive to a sense of security and wellbeing is an essential human need. Yet this need goes unmet for a great number of individuals diagnosed with schizophrenia, the most common serious mental disorder among the homeless (Teesson and Buhich, 1990). Studies have shown that mental disorder and homelessness are interrelated in a number of ways. First, with a disorder like schizophrenia, the positive symptoms often result in disruption of home life and destruction of relationships. Positive symptoms may affect the relationship between an individual with schizophrenia who is a tenant and the owner of a property, in some cases resulting in eviction of the individual with the disorder. Secondly, negative symptoms often affect the individual's ability to form and maintain attachments with others (Opler et al., 1995). Coupled with negative symptoms is the inability to work, which may result in failure to meet commitments associated with tenancy and mortgage repayments.

However, this is not the only way in which mental disorder and homelessness are related. For some, mental disorder develops after the person becomes homeless and is probably associated with the immense stress associated with the conditions of homelessness: frequent assaults, rapes, robberies, malnourishment, lack of supports and lack of access to health services, to name a few. Clearly, suffering from the symptoms of schizophrenia and being homeless is destructive. According to the literature, death rates for those who find themselves in both situations is four times that of the general population and twice that of those experiencing schizophrenia but who have a home (Folsom and Jeste, 2002). The great challenge for mental health policy makers and clinicians is to provide comprehensive healthcare to the homeless group with mental health problems and to promote access to housing and health agencies for individuals suffering from symptoms of schizophrenia.

Work

Work, education and socioeconomic status are key aspects of most people's lives and those who have experiences with schizophrenia often suffer significant disruption and disadvantage. Lack of employment opportunities represents yet another form of social exclusion facing those experiencing the effects of schizophrenia (Marwaha and Johnson, 2004). Unemployment rates run as high as 70% in those who experience psychoses (Office for National Statistics, 2001). Of those who are engaged in employment, when ill a significantly large period of time is lost to sick leave. There is a great need for research into the area of the beneficial effects of work on those who have been diagnosed with schizophrenia as well as the factors that either facilitate or inhibit finding work or returning to work.

Many people who have experienced severe breakdown as a result of schizophrenia have resumed their lives and returned to work. This is not easy to achieve but it can be facilitated by easing back into work on a part-time basis. Often the transition back into work is easier if voluntary work is undertaken initially. In most cases the employer is responsible for the provision of a workplace that is both safe and free from adverse responses from the employer and other employees. This is often difficult given the societal stigma that a disorder such as schizophrenia carries.

Labelling and stigma

The stigma associated with mental disorder is profoundly debilitating to the individual with schizophrenia. Those experiencing the effects of stigma have been known to say that they are as bad as the effects of the disorder itself (Access Economics, 2002). Mental disorder continues to bring a sense of shame on the individual and, in some cases, their family, and the family is often blamed for its development. Phil Barker makes some sound philosophical statements regarding this issue when he states that '…people are not the problem—the problem is the problem' and 'the person who has a problem with schizophrenia, or depression, or obsessional thoughts, is neither morally responsible for the problem, nor possessed of some fundamental flaw' (Barker, 1999, p. 119). Stigma and discrimination also serve as barriers to enjoying aspects of a fulfilling life, such as being in paid employment (Marwaha and Johnson, 2004). In Western society, despite major education campaigns people still consider individuals diagnosed with schizophrenia as unpredictable and dangerous. Although those diagnosed with schizophrenia are more likely to be violent than those without such a diagnosis (Citrome and Volavka, 1999; Walsh et al.,

2002), the overall contribution to the violence found in society by those diagnosed with schizophrenia is small. Furthermore, studies have shown that violence is more closely linked to other mental disorders such as personality disorders and mood disorders than to schizophrenia (Harris et al., 1993).

Even when no harm is intended, the word 'schizophrenia' is often misused and misrepresented. Attempts have been made, however, to challenge public perception of mental health problems. For example the Time to Change campaign, led by the UK mental health charities Mind and Rethink Mental Illness, has sought to increase the public's awareness of issues relating to mental health and to challenge stigma, discrimination and prejudice (see http://www.time-to-change.org.uk/home). While medical and nursing organizations and governments attempt to demystify the disorder, various media portrayals often use the term 'schizophrenic' to describe difficult and socially inappropriate behaviours that happen in the community. The term is used by the layperson as a way of conceptualizing aberrant behaviour that they may not fully understand. This is a means of explaining behaviours that they find difficult or impossible to understand by any other means.

Unfairly, when an individual diagnosed with schizophrenia shows symptoms during a public incident, the media tend to emphasize this. For example, when an individual is experiencing psychotic behaviour (such as hallucinations and delusions) in a way that affects others in the community (intrusive or aggressive) the media tend to sensationalize such events. Furthermore, Nairn (2005) analysed mass media in a study and found that few ever reported the views of those with a mental disorder. According to the authors the consumers' views are seldom heard. Lee (2002) notes that even if psychiatric stigma is concealed, it remains a constant source of psychic pain to individuals diagnosed with schizophrenia. In the depths of their disorder the individual rarely has the opportunity to concentrate on societal norms such as appropriate dress, social etiquette and personal hygiene because of the intensity of their symptoms. In addition, some of the medications used to treat schizophrenia have adverse effects which affect the person's gait, for example, serving to further identify and alienate the individual experiencing the disorder.

CRITICAL THINKING CHALLENGE 14.5

There appears to be an historical, ingrained societal perception that individuals diagnosed with schizophrenia are violent or otherwise dangerous. In the past, attempts have been made to explain the behaviours of society's most dangerous members as having a basis in mental

disorder (for example, the killings by Thomas Hamilton in Dunblane, Scotland, in 1996). In more recent times, on 16 April 2007, Seung-Hui Cho, a Korean student studying in the USA who was allegedly armed with a firearm, opened fire at Virginia Tech, a US university campus, killing 32 and wounding a further 25 before turning the gun upon himself. Having come to the attention of mental health professionals previously, this action by Seung-Hui Cho added fuel to the debate about the dangerousness or otherwise of those with mental disorders.

While those diagnosed with disorders such as paranoid schizophrenia can be and often are responsible for violence and aggression (Milton et al., 2001), the reality is that those members of our society who suffer from psychoses are at great risk of becoming victims of violence (Hiday et al., 2002).

♦ What are some of the reasons why people with mental health problems continue to be feared?

♦ Reflect on your own fears that you hold/have held as you think about your exposure to mental health nursing.

♦ Identify some occasions where popular film or television has perpetuated the stigma attached to sufferers of mental health problems.

General health

To live with the experience of schizophrenia is to experience poorer physical health and have a life expectancy that is significantly shorter than the prevailing average of the society to which the affected individual belongs (Bradshaw et al., 2005; Fontaine et al., 2001; Phelan et al., 2001). Fontaine's study stresses that early death stems largely from suicide, while Bradshaw et al. (2005) explain loss of life as arising from poor physical health (natural causes). The most common natural causes tend to be cardiovascular diseases related to obesity, hypertension, lack of physical exercise and smoking (Goff et al., 2005). It is noteworthy that the issue of obesity is compounded by drugs such as clozapine, which can be responsible for significant weight gain.

The physical health of people with a diagnosis of schizophrenia should be monitored at least once a year. Particular emphasis should be placed on assessing cardiovascular disease as people with a diagnosis of schizophrenia are at an elevated risk of this disease compared to the general population (NICE, 2009). However, there is also an increased incidence of infections and endocrine disorders (such as diabetes and galactorrhoea, or milk secretion from the breasts among men and women who are not breastfeeding) within this service user group (NICE, 2009). The national mental health charity Rethink Mental Illness has developed an annual Physical Health Check (PHC) which assesses general health and lifestyle issues, general screening for physical illness and action plans to address identified areas of concern. The PHC is recommended to all mental health nurses as an integral part of overall care. The PHC can be obtained from Rethink Mental Illness at http://www.rethink.org/how_we_can_help/research/service_evaluation_and_outcomes/physical_health_check/physical_health_chec.html.

RESEARCH BRIEF: PHYSICAL HEALTH

Two Australian nurse researchers, Margaret Fogarty and Brenda Happell, conducted a qualitative study into the effects that a structured physical exercise programme would have on a small group of six people diagnosed with schizophrenia. Each participant had a programme tailored to their needs and the duration of the programme was 3 months. At the conclusion of the programme participants revealed in focus group interviews that they found the programme to be beneficial. They reported that the programmes:

- allowed for a sense of achievement,
- provided a means by which weight loss and increased fitness could be achieved,
- created a sense of group support and encouragement,
- motivated the participants to incorporate physical activity into their future daily life.

Source: Fogarty and Happell (2005).

A THOUGHT FROM A SERVICE USER

I have a vision that goes like this: in this new century, mentally ill people will have the science, the organized voting strength and the means to leave our ghettos of isolation behind us. We will finally join with the mainstream community, where we'll be able to live as individuals and not as a group of people who are known and feared by the names of our illness (Steele and Berman, 2001, p. 252).

CRITICAL THINKING CHALLENGE 14.6

Nurses have an educative and supportive role in assisting people in their transition back to work.

- How might nurses assist in this process?
- Who would require education and support?
- What information would be required in an education programme designed to assist the individual's return to work?

CONCLUSION

Schizophrenia is a group of severe and often debilitating disorders that strikes 4 in 1000 people in the UK. It often strikes those aged 18–24 years and results in severe alterations in a person's perception, behaviour, mood, thinking ability, and social and occupational functioning. It has a major impact on national health expenditure and is one of the most expensive of all disorders facing Western economies.

Despite its prevalence and impact, schizophrenia remains misunderstood and its sufferers maligned. The disorder continues to be erroneously associated with 'split personality' or 'multiple personality', and individuals with this disorder are often mistrusted, feared and discriminated against. The stigma of violence and dangerousness is over-emphasized by a great many in society and this further compounds the difficulties faced by the individual experiencing the clinical manifestations of this disorder.

Schizophrenia is a cluster of disorders with a number of similarities and differences. This cluster of disorders includes paranoid, disorganized, catatonic, residual and undifferentiated schizophrenia. Causation remains complex and inconclusive but research points to neurobiological explanations. To be more specific, brain anatomy, brain biochemistry and genetics are the key areas of current research and theory development. The relationship between stress and schizophrenia is a further area of theory development.

Modern mental healthcare now offers hope, whereas in the past, prior to effective drug-based therapies, there was none. Effective care and treatment for schizophrenia now includes a range of medications as well as a variety of nonpharmacological treatments. Modern drugs such as the typical and atypical antipsychotics enable a great number of individuals diagnosed with schizophrenia to recover from their disorder. Nonpharmacological therapies such as CBT enable an individual to learn about their disorder and ways of living with its effects. Both forms of therapy can minimize the symptoms of schizophrenia and prevent further relapses.

Nurses play an important role in assisting the individual experiencing schizophrenia to recover from the disorder, maintain their health and achieve their optimal level of wellness. Nurses use the information gained from mental status assessment, including both subjective and objective data, to plan and implement care designed to assist individuals to maintain their own and others' safety and to accurately interpret reality.

The great challenge to improve the lives of those who experience this disorder is far from over. Understanding schizophrenia and its effects enables the nurse to assist in meeting this challenge.

EXERCISES FOR CLASS ENGAGEMENT

You are nursing a service user diagnosed with paranoid schizophrenia in an inpatient treatment facility. The individual expresses the belief that the water is poisoned and consequently refuses to drink.

- Devise strategies that may assist the service user to drink the volume required to maintain physical health.
- They also believe that you and the other nurses involved in their care are assassins. How will you respond to this expression of belief?

Brainstorm this issue in small groups, then conduct it as a role play.

Make a list of adverse reactions to antipsychotic medications that are considered to be extrapyramidal. Share your list with the group, then brainstorm with the group to develop as many strategies as you can that could contribute to greater levels of medication adherence in a person diagnosed with schizophrenia and treated with antipsychotic medication.

REFERENCES

Access Economics, 2002. Schizophrenia Costs: an Analysis of the Burden of Schizophrenia and Related Suicide in Australia. SANE, Australia.

American Psychiatric Association 2000. Diagnostic and statistical manual of mental disorders: DSM-IV TR, fouth ed. text revision. American Psychiatric Association, Washington DC.

Andreasen, N., 1999. A unitary model of schizophrenia: Bleuler's 'Fragmented Phrene' as schizencephaly. Arch. Gen. Psychiatry 56 (9), 781–787.

Barker, P., 1999. The Philosophy and Practice of Psychiatric Nursing. Churchill Livingstone, Edinburgh.

Birtwistle, J., Baldwin, D., 1998. Role of dopamine in schizophrenia and Parkinson's disease. Br. J. Nurs. 7 (14), 832–841.

Blin, O., Azorin, J., Bouhours, P., 1996. Antipsychotic and anxiolytic properties of risperidone, haloperidol, and methotrimeprazine in schizophrenic patients. J. Clin. Psychopharmacol. 16 (1), 38–44.

Bradshaw, T., Lovell, K., Harris, N., 2005. Healthy living interventions and schizophrenia: a systematic review. J. Adv. Nurs. 49 (6), 634–654.

British Psychological Society and Royal College of Psychiatrists, 2010. Schizophrenia core interventions in the treatment and management of schizophrenia in adults in primary and secondary care (updated

edition). <http://www.nice.org.uk/nicemedia/pdf/CG82FullGuideline.pdf>.

Brown, A., 2006. Prenatal infection as a risk factor for schizophrenia. Schizophr. Bull. 32 (2), 200–202.

Caton, C., 1997. Mental health service use among homeless and never-homeless men with schizophrenia. Year Book Psychiatry Appl. Ment. Health Ann. 7, 291–292.

Citrome, L., Volavka, J., 1999. Schizophrenia: violence and comorbidity. Curr. Opin. Psychiatry 12 (1), 47–51.

Coffey, M., 1998. Schizophrenia: a review of current research and thinking. J. Clin. Nurs. 7 (6), 489–498.

Cotter, D., Pariante, C.M., 2002. Stress and the progression of the developmental hypothesis of schizophrenia. Br. J. Psychiatry 181, 363–365.

Davidson, M., Reichenberg, A., Rabinowitz, J., et al., 1999. Behavioral and intellectual markers for schizophrenia in apparently healthy male adolescents. Am. J. Psychiatry 156 (9), 1328–1335.

Farrison, P., 2000. Dopamine and schizophrenia—proof at last? Lancet 356 (9234), 958–959.

Fogarty, M., Happell, B., 2005. Exploring the benefits of an exercise program for people with schizophrenia: a qualitative study. Issues Ment. Health Nurs. 26 (3), 341–351.

Folsom, D., Jeste, D., 2002. Schizophrenia in homeless persons: a systematic review of the literature. Acta Psychiatr. Scand. 105 (6), 404–413.

Fontaine, K., Heo, M., Harrigan, E., et al., 2001. Estimating the consequences of anti-psychotic induced weight gain on health and mortality rate. Psychiatry Res. 10 (3), 277–288.

Gardner, D., Baldessarini, R., Waraich, P., 2005. Modern antipsychotic drugs: a critical overview. Can. Med. Assoc. J. 172 (13), 1703–1711.

Geddes, J., Lawrie, S., 1995. Obstetric complications and schizophrenia: a meta-analysis. Br. J. Psychiatry 167 (6), 786–793.

Goff, D., Sullivan, L., McEvoy, J., et al., 2005. A comparison of 10-year cardiac risk estimates in schizophrenia patients from the CATIE study and matched controls. Schizophr. Res. 80 (1), 45–53.

Hammen, C., Henry, R., Daley, S., 2000. Depression and sensitization to stressors among young women as a function of childhood adversity. J. Consult. Clin. Psychol. 68 (5), 782–787.

Harris, G., Rice, M., Quinsey, V., 1993. Violent recidivism of mentally disordered offenders: the development of a statistical prediction instrument. Crim. Justice Behav. 20 (4), 315–335.

Haukka, J., Suvisaari, J., Varilo, T., et al., 2001. Regional variation in the incidence of schizophrenia in Finland: a study of birth cohorts born from 1950 to 1969. Psychol. Med. 31 (6), 1045–1053.

Healy, D., Savage, M., Michael, P., et al., 2001. Psychiatric bed utilization: 1896 and 1996 compared. Psychol. Med. 31 (5), 779–790.

Hiday, V., Swartz, M., Swanson, J., et al., 2002. Impact of outpatient commitment on victimization of people with severe mental illness. Am. J. Psychiatry 159 (8), 1403–1411.

Jarboe, K., Littrell, K., Tugrul, K., 2005. Long-acting risperidone: an emerging tool in schizophrenia treatment. J. Psychosoc. Nurs. Ment. Health Serv. 43 (12), 25–33.

Kane, J., Davis, J., Schooler, N., et al., 2002. A multidose study of haloperidol decanoate in the maintenance treatment of schizophrenia. Am. J. Psychiatry 159 (4), 554–560.

Kaplan, H., Sadock, B., 2005. Kaplan and Sadock's Comprehensive Textbook of Psychiatry, eighth ed. Lippincott Williams & Wilkins, Baltimore.

Kapur, S., Seeman, P., 2001. Does fast dissociation from the dopamine D2 receptor explain the action of atypical antipsychotics? A new hypothesis. Am. J. Psychiatry 158 (3), 360–369.

Keltner, N., Folks, D., 2005. Psychotropic Drugs, fourth ed. Mosby, St Louis.

Kety, S., Wender, P., Jacobsen, B., et al., 1994. Mental illness in the biological and adoptive relatives of schizophrenic adoptees: replication of the Copenhagen study in the rest of Denmark. Arch. Gen. Psychiatry 51 (6), 442–455.

Kopelowicz, A., Liberman, R., Wallace, C., 2003. Psychiatric rehabilitation for schizophrenia. Int. J. Psychol. Psychol. Ther. 3 (2), 282–298.

Lawrie, S., Whalley, H., Abukmeil, S., et al., 2002. Temporal lobe volume changes in people at high risk of schizophrenia with psychotic symptoms. Br. J. Psychiatry 181 (2), 138–143.

Lee, S., 2002. The stigma of schizophrenia: a transcultural problem. Curr. Opin. Psychiatry 15 (1), 37–41.

Levinson, D., Mahtani, M., Nancarrow, D., et al., 1998. Genome scan of schizophrenia. Am. J. Psychiatry 155 (6), 741–750.

McCabe, S., 2002. Psychopharmacology and Other Biological Treatment: Psychiatric Nursing: Contemporary Practice. Lippincott, Philadelphia.

McGrath, J., Davies, J., 1999. Schizophrenia: new aspects of management. Curr. Ther. (Seaforth) 40 (8), 14–22.

Marwaha, S., Johnson, S., 2004. Schizophrenia and employment: a review. Soc. Psychiatry Psychiatr. Epidemiol. 39 (5), 337–349.

Milton, J., Amin, S., Singh, S., et al., 2001. Aggressive incidents in first-episode psychosis. Br. J. Psychiatry 178, 433–440.

Muller, M., Wetzel, H., Eich, F., et al., 2002. Dose-related effects of amisulpride on five dimensions of psychopathology in patients with acute exacerbation of schizophrenia. J. Clin. Psychopharmacol. 22 (6), 554–560.

Munk-Jorgensen, P., Ewald, H., 2001. Epidemiology in neurobiological research: exemplified by the influenza–schizophrenia theory. Br. J. Psychiatry 178 (40), 30–32.

Murty, R., Mistry, S., Chacko, R., 2002. Neuroleptic malignant syndrome with ziprasidone. J. Clin. Psychopharmacol. 22 (6), 624–626.

Nairn, R., 2005. People never see us living well: an appraisal of the personal stories about mental illness in a prospective print media sample. Aust. N. Z. J. Psychiatry 39 (4), 281–287.

National Institute of Mental Health 2009. Schizophrenia. <http://www.nimh.nih.gov/health/publications/schizophrenia/schizophrenia-booket-2009.pdf>.

NICE (National Institute for Health and Clinical Excellence) 2009. Core interventions in the treatment and management of schizophrenia in adults in primary and secondary care. Schizophrenia (update) CG82. <http://www.nice.org.uk/CG82>.

O'Connor, F., 1998. The role of serotonin and dopamine. J. Am. Psychiatr. Nurses Assoc. 4 (4), 32–34.

Office for National Statistics 2001. Psychiatric morbidity among adults living in private households, 2000. <http://www.statistics.gov.uk/statbase/Product.asp?vlnk=8258&More=N>.

Opler, L., Caton, C., Shrout, P., et al., 1995. Symptom profiles and homelessness in schizophrenia. Year Book Psychiatry Appl. Ment. Health Ann. 1995 (7), 250–251.

Oyewumi, L., Al-Semaan, Y., 2000. Olanzapine: safe during clozapine-induced agranulocytosis. J. Clin. Psychopharmacol. 20 (2), 279–281.

Phelan, N., Stradins, L., Morrison, S., 2001. Physical health of people with severe mental illness. Br. Med. J. 322, 442–444.

Rivas-Vazquez, R., 2003. Aripiprazole: a novel antipsychotic with dopamine stabilizing properties. Prof. Psychol. Res. Pr. 34 (1), 108–111.

Salokangas, R., Cannon, T., Van Erp, T., et al., 2002. Structural magnetic resonance imaging in patients with first-episode schizophrenia, psychotic and severe non-psychotic depression and healthy controls: results of the Schizophrenia and Affective Psychoses (SAP) Project. Br. J. Psychiatry 181 (43), 58–65.

Schulze, B., Angermeyer, M., 2005. What is schizophrenia? Secondary school students' associations with the word and sources of information about the illness. Am. J. Orthopsychiatry 75 (2), 316–323.

Sharma, T., Murray, R., 1993. Aetiological theories in schizophrenia. Curr. Opin. Psychiatry 6 (1), 80–84.

Steele, K., Berman, C., 2001. The Day the Voices Stopped: A Memoir of Madness and Hope. Basic Books, New York.

Suvisaari, J., Haukka, J., Lonnqvist, J., 2002. Seasonal fluctuation in schizophrenia. Am. J. Psychiatry 159 (3), 500.

Teesson, M., Buhich, N., 1990. Prevalence of schizophrenia in a refuge for homeless men: a five-year Australian follow-up. Psychiatr. Bull. 14, 597–600.

Turkington, D., Kingdon, D., Turner, T., 2002. Effectiveness of a brief cognitive–behavioural therapy intervention in the treatment of schizophrenia. Br. J. Psychiatry 180, 523–527.

US Department of Health and Human Services, 1999. Mental Health: Report of the Surgeon General. US DHHS, Rockville, MD.

van Heeringen, K., 2000. A stress-diathesis model of suicidal behavior. Crisis: J. Crisis Interv. Suicide 21 (4), 192.

van Os, J., 2000. Social influences on risk for disorder and natural history. Curr. Opin. Psychiatry 13 (2), 209–213.

Venables, P., Liu, J., Raine, A., et al., 2007. Prenatal influenza exposure and delivery complications: implications for the development of schizophrenia. Fam. Community Health 30 (2), 151–159.

Walsh, E., Buchanan, A., Fahy, T., 2002. Violence and schizophrenia: examining the evidence. Br. J. Psychiatry 180, 490–495.

Weisman, A., 2005. Integrating culturally based approaches with existing interventions for Hispanic/Latino families coping with schizophrenia. Psychotherapy 42 (2), 178–197.

Wilson, C., Coverdale, J., Panapa, A., 2000. How mental illness is portrayed in children's television: a prospective study. Br. J. Psychiatry 176, 440–443.

Yellowlees, P.M., Cook, J.N., 2006. Education about hallucinations using an internet virtual reality system: a qualitative survey. Acad. Psychiatry 30 (6), 534–539.

Zubin, J., Spring, B., 1977. Vulnerability: a new view of schizophrenia. J. Abnorm. Psychol. 86 (2), 103–126.

Chapter | 15 |

Mood disorders

Peter Athanasos

CHAPTER CONTENTS

DOI: http://dx.doi.org/10.1016/B978-0-7020-4493-9.00015-9

- psychomotor retardation
- suicide-prevention contract

CHAPTER POINTS

- While each person is unique, there are key nursing principles and interventions for working with people experiencing a mood disorder.
- Depression is associated with an increased risk of attempting and completing suicide.
- The establishment of a therapeutic relationship is critical to treatment success.
- Mood disorders are responsive to a variety of psychological, sociocultural and biological interventions.
- Theories relevant to nursing people with depression and bipolar disorder do not fully explain mood disorders, but serve to guide and support nursing interventions.
- The major classes of medication used in the treatment of mood disorders are antidepressants and mood stabilizers.

KEY TERMS

- affect
- bipolar disorder
- cyclothymia
- dysthymia
- egocentricity
- elation
- grief
- hypomania
- impulsivity
- major depressive disorder
- mania
- mood
- observation

INTRODUCTION

This chapter examines the nature of mood disorders. It also explores mental health nursing assessment, and the interventions, knowledge and attitudes that one needs to work effectively with people with mood disorders. A holistic view is essential. Mood disorders can and often do affect most aspects of a person's existence, from feelings to thoughts to behaviours. Basic requirements such as eating, sleeping and communication may all be affected and should be taken into consideration.

Changes in mood such as depression and elation are common in most mental health disorders. This chapter considers disorders where mood change is the predominant condition and is disabling. With mood disorder, the changes in mood are more intense and persistent than common variations in mood and may affect functioning at work and at home. Also associated are a range of disturbances in such areas as behaviour, cognition, communication and physical functioning. The effective nurse will consider all these areas when collaborating with the service user.

As always in mental health nursing, the key to working effectively with someone with a mood disorder is a collaborative relationship characterized by openness and respect, in which the nurse is seen as a partner in the service user's recovery.

COMORBIDITY

Comorbidity is the coexistence of two or more disorders. A mood disorder, for example, rarely occurs in isolation. Mood disorders often occur in conjunction with other conditions such as personality disorders, eating disorders, anxiety disorders and especially substance abuse disorders (Hussein Rassool, 2006). Similarly, service users diagnosed with schizophrenia often have mood disturbances. It is not clear why these conditions occur together. Does one disorder cause another or do they share the same original disruptive mechanism? Does someone with diagnosed depression use alcohol to excess in an attempt to self-medicate, or are service users diagnosed with a severe mental health problem more 'sensitive' to small amounts of alcohol or drugs (Hall and Queener, 2007; Khantzian, 1997; Mueser et al., 1995)? A number of theories have been proposed but there is little consensus. In addition, service users diagnosed with mental health disorders have an increased exposure to health risk factors, poorer physical health and higher rates of death from many causes, including suicide.

As nurses, the important principle is that we care for our service users holistically, in many aspects of their lives, and do not treat a service user as a single, abstract disorder.

EPIDEMIOLOGY AND ECONOMIC COST OF MOOD DISORDERS

Mood disorders are common in the UK. About 1% of adults develop bipolar disorder (also known as *bipolar affective disorder* or *manic depression*) at some point in their life. It usually originates during teenage years, often with a first episode before the age of 30 years, and men and women are affected equally (BPS and RCP, 2006; National Institute for Health and Clinical Excellence, 2006). There appears to be an increased incidence among black and ethnic minorities (BPS and RCP, 2006) with social exclusion and a lack of social support being cited as possible aetiological factors (Bentall, 2004).

Almost 50% of people will experience at least one episode of depression in their life (Andrews et al., 2005). Over 15% of the population will experience a depressive episode during the course of their lifetime, the average duration of episodes being between 6 and 8 months. Thirty per cent of such depressive episodes will be, for many, moderate or severe in nature and will impact on their general functioning and daily lives. There is also a likelihood that the depressive episode will reoccur as over 50% experience a recurrence of depressive symptoms after a first episode, while 70 and 90% of people experience a recurrence after a second or third episode respectively (BPS and RCP, 2010).

Among older people, approximately 11% experience minor depression while 2% will have major depression (BPS and RCP, 2010). While rates of depression do not vary greatly across males in ethnic groups in the UK, for women there are much higher rates of depression, particularly women of Asian and Oriental family origin or background. However, the lowest rates are to be found in women of West Indian or African family origin or background (BPS and RCP, 2010).

Depression is also associated with increased exposure to health risk factors, poorer physical health and higher rates of death from many causes, including suicide (Begg et al., 2007). For example, depression doubles the risk of coronary heart disease (BPS and RCP, 2010). Twenty per cent of people with coronary heart disease are clinically depressed (Glassman et al., 2002).

The societal cost of depression to the UK is significant. The direct treatment costs of depression have been estimated at £370 million, of which over 80% is accounted for by the prescription of antidepressant medication. Indirect costs (including lost productivity and so forth) account for a further £8 billion (Office for National Statistics, 2001). The annual societal cost to the UK of bipolar disorders is estimated at £2 billion (BPS and RCP, 2006). However, while mood disorders place significant demands on the healthcare system the heaviest burden will be experienced by individuals and their carers, friends and families.

SERVICE RESPONSE

People with symptoms of depression account for approximately 5% of attendees at GP practices (BPS and RCP, 2010; Thompson C et al., 2004). There are clear regional differences in hospital admission rates, but overall depression and anxiety are the most common reasons for admission, accounting for almost 30% of admissions (Thompson A et al., 2004). The National Institute for Health and Clinical Excellence (NICE) recommends an escalating 'stepped' approach to the care of people with depression (National Institute for Health and Clinical Excellence, 2009) based on the complexity or severity of the disorder. This approach seeks to formalize the delivery of care as the patient progresses through the system (BPS and RCP, 2010). During the initial stages (Steps 1 and 2; usually, but not always, in primary care and general hospital settings) the emphasis is placed on the initial recognition and nonpharmacological treatment of a depressive episode, including general advice about the contribution that sleep, exercise and healthy eating can make to alleviating symptoms. Low-intensity psychosocial interventions and self-help using cognitive behavioural techniques are also recommended. For people with persistent symptoms of depression (Step 3), an antidepressant (usually a selective serotonin-reuptake inhibitor or SSRI) may be prescribed with a stepping of the intensity of psychological treatments. If the person presents with severe and complex depression, or where there is a risk to self-harm or suicide or severe self-neglect, then referral to specialist secondary care services may be appropriate (Step 4). Here, emphasis is placed in treatments not previously used in primary care using a specialist multiprofessional mental health team approach including possible hospitalization if appropriate (National Institute for Health and Clinical Excellence, 2009).

For bipolar disorder, National Institute for Health and Clinical Excellence (2006) recommends that all new or suspected presentations are refered to specialist secondary mental health services, particularly if the person has experienced a period of overactivity lasting for 4 days or more. If a person with a diagnosis of bipolar disorder is supported solely in primary care, then arrangements must be made for urgent referral to secondary services if the person's condition deteriorates or if adherence to medication is problematic or if the person uses alchol and drugs. If the person is at significant risk of harm then admission to hospital must be considered (National Institute for Health and Clinical Excellence, 2006). Such support will require regular monitoring and input by primary care staff.

DEPRESSION

Depressive symptoms may range from mild, such as 'feeling blue', to very severe, where there is extraordinary sadness and dejection, and an inability to take pleasure in activities. The disorder is described as *major depressive disorder* if the depressive symptoms are all-pervasive and debilitating in most areas of the service user's existence. If the service user describes 'feeling blue' for a prolonged period of time and shows symptoms of mild depression, their mental health problem could be characterized as *dysthymia*.

The important differentiating factors are: number of symptoms, degree of severity and duration of symptoms. It is also important to recognize that, depending on life events, periods of transitory sadness and grief are part of normal human functioning and we should not see these periods as disease states.

Mild depression

Mild depression is more common than major depression. It can be seen as an exaggeration of ordinary unhappiness.

The service user may complain of 'the blues' but not show the features that would describe major depression. Mild depression includes the following features: tearfulness, anxiety, low mood, lack of energy and interest, irritability and sleep disturbance.

In mild depression, the sleep disturbance would not be the early morning waking of major depressive disorder but rather difficulty in falling asleep and frequent waking through the night, with sleep finally coming at the end of the night.

With mild depression the somatic symptoms (physical symptoms that have a psychological rather than a physiological basis) are not prominent, and delusions and hallucinations do not occur.

Major depression

Major depression is characterized by seven main features: low mood, lack of energy, lack of pleasure or interest in activities (called *anhedonia*), negative thinking, disturbed sleep, difficulty concentrating and recurring thoughts of death and suicide. It is a disorder that may often go unrecognized when the service user presents with a concurrent range of physical ailments. It is important that the disorder does *not* go unrecognized, as depression is one of the primary causes of self-harm and suicide, and may have a profound effect not only on the service user but also on their family and friends (Gelder et al., 2005a).

A number of features central to major depressive disorder differentiate it from milder forms of depression. These include alterations in appearance and behaviour, thinking (such as poor concentration and decision-making), mood, perception and neurovegetative symptoms and weight loss. Service users may exhibit some, but not necessarily all, of these symptoms.

Appearance and behaviour

Psychomotor retardation is a slowing of mental and physical activity, and is a characteristic of major depressive disorder. Interestingly, and in contrast, agitation and a feeling of restlessness is also a characteristic of major depressive disorder. This condition is described as *agitated depression*. Frequently, the service user finds it hard to remain still for an extended period of time and may pace around the room.

Mood

The service user who experiences depression usually appears sad and anguished and may describe a sense of hopelessness and powerlessness about their situation. They also describe a different quality to their low mood compared to ordinary sadness. The severity of the mood changes with the time of day. The service user may wake early. The mood is usually worse in the morning, with pessimistic thoughts about the coming day and a focus on past perceived failures. As the day wears on, the person's mood becomes lighter.

The service user may be irritable and anxious. They may withdraw both socially and emotionally from contact with others. There is a marked decrease in pleasure or interest in previously enjoyed activities (Gelder et al., 2005a).

Thinking and speech

The person experiencing symptoms of depression may be increasingly egocentric in that they may focus on themselves and fail to realize that others may have needs as well. A gloomy, negative outlook pervades all their thinking. The person thinks about themselves as incompetent, unlovable and a failure. They will also think of the world as incompetent and unlovable. Others will be thought of as uncaring and unhelpful. The depressed person's thinking becomes catastrophic and their emotional state is crippled with inappropriate guilt.

Poor concentration and poor memory are important characteristics of major depression. The person may have difficulty reading or focusing on a problem. They become immobilized by the cognitive difficulties involved in making a simple decision. Their outlook becomes dominated by negative self-absorption, poor energy and a lack of interest in others. They may be reluctant to initiate a conversation. When asked a question, they will take a long time to answer and then give a short and perfunctory reply.

The spectrum of thinking of the depressed person also narrows. The person focuses on negative thoughts and ideas to the exclusion of all else. These thoughts and ideas become repetitive and fixed, and the rumination eventually interferes with ordinary thought processes.

Thinking about the past, present and future

In thinking about the present, the person will tend to see the unhappy side of everything that happens. They may be convinced that others think of them as a failure, and if something positive happens, they may attribute it to a lucky chance that will never happen again.

In thinking about the past, the person may be consumed with inappropriate guilt, often over a small matter. They may feel that they have let someone down and contributed to their misfortune. The depressed person may not have considered these matters for many years but in the midst of their depression these thoughts will come flooding back and overwhelm them.

In thinking about the future, their outlook can be unremittingly grim. They may foresee catastrophe in their work, failure in their relationships with family members and friends, and an inevitable deterioration in their physical health. This preoccupation with a bleak future and a sense of doom often leads to thoughts of death and suicidal ideation, and should be considered with care (Gelder et al., 2005a).

Perception

Major depressive disorders may also be accompanied by delusions and hallucinations. While people with moderate depressive disorders may suffer from feelings of inappropriate guilt, people with more severe depressive disorders will experience delusions of guilt. These are described as psychotic symptoms and when these symptoms are combined with depression, the condition is called *psychotic depression* or *major depression with psychotic features*.

The same themes that present as inappropriate emotions in moderate depression are present in a more severe, psychotic form in major depression: for example, feelings of worthlessness, failure or incompetency. When hallucinations are present, they usually manifest as negative, derisory voices echoing the nihilistic themes of, 'You're a failure, you're incompetent, you're evil' and so on.

Biological symptoms

Sleep disturbances and, in particular, problems in falling asleep and early morning waking, are common features of depression. Service users with depression will also feel unrefreshed in the morning when they wake. Fatigue, lack of appetite, decreased sexual interest and decreased care with hygiene are all common signs of major depression. A decrease in weight is often a good indication of a possible depressive disorder, but it is important not to exclude other possibilities or the fact that the person may have elected to lose weight. A proportion of the population, often from non-Western backgrounds, may not describe a depressed mood. Rather, these depressed people will describe a range of pain conditions or other physical symptoms. This is called *somatization* and should be carefully noted.

CRITICAL THINKING CHALLENGE 15.1

Why do you think people are so reluctant to admit that they are depressed and need help?

What would be your first reaction if you were diagnosed with depression, initiated weekly counselling and were prescribed antidepressants?

Aetiology of depression

Biopsychosocial model of causation

What causes depression? As with many diseases in mental health, researchers have focused on the influence of three main areas: biological, psychosocial and sociocultural factors. Each of these areas has been studied in detail to assess how they contribute to this mood disorder. To accurately assess what causes depression, we need to understand that there is unlikely to be any one factor that is wholly responsible. Rather, it is a combination of factors interacting that causes the mental health problem. This combination of factors is called the *biopsychosocial model of causation*.

Genetic factors

Sullivan et al. (2000) examined a number of twin studies (more than 21 000 twins studied in total) and found that an identical twin was approximately twice as likely to suffer from major depression as a nonidentical twin. Sullivan et al. (2000) concluded that genetic factors accounted for 31–42% of the likelihood of developing major depression.

Gene–environment interaction

Much research has been devoted to identifying the specific genes involved in depression. So far there has been limited success, but a number of approaches have shown promise. One of these is the concept of the *gene–environment interaction*. Researchers have found that, while some people had a genetic predisposition to depression (in the serotonin transporter gene), if they had also had stressful life events in the past 5 years or had been severely maltreated as children, they were far more likely to develop depression than those with the gene only or stressful life events/maltreatment as children only (Caspi et al., 2003; Moffitt et al., 2005). This suggests that searching for the genes involved in depression would be more fruitful if the gene–environment interaction was also examined.

Neurochemical factors

The idea that depression is a result of a complex interaction between neurotransmitters and other systems in the brain originated in the 1960s and has gained influence since. It should be emphasized that depression is not simply a consequence of low levels of serotonin or other neurotransmitters (monoamines) in the brain. This was the 'monoamine hypothesis' and originated in 1965, but by the 1980s researchers had concluded that this approach was too simplistic. For example, a number of studies have found that people diagnosed with severe depression had increased levels of neurotransmitters such as noradrenaline and that only a small proportion had decreased levels of serotonin (Thase et al., 2002). More recently, researchers have suggested that the causes of depression are more complex and probably depend on an interaction between neurotransmitters and disturbances in hormonal, neurophysiological and biological systems in the body (Southwick et al., 2005). Although this is a more accurate description, it is not easy to explain it as a single mechanism or process.

Hormone systems and circadian rhythms

It has been suggested that hormonal systems, and specifically the hypothalamic–pituitary–adrenal (HPA) axis and the cortisol and thyroid hormones, are implicated in depression (Marangell et al., 1997; Thase et al., 2002). Also implicated are low levels of brain activity in key regions of the brain (Davidson et al., 2002), the qualities of rapid-eye-movement (REM) sleep and disturbances in circadian rhythms (24-hour body cycles) (Thase et al., 2002).

NURSE'S STORY: A DEPRESSED YOUNG MAN

Branko had been the main support for his family since his father died when Branko was 15. He lived with his mother and two younger sisters in an inner-city suburb and worked as a storeman at a local supermarket.

His mother had suffered from depression for as long as Branko could remember. Antidepressants and counselling from their local priest seemed to help his mother, but much of the time Branko worked, paid the bills, cooked the meals and organized his sisters for school each day. His position at the supermarket had some flexibility and so he would pick his sisters up from school and then return to work in the evening when his family was settled.

The eldest daughter, a 14-year-old, had called into the local health centre, concerned that her mother had become 'unwell' again. She asked if a nurse could come to their house to see her. That's where I came in.

When I arrived at their house the next day I was surprised to find Branko at home and still in his dressing gown. He told me that his mother had remained in bed for these last 2 weeks and was eating poorly. He was worried for her. His mother and I talked, I made an assessment and then spent the next half hour organizing her admission to an acute mental healthcare ward.

While we waited for the ambulance I sat down with Branko. He seemed very flat. There was little animation in his voice. I asked him why he wasn't at work and he replied rather vaguely that he just wasn't feeling very well. It was obvious that he didn't want to talk and so we sat for a little while in silence. The ambulance eventually came and before I left I made an appointment to catch up with him a week later.

I had known Branko superficially for a number of years in the context of providing care for his mother. I suspected that he was under strain but had hoped that he was coping. I had never seen him so flat before and sensed he was in some distress. My first priority was to visit him regularly to try to develop a therapeutic relationship. This was partly in the context of planning for his mother's discharge from hospital but also because I wanted to engage with him and develop a sense of trust between us. I hoped that he would open up and talk about how he felt. This happened very slowly. Much of the time we would sit quietly together each time I visited. At all times I tried to be as genuine and honest with him as I could. As a consequence he gradually opened up to me.

Branko described how he had lost his appetite and felt constant fatigue. He was also irritable much of the time with the long hours at work and burdens at home. He recognized his irritability and hated himself for it. He didn't like being irritable with his family. He'd had a girlfriend for a couple of months the year before, but there was little time in his life to devote to another relationship and it soon ended. He then found himself lacking energy and more irritable than before. At times during our interactions Branko was angry with himself. At other times he turned his anger on me. I realized he wasn't targeting me personally and that it was a symptom of his illness. He would always apologize after the anger had passed and we would be relaxed with each other again.

All the time I was with him I expressed hope to him that his spirits would lift. I focused on what a good, caring son and brother he was. He regularly visited his mother in hospital. I also praised him on how his sisters were turning out with his help. They were well respected at the school and getting good marks in their studies.

Finally his mother did return from hospital. This seemed to be a turning point for him. Branko had missed his mother keenly. She was brighter and able to help more around the house and with the two girls. Branko himself seemed to be coping better and was taking less time off from work. He agreed to trial some antidepressant medication. He had also mentioned during my last visit that he was thinking of getting in touch with his ex-girlfriend to see if she wanted to spend some time with him.

On my final visit a couple of weeks later it was obvious that he was better. He'd recently gained a promotion at work and his girlfriend was coming around that night for dinner with his family. He thanked me for my efforts over the past couple of months and spoke in positive terms about his future. I was glad.

It has been argued that psychosocial factors play as strong a part in the development of depression as biological factors. However, it is likely that it is the impact of stressful life events on the biochemical hormonal and circadian systems that causes depression (Hammen, 2005; Howland and Thase, 1999).

Gender differences

It has long been established that women are more than twice as likely to develop depression as men (Nolan-Hoeksema, 2002). The theories that have been proposed to explain this range from biological (hormonal and genetic factors) to social and psychological (Helgeson, 2002; Nolan-Hoeksema, 2002). One approach suggests that depression is largely a consequence of women's roles in society. These researchers argue that women regularly experience a lack of control over negative life events and that this contributes to the development of depression. These events include poverty, discrimination in the workplace, unemployment, imbalance of power in relationships with men, high rates of abuse (sexual and physical) and overload in role expectation (e.g. wife, work, children) (Ben Hamida et al., 1998; Heim et al., 2000; Nolan-Hoeksema, 2002). Again, it is likely that these life events affect hormonal and neurophysiological systems to produce depression.

MANIA AND BIPOLAR DISORDER

Mania is classified as an elevated, expansive or irritable mood for at least 1 week. There is also significant impairment in social or occupational functioning. *Mania* is characterized by three main features: persistently elevated mood, which may be one of elation or irritability; increased activity; and poor quality of judgement. Also present may be inflated self-esteem or grandiosity, a decreased need for sleep, flight of ideas and racing thoughts, talkativeness with pressure of speech, and distractibility. There may be an increase in the amount of goal-directed activities (such as work, social and/or sexual activities) and there may be reckless behaviour (that is, involvement in activities with little or no awareness of consequences, such as spending, sexual behaviour or business activities). The occurrence of manic episodes with a depressive disorder is called *bipolar disorder, bipolar affective disorder* or *manic depression*. Mania is less common than depression. Again, it is important that the disorder not go unrecognized because as the mental health problem progresses the service user may become less and less inclined to accept treatment, and the consequences of the mental health problem (increased activity, poor judgement) may become more serious.

Hypomania has similar symptoms to mania, with the following exceptions: there is no significant impairment in social or occupational function, there are no psychotic features and there is generally no need for hospitalization.

Although the name bipolar disorder suggests two categories of symptoms – depression and mania – it does not require a depressive episode for the diagnosis to be made. There are individuals suffering from bipolar disorder who have never had a depressive episode. In general, however, the disorder is characterized by a cycling between depression and normal mood and mania. This may occur over periods of time from days to weeks to months.

As with depression, the more severe form of mania is accompanied by delusions and hallucinations (Gelder et al., 2005a).

Appearance and behaviour

The behaviour of a person experiencing symptoms of mania is characterized by four main factors: increased activity, impulsivity, disinhibition and inflated ideas. The increased activity, often for long periods, leads to physical exhaustion. People diagnosed with mania may spend money excessively and dramatically increase their intake of drugs and alcohol. They become sexually hyperactive and disinhibited. As a result, their behaviour is considered inappropriate by others. It is important to remember that such activities are often out of character for the person and may later cause embarrassment and problems at work and in their social circle.

When their condition is more severe they may be dishevelled and malodorous. They are often distractible, which leads to them initiating and then leaving unfinished a series of activities. As they become more manic, their behaviour becomes more disorganized and they have trouble completing even the simplest tasks (Gelder et al., 2005a).

Mood

The person's mood is often elated. They may appear as euphoric, excessively optimistic and may display infectious gaiety. At other times they may be irritable and aggressive. They can be quite labile through the day but there is not the same clear pattern of change in outlook as is associated with depression.

Thinking and speech

The person's thoughts are unusually rapid, abundant and varied. Their speech reflects these rapid changes in thoughts and this is described as *pressure of speech*. As they become more activated, their speech may consist of puns, jokes, rhymes and irrelevancies. At the next level they exhibit looseness of associations between ideas, and the ability to concentrate diminishes. At its most severe, acute manic speech is indistinguishable from the speech of someone with acute schizophrenia.

Most service users who experience mania have delusions: the person thinks their ideas are novel, their opinions profound and their work of outstanding genius. Their delusions may have a religious, persecutory or paranoid flavour. They may believe that they are extremely wealthy or powerful and become irritable when their thoughts are challenged.

Perception

Hallucinations might occur with mania. Their content is congruent with the person's fluctuations in mood. For example, the service user may hear voices that have religious or persecutory content when they are in a negative mood and praise them excessively when their mood is positive.

Biological symptoms

When experiencing a manic episode, service users may have little time for sleep. They may wake very early, feeling energetic, become active and disturb others. This increased activity may lead to exhaustion. In some cases, appetite increases and they may consume food quickly, with little concern for social etiquette. In other cases, the person is too distracted to take interest in eating. Libido increases, and may bring with it recklessness and behaviour that is out of character (Gelder et al., 2005a).

CASE STUDY: SERVICE USER DIAGNOSED WITH BIPOLAR DISORDER

Sarah's husband threatened to divorce her if she did not go with him to the accident and emergency department of the local general hospital for assessment. She was 39 years old, sporadically unemployed and had been functioning poorly for a number of years. During the past week Sarah had been partying all night with some new friends of hers and shopping during the day. She was an attractive woman, fast-talking, cheerful and casually flirtatious. She easily became irritable when challenged.

About 5 years before, Sarah had experienced some mild depressive symptoms. She was listless, had trouble getting out of bed, and experienced intermittent insomnia and loss of appetite. This lasted for 2 months and then Sarah became well again.

Two years later, Sarah's father died. She had been very close to her father and felt his death harshly. She believed that she had not been a good enough daughter. Sarah's husband saw a dramatic change in his wife following her father's death. She had 3 weeks of remarkable energy, hyperactivity and euphoria. She would stay awake cleaning the house every night. She had a strong sexual interest in her husband and was bright, self-confident company. This was then followed by 1 week where she could barely lift herself out of bed. She slept for long periods and complained of exhaustion.

When Sarah was in one of her energetic periods, she was bright, energetic and brimming with self-confidence. She had worked in a car yard for many years and had months when she was the most successful dealer among her coworkers. She would spend excessively during these energetic periods, on such things as wide-screen televisions, hi-fi equipment and hundreds of pairs of shoes. Her husband also suspected her of having impulsive sexual encounters with her coworkers. On two occasions she was fired from her job for her erratic behaviour. She was then rehired by other firms soon after. However, towards the end of her energetic periods she became irritable and caustic, and she received complaints from her customers. Following these episodes she would go to bed for weeks at a time to try to deal with the depressive symptoms. She would not shower during these periods and would eat very little.

This pattern of alternating periods of excessive energy followed by depression, with a few 'normal functioning' days, repeated itself over the next few years. It occurred most often near the anniversary of her father's death or when she felt under pressure at work.

However, on this last occasion, she had been without work for 3 months. She was out at night with a new circle of friends and shopping most of the day, running up debt. Her husband suspected she was using drugs.

Sarah's husband felt very frustrated and gave her the ultimatum. Though angry at first and denying that anything was wrong, Sarah agreed to be seen by the doctor. He prescribed her a mood stabilizer, sodium valproate, which she was reluctant to take. After many false starts and much fighting between Sarah and her husband, Sarah was finally stabilized on the medication. She got her job back at the car dealership and was moderately successful. She stated that she missed the highs of her illness very much but was relieved she didn't have to experience the lows as well.

Aetiology of bipolar disorder

Genetic factors

Interestingly, researchers have concluded that there is a far greater genetic contribution to bipolar disorder than to depression. McGuffin et al. (2003) found that 67% of identical twins diagnosed with bipolar disorder had a co-twin who also had the disorder, compared with 19% of nonidentical twins. From this and other studies it has been calculated that genetic factors account for 80–90% of the likelihood of developing bipolar disorder. This means that genetic factors contribute more to the likelihood of developing bipolar disorder than to depression or any of the other psychiatric disorders such as schizophrenia (Torrey et al., 1994).

Neurochemical factors

Interestingly, the monoamine hypothesis for depression was originally extended to account for bipolar disorder. It was argued that, as decreases in monoamines (the neurotransmitters serotonin, noradrenaline and dopamine) caused depression, increases in the monoamines caused mania. This was supported by evidence that drugs such as cocaine and amphetamines stimulate dopamine activity and mimic the symptoms of mania (Manji and Lenox, 2000). However, as with depression, while neurotransmitter imbalances are important the process is more complex than a simple increase in monoamines. For example, serotonin activity has found to be decreased in both depressive and manic episodes.

Hormone systems and circadian rhythms

Similarly to depression, there has been significant research into imbalances in the HPA axis and the pituitary gland. Cortisol and thyroid hormone levels have been found to be elevated during manic episodes in service users (Watson et al., 2004). Other researchers have found differences in structural brain function (blood flow from one part of the brain to another) during disturbances of mood compared to periods of normal functioning. During depression, blood flow to the left frontal cortex is reduced. During mania, blood flow is reduced to the right frontal and temporal regions. During normal mood, blood flow across the two brain hemispheres is approximately equal. This indicates that there may be shifting patterns of brain activity during depressed, manic and normal moods (Howland and Thase, 1999; Whybrow, 1997). Again, it should be noted that while this disturbance in blood flow may happen in mood disturbances, it may reflect the mood disturbance rather than be a cause.

There has also been evidence to support the influence of circadian rhythms. One of the prominent features of the manic stage of bipolar disorder is a lack of sleep. Some researchers argue that service users diagnosed with bipolar disorder in particular are sensitive to disturbances in their 24-hour circadian cycles and that this is a prominent feature of the disorder, even during manic and depressive episodes (Harvey et al., 2005; Jones et al., 2005).

Psychosocial factors

Similarly to depression, it is likely that stressful life events play a significant part in the development of bipolar disorder, by causing disequilibrium in the hormonal and neurophysiological systems. Progression of the disorder then disrupts the balance further.

CRITICAL THINKING CHALLENGE 15.2

Many service users describe hypomania as an intoxicating state that gives rise to ceaseless energy and great pleasure. At what stage do these service users need treatment?

DYSTHYMIA AND CYCLOTHYMIA

Dysthymia describes chronic mild depression. *Cyclothymia* describes chronic instability of mood, with mild depression and mild manic symptoms.

Dysthymia and cyclothymia are less severe mood disorders of longer duration than major depression or manic episodes. A diagnosis of major depressive disorder requires a minimum of 2 weeks of symptoms, and manic episodes require 1 week of symptoms. A diagnosis of dysthymia or cyclothymia requires 2 years of symptoms (American Psychiatric Association, 2000).

CHILDBIRTH AND MOOD DISORDERS

Postpartum 'blues'

The birth of a child is generally seen as a happy event. However, many women and some men experience symptoms of depression 4–6 weeks following childbirth. Many parents have difficulty understanding why they are depressed, because they assume that this is a joyous time. Most of these people are experiencing what is known as *postpartum 'blues'*. Postpartum 'blues' are a normal response to the stresses of childbirth and disappear quickly, generally within days to weeks.

Postpartum 'blues' is a transient disturbance in mood and is characterized by a labile mood, sadness, dysphoria and subjective confusion (Brockington, 2000). The mother may burst into tears and be puzzled by such uncharacteristic weeping. Somewhat incongruously, these feelings are often interrupted by happy feelings (Miller, 2002; O'Hara et al., 1990, 1991). These symptoms may occur in as many as 50–70% of women and usually subside on their own (Miller, 2002).

A number of explanations have been proposed for postpartum 'blues', including physical exhaustion, the stress of childbirth, awareness of the increased responsibility that motherhood brings and changes in women's hormone regulation and immune system function (Groer and Morgan, 2007).

The main nursing intervention for postpartum 'blues' is education and support for the new mother. If the symptoms of postpartum 'blues' last for more than 2 weeks the service user needs to be assessed for postpartum depression.

Postpartum depression

Postpartum depression is characterized by a depressed mood, excessive anxiety, insomnia and change in weight. Symptoms often occur within 12 weeks after delivery and if the disorder is untreated it may last from months to years (Sadock and Sadock, 2007). Interestingly, it has been argued that major depression occurs no more frequently in the postpartum period than in women of similar age and sociocultural status who have not given birth (Hobfoll et al., 1995; O'Hara et al., 1990, 1991). Additionally, a number of studies have found essentially no differences between postpartum major depression and traditional major depression, in aetiology or treatment approaches (Gotlib et al., 1991; Whiffen, 1992; Whiffen and Gotlib, 1993; Wisner et al., 2002). However, one treatment approach that has not been well studied is that of antidepressants, because of concerns that these medications may be transmitted to the newborn through lactation. The NICE guidelines *Antenatal and Postnatal Mental Health* (National Institute for Health and Clinical Excellence, 2007) provide details of recommended care, including the use of antidepressants and other medications during pregnancy and breastfeeding.

The causes of postpartum depression are similar to the causes of depression in all ages, and include heredity, a history of previous depression, adverse events or social conditions, difficult relationships and social isolation (Brockington, 2000).

Interventions

Nursing interventions for postpartum depression include regular counselling and education with the mother. These can be provided as part of the regular postpartum care of mother and child, or as additional visits as required.

It is also important to work with the significant other in the relationship. This is often the child's father, but not necessarily so. This person may be the main support person and mood changes can occur for this person as well as for the mother, with significant impact on the family unit. Several factors may be involved: added responsibility, diminished sexual outlet, decreased attention from the mother and the belief that their child is a binding force in an unsatisfactory partnership. Regular counselling and education are good nursing interventions in this instance (Dennis, 2005).

Postpartum psychosis

Postpartum psychosis is a rare psychotic disorder among women who have recently had a baby. The syndrome is often characterized by the mother's depression, delusions and thoughts of harming herself or her infant. It is important that such ideation be carefully monitored by nursing staff.

The incidence of postpartum psychosis is about 1 in 1000 pregnancies. It has been argued that an episode of postpartum psychosis is actually an episode of a mood disorder, usually a bipolar disorder but occasionally a depressive disorder. The delivery process is the nonspecific stress that causes the development of the major mood disorder. There is also evidence that the steroid hormones involved in menstruation and childbirth may be involved (Zonana and Gorman, 2005).

Infant loss

There are a number of reasons that a child may be lost. These include termination of pregnancy at the behest of the mother; miscarriage, ectopic pregnancy and late termination of a wanted child for medical reasons; foetal death *in utero*, stillbirth, neonatal death and sudden infant death syndrome (SIDS, or 'cot death'); and relinquishment to adoption (Brockington, 2000). Each of these circumstances (termination of pregnancy, miscarriage, foetal death and adoption) carries with it a complex range of grieving. Counselling plays an important part in healing, as does consideration of the feelings of the surviving family. For instance, surviving children may be confused by their parent's grief, upset by family turmoil and deprived of attention and care; they are also grieving and preoccupied with their own search for the meaning of death and should be included in any therapy (Brockington, 2000).

GRIEF AND MOOD DISORDERS

Grief can be considered the normal psychological process that a person goes through following the death of a loved one. Bowlby (1980) describes four phases of normal response to the death of a spouse or close family member.

- Shock and protest: a numbing of emotions and disbelief punctuated by outbursts of intense distress, panic or anger. This may last from a few hours to a week.
- Preoccupation: a yearning for and searching preoccupation with the loved one. This may last for weeks or months. A variety of symptoms accompany these feelings, including insomnia and restlessness. Anger towards the loved one for leaving or unresolved issues is not uncommon. In time, this yearning diminishes and is replaced by disorganization and despair.
- Disorganization: when the service user begins to accept the loss of the loved one and begins to establish a new identity independent of the loved one, there is disorganization of previous emotions, and despair diminishes. The service user may begin to accept that they are now a widow or widower.
- Resolution: the service user begins to rebuild their life, there is a decrease in sadness and an enjoyment of life returns. The service user reorganizes themself.

Importantly, where is the point at which grief ceases to be grief and should be described as a major depressive disorder? Service users diagnosed with major depressive disorder often become fixed in the disorganization and despair stage of the grief response and cannot move on. However, it is important to recognize that it is normal to show signs of depression following the bereavement of a spouse or close family member. As a consequence, even if all the symptoms of major depressive disorder are met, a person cannot be diagnosed with the disorder until more than 2 months have passed since the death of a loved one.

OLDER ADULTS AND MOOD DISORDERS

Major depression and dysthymia in older adults is a major health problem (Beekman et al., 2004). It is often difficult to detect among older people because many of the symptoms associated with depression are also associated with common medical illnesses or symptoms of dementia (Alexopoulos et al., 2002). For instance, it has been estimated that perhaps as many as 50% of service users diagnosed with Alzheimer's disease also suffer from depression, which increases the burden on families even further (Lyketsos and Olin, 2002).

Symptoms associated with late-onset depression include marked sleep difficulties, hypochondriasis and agitation. While there are many adverse consequences for the service user's health if depression goes untreated, no matter what their age, there are particular dangers for the older person. For example, Schulz et al. (2002) found that depression could double the risk of death in older people who had had a heart attack or stroke, as it impedes their ability to recover.

Baldwin (2000) describes a number of factors that may influence the presentation of depression among older people. These include:

- an overlap between the symptoms of the physical disorder with the somatic symptoms of depression,
- the tendency of older people to minimize a complaint of sadness and instead complain of a physical illness,
- newly presenting neurotic symptoms such as severe anxiety, obsessive–compulsive symptoms and so on, which 'mask' depression,
- any act of deliberate self-harm may indicate depression, even ostensibly 'trivial' overdoses,
- 'pseudo-dementia': the service user appears confused upon presentation but the onset of the confusion is acute and accompanied by nonverbal despair. Unlike service users diagnosed with degenerative dementia, these service users complain loudly about their loss of memory,
- behavioural disturbances such as alcohol abuse or shoplifting: these may also reflect underlying depression.

CULTURAL CONSIDERATIONS

We live in increasingly multicultural societies and so it is common for nurses to care for members of ethnic minorities. For this reason it is important that mental health nursing practice be transcultural in approach. There is a rich variety of experience of illness and distress across the world. The Western biomedical model of disease is only one approach among many different ways of dealing with the experience of illness and loss.

How does each culture develop its own methods of dealing with loss and emotional pain (Obeyesekere, 1985)? The Buddhists of Sri Lanka see the world of sense, pleasure and domesticity as illusory in nature and lacking permanency. The Kaluli tribe of New Guinea express their grief in anger. When a member of the tribe suffers a loss there is a strong expectation that others in the community will compensate them. In this way, blame is externalized and the community is held responsible for the support of the aggrieved individual (Schieffelin, 1985). Good et al. (1985) describe the situation in Iranian society where children are taught to grieve in the context of religious ceremonies for Iranian martyrs. The personal response to loss is in this way assimilated into the wider communal experience of a historical tragedy.

Obeyesekere (1985) sees these coping measures as an integral part of the culture in which they originate. He contends that what we in the West call depression is a 'disease' construction, originating from within a narrow Western viewpoint and then imposed on the rest of the world as a universal condition. It has been argued that if a biochemical basis for the neuroses was firmly established, the conception of depression as a universal condition would be justified (Leff, 2000). However, the efficacy of nonbiological treatments for depression and anxiety, such as cognitive therapy, marital therapy and behavioural therapy, suggests that Obeyesekere's view warrants serious consideration. It is important that in the field of mental health we remain open to the means that other cultures have developed for helping people with what we would term mental 'illness' or 'disorder' (Leff, 2000).

MEDICAL CONDITIONS AND DRUG REACTIONS

Many medical conditions or drug reactions can produce symptoms of depression or mania identical to those found with major depression or bipolar mood disorder. It is important for nurses to be able to rule out the possibility of these factors being the underlying cause of a mood disorder.

Medical conditions that cause depression and mania

Depression can be an integral feature of a number of medical conditions, including:

- neurological disorders: such as Parkinson's disease, dementia, multiple sclerosis,
- endocrine disorders: such as hypothyroidism,
- virus infections: such as influenza,
- deficiencies of vitamins: such as vitamin B_{12} and folate.

Manic episodes could be due to a range of organic brain lesions, particularly in the frontal lobe, and endocrine disorders such as thyrotoxicosis or Cushing's syndrome (Gill, 2007).

Drug reactions that cause depression and mania

Drugs that can precipitate depression include:

- antihypertensives: especially reserpine and methyldopa,
- corticosteroids and possibly sex hormones,
- levodopa,
- digitalis,
- certain cytotoxics,
- certain antimalarials,
- sulphonamides,
- antipsychotics,
- cholesterol-lowering drugs.

Drugs that can instigate a manic episode include corticosteroids, antidepressants, levodopa, LSD, cocaine and amphetamines (Gill, 2007).

Overview of causation

One of the most important concepts to consider when reviewing the causal factors of depression and bipolar disorder is that of cause and effect. For example, with depression we know that antidepressants such as sertraline (Lustral) can help correct the functioning of neurotransmitters in the brain. This does not mean that disturbances in neurotransmitter functioning alone cause depression. Some unknown mechanism may have caused the imbalance in neurotransmitter functioning, and then the imbalance caused the mental health problem. While antidepressants help treat the disorder, they may have no effect on the original unknown and debilitating mechanism.

SUICIDE

Epidemiology

Suicide is a serious risk in all kinds of depression. While some people commit suicide for reasons other than depression, two-thirds of people who commit suicide are thought to be depressed, making depression the leading cause of suicide in the UK. Interestingly, clinical experience tells us that people are most at risk when they are emerging from the most debilitating phase of their depression.

The overall incidence of suicide in the UK has decreased in recent years. In 2009 there were 5675 suicides in the UK (4304 male suicides [17.5 per 100 000 population] and 1371 female suicides [5.2 per 100 000]; Office for National Statistics 2011). Globally, the rate of suicide mortality is estimated at 16 per 100 000 population (World Health Organization, 2005). Although the current downward trend is encouraging, there is no reason for complacency (Goldney, 2006).

Aetiology of suicide

Psychosocial factors

A number of factors may contribute to a person taking their own life. These include relationship breakdown, severe financial reversal, imprisonment or other severe personal crisis. Some researchers suggest that different factors influence suicide in the short term than in the long term. In the short term, for service users experiencing major depression, symptoms that may reliably predict suicide are severe psychic anxiety, panic attacks, severe anhedonia, global insomnia, delusions and alcohol abuse (Busch et al., 2003). In the longer term, a sense of hopelessness about the future may be a more reliable predictor (Coryell and Young, 2005; Stolberg et al., 2002).

But what causes people to reach this state of desperation? The answer to this question is not unexpected. People who take their own lives often have a family background characterized by family psychopathology, child mistreatment and family instability (Molnar et al., 2001). The child then makes the adult. These early childhood experiences of low self-esteem, hopelessness and difficulties with problem-solving are carried into adulthood, with subsequent emotional and cognitive deficits. The emotional and cognitive deficits are the bridge that adults can negotiate to suicidal ideation (Yang and Clum, 1996).

Biological factors

There is strong evidence that genetic factors contribute to many mental health problems. Suicide is no exception, and there has been a substantial amount of research in

this area (Baldessarini and Hennen, 2004). For example, the likelihood that one twin will commit suicide if the other does is approximately 19 times higher with identical twins than with fraternal twins (Roy et al., 1999). There is research to suggest that the risk of suicide may even be partly independent of other psychiatric diagnosis such as depression or schizophrenia and be a consequence of poor serotonin functioning. However, this theory requires further supportive evidence (Mann et al., 2001).

Nursing interventions for suicide prevention

The following is an outline of key principles and issues for ongoing assessment and prevention of suicide in people who are depressed.

- Assess active suicidality by asking the service user if they plan to hurt themselves. The main barrier for nurses asking a person about suicide is personal discomfort or fear. It is not a pleasant activity. However, it is the nurse's role to prevent suicide if possible. The simple process of asking a service user about their intentions is an extremely effective means of making a mental health nursing assessment. Always remember: talking to a service user about suicide or death will not put the idea into their heads or increase the likelihood that they will act upon the idea.
- Always take seriously all service users' suicidal feelings, ideas and plans. The more lethal, detailed and practicable the suicide plan, the more the person is at risk.
- If there have been previous suicide attempts, and the ongoing issues have not been resolved, there is a higher risk of suicide in the future.
- Examine the local unit, ward, hospital or health service for the policies and protocols that are to be followed when a person is assessed to be at risk for attempting suicide.
- The best means of preventing suicide is to develop a therapeutic relationship with the potentially suicidal service user.
- It is important to allow the person to tell his or her story about events that have led to their present feelings of hopelessness and desperation.
- Try to determine who is in the person's social network and ask the service user if a person may be available to support them in a particular way.
- Another simple nursing approach is to ask the service user what their most pressing problems are, and little by little problem-solve those that can be changed.
- Encourage the service user at risk to write down the name of a person they can call in a crisis. Encourage them to describe what they will say to this person. In this way, the service user will have a strategy to follow when they are at risk.

These interventions have been drawn and adapted from a range of sources, including Drew (2001), Fontaine (2003), Horsfall et al. (2000), Keltner (2007) and Valente (2002).

Suicide-prevention contracts and observation

Two of the most widely and internationally used nursing interventions for the prevention of suicide are suicide-prevention contracts between nurse and service user, and observation. Both approaches have been criticized as lacking evidence for their efficacy. However, they have been used in practice and, in the absence of other interventions, have their advocates.

Suicide-prevention contracts

Suicide-prevention contracts (or, more commonly, contracts not to self-harm) are agreements between a particular nurse and a specific service user. They may be verbal agreements or written agreements and are generally reviewed at the change of each shift. The nurse discusses with the service user the safe actions the service user will take if the service user's suicidal ideation increases. These actions are agreed upon by the nurse and service user.

The first reported study describing a form of suicide-prevention contract was published in 1973 by Drye et al. (1973). Originally it was in a form of assessment of suicidal ideation. The therapist would have the service user state verbally that they would not harm themselves. The service user then reported to the therapist how making the statement made them feel. The therapist would then assess for incongruence or reluctance on the part of the service user to make the unqualified statement (Edwards and Harries, 2007).

From this beginning the suicide-prevention contract has taken on its own life in clinical practice and has moved from the function originally prescribed to it – that of assessment – and has become focused on medi-conursing legal protection in the event of adverse clinical outcomes. That is, if a service user attempts to take their own life, and the nurse or doctor has entered into a verbal or written contract with them not to harm themselves (and it has been documented), then the nurse or doctor is partly absolved of responsibility for the act. Unfortunately, the technique is used widely by practitioners in the absence of any evidence of its efficacy. Studies are presently under way to rectify this obvious knowledge gap (Edwards and Harries, 2007).

CRITICAL THINKING CHALLENGE 15.3

In your experience, are verbal or written suicide-prevention contracts effective?

Constant observation

Constant observation (sometimes informally known as 'specialling') is uninterrupted, one-to-one, constant mental health nursing care and usually applies to service users who are suicidal. This procedure is generally prescribed by senior healthcare staff and carried out by nursing staff. Like suicide-prevention contracts, there is a great deal of debate about its efficacy and whether it is appropriate ethically (Cutcliffe and Barker, 2007; Ward and Jones, 2007).

Some authors suggest that it amounts to little more than gatekeeping on the part of the mental health nurse and should be supplanted by shorter, more therapeutic interactions that 'engage with the service user and inspire hope' (Cutcliffe and Barker, 2007). Others suggest that there is little wrong with observations as such, as long as there is positive interaction between nurse and service user (Ward and Jones, 2007). They argue that the criticism of constant observation has turned the practice into a scapegoat for criticisms that should be directed at poor mental health nursing care. Again, further evidence in this area is required.

CRITICAL THINKING CHALLENGE 15.4

In your experience, is constant observation (or 'specialling') an effective mental health nursing intervention or are we simply fulfilling the role of gatekeepers?

In your experience, is constant observation effective in reducing the incidence of successful suicide?

PHARMACOLOGY

Effective psychopharmacology began with the introduction of mood stabilizers in 1948 (John Cade, lithium carbonate), antipsychotics in 1951 (Henri Laborit [among others], chlorpromazine) and antidepressants in 1956 (Roland Kuhn, the tricyclic imipramine) (Spiegel, 2003).

The major classes of medication used in the treatment of major depressive and bipolar disorders are antidepressants and mood stabilizers. When psychotic features are evident (either with major depression or bipolar disorder), an antipsychotic may be required. SSRIs are the more popular class of antidepressants, and lithium is one of the most popular mood stabilizers, and the actions and side effects of these drugs are discussed in detail below.

Drugs used in the treatment of depression

Antidepressants

Antidepressants generally have a long half-life and can be taken once a day. Action generally occurs within 10–14 days after the drug is first taken. If therapy is discontinued, the process should occur slowly, as sudden cessation may lead to restlessness, insomnia, anxiety and nausea.

The main types of antidepressant are:

- SSRIs: these include sertraline (Lustral), paroxetine (Seroxat), fluvoxamine (Faverin), fluoxetine (Prozac), escitalopram (Cipralex) and citalopram (Cipramil),
- selective noradrenaline-reuptake inhibitors: these include reboxetine (Edronax),
- serotonin- and noradrenaline-reuptake inhibitors: these include venlafaxine (Efexor),
- tricyclic antidepressants: amitriptyline and imipramine,
- monoamine oxidase inhibitors: phenelzine (Nardil) and moclobemide (Manerix),
- atypical antidepressants: these include mirtazapine.

These drugs have not been shown to differ substantially in effectiveness or speed of action. They differ in their side-effect profiles (Lehne, 2007).

Selective serotonin-reuptake inhibitors (SSRIs)

At present the first-line pharmacological treatment for depression is the SSRIs. This class of drugs was first introduced in 1987 and has since become the most commonly prescribed group of antidepressants. These drugs are as effective as tricyclic antidepressants but do not cause hypotension, sedation or anticholinergic effects (dry eyes, dry mouth, blurred vision, constipation and urinary retention) (Lehne, 2007).

Side effects

Common side effects of SSRIs include:

- gastrointestinal: nausea, flatulence, diarrhoea,
- central nervous system: insomnia, restlessness, irritability, agitation, tremor and headache,
- sexual: ejaculatory delay and anorgasmia (Gelder et al., 2005b).

More recent generations of antidepressants such as the serotonin and noradrenaline reuptake inhibitors (venlafaxine, or Efexor) are gaining in popularity. Tricyclic antidepressants are still often prescribed (e.g. amitryptyline). Monoamine oxidase inhibitors (phenelzine, or Nardil) are prescribed as a last resort because of their interactions with food rich in tyramine such as many pickled, smoked, brewed, dried or fermented foods (e.g. red wine (especially Chianti), coffee and soy sauce) (Gelder et al., 2005b).

Drugs used in the treatment of bipolar disorder

Bipolar disorder is treated with three main groups of drugs: mood stabilizers, antipsychotics and antidepressants. The term *mood stabilizer* describes a group of drugs, not a specific pharmacological class. These drugs help prevent the recurrence of bipolar affective disorder and also can be effective in treating the acute episodes of mania and depression that occur with the disorder. The main mood

stabilizers are lithium carbonate and the antiepileptic drugs, including sodium valproate and carbemazepine. The only other drugs licensed for use in the UK for mania are olanzapine, quetiapine and risperidone (National Institute for Health and Clinical Excellence, 2006).

Lithium carbonate

Lithium carbonate is one of the most popular agents for the long-term treatment of bipolar disorder. However, caution should be exercised: the dose that is therapeutic and the dose that is toxic are close, and so it is important to measure plasma concentrations of lithium regularly during treatment. Service users should be monitored regularly by nursing staff for both side effects and toxic effects of the drug.

Side effects of lithium:

- early effects: polyuria (increased urination), tremor, dry mouth, metallic taste, weakness and fatigue,
- later effects: fine tremor (coarse tremor is a sign of toxicity), polyuria and polydipsia (increased thirst), hair loss, thyroid enlargement, hypothyroidism, impaired concentration, weight gain, gastrointestinal distress, sedation, acne and electrocardiogram (ECG) changes (T-wave flattening and QRS-interval widening).

Toxic effects are nausea and vomiting, diarrhoea, coarse tremor, ataxia (disjointed movement), muscle twitching, confusion, coma, convulsions, renal failure and cardiovascular collapse. It is important that lithium level checks are undertaken every 3–6 months and a blood test for thyroid and kidney function at least every 15 months. The service user should be encouraged to manitian good hydration.

One of the most persistent challenges nurses face is encouraging adherence with medication. A good strategy to encourage compliance is to have a solid knowledge of medications (effects and side effects) and the implications of discontinuing treatment. By educating our service users about these matters, we can ensure that they are well informed about their treatment and realize the risks they take when noncompliant. A good knowledge of the pharmacology of these medications also ensures that we can properly monitor our service users for signs that they may be noncompliant, or that the medications are becoming toxic or are having a therapeutic effect.

OTHER TREATMENTS

Psychotherapy

A number of psychotherapies have proved effective in the treatment of mood disorders and should always be considered with service users. These include planned short-term psychotherapy, cognitive behavioural therapy, family therapy, narrative therapy and motivational interviewing.

Light therapy

Light therapy is a treatment that consists of using artificial light therapeutically for 30–180 min once or twice daily. It has been shown to be most effective for service users with mild to moderate symptoms of depression associated with a seasonal pattern, called *seasonal affective disorder*, which, it is suggested, is related to a lack of light in certain seasons and decreased melatonin production (Westrin and Lam, 2007). It has also been argued that alterations in brain serotonin systems also contribute to seasonal affective disorder and that phototherapy may compensate for this imbalance (Neumeister et al., 1999). Nurses can promote health in service users with a propensity for seasonal affective disorder by educating them about the relationship of sunlight to mood and the benefits of daily exposure to the sun (Mohr, 2006).

Electroconvulsive therapy

Electroconvulsive therapy (ECT) is a treatment for depression in the following circumstances:

- when an urgent response is needed: this can occur when life is threatened in a severe depressive disorder by a refusal to drink or eat, or when the service user is experiencing treatment-resistant, intense suicidal ideation;
- for a resistant depressive disorder, following failure to respond to treatment with antidepressant medication.

ECT works more quickly than antidepressant drugs, although the outcome after 3 months is similar. It involves the administration of an electric current to the head of an anaesthetized service user to produce seizure activity while motor effects (uncontrolled movements of torso and limbs) are prevented with a muscle relaxant (Gelder et al., 2005a).

Because the service user is put under general anaesthesia, they have no memory of the experience. Adverse effects include a brief period of headache following treatment, and brief memory and cognitive impairment (which clears rapidly for most service users). It should be noted that cognitive impairment and memory loss also occur with depressive disorder alone.

While its use remains controversial, on the basis of the evidence, ECT is widely accepted as an effective intervention in the treatment of severe depression (Bray, 2003; Loo et al., 2006).

Tables 15.1 and 15.2 list suggested interventions for service users diagnosed with depression and mania.

Table 15.1 Nursing interventions for service users diagnosed with depression

Intervention	Rationale
Be genuine and honest with service users. Accept them for who they are (both negative and positive aspects).	Depressed people have chronically low self-esteem. Genuine acceptance by others is a first step to recovery.
Treat anger and negative thinking as symptoms of the disorder, not as personally targeted at the nurse.	Depressed people are often negative and angry. By identifying that negativity and anger are aspects of the disorder, the nurse can encourage the service user to move on from these issues to express more appropriate emotions.
Never reinforce hallucinations, delusions or irrational beliefs.	It is not appropriate to agree with the service user's perceptual abnormalities. Equally, arguing that they do not exist serves little purpose. The nurse should state their perception of the situation. The nurse should state that there is a discrepancy between what is perceived by the service user and what is perceived by the nurse. The nurse should then steer the conversation to discussing real people and real events.
Spend time with withdrawn service users, even if no words are spoken.	Withdrawn people are still very aware of where they are and who they are with. Simply by spending time with withdrawn service users, nurses can help the service users emerge from their isolation by providing a nonthreatening one-on-one relationship, practising assertive interactions and providing positive regard.
Make positive decisions for service users if they are unwilling to make decisions for themselves, e.g. it is time to get out of bed.	Depressed people can have difficulties making even the simplest of decisions. By using problem-solving techniques, i.e. identifying options, the advantages and disadvantages of each option available, and exploring the consequences of taking these actions: the nurse can guide the service user to appropriate decisions.
Express hope that they will get better. Focus on their strengths, however small these seem.	By identifying their strengths and giving them hope and positive regard, we encourage them to regain a sense of self-worth.

(continued)

Table 15.1 Continued

Intervention	Rationale
Identify and involve service users in activities where they can enjoy success.	It is important for service users to feel good about themselves. By involving service users in activities that they can accomplish, they may begin to improve their sense of self-worth.

Table 15.2 Nursing interventions for service users diagnosed with mania

Intervention	Rationale
Speak in a calm, supportive tone.	Using this tone of voice encourages the service user to respond positively, not defensively. A clear, calm tone discourages the service user's need to engage in power struggles. The tone conveys to the service user that they are supported and that events are under control.
Give firm, simple directions and comments. Limit-setting may be required.	Manic service users have flight of ideas, pressure of speech and are easily distracted. Nurses need to take control of the situation by politely but firmly interrupting excessively talkative service users. This is particularly important when the nurse is leading a group and the manic service user is disrupting others.
Do not argue or engage in debate about the rules and limits of the ward.	Argument and debate may encourage a power struggle between the nurse and service user. It may also provoke the service user to become defensive. It is more appropriate to simply state the ward policy and then move on.
Never reinforce hallucinations, delusions or irrational beliefs. Reinforce reality and redirect conversation.	The same policies apply to service users diagnosed with mania as to service users diagnosed with depression. It is not appropriate to agree with the service user's perceptual abnormalities. Equally, arguing that they do not exist serves little purpose. The nurse should state their perception of the situation. The nurse should state that there is a discrepancy between what is perceived by the service user and what is perceived by the nurse. The nurse should then steer the conversation to discussing real people and real events.
Always respond to legitimate complaints.	Service users diagnosed with mania may often make many frivolous complaints. However, nurses must always respond to legitimate complaints appropriately, to defuse irritability and develop trust.

Reprinted from Keltner N, Schweke L, Bostrom C, 2007, Psychiatric Nursing, Mosby, with permission from Elsevier.

CASE STUDY: SERVICE USER AT RISK

Julia was a woman in her late thirties who had been hospitalized a number of times with depression. She had a caring and supportive family, but had a history of physical abuse in her childhood. Over the past few years she had been trialled on a series of antidepressants, with little success. Her husband and two teenage daughters wanted Julia to get well but were unsure as to what to do.

Her husband called the on-call Approved Mental Health Professional (AMHP) who convened a Mental Health Act assessment. Her husband explained that for the previous 3 weeks she had become increasingly withdrawn. She was spending much of the day in her room, and rarely emerged except to eat and drink. In the previous 2 days, despite his encouragement, she had refused to eat and had taken little fluid.

She was placed under Section 2 of the Mental Health Act 1983, amended 2007, and taken to hospital. She did not resist but found it difficult to walk, because of her malnutrition. On the ward, she lay on her bed and continued to refuse to eat or drink. Any food or liquid that was put into her mouth was spat out. She was put on intravenous fluids.

Julia was assessed by two psychiatrists and a mental health nurse. A full psychological and physical assessment was carried out. A decision was made that she required emergency ECT before her condition deteriorated.

Treatment was therefore undertaken in accordance with Section 58A of the Mental Health Act 1983, amended 2007. The procedure was explained to her along with the reasons that it was required. The mental health nurse also described the possible adverse effects of cognitive impairment and short-term memory loss. Julia refused to give consent. It was decided that the treatment was necessary to prevent serious damage to Julia's health.

The next morning Julia was taken to the ECT suite, where ECT was carried out. The nursing and medical staff in the room greeted Julia but she was unable to speak. She was placed under anaesthetic and the procedure was carried out. She then returned to the ward and remained on her bed without moving. The next morning Julia consented to drinking a little water but remained in bed.

The ECT procedure was performed six times over the next 2 weeks. The change was dramatic. When the recovery staff had first encountered Julia, she was unable to speak and had difficulty lifting herself from the recovery trolley. By the end of the second week, Julia was greeting the recovery staff by name and smiling. By the end of the third week, Julia was given antidepressants, observed for a further week and then discharged home to her grateful family. She told her family that she was going to do her best to stay out of hospital, but that if she ever did get so unwell again, she wanted ECT.

CONCLUSION

Variations in mood are a natural part of life. They indicate that a person is connecting with the world around them. Extremes in mood are associated with normal reactions to joy, ecstasy, grief, loss and despair. When these extremes in mood become debilitating and disordered, our service users require our help.

Mood disorders are one of the most common groups of mental disorders in the community. This chapter has drawn on a range of mental health sources to provide a brief overview of our present understanding of mood disorders, their signs and symptoms and a variety of postulated aetiologies. Particular conditions associated with mood disorders were considered, including the nature of childbirth and mood disorders, infant loss, grief, old age and non-Western perspectives on depression and suicide.

Practical nursing interventions were described, with an emphasis on caring for the service user holistically, not as an abstract mental health problem. Other major therapeutic interventions described include medication, psychotherapy, light therapy and, for particular cases of treatment-resistant depression, ECT. With good nursing care and prescribed medication, service users with mood disorders generally respond to treatment and regain their former level of abilities.

EXERCISES FOR CLASS ENGAGEMENT

According to Boyd (2002), many people from China, Japan, Korea, the Philippines and Vietnam consider mental health problems to be caused by character weakness, emotional strain, lack of self-discipline, physical exhaustion, unrequited love or Yin-Yang imbalance. Mental health problems may be viewed as shameful among immigrants from these countries. It is not surprising, therefore, that family members with mental health problems are often hidden, and assistance from health professionals is only sought when behaviours become extreme or unmanageable. Working in groups, discuss the following questions.

♦ What consequences would arise for a depressed person from the anticipation of family shame and the fear of cultural insensitivity from healthcare providers?

♦ Define *stereotyping*. How might cultural stereotyping affect a depressed person in an inpatient unit?

♦ European or Westernized cultures value autonomy, independence and individualism, but many African, Asian, Aboriginal Australian and Pacific Island cultures value the collective over the individual. For these groups, family obligation and commitment to the community are central precepts for living. The aim of most psychological treatments for depression is to enhance personal autonomy: what difficulties may then arise for a depressed person from a culture that prizes the group as a whole? (See Donnelly [2002]) for further discussion.)

Chronic low self-esteem is a nursing diagnosis associated with depression and some other mental illnesses. The evidence for low self-esteem includes expression of inappropriate guilt, self-negating statements and passivity in relation to others (Bailey et al., 2002).

In a group, develop at least six detailed nursing interventions and rationales to improve a depressed person's self-esteem over 12 months.

Blame can be understood as under-responsibility for self; and *guilt* may be defined as over-responsibility for others. During the next week, listen to conversations within your family and friends for expressions of inappropriate blame and guilt. Share your findings with your group and discuss how such cognitions impede recovery from depression, and what strategies can be used to ameliorate them.

REFERENCES

Alexopoulos, G.S., Abrams, R.C., Young, R.C., et al., 2002. Assessment of late life depression. Biol. Psychiatry 52 (3), 164–174.

American Psychiatric Association, 2000. Diagnostic and Statistical Manual of Mental Disorders, fourth ed., text rev. American Psychiatric Association, Washington DC.

Andrews, G., Poulton, R., Skoog, I., 2005. Lifetime risk of depression: restricted to a minority or waiting for most? Br. J. Psychiatry 187, 495–496.

Bailey, K.P., Sauer, C.D., Herrell, C., 2002. Mood disorders. In: Boyd, M. (Ed.), Psychiatric Nursing. Contemporary Practice, second ed. Lippincott, Philadelphia, pp. 410–451.

Baldessarini, R.J., Hennen, J., 2004. Genetics of suicide: an overview. Harv. Rev. Psychiatry 12 (1), 1–13.

Baldwin, R., 2000. Mood disorders in the elderly. In: Gelder, M., Lopez-Ibor, J., Andreasen, N. (Eds.), New Oxford Textbook of Psychiatry. Oxford University Press, Oxford.

Beekman, A.T., Deeg, D., Smit, J., et al., 2004. Dysthymia in later life: a study in the community. J. Affect. Disord. 81 (3), 191–199.

Begg, S., Vos, T., Barker, B., et al., 2007. The Burden of Disease and Injury in Australia 2003. Australian Institute of Health and Wellbeing, Canberra.

Ben Hamida, S., Mineka, S., Bailey, J.M., 1998. Sex differences in perceived controllability of mate value: an evolutionary perspective. J. Pers. Soc. Psychol. 75 (4), 953–966.

Bentall, R., 2004. Madness Explained: Psychosis and Human Nature. Penguin, London.

Bowlby, J., 1980. Attachment and Loss, 3. Loss, Sadness and Depression. Basic Books, New York.

Boyd, M., 2002. Cultural issues related to mental health care. In: Boyd, M. (Ed.), Psychiatric Nursing. Contemporary Practice, second ed. Lippincott, Philadelphia, pp. 16–28.

BPS and RCP (British Psychological Society and Royal College of Psychiatrists), 2006. Bipolar Disorder: The Management of Bipolar Disorder in Adults, Children and Adolescents, in Primary and Secondary Care. <http://guidance.nice.org.uk/CG38/Guidance>.

BPS and RCP (British Psychological Society and Royal College of Psychiatrists), 2010. Depression: The NICE Guideline on the Treatment and Management of Depression in Adults (updated edition). <http://guidance.nice.org.uk/CG90/Guidance>.

Bray, J., 2003. The nurse's role in the administration of ECT. In: Barker, P. (Ed.), Psychiatric and Mental Health Nursing. The Craft of Caring. Hodder Arnold, London.

Brockington, I., 2000. Obstetric and gynaecological conditions associated with psychiatric disorder. In: Gelder, M., Lopez-Ibor, J., Andreasen, N. (Eds.), New Oxford Textbook of Psychiatry. Oxford University Press, Oxford.

Busch, K.A., Fawcett, J., Jacobs, D.G., 2003. Clinical correlates of inpatient suicide. J. Clin. Psychiatry 64 (1), 14–19.

Caspi, A., Sugden, K., Moffitt, T.E., et al., 2003. Influence of life stress on depression: moderation by a polymorphism in the 5-HTT gene. Science 301 (5631), 386–389.

Coryell, W., Young, E.A., 2005. Clinical predictors of suicide in primary major depressive disorder. J. Clin. Psychiatry 66 (4), 412–417.

Cutcliffe, J., Barker, P., 2007. Considering the care of the suicidal client and the case for 'engagement and inspiring hope' or 'observations'. In: Cutcliffe, J.R., Ward, M. (Eds.), Key Debates in Psychiatric/ Mental Health Nursing. Churchill Livingstone, Elsevier, London.

Davidson, R.J., Pizzagalli, D., Nitschke, J.B., et al., 2002. Depression: perspectives from affective neuroscience. Annu. Rev. Psychol. 53, 545–574.

Dennis, C.L., 2005. Psychosocial and psychological interventions for prevention of postnatal depression: systematic review. Br. Med. J. 331 (7507), 15.

Donnelly, T.T., 2002. Contextual analysis of coping: implications for immigrants' mental health care. Issues Ment. Health Nurs. 23 (7), 715–732.

Drew, B.L., 2001. Self-harm behavior and no-suicide contracting in psychiatric inpatient settings. Arch. Psychiatr. Nurs. 15 (3), 99–106.

Drye, R., Goulding, R.L., Goulding, M.E., 1973. No-suicide decisions: patient monitoring of suicidal risk. Am. J. Psychiatry 130, 171–174.

Edwards, S., Harries, M., 2007. No-suicide contracts and no-suicide agreements: a controversial life. Australas. Psychiatry 15 (6), 484–489.

Fontaine, K., 2003. Mental Health Nursing, fifth ed. Pearson, Prentice Hall, New Jersey.

Gelder, M., Mayou, R., Geddes, J., 2005a. Mood disorders. In: Gelder, M., Mayou, R., Geddes, J. (Eds.), Psychiatry, third ed. Oxford University Press, Oxford, pp. 97–118.

Gelder, M., Mayou, R., Geddes, J., 2005b. Drugs and other physical treatments. In: Gelder, M., Mayou, R., Geddes, J. (Eds.), Psychiatry, third ed. Oxford University Press, Oxford, pp. 231–254.

Gill, D., 2007. Hughes Outline of Modern Psychiatry, fifth ed. John Wiley and Sons, Chichester.

Glassman, A.H., O'Connor, C.M., Califf, R.M., et al., 2002. Sertraline treatment of major depression in patients with acute MI or unstable angina. J. Am. Med. Assoc. 288, 701–709.

Goldney, R.D., 2006. Suicide in Australia: some good news. Med. J. Aust. 185 (6), 304.

Good, B.J., Good, M., Moradi, R., 1985. The interpretation of human depressive illness and dysphoric affect. In: Kleinman, A., Good, B. (Eds.), Culture and Depression: Studies in the Anthropology and Cross-Cultural Psychology of Affect and Disorder. University of California Press, Berkeley, CA, pp. 369–428.

Gotlib, I., Whiffen, V.E., Wallace, P.M., 1991. Prospective investigation of postpartum depression: factors involved in onset and recovery. J. Abnorm. Psychol. 100 (2), 122–132.

Groer, M.W., Morgan, K., 2007. Immune, health and endocrine characteristics of depressed postpartum mothers. Psychoneuroendocrinology 32 (2), 133–139.

Hall, D.H., Queener, J.E., 2007. Self-medication hypothesis of substance use: testing Khantzian's updated theory. J. Psychoactive Drugs 39 (2), 151–158.

Hammen, C., 2005. Stress and depression. Annu. Rev. Clin. Psychol. 1, 293–319.

Harvey, A.G., Schmidt, A., Scarna, A., et al., 2005. Sleep-related functioning in euthymic patients with bipolar disorder, patients with insomnia, and subjects without sleep problems. Am. J. Psychiatry 162 (1), 50–57.

Heim, C., Graham, Y.P., Miller, A.H., 2000. Pituitary-adrenal and autonomic responses to stress in women after sexual and physical abuse in childhood. J. Am. Med. Assoc. 284 (5), 592–597.

Helgeson, V., 2002. The Psychology of Gender. Pearson, New Jersey.

Hobfoll, S., Ritter, C., Lavin, J., et al., 1995. Depression prevalence and incidence among inner-city pregnant and postpartum women. J. Consult. Clin. Psychol. 3, 445–453.

Horsfall, J., Stuhlmiller, C., Champ, S., 2000. Interpersonal Nursing for Mental Health. McLennan & Petty, Sydney.

Howland, R., Thase, M., 1999. Affective disorders: biological aspects. In: Millon, T., Blaney, P. (Eds.), Oxford Textbook of Psychopathology. Oxford University Press, New York, pp. 166–202.

Hussein Rassool, G., 2006. Dual Diagnosis Nursing. Blackwell, Oxford.

Jones, S.H., Hare, D.J., Evershed, K., 2005. Actigraphic assessment of circadian activity and sleep patterns in bipolar disorder. Bipolar Disord. 7 (2), 176–186.

Keltner, N., 2007. Depression. In: Keltner, N., Schweke, L., Bostrom, C. (Eds.), Psychiatric Nursing. Mosby, St Louis.

Khantzian, E.J., 1997. The self-medication hypothesis of substance use disorders: a reconsideration and recent applications. Harv. Rev. Psychiatry 4 (5), 231–244.

Leff, J., 2000. Transcultural psychiatry. In: Gelder, M., Lopez-Ibor, J., Andreasen, N. (Eds.), New Oxford Textbook of Psychiatry. Oxford University Press, Oxford.

Lehne, R., 2007. Antidepressants. In: Lehne, R. (Ed.), Pharmacology for Nursing Care, sixth ed. Elsevier, St Louis.

Loo, C.K., Schweitzer, I., Pratt, C., 2006. Recent advances in optimizing electroconvulsive therapy. Aust. N. Z. J. Psychiatry 40 (8), 632–638.

Lyketsos, C.G., Olin, J., 2002. Depression in Alzheimer's disease: overview and treatment. Biol. Psychiatry 52 (3), 243–252.

McGuffin, P., Andrew, M., Cardno, A., 2003. The heritability of bipolar affective disorder and the genetic relationship to unipolar depression. Arch. Gen. Psychiatry 60 (5), 497–502.

Manji, H.K., Lenox, R.H., 2000. The nature of bipolar disorder. J. Clin. Psychiatry 61 (Suppl. 13), 42–57.

Mann, J.J., Brent, D.A., Arango, V., 2001. The neurobiology and genetics of suicide and attempted suicide: a focus on the serotonergic system. Neuropsychopharmacology 24 (5), 467–477.

Marangell, L.B., Ketter, T.A., George, M.S., et al., 1997. Inverse relationship of peripheral thyrotropin-stimulating hormone levels to brain activity in mood disorders. Am. J. Psychiatry 154 (2), 224–230.

Miller, L., 2002. Postpartum depression. J. Am. Med. Assoc. 287 (6), 762–765.

Moffitt, T.E., Caspi, A., Rutter, M., 2005. Strategy for investigating interactions between measured genes and measured environments. Arch. Gen. Psychiatry 62 (5), 473–481.

Mohr, W., 2006. Psychiatric Mental Health Nursing, sixth ed. Lippincott, Williams & Wilkins, Philadelphia.

Molnar, B.E., Berkman, L., Bulka, S., 2001. Psychopathology, childhood sexual abuse and other childhood adversities: relative links to subsequent suicidal behaviour in the US. Psychol. Med. 31 (6), 965–977.

Mueser, K., Bennet, M., Kushner, M., 1995. Epidemiology of substance use disorders among persons with chronic mental illness. In: Lehman, A., Dixon, L. (Eds.), Chronic Mental Illness and Substance Abuse Disorders. Harwood Academic, Chur.

National Institute for Health and Clinical Excellence, 2006. Bipolar Disorder: The Management of Bipolar Disorder in Adults, Children and Adolescents, in Primary and Secondary Care. <http://guidance.nice.org.uk/CG38/NICEGuidance/pdf/English>.

National Institute for Health and Clinical Excellence, 2007. Antenatal and Postnatal Mental Health. <http://www.nice.org.uk/nicemedia/live/11004/30433/30433.pdf>.

National Institute for Health and Clinical Excellence, 2009. Depression: The Treatment and Management of Depression in Adults. <http://guidance.nice.org.uk/CG90/NICEGuidance/pdf/English>.

Neumeister, A., Praschak-Rieder, N., Willeit, M., et al., 1999. Monoamine depletion in non-pharmacological treatments for depression. Adv. Exp. Med. Biol. 467, 29–33.

Nolan-Hoeksema, S., 2002. Gender differences in depression. In: Gotlib, I., Hammen, C. (Eds.), Handbook of Depression. Guilford, New York, pp. 492–509.

Obeyesekere, G., 1985. Depression, Buddhism and the work of culture in Sri Lanka. In: Kleinman, A., Good, B. (Eds.), Culture and Depression: Studies in the Anthropology and Cross-Cultural Psychology of Affect and Disorder. University of California Press, Berkeley, CA, pp. 134–152.

Office for National Statistics, 2001. Psychiatric Morbidity among Adults Living in Private Households, 2000. <http://www.statistics.gov.uk/statbase/Product.asp?vlnk=8258&More=N>.

O'Hara, M., Zekoski, E., Philipps, L., et al., 1990. Controlled prospective study of postpartum mood disorders: comparison of childbearing and non-childbearing women. J. Abnorm. Psychol. 99, 3–15.

O'Hara, M., Schlechte, J., Lewis, D., et al., 1991. Controlled prospective study of postpartum mood disorders: psychological, environmental and hormonal variables. J. Abnorm. Psychol. 100, 63–73.

Roy, A., Nielsen, D., Rylander, G., et al., 1999. Genetics of suicide in depression. J. Clin. Psychiatry 60 (Suppl. 2), 12–17. [discussion 18–20:113–116].

Sadock, B., Sadock, V., 2007. Classification in psychiatry and psychiatric rating scales. In: Sadock, B., Sadock (Eds), Kaplan and Sadock's Synopsis of Psychiatry. Lippincott, Williams & Wilkins, Philadelphia, pp. 284.

Schieffelin, E., 1985. The cultural analysis of depressive affect: an example from New Guinea. In: Kleinman, A., Good, B. (Eds.), Culture and Depression: Studies in the Anthropology and Cross-Cultural Psychology of Affect and Disorder. University of California Press, Berkeley, CA, pp. 101–133.

Schulz, R., Drayer, R., Rollman, B., 2002. Depression as a risk factor for non-suicide mortality in the elderly. Biol. Psychiatry 52 (3), 205–225.

Southwick, S.M., Vythilingam, M., Charney, D.S., 2005. The psychobiology of depression and resilience to stress: implications for prevention and treatment. Annu. Rev. Clin. Psychol. 1, 255–291.

Spiegel, R., 2003. Psychopharmacology. An Introduction, fourth ed. John Wiley & Sons, Chichester.

Stolberg, R.A., Clark, D.C., Bongar, B., 2002. Epidemiology, assessment and management of suicide in depressed patients. In: Gotlib, I., Hammen, C. (Eds.), Handbook of Depression. Guilford, New York, pp. 581–601.

Sullivan, P.F., Neale, M.C., Kendler, K.S., 2000. Genetic epidemiology of major depression: review and meta-analysis. Am. J. Psychiatry 157 (10), 1552–1562.

Thase, M.E., Jindal, R., Howland, R.H., 2002. Biological aspects of depression. In: Gotlib, I., Hammen, C. (Eds.), Handbook of Depression. Guilford, New York.

Thompson, A., Shaw, M., Harrison, G., et al., 2004. Patterns of hospital admission for adult psychiatric illness in England: analysis of Hospital Episode Statistics data. Br. J. Psychiatry 185, 334–341.

Thompson, C., Thompson, S., Smith, R., 2004. Prevalence of seasonal affective disorder in primary care: a comparison of the seasonal health questionnaire and the seasonal pattern assessment questionnaire. J. Affect. Disord. 78, 219–226.

Torrey, E.F., Bowler, A.E., Taylor, E.H., et al., 1994. Schizophrenia and Manic-Depressive Disorder: The Biological Roots of Mental Illness as Revealed by the Landmark Study of Identical Twins. Basic Books, New York.

Valente, S., 2002. Overcoming barriers to suicide risk management. J. Psychosoc. Nurs. Ment. Health Serv. 40 (7), 22–33.

Ward, M., Jones, J., 2007. Close observation: the scapegoat of mental health nursing. In: Cutcliffe, J.R., Ward, M. (Eds.), Key Debates in Psychiatric/Mental Health Nursing. Churchill Livingstone, London.

Watson, S., Gallagher, P., Ritchie, J.C., et al., 2004. Hypothalamic-pituitary-adrenal axis function in patients with bipolar disorder. Br. J. Psychiatry 184, 496–502.

Westrin, A., Lam, R.W., 2007. Long-term and preventative treatment for seasonal affective disorder. CNS Drugs 21 (11), 901–909.

Whiffen, V., 1992. Is postpartum depression a distinct diagnosis? Clin. Psychol. Rev. 12 (5), 485–508.

Whiffen, V., Gotlib, I., 1993. Comparison of postpartum and non-postpartum depression: clinical presentation, psychiatric history, and psychosocial functioning. J. Consult. Clin. Psychol. 61 (3), 485–494.

Whybrow, P.C., 1997. A Mood Apart: Depression, Mania and Other Afflictions of the Self. Basic Books, New York.

Wisner, K.L., Parry, B.L., Piontek, C.M., 2002. Postpartum depression. N. Engl. J. Med. 347, 194–199.

World Health Organization, 2005. International Suicide Prevention. <http://www.who.int/mental_health/prevention/suicide/suicideprevent/en/suicidestatisticsresource>.

Yang, B., Clum, G., 1996. Effects of early life experience on cognitive functioning and risk for suicide: a review. Clin. Psychol. Rev. 16 (3), 177–195.

Zonana, J., Gorman, J.M., 2005. The neurobiology of postpartum depression. CNS Spectr. 10 (10), 792–799. [805].

Chapter | 16 |

Personality disorders

Christina Campbell and Gerald Farrell

CHAPTER POINTS

- People diagnosed with personality disorders are considered by nurses and others to be among the most challenging service users to care for.
- Although personality characteristics are formed early in life and evolve over time, once established they are resistant to change.
- People diagnosed with personality disorder have problems relating to others at home, work, school and in the community.
- Personality disorders are longstanding, pervasive and maladaptive behaviours that are resistant to treatment and are not caused by another psychiatric disorder, but may coexist with another psychiatric disorder.
- There are several theories of personality disorder with varying degrees of explanatory power.
- Evolution-based theory provides a broad base for understanding personality disorder by addressing fundamental developmental processes.
- People diagnosed with personality disorders may exhibit self-destructive behaviours such as self-mutilation, eating disorders, alcohol or substance abuse or even shoplifting.
- Improvement can only be achieved when the person with the disorder commits to exploring and re-evaluating their behaviour and relationships and then formulates realistic expectations, although, given the symptoms of personality disorder, this may be a very lengthy process.
- People diagnosed with personality disorder fall into psychiatry's grey area: they are often complained about for exhibiting the behaviours that led to their hospitalization in the first place.
- There is an urgent need for nursing practice in this field to be based on evidence that demonstrates and validates the contribution that nurses make to the care of these service users.

KEY TERMS

- agenda setting
- antisocial
- avoidant
- borderline
- dependency
- dependent
- histrionic
- limit-setting
- narcissistic
- obsessive–compulsive
- paranoid
- personality
- personality disorder
- personality traits
- schizoid personality disorder
- schizotypal personality disorder
- self-harm
- splitting

LEARNING OUTCOMES

The material in this chapter will assist you to:

- differentiate between a personality trait and a personality disorder,
- identify the main characteristics of each of the three clusters of personality disorders,
- develop an awareness of the feelings that may be experienced by nurses and other healthcare workers when working with people who have a personality disorder,
- understand the importance of maintaining clear professional boundaries when working with people who have a personality disorder,
- identify appropriate nursing interventions and treatments for the care of people with personality disorder,
- comprehend the evolutionary theory of personality disorder,
- appreciate the need for research into the study and treatment of personality disorder.

INTRODUCTION

People diagnosed with personality disorders exhibit attitudes and behaviours that can be difficult to change and which may coexist with another psychiatric disorder.

Indeed the individual who has any one of the recognized personality disorders may have no desire to change. These people tread an uneasy path between being seen as deserving treatment and being seen as not having a 'real' mental health problem. Nurses caring for such service users need appropriate education and support to be able to engage therapeutically with them. This chapter explains the main categories of personality disorders and their diagnosis. Nursing interventions are described, and challenges in working with people who have been diagnosed with a personality disorder are discussed. Limitations in our understanding of personality disorders and problems of categorization, diagnosis and treatment are also discussed.

'TRAIT' VERSUS 'DISORDER'

Each of us has a personality and a common sense understanding of what that means. We describe others as 'outgoing' or 'assertive' or maybe 'withdrawn' or 'shy'. Sometimes the ones we might choose to describe ourselves would not be chosen by those who know us. Some individuals have personalities that seem to draw people to them. They may be described as charismatic, outgoing, friendly, good team players, helpful or kind. Others seem to have difficulty attracting others or maintaining relationships. They appear unreceptive, cold, aloof, isolative, eccentric or perhaps are moody, aggressive or reckless. Our personality may be thought of as the expression of our feelings, thoughts and patterns of behaviour that evolve over time. Our genetics, life experiences and the environment to which we are exposed all serve to shape our personality. Our personality manifests in our moods, attitudes and opinions and is clearly expressed when we interact with others.

Enduring aspects or features of our personality are referred to as *personality traits*. These traits are what make us unique and interesting and they differentiate us from each other. Social mores provide unwritten boundaries for what constitutes a 'normal' personality trait. For example, if a student expresses concern at having to present their work to the class because they are shy, and public speaking makes them anxious, we regard that as being within the bounds of normal behaviour. It is very common for people to feel uncomfortable at the prospect of standing up in front of an audience, even one composed of their peers. With encouragement and support, most people are able to jump this particular hurdle. However, some individuals feel so strongly about appearing in public that they avoid all social situations where this may be required of them, to the point where they will withdraw from an enjoyable course of study or well-paid employment or even contact with their family. This behaviour is beyond what is socially regarded as shyness. The personality trait has moved beyond normal boundaries to a point where it may be understood in terms of psychopathology. Some individuals display personality traits that seem to be beyond the scope of what is considered reasonable as observed by their behaviour and attitudes to others, and, as in the foregoing example, will do almost anything to avoid feeling ridiculed, rejected or embarrassed.

When these manifestations of personality start to interfere negatively with a person's life or with the lives of those close to them, the person is diagnosed as suffering from a *personality disorder*. The challenge for nurses, and indeed for anyone involved with such an individual, lies in determining appropriate behaviour, given that norms relating to behaviour are socially and culturally constructed. When is the expression of someone's personality to be considered disordered? Let us set the scene for our contemplation of this question by considering the case study of Jodie.

CASE STUDY: JODIE

Jodie is 28 years old. She is an only child and still lives at home with her parents. She is particularly close to her mother. Jodie works as an administrative assistant for a small law firm where she is considered to be very good at her job. She is highly productive and has always been reliable. However, her colleagues state that they don't know 'what to do with her'. She has a fixation on her boss John, the senior partner in the firm. She believes, despite her feelings not being reciprocated, despite the considerable difference in their ages and despite their working together, that there are no barriers to their having a relationship. She is in love with him and believes they are meant to be together. She talks at length about him to her work mates. She becomes tearful and despondent and has been sent home 'sick' on a number of occasions by Laura, the office manager. Jodie blames her boss's inability to see how perfect they are for each other for her inability to function at work on these occasions.

The situation reached crisis point at the firm's Christmas party. Everyone from the office was treated to a dinner cruise with food, wine and music. Initially, Jodie appeared to be having a great time, laughing, flirting and expending a lot of energy on trying to get John to dance with her. After a while, however, Laura noticed that Jodie was missing. Laura found Jodie sitting apart from the main group, crying and sobbing, 'Why won't he come to his senses? How can he do this to me?' Jodie was clutching a handful of tablets. She told Laura that she had already swallowed a handful and she refused to say what they were. The boat had to return prematurely to port and an ambulance was called. The guests felt uncomfortable about eating the beautiful food that had been hurriedly presented to them and fell silent. Some were angry, while others were also confused. The party was ruined. In Jodie's opinion it was all John's fault.

Clearly, Jodie has some problems. In particular, she seems to have trouble with her relationships and with discerning appropriate ways of dealing with disappointment. It is one thing to have unrequited feelings for someone and to feel sad. It is quite another to deal with the situation as Jodie did. Jodie may be exhibiting the features of a personality disorder. In order to determine whether Jodie does have such a disorder, an assessment would need to be conducted that considered more than the events that triggered her attempted overdose and ensuing admission. A full psychosocial history would be obtained to enable clinicians to detect patterns in Jodie's behaviour over time. Without a comprehensive assessment, Jodie's behaviour may be interpreted as resulting from a fixed delusion on her boss. The problem is compounded by the fact that we believe that these behaviours are usually enacted unconsciously; that is, sufferers have little or no conscious awareness of their disorder.

However, it is rare for a person who has a diagnosis of a personality disorder to present with problems associated with the disorder as people tend to report secondary mental health issues such as depression, feeling unable to cope or because of the effects of a situational crisis in which they may find themselves.

CLASSIFICATION OF PERSONALITY DISORDERS

While each of the personality disorders described in the *ICD-10 Classification of Mental and Bhevaioural Disorders;* (World Health Organisation (WHO) 1992), has particular characteristics, they also have certain features in common. Personality disorders are recognized by persistent and enduring patterns of behaviour that are often destructive and nearly always characterized by maladaptive and inflexible ways of coping with stress (such as Jodie's response to John's rejection). As a result, those affected experience significant impairment in their ability to relate satisfactorily to others at work or socially. People diagnosed with personality disorder also seem to have an outsized capacity to evoke interpersonal conflict and therefore have an intense, often negative, impact on those around them.

One of the difficulties of caring for these people is that they tend to have very little or no insight into their condition. Clinicians often comment that the trouble with working with people with a personality disorder is that as far as they are concerned the problem is yours, not theirs! This lack of insight stems from an inability to empathize with others, which can be seen to be related to impaired cognition, affect, interpersonal functioning and impulse control (American Psychiatric Association, 2000). Of course we have to acknowledge that this view is the orthodox one and it may simply be that service users are unwilling to share with us how they feel and what they believe.

Box 16.1 summarises the diagnostic criteria used in clinical settings. It should be noted that the ICD-10 also provides a category to accommodate the diagnosis of people whose personality disorders do not fit the criteria for any specific disorder, which is referred to as 'unspecified'.

PROBLEMS OF DIAGNOSIS

The rise of evidence-based practice cautions health professionals to acknowledge the individual determinants of health and illness. Health professionals are urged to look at service users holistically and not reduce them to a label based purely on a collection of signs and symptoms. This is because the application of diagnostic categories has the potential to have a stigmatizing effect. That is, people may be treated in a negative way socially and within healthcare systems because of their diagnosis. Markham (2003, p. 595) conducted a study in which he evaluated the effect of the label 'borderline personality disorder' on registered mental health nurses' attitudes and perceptions of service users with that diagnosis. Markham (2003, p. 595) concluded that such nurses were least optimistic about service users diagnosed with a borderline personality disorder label and more negative about their experience working

---

Box 16.1 Diagnostic criteria for personality disorders

These types of condition comprise deeply ingrained and enduring behaviour patterns, manifesting themselves as inflexible responses to a broad range of personal and social situations. They represent either extreme or significant deviations from the way the average individual in a given culture perceives, thinks, feels, and particularly relates to others. Such behaviour patterns tend to be stable and to encompass multiple domains of behaviour and psychological functioning. They are frequently, but not always, associated with various degrees of subjective distress and problems in social functioning and performance.

Personality disorders differ from personality change in their timing and the mode of their emergence: they are developmental conditions, which appear in childhood or adolescence and continue into adulthood. They are not secondary to another mental disorder or brain disease, although they may precede and coexist with other disorders. In contrast, personality change is acquired, usually during adult life, following severe or prolonged stress, extreme environmental deprivation, serious psychiatric disorder, or brain disease or injury.

Each of the conditions in this group can be classified according to its predominant behavioural manifestations. However, classification in this area is currently limited to the description of a series of types and subtypes, which are not mutually exclusive and which overlap in some of their characteristics. Personality disorders are therefore subdivided according to clusters of traits that correspond to the most frequent or conspicuous behavioural manifestations. The subtypes so described are widely recognized as major forms of personality deviation. In making a diagnosis of personality disorder, the clinician should consider all aspects of personal functioning, although the diagnostic formulation, to be simple and efficient, will refer to only those dimensions or traits for which the suggested thresholds for severity are reached.

A specific personality disorder is a severe disturbance in the characterological constitution and behavioural tendencies of the individual, usually involving several areas of the personality, and nearly always associated with considerable personal and social disruption. Personality disorder tends to appear in late childhood or adolescence and continues to be manifest into adulthood. It is therefore unlikely that the diagnosis of personality disorder will be appropriate before the age of 16 or 17 years.

General diagnostic guidelines

Conditions not directly attributable to gross brain damage or disease, or to another psychiatric disorder, meeting the following criteria:

(continued)

a. markedly disharmonious attitudes and behaviour, involving usually several areas of functioning, e.g. affectivity, arousal, impulse control, ways of perceiving and thinking, and style of relating to others;

b. the abnormal behaviour pattern is enduring, of long standing, and not limited to episodes of mental illness;

c. the abnormal behaviour pattern is pervasive and clearly maladaptive to a broad range of personal and social situations;

d. the above manifestations always appear during childhood or adolescence and continue into adulthood;

e. the disorder leads to considerable personal distress but this may only become apparent late in its course;

f. the disorder is usually, but not invariably, associated with significant problems in occupational and social performance.

For different cultures it may be necessary to develop specific sets of criteria with regard to social norms, rules and obligations. For diagnosing most of the subtypes listed here, clear evidence is usually required of the presence of at least three of the traits or behaviours given in the clinical description.

Paranoid personality disorder

Paranoid personality disorder is characterized by:

a. excessive sensitiveness to setbacks and rebuffs;

b. tendency to bear grudges persistently, e.g. refusal to forgive insults and injuries or slights;

c. suspiciousness and a pervasive tendency to distort experience by misconstruing the neutral or friendly actions of others as hostile or contemptuous;

d. a combative and tenacious sense of personal rights out of keeping with the actual situation;

e. recurrent suspicions, without justification, regarding sexual fidelity of spouse or sexual partner;

f. tendency to experience excessive self-importance, manifest in a persistent self-referential attitude;

g. preoccupation with unsubstantiated 'conspiratorial' explanations of events both immediate to the patient and in the world at large.

Schizoid personality disorder

This is a personality disorder meeting the following description:

a. few, if any, activities, provide pleasure;

b. emotional coldness, detachment or flattened affectivity;

c. limited capacity to express either warm, tender feelings or anger towards others;

d. apparent indifference to either praise or criticism;

e. little interest in having sexual experiences with another person (taking into account age);

f. almost invariable preference for solitary activities;

g. excessive preoccupation with fantasy and introspection;

h. lack of close friends or confiding relationships (or having only one) and of desire for such relationships;

i. marked insensitivity to prevailing social norms and conventions.

Dissocial personality disorder

Dissocial personality disorder usually comes to attention because of a gross disparity between behaviour and the prevailing social norms, and is characterized by:

a. callous unconcern for the feelings of others;

b. gross and persistent attitude of irresponsibility and disregard for social norms, rules and obligations;

c. incapacity to maintain enduring relationships, though having no difficulty in establishing them;

d. very low tolerance to frustration and a low threshold for discharge of aggression, including violence;

e. incapacity to experience guilt or to profit from experience, particularly punishment;

f. marked proneness to blame others, or to offer plausible rationalizations, for the behaviour that has brought the patient into conflict with society.

Emotionally unstable personality disorder

This is a personality disorder in which there is a marked tendency to act impulsively without consideration of the consequences, together with affective instability. The ability to plan ahead may be minimal, and outbursts of intense anger may often lead to violence or 'behavioural explosions'; these are easily precipitated when impulsive acts are criticized or thwarted by others. Two variants of this personality disorder are specified, and both share this general theme of impulsiveness and lack of self-control.

Impulsive type

The predominant characteristics are emotional instability and lack of impulse control. Outbursts of violence or threatening behaviour are common, particularly in response to criticism by others.

Borderline type

Several of the characteristics of emotional instability are present; in addition, the patient's own self-image, aims, and internal preferences (including sexual ones) are often unclear or disturbed. There are usually chronic feelings of emptiness. A liability to become involved in intense and unstable relationships may cause repeated emotional crises and may be associated with excessive efforts to avoid abandonment and a series of suicidal threats or acts of self-harm (although these may occur without obvious precipitants).

(continued)

Histrionic personality disorder

Histrionic personality disorder is characterized by:

a. self-dramatisation, theatricality, exaggerated expression of emotions;
b. suggestibility, easily influenced by others or by circumstances;
c. shallow and labile affectivity;
d. continual seeking of excitement and activities in which the patient is the centre of attention;
e. inappropriate seductiveness in appearance or behaviour;
f. over-concern with physical attractiveness.

Associated features may include egocentricity, self-indulgence, continuous longing for appreciation, feelings that are easily hurt, and persistent manipulative behaviour to achieve own needs.

Anankastic personality disorder

This is a personality disorder characterized by:

a. feelings of excessive doubt and caution;
b. preoccupation with details, rules, lists, order, organization, or schedule;
c. perfectionism that interferes with task completion;
d. excessive conscientiousness, scrupulousness, and undue preoccupation with productivity to the exclusion of pleasure and interpersonal relationships;
e. excessive pedantry and adherence to social conventions;
f. rigidity and stubbornness;
g. unreasonable insistence by the patient that others submit to exactly his or her way of doing things, or unreasonable reluctance to allow others to do things;
h. intrusion of insistent and unwelcome thoughts or impulses.

Anxious (avoidant) personality disorder

This personality disorder is characterized by:

a. persistent and pervasive feelings of tension and apprehension;
b. the belief that one is socially inept, personally unappealing, or inferior to others;
c. excessive preoccupation with being criticized or rejected in social situations;
d. unwillingness to become involved with people unless certain of being liked;
e. restrictions in lifestyle because of the need to have physical security;
f. avoidance of social or occupational activities that involve significant interpersonal contact because of fear of criticism, disapproval or rejection.

Associated features may include hypersensitivity to rejection and criticism.

Dependent personality disorder

Dependent personality disorder is characterized by:

a. encouraging or allowing others to make most of one's important life decisions;
b. subordination of one's own needs to those of others on whom one is dependent, and undue compliance with their wishes;
c. unwillingness to make even reasonable demands on the people one depends on;
d. feeling uncomfortable or helpless when alone, because of exaggerated fears of inability to care for oneself;
e. preoccupation with fears of being abandoned by a person with whom one has a close relationship, and of being left to care for oneself;
f. limited capacity to make everyday decisions without an excessive amount of advice and reassurance from others.

Associated features may include perceiving oneself as helpless, incompetent and lacking stamina.

Adapted from World Health Organisation (1992) The ICD-10 Classification of Mental and Behavioural Disorders, pp. 156–161 with permission.

with this group compared to other service user groups. For example, nurses expressed higher levels of social rejection of service users with borderline personality disorder than of those with a diagnosis of schizophrenia (Markham, 2003, p. 608). They also attributed higher levels of dangerousness to those with the borderline personality disorder label than those diagnosed with schizophrenia (Markham, 2003, p. 602). The application of a diagnostic label may also affect the way the service user behaves. That is, when people are treated in a particular way they may respond in kind. A person may take the labels they have been given and behave in the way that the label suggests is expected of them (Haywood and Bright, 1997).

Individual service user predicaments and concerns should be given equal weight alongside what the research/diagnostic evidence says, so that together clinicians and service users can make informed choices about what might be the optimum care in a given situation (Farrell, 1997, p. 1). Psychologists remind us also of the interplay between psychological and physical determinants of illness and treatment outcomes. Yet it appears that psychiatry is moving ever more towards a reductionist approach to illness, whereby mental disorders are categorized into discrete entities, based on the presence of specific symptoms or signs.

Whereas the layperson may be forgiven for thinking that psychiatric diagnoses are reliable and valid, the mental health nurse should be aware that psychiatric diagnosis is problematic at best and flawed at worst. The DSM-IV TR (American Psychiatric Association, 2000) issues a cautionary statement to clinicians regarding the interpretation of its diagnostic categories; indeed, they are advised that specific diagnostic criteria serve only to inform professional judgement, not to override it. This is especially the case in personality disorder, where the diagnosis is often subject to heated debate. It acknowledges that:

> *...there is no assumption that each category of mental disorder is a completely discrete entity with absolute boundaries dividing it from other mental disorders or from no mental disorder. There is also no assumption that all individuals described as having the same mental disorder are alike in all important ways. The clinician using DSM-IV TR should therefore consider that individuals sharing a diagnosis are likely to be heterogeneous even in regard to the defining features of the diagnosis and that boundary cases will be difficult to diagnose in any but a probabilistic fashion.*

(American Psychiatric Association, 1994, p. xxii)

The DSM-IV TR (American Psychiatric Association, 2000) issues a cautionary statement to clinicians regarding the interpretation of its diagnostic categories; indeed, they are advised that specific diagnostic criteria serve only to inform professional judgement, not to override it. This is especially the case in personality disorder, where the diagnosis is often subject to heated debate.

The diagnosis of personality disorder clearly shows the weakness in relying on 'soft' or nebulous criteria for its diagnosis that are not usually generated by evidence-based research. The formulations of personality disorders in the DSM-IV TR and ICD-10 are atheoretical: they are simply lists of signs and symptoms and provide little in the way of explanation. The fact that service users are often diagnosed with four or more personality disorders illustrates the difficulties in providing a clear formulation of the disorder (Sadock and Sadock, 2003). Tyrer and Simonsen (2003, p. 41) quote work by Livesly (1986, 1991) that demonstrates that the key components of personality disorder are distributed among many individual categories and so it is not surprising that comorbidity of personality disorder is so common. In trying to gain an understanding of personality disorder, as with much of psychiatry, we are dealing with open concepts (Pap, 1953,

p. 41); that is, concepts that are subject to conceptual stretch. These concepts are over-used to the point of rendering them useless due to their breadth of application, thereby leading to confusion or misunderstanding. For instance, where does assertion end and aggression begin?

Personality disorders present problems not only of diagnosis but also of care, treatment and management. Nurses undertaking care of such individuals are advised to base their approach on four key areas of disturbance for such service users:

- cognition: the mental process of knowing, thinking, learning, understanding and judging,
- affect: one's expressed feeling or emotions,
- interpersonal functioning: interactions with others,
- impulse control: self-restraint (Anderson et al., 2002).

EPIDEMIOLOGY

The prevalence of a disorder refers to the estimated number of people in the population affected by it. Prevalence represents the number of new and pre-existing people with the disorder alive on a certain date. In the UK general population, the prevalence of personality disorder is estimated at 10–13% (Department of Health, 2003) although a more recent study has estimated this rate at 4.4%, with higher rates in urban areas, and among men (except for schizotypal personality disorder) (Coid et al., 2006). Personality disorders are diagnosed more often among white people (Department of Health, 2003).

In general, studies that are available on the prevalence of personality disorder are narrow in focus and lack the robustness of formal epidemiological research (Mattia and Zimmerman, 2001, p. 107). According to Mattia and Zimmerman (2001) no epidemiological survey of the full range of personality disorders has been conducted since the release of DSM-III. The studies that do exist suffer from problems of definition. Estimating the prevalence of suffers from the unavailability of standardized assessment tools, as well as the costs associated with conducting broad-based research.

Of all the personality disorders, antisocial personality disorder has received the most attention in epidemiological research. It appears that the median prevalence rate of antisocial personality is 1.2%, with a range of 0–3.7%. Table 16.2 summarizes the median prevalence rates for the other types of personality disorders. Note that the medians presented in Table 16.2 are those obtained across all studies reported by Mattia and Zimmerman (2001). These studies were conducted primarily in North America from 1985 to 1995.

From Table 16.1 it can be seen that the narcissistic personality is the least prevalent personality disorder. Most studies so far reported failed to find participants who

Table 16.1 Prevalence of personality disorders		
Type		**P (%)**
A Odd/eccentric	Paranoid	1.1
	Schizoid	0.6
	Schizotypal	1.8
B Dramatic	Histrionic	2.0
	Antisocial	1.2
	Borderline	1.1
	Narcissistic	0
C Anxious/fearful	Avoidant	1.2
	Dependent	2.2
	Passive–aggressive	2.1
	Obsessive–compulsive	4.3

Source: Adapted from Mattia and Zimmerman (2001), p 112.
P=Median prevalence.
Most studies report low numbers of subjects or none meeting the criteria for narcissistic personality disorder.

merited the diagnosis. Overall, community-based surveys from the USA, Canada, Scandinavia and New Zealand report a lifetime prevalence rate for all personality disorders of 10–13% (Falconer, 2001, p. 315). In both men and women the prevalence of personality disorders decreases with age (Andrews et al., 1999, p. 31; Samuels et al., 2002).

The person diagnosed with a personality disorder often experiences considerable impairment in activities of daily living, such as disturbance in relationships and impulsivity. Fifteen per cent of people had experienced at least 2 days of impaired functioning in the previous month; more than twice that of the rest of the population (Andrews et al., 1999, p. 31).

Anecdotally, clinicians report that their caseload of service users diagnosed with personality disorder is on the rise. While the majority of people diagnosed with a personality disorder will be treated and cared for in primary care (Department of Health, 2003), one Scottish study found that personality disorder occurs in 7% of all acute inpatient admissions, many of whom have additional diagnoses of other mental health problems and/or substance misuse, which further complicates their care and treatment (Dasgupta and Barber, 2004).

AETIOLOGY

There is consensus among researchers that when disorders are so entwined with temperament, it is reasonable to assume at least some genetic component in their aetiology (Sadock and Sadock, 2003, p. 800). The borderline personality has an estimated 69% level of heritability. This confirms the observations of practitioners who have long noted higher rates of personality disorder among descendents of those with the diagnosis than among those who do not have such a family history. However, the explanatory power of genetics is limited. Childhood abuse or other trauma that may result in low self-esteem or even self-loathing often appears in the histories of many people with a Cluster B disorder. Childhood abuse and neglect may contribute to the onset of some personality disorders. It would appear that people who have experienced childhood abuse or neglect are considerably more likely than those who have not been abused or neglected to have personality disorders and elevated personality disorder symptom levels during early adulthood (Johnson et al., 1999).

Evolution-based theory of personality

Theories should sharpen our focus and deepen our understanding of the development of phenomena. In psychiatry, they should provide a substantial explanation for the occurrence of disorders and for their treatment. However, when it comes to personality disorder we have a plethora of partial views. Contemporary explanations are predicated on a combination of biological, psychological and social risk factors such as genetic components, life experiences, and the influence of environmental factors that determine whether or not strong personality traits develop into personality disorders. Further, we lack a valid and reliable taxonomy of the personality disorders. (Readers interested in further discussion on the parlous state of our understanding of personality disorders should consult Millon et al. (2001). These authors provide an excellent overview of the difficulty in developing clear and substantive formulations on the complex composition of personality and psychopathological disorders, and the diversity of practical and theoretical approaches and frames of references that exist.)

In order to make sense of the theories that attempt to account for personality disorder we are going to discuss Millon et al.'s (2001) evolution-based theory, which transcends other theories in its fundamental inclusiveness of developmental factors. Millon et al. (2001) acknowledge the role of other theories, such as intrapsychically based theories (see Freud, 1915, 1931), behaviour-based theories (see, for example, Lang, 1968), interpersonally based theories (see, for example, Benjamin, 1974), cognitively based theories (see, for example, Alford and Beck, 1997) and neurobiologically based theories (see, for example, Cloninger, 1986), but make a convincing argument for the adoption of the evolution-based theory.

An evolution-based theory recognizes that personality is the aggregate of behaviour, cognition and interpersonal aspects of humans, thereby providing a way of understanding the total phenomenon of personality (and, by implication, personality disorder) in an integrated way. This theory tries to encompass all the variables that are thought to be the component parts of people, including their personality. It is an attempt to unify competing theories by providing a framework that is transposable to other existing explanations, such as interpersonal theory and neurobiological theory.

This theory is premised on the idea of focusing on the whole organism (the person). It is proposed that the principles of evolution should be applied to formulate a theory of personality, precisely because they are outside personality proper and can therefore accommodate the conflation of various schools of thought through the ages, thereby circumventing the dogma of the past (Millon et al., 2001). Millon et al. (2001) suggest that evolution is a logical choice in developing an understanding of personality as it allows us to apply the known developmental tasks of evolution to another phenomenon, that of personality. Personality development is therefore considered in relation to three universal evolutionary tasks: reproduction, survival in the ecosystem and homeostasis in the ecosystem.

Reproduction

The goal of reproduction is to maximize diversification and selection within a species. To evolve, a species must reproduce. Biologists describe two strategies for achieving this. First is the r-strategy, where many offspring, even hundreds, are produced, but are left to fend for themselves. Examples are mosquitoes and fish. Second is the K-strategy, where few offspring, perhaps one or two, are produced and are closely cared for by one or both parents for a time. Humans are an example.

While evolutionary theorists acknowledge exceptions to this, they regard the r-strategy as being more masculine – that is, self-orientated – while the K-strategy is more feminine or 'other nurturing'. For example, the rather selfish, narcissistic personality tends to be the former, while dependent types are closer to the latter.

Thus, evolutionary theory proposes three content polarities: pleasure–pain, active–passive and self–other. This theory of personality suggests that an individual may develop a personality disorder if they experience or encounter challenges to the balance of these polarities in their lives. Challenges may be in the form of neurological defects, genetic predisposition, childhood abuse or other traumatic experiences, which provide a way to explain how various personality styles develop and change.

Survival

Survival tasks are related to life enhancement as well as preservation of the individual; for example, pleasurable activities tend to be repeated, whereas painful ones tend to be avoided. Some people fail to develop this aspect of their personality. For example, most people who experience pain seek to avoid it. In the case of masochism, this survival response is distorted, as the person invites and enjoys pain. This would be contrary to the normal will to survive.

Homeostasis

Homeostasis requires the organism to adapt to its surroundings, or, as is more often the case in humans, adapt the environment to accommodate their needs. This may be regarded as a tension between a passive and an active orientation. Beings who fail to achieve adaptation of themselves or their environment tend to be selected out in evolutionary terms; an example is antisocial personalities, including extreme risk-takers and lawbreakers, who impulsively affect their environment with no thought or care for the consequences of their actions.

ASSESSMENT

People are rarely admitted to inpatient or acute mental health settings purely on the basis of a diagnosed personality disorder. Rather, they are admitted because of conditions coexisting with their disorder, such as depression or substance abuse, or for assessment due to some behavioural disturbance. Blackburn (2000) contends that more than half the service users in general psychiatric samples have a diagnosis of a coexisting personality disorder. Individuals with a diagnosis from Cluster A, odd and eccentric personality disorders, are the least likely to seek treatment. Those with Cluster C, anxious and fearful disorders, more frequently require treatment. It is the Cluster B, dramatic and emotional, personality disorders that most frequently find themselves the recipients of care by mental health clinicians. When one reviews the characteristics of people who have these disorders, it is easy to appreciate why this may be so. Reckless, irresponsible behaviour, impulsivity, sexually inappropriate behaviour and self-harming and self-mutilating behaviour tend to bring them into contact with the legal or healthcare services. Other behaviours that may draw attention include a propensity to litigious behaviours, shoplifting and abuse of drugs and alcohol. Very often their admissions are accompanied by a sense of drama, broken relationships and the consequences of dealing so poorly with the stresses of life.

Tredget (2001) notes that although symptoms vary in severity, people with personality disorder commonly present as being devoid of concern for others and as extremely egocentric; they will also lie to either explain or excuse their own behaviour or to gain sympathy.

Box 16.2 Assessment of a service user with a potential personality disorder

Drug and alcohol use
Self-harm or mutilation
Suicidal ideation and/or attempts
Instances of aggression or violence
Unexplained, visible injuries to body
Sexual activity
Family relationships

Source: Adapted from World Health Organisation (1992)
The ICD-10 Classification of Mental and Behavioural Disorders,
pp. 156–161 with permission.

Given that these people characteristically have no or little insight into their problems, they have a pronounced tendency to blame others for problems of their own making, which further rattles their already strained relationships with others. As they also tend not to learn from their mistakes in their relationships and in other aspects of life, they are doomed to repeat these errors over and over. So, for example, people with a borderline personality disorder fear being abandoned, yet they continue to behave in ways that tend to repel others. This, coupled with the fact that their tolerance for emotional pain is low, inevitably leads many to experience low self-esteem, which they may deal with by self-medicating with alcohol or other drugs, indulging in self-harming behaviour such as cutting, or they may develop eating disorders or be sexually promiscuous. These maladaptive behaviours are all examples of ways in which these service users may deal with the feelings they experience. The areas that need to be assessed are listed in Box 16.2.

An established pattern in one or more of the high-risk behaviours, such as illicit drug abuse or violence, may indicate that the service user has come to the attention of the police. Outstanding fines or impending legal proceedings further complicate the life of the person who has been diagnosed with a personality disorder.

The assessment should also be used to negate the existence of other conditions that could explain the presentation, such as hyperthyroidism, Cushing's syndrome, mood or anxiety disorder, post-traumatic stress disorder, substance abuse or an organic disorder. If an organic cause is suspected, a computerized axial tomography (CAT) scan may be ordered and blood collected and analysed for hormone levels (e.g. thyroid hormones or adenocorticotropic hormone). In some cases, testing of blood alcohol levels and a drug screen may be indicated. Indeed, substance or alcohol abuse often coexists with personality disorders and with borderline personality disorder in particular (Glod, 1998). The ingestion of these substances has the potential to alter behaviour. This may be particularly evident during withdrawal from these substances when aggressive, hostile, agitated or swinging mood states (lability) may be misinterpreted as signs of personality disorder. Another example is the side effects of steroid abuse, which may manifest in similar behaviour. The single most significant criterion for differentiating medical conditions, substance abuse or unwanted side effects of prescription medication is the comparison of the service user's presenting behaviour with their previous behaviour prior to the current episode. As stated above, personality disorders are characterized by enduring, pervasive patterns of behaviour over time, whereas in these alternative states there is usually a rapid, abrupt change in the individual that contrasts with their usual behavioural pattern.

The nurse needs to be aware of all these potentialities when assessing and caring for individuals diagnosed with personality disorders. Assessment often requires a lengthy interview and the clinician will need to observe keenly and demonstrate high-level assessment skills. Even then, the findings may be best considered provisional rather than definitive, at least until further corroborating material is gathered.

Marshall and Turnbull (1996) recommend the International Personality Disorder Examination (IPDE) (Loranger et al., 1994) as a useful standardized tool for assessment. Although the length of the instrument is problematic in some settings, its strength lies in the fact that it is a structured interview that accommodates cultural differences (Davison and Neale, 1998). This is the only personality disorder interview based on worldwide field trials. It has two parts: a self-administered screening questionnaire, which takes about 15 min to complete, and a semi-structured interview booklet with scoring materials, which takes up to 2 h to administer.

Given the multicultural nature of contemporary society, it is very important for the nurse to be sensitive to cultural differences. A behaviour that seems incongruent to a nurse of Anglo-Celtic origins may in fact be the norm for the cultural background of the service user. For example, in some cultures interactions between women and men, the young and the elderly, are governed by certain conventions that serve to maintain respect and that mirror the power differentials in relationships.

Their behaviours, such as eye contact, physical proximity and turn-taking during interactions, may be different from what you are accustomed to, and yours may seem odd to them!

CRITICAL THINKING CHALLENGE 16.1

Think about the community you live and work in, and identify some examples of cultural diversity. Can you incorporate this knowledge usefully into your own nursing practice?

INTERVENTIONS

Despite the prevalence of personality disorders, they are notoriously frustrating to treat. However, effective interventions do exist to alleviate symptoms and reduce the problematic behaviours that accompany personality disorders. Although people usually improve in terms of clinical and statistical significance, they might not reach 'normalcy' (Sanislow and McGlashan, 1998). From the service user's perspective this may mean dealing with their personality disorder to some degree for the rest of their lives. Therefore, long-term management plans need to be instituted for these people to promote their quality of life, including their relationships.

When planning care for a person diagnosed with a personality disorder, some factors require consideration regardless of which disorder the person may have. These factors relate to culture, insight, comorbidity and self-destructive behaviours. Cultural factors, including religion and ethnicity, must always be recognized, as a failure to do so could undermine any therapeutic intention the treatment team or therapist may have.

Given the intrinsic nature of personality, it is difficult to effect change if the service user does not acknowledge the need for it. Given that many of these service users will exhibit very low levels of insight, and are prone to nonadherence due to their inability to appreciate the need for intervention, the challenge is obvious for both service user and clinician. Altering aspects of personality takes place over extended periods of time and, though the gains may be very limited, they should be celebrated. So while the coexisting disorder may respond to the standard treatments for that condition, the underlying personality disorder may remain resistant to change. The principles of caring for the service user with a personality disorder are listed in Box 16.3.

The nurse must monitor the service user for signs of self-harm and suicidality. Although such behaviours may on occasion be dismissed by members of the treatment team as attention seeking or nonlethal manipulation, they are nonetheless an aspect of the service user's disorder and may well have been the motivating factor in admission. There must be consensus among team members as to how these behaviours are to be managed. Clear and frequent communication among team members will assist in this regard. Firm, fair and consistent limit-setting enacted with a nonjudgemental attitude should be continually strived for. Limit-setting aims to offer service users a degree of control over their behaviour. Whenever limit-setting is employed, the service user should know in advance the behaviours expected (for example, attend group therapy daily), as well as the consequences of breaches (for example, forfeit attendance at the late-night cinema). As far as practicable, the service user should be involved in setting the limits and determining the consequences. The use of contracts (where the service user and staff both sign a written agreement that sets out acceptable standards of behaviour) and time out (where the service user is offered monitored time in a quiet, private, low-stimulus environment until the urge to self-harm passes) have both been found to be useful tools in practice. The first gives the service user boundaries within which to operate and concrete consequences for behaviour. The second encourages the service user to attempt to deal with maladaptive behaviours in a more positive and acceptable way. Carried out consistently by a team that communicates well, the behaviours (see Box 16.4) of seduction, dependency, rejection, agenda setting, collusion and staff splitting (Tredget, 2001) may be avoided.

Such manipulative behaviour is analogous to the service user's propensity for dividing the world into 'good' and 'bad' with no individual or thing having both qualities at the same time. In an attempt to overcome some of these difficulties it is worth remembering that, as a nurse, your task is to accept that your role is to establish a relationship with a person who needs relief from feelings, has no reason to trust

---

Box 16.3 **Principles of care**

- Monitor for signs of self-harm and suicidality.
- Ensure consistency of care among treatment team members.
- Communicate frequently and clearly with the treatment team.
- Enact firm, fair and consistent limit-setting on service user.
- Involve service user in setting limits and determining consequences.

Box 16.4 **Definition of terms**

- Seduction: the service user engages in behaviours that can range from simple flattery to sexual seduction.
- Dependency: the nurse experiences gratification from the service user's perceived dependency on them.
- Rejection: the service user rejects the nurse(s) because they feel it is inevitable that the nurse(s) will reject them.
- Agenda setting: the service user is allowed to control the therapeutic relationship and the treatment regimen.
- Collusion: the service user attempts to persuade individual staff members to endorse their way of behaving.
- Staff splitting: the service user attempts to split the treatment team by appealing to individual members by sharing 'secrets' and suggesting that the staff member is the 'only one' who understands or is approachable.

you, has experienced a lifetime of betrayal, lives in a state of chronic arousal and cannot comfort or soothe themselves (Gallop, 2002). Gallop (2002) suggests that nurses need to set modest, service user-centred, short-term goals so that success can be easily recognized and experienced.

As with all people with mental health problems, it is vital for nurses to work in a spirit of collaboration and partnership with the person diagnosed with a personality disorder, encouraging them to find solutions to their own problems and to consider the options and consequences of the life choices that they make (NICE, 2009a).

Interactive therapies

The most appropriate psychological therapy for a service user with a diagnosis of personality disorder is likely to involve consideration of:

- the choice and preference of the service user,
- the degree of impairment and severity of the disorder,
- the person's willingness to engage with therapy and their motivation to change,
- the person's ability to remain within the boundaries of a therapeutic relationship,
- the availability of personal and professional support (NICE, 2009a, p. 20).

Increasingly, mental health nurses have been trained in *cognitive behavioural therapy* (CBT). CBT uses aspects of both cognitive therapy, which primarily seeks to identify and alter unhelpful patterns of belief, and behaviour therapy, which seeks to identify unhelpful patterns of behaviour and to implement strategies to break these patterns. CBT aims to help people to develop more efficient coping mechanisms by equipping them with strategies that promote logical ways of thinking about and responding to everyday situations (see Ch 23). *Cognitive analytic therapy* (CAT) is also an approach which has been used as therapy for personality disorders. The approach focuses on the development of relationships. It is an approach which stresses the importance of the active involvement of the patient in the therapeutic process and seeks to ensure collaboration between the therapist and patient (Ryle, 1997). The treatment process emphasizes the importance of the accurate description of the service user's styles of relating and thinking (Warren et al., 2003).

Dialectical behaviour therapy (DBT) is similar to CBT, but it also actively incorporates social skills training. The focus of this therapy is: first, the attenuation of parasuicidal and life-threatening behaviours; second, the attenuation of behaviours that hinder therapy; and third, the attenuation of behaviours that frustrate the service user's ability to improve their quality of life. Essentially this therapy, developed by Linehan (1998, 2000), moves between validation and acceptance of the person. Therapeutic procedures include attention to the present moment, being nonjudgemental and focusing on

effectiveness. Change strategies include behavioural analysis of maladaptive behaviours and problem-solving techniques, such as skills training, contingency management (using reinforcers and punishment), cognitive modification and exposure-based strategies (assisting service users to confront difficult situations) (Linehan, 1998, 2000).

In a meta-analysis of the effects of the two most frequently applied forms of psychotherapy in the treatment of personality disorders, psychodynamic therapy and CBT, it was found that both these therapies can be effective treatments for personality disorder. However, these results should be regarded as preliminary due to the limited number of studies that were included in the meta-analysis (Leichsenring and Leibing, 2003). Both these therapies are discussed in Chapter 23.

Pharmacological intervention

Medication has been of limited use in the treatment of personality disorder. In the UK, for example, there are no licensed drugs for the treatment of borderline personality disorder (NICE, 2009a) or antisocial personality disorder (NICE, 2009b). However, medication may help to control some of the comorbid symptoms that a person diagnosed with a personality disorder may experience, such as insomnia, anxiety and depression. Mood stabilizers such as lithium, anticonvulsants such as carbamazepine and sodium valproate, and selective serotonin-reuptake inhibitors such as sertraline hydrochloride or fluoxetine, may help to control the compulsive element of the dramatic disorders. Although antidepressant and anti-anxiety medications may have little effect on something as fundamental as personality, medical practitioners and psychiatrists find that if they prescribe medication that relieves the stress that comes with living such disordered lives, then some service users may be motivated or enabled to undertake the therapies described above. There is also some indication that antipsychotic medications may alleviate paranoid, schizoid and schizotypal symptoms (Sadock and Sadock, 2003, p. 804). Chapter 24 provides more information about these medications.

Therapeutic community

Tredget (2001) defines a therapeutic community as a setting where a conscious effort is made to ensure that the potential of all service users and staff is used to create a social environment that is conducive to personal development. This style of care seeks to minimize hierarchical power relationships so that there is equality between service users and staff in relation to decisions concerning treatment and the running of the community. One of the most prominent exponents of this style of care is the Richmond Fellowship. Originally founded by a social worker in England, the Fellowship maintains many residences offering the opportunity for personal growth and development to young people with a range of mental disorders. Chapter 21 offers further discussion of the therapeutic community.

Team or triumvirate nursing interventions

Given the propensity for people diagnosed with a personality disorder to split staff, this form of care delivery might be useful, particularly in the inpatient setting, although empirical evidence to substantiate its degree of efficacy is lacking. It involves nurses working in teams of three, each with equal responsibility for the provision of care to the service users assigned to them. Two nurses of the team of three conduct sessions with the service user. A debriefing session is conducted with the third nurse after each occasion. Tredget (2001) describes this role as the clinical coordinator role, as this person attempts to constructively challenge what has transpired in the therapy sessions with the service user. This provides an appropriate, professional forum for dealing with any issues that may have arisen and facilitates reflective practice. The nurses' roles are interchangeable, so that no one nurse is always the clinical coordinator. For this system to work well, staffing and rostering issues must be taken into account to maintain viable teams. The point of this exercise is to ensure that all staff involved in the service user's care, regardless of whether they are full-time or part-time workers, are privy to the same information in relation to the service user's management while at work.

WORKING WITH PEOPLE DIAGNOSED WITH PERSONALITY DISORDER

Given the discussion thus far, it will not surprise you to learn that working with people who have a diagnosis of a personality disorder can be very challenging for all concerned. This particular diagnosis is especially prone to having a loaded label. By 'loaded label' we mean that the very term itself carries negative connotations. Listen to the way people say 'PDs' and in what context and ask yourself what images it conjures up for you. The nurse and indeed all those involved with such service users must resist the temptation to respond to these service users in a way that may negatively affect their care.

A significant challenge when working with people with a diagnosis of personality disorder is the care, management and support of the person during a time of crisis. At such times, for example, a person with borderline personality disorder may benefit from interventions where the nurse:

- maintains a calm and nonthreatening attitude,
- tries to understand the crisis from the person's point of view,
- explores the person's reasons for distress,

- uses empathic open questioning, including validating statements, to identify the onset and the course of the current problems,
- seeks to stimulate reflection about solutions,
- avoids minimizing the person's stated reasons for the crisis,
- refrains from offering solutions before receiving full clarification of the problems,
- explores other options before considering admission to a crisis unit or inpatient admission,
- offers appropriate follow-up within a time frame agreed with the person (NICE, 2009a, 23–24).

One of the behaviours that is particularly difficult to work with is that of self-harm/self-mutilation. Self-harming behaviours may be regarded as occurring along a continuum from pulling out one's own hair, cutting, piercing or burning oneself, through to suicide. People diagnosed with borderline personality disorder are particularly at risk of self-harm and suicide (NICE, 2009a). As Smyth (1989) suggests, human beings are creatures of habit, and even bad habits can feel safe and familiar. Therefore, self-harming behaviours such as the above may be difficult to understand yet are comforting and confirming for the service user. Gallop (2002) suggests that self-harm fulfills many functions for the service user:

- it communicates feelings,
- it recreates chaos and provides stimulation,
- it re-enacts past trauma,
- it provides a distraction from painful emotions.

As Gallop (2002) suggests, the self-harming behaviour is the service user's 'best friend' in a world that is out of control from their perspective. In terms of management, the nurse must be cognisant of the fact that asking service users to 'let go' of self-harming behaviours can precipitate intense panic and anxiety. In effect, the service user is asked to give up a familiar mode of self-regulation, to give up a way of numbing, a way of containing fear, rage and shame, and a way of not feeling alone (Gallop, 2002).

It must also be noted that criminality is not uncommon among people diagnosed with antisocial personality disorder, but a history of aggression, unemployment and promiscuity are more common than serious criminal behaviour among this client group (NICE, 2009b). People in prisons and forensic mental healthcare settings in particular have a greater chance of being diagnosed with antisocial personality disorder (Department of Health, 2003). The care, treatment and risk management of people with such diagnosis are likely to involve liaison with the criminal justice system (NICE, 2009b).

As indicated in the research, change is likely to be slow and piecemeal, and nurses will need advanced clinical skills and staying power to effect change in the lives of these service users. Establishment of a therapeutic relationship with these service users underpins all the therapeutic approaches to care discussed above. Time and high-level interpersonal skills are needed to create a safe relationship in order to understand the intimate details of the underlying emotions and thoughts that trigger service users' behaviour.

Research suggests that service users with a diagnosis of borderline personality disorder have higher rates of childhood sexual and childhood physical abuse than other clinical populations (Gallop, 2002). A survey conducted by Cleary et al. (2002, p. 188) of mental health staff in a public area mental health service in New South Wales illustrates the degree to which nurses in this area of practice have difficulty. Results indicate that 80% of nurses surveyed admitted to finding service users who have borderline personality disorder moderately to very difficult to deal with, and 84% admitted that dealing with this service user group was more difficult than dealing with other service users.

An earlier phenomenological study by O'Brien and Flöte (1997) of a group of nurses caring for a service user with borderline personality disorder on an acute inpatient unit provides a rich description of the experience of caring for such impulsive and self-destructive individuals. Following is the brief description of the service user that appears in the published article.

The client in this study ... was in her early thirties. Her childhood was marked by physical and sexual abuse from a very early age. She left home at thirteen, was admitted to various residential institutions in her adolescent years, and had psychiatric admissions from late adolescence. She had periods of relative stability when she was in psychotherapy but disruption to this process inevitably led to further acts of self-harm. Despite this background she was seen as capable of change, intelligent, and psychologically minded. Her admissions to the unit, where the study was conducted, were marked by difficulty. She was usually admitted in crisis following periods of self-harm and, although she settled upon admission, the self-harm behaviour subsequently escalated and there was difficulty in effecting her discharge.

(O'Brien and Flöte, 1997, pp. 137–138)

Whereas Cleary et al. (2002) administered a postal, structured questionnaire for respondents to complete and return, O'Brien and Flöte (1997) conducted face-to-face interviews with a small group of staff to collect their data. The analysis of the transcribed tape-recorded interviews revealed several key points or themes in what the nurses had to say. Three of these themes were:

- being unsure,
- being in conflict,
- struggling to make sense of the service user's experience.

The theme of being unsure meant that staff felt unsure of treatment and interventions or how to proceed with the service user's care. The staff felt pessimistic about the service user's prognosis, and therefore also felt helpless and hopeless. The theme of being in conflict relates to being in conflict with other staff about the service user's care and also having conflicting feelings towards the service user herself. On the one hand, staff described feelings of compassion and empathy for the service user; on the other, they felt manipulated. The nurses felt they had to be guarded in their interactions with the service user, a feeling that was bound up with their distrust of her. The interviews revealed that this service user evoked such strong emotions in the staff that there was conflict over her treatment, even her right to treatment, before she arrived on the ward. The theme of struggling to make sense of the service user's experience refers to struggling to understand her impulsive self-harming behaviour, her motivations for treating herself in such a violent way. The notion was expressed that it felt like being involved in some mystery where the line between truth and fiction couldn't be drawn, particularly in relation to her history of having been sexually abused, and being traumatized. This latter theme emerged from the nurses' experiences of listening to the service user's dreadful stories and dealing with the constant threat of more trauma occurring. Their feelings were compounded by the difficulty of maintaining appropriate professional distance with someone they had to work so physically closely with in order to prevent more trauma (self-harm). They felt professionally under threat in other ways. Dilemmas arose for the nurses out of certain interventions. For example, seclusion had such a distressing effect on the service user that the nurses questioned who it was intended to be good for.

NURSE'S STORY: AIDAN, BY RICHARD

I will never forget the impact that nursing Aidan had on my professional life. It started early one Sunday morning while I was on night duty on an acute adult psychiatric unit in a large hospital in an inner-city suburb. I had taken a call from the registrar on duty in the accident and emergency department who said he wanted to admit a 23-year-old male who had been brought in by police, who had found him 'playing chicken' with the cars on the freeway while wailing about having been abandoned by Kevin, 'the absolute darling, love of my life!'. The client had a history of short to medium/long admissions, with a diagnosis of depression and a diagnosis of histrionic personality disorder.

When Aidan arrived on the ward, I remember thinking, 'What a tragic, over-the-top mess'. Aidan was resplendent in an old pink voile and organza evening frock, something like Audrey Hepburn used to wear, accessorized with the longest pair of shoes I, or indeed any of the staff on the ward, had ever seen. They were high-heeled, silver, beaded pumps. Now scuffed and worn, they added another three inches to Aidan's already substantial height of 190 cm. He was also wearing a matted, tatty ash blonde wig that kicked up around the bottom, Doris Day style. The once elaborate make-up was smudged and tear-stained, which gave Aidan's face a 'melted' look. The three of us nurses looked at each other with raised eyebrows. Someone whispered, 'I've seen drama queens before, but this guy is too much!'. It wasn't just Aidan's appearance, it was his whole manner. The theatrical way he would throw his arms around while he talked, the way he swung his hips to and fro while he walked and the tears he managed to produce, seemingly at will. I was the only male nurse on the shift and Aidan zeroed in on me.

I admitted Aidan to the ward, adhering to all the standard procedures. Despite my professional manner, however, Aidan seemed to read much more into the nascent nurse–client relationship. Aidan didn't reside on the ward, he performed on it. Every interaction was like a stage performance on his part. He seemed to crave being the centre of attention and became very frustrated when he wasn't. This was particularly so if I wasn't taking notice of him. If I was attending to another client, Aidan would sidle up behind me in a seductive manner, calling me 'Angel of Mercy' or 'My darling one' and so on. After a short time this tried my patience. I am a happily married man, but other staff on the ward started to make jokes about my sexuality, which I detested. It wasn't homophobia; it was more that they were not always discreet when they made these jibes, so other clients often heard them.

Aidan proved to be disruptive in other ways as well. He started to refuse to cooperate with the general milieu of the ward. He wouldn't take his medication, bathe or attend group activities unless I asked him to. This resulted in the ward staff having disagreements about Aidan's management. Some felt this behaviour was inappropriate and that limit-setting should be incorporated into Aidan's care plan, while others trivialized it, and said they had no problem with 'leaving the queen' to me. During this time I became increasingly stressed by the continued pressure being placed on me by Aidan. Aidan dominated my work, which made me feel that I was not giving my other clients the attention they deserved.

It all came to a head when another staff member mistakenly opened a letter from Aidan that was intended for me. There was a greeting card inside and in it, Aidan had not only declared his undying love for me, but had also expressed a desire to repeat some 'performances' of a sexual nature with me. The letter read as if Aidan and I had been engaging in such behaviour while I was rostered on night duty. The next time I presented for duty, the nurse manager took me aside and asked me to give my account of the situation. I was mortified. I felt that my professional integrity had been challenged. I was stunned: while some nursing staff were supportive of me and rejected Aidan's insinuations, others delighted in casting aspersions. Some made comments like, 'Where there's smoke there's fire' and 'Now we know what you get up to on nights' and

other inflammatory statements. I decided this all had to stop: the division and dissension caused by this one client was having a negative impact on the whole ward. At this point it was likely that Aidan would soon be discharged, although, given his history, it was also likely that he would be readmitted in the future, and so it would be useful to have already formulated workable strategies for dealing with Aidan and clients like him. To this end, I volunteered to present Aidan as a case history at the next Grand Round (multidisciplinary meeting where case studies are presented and discussed). This proved to be very worthwhile and as a result the ward staff, including nonnursing staff, agreed that they had to function as a cohesive team. Consistency of approach had to be used with Aidan, and limit-setting strategies were discussed. Further, I became one of three staff members who took responsibility for planning Aidan's care. We all agreed to communicate with each other and with Aidan in a clear and respectful manner. I no longer spent time alone with Aidan.

The nurse's story about Aidan starkly yet sensitively encapsulates many of the challenges potentially presented by service users who have a diagnosis of a personality disorder. That is not to say that all present with such intensity. The story illustrates how quickly staff abrasions and fractured service user care can occur when nursing staff fail to act with a common purpose and resolve. Richard, the nurse in the story, shows how important it is to quickly bring issues out into the open and to act proactively for the future. Staff need to pull together if they are to effect change in the service user's behaviour and maintain their own composure. Being able to recognize your responses to the service user for what they are, and deal with them appropriately by using reflection and professional discussion with colleagues, is the best way to cope with service users who have this disorder.

CRITICAL THINKING CHALLENGE 16.2

Has reading this chapter changed your attitude towards people who self-harm? If so, how? If not, why not?

CONCLUSION

People diagnosed with personality disorder pose major challenges for mental health service providers. Working with these service users often instils negative feelings in nurses and others. Finding it hard to empathize with these service users will impair the nurse's ability to work with them therapeutically. Ironically, the very reasons for their admission are often the catalyst for some nurses seeking their discharge. Nurses need education, supervision and staff support to deal with the challenges posed by this service user group (NICE, 2009a). Any issues of disagreement over the service user's care should be openly discussed and ways found to support staff so that workplace relations and service user management are not compromised.

Finally, there is an immediate need for nursing research in the management of personality disorder. As the single largest group of mental healthcare providers, nurses are ideally placed to make a significant contribution to improvements in the delivery of care to those with personality disorder. However, a review of the research literature shows that there is a weak evidence base for what constitutes effective nursing care and management of personality disorder. There is stronger evidence to support multidisciplinary approaches to management rather than nursing approaches alone (Woods and Richards, 2002). Studies need to be developed around structured and systematic strategies to provide empirical evidence upon which to base practice.

EXERCISES FOR CLASS ENGAGEMENT

Re-read Jodie's scenario at the beginning of the chapter and discuss the following questions with your group.

♦ What possible diagnoses would you consider for Jodie?
♦ What other information would be needed to make a diagnosis?
♦ What potential problems might a service user like Jodie present for nursing staff in terms of her care?

When you arrive for your evening shift you receive a handover for a new service user. The service user is a 21-year-old female who has been admitted as an inpatient via the accident and emergency department following an apparent suicide attempt. Her name is Kylie. Both her forearms are bandaged and you are told that Kylie has inflicted significant though not life-threatening wounds to herself. It seems that her self-harming was a response to the break-up of her relationship with her partner. The relationship was only 6 weeks old. You talk to her and find that despite your misgivings due to her self-harming, you easily establish rapport with Kylie. You are about the same age and it turns out that she was in your younger brother's class at school. You feel buoyed by the experience, especially given the negative comments the other staff made about the new 'PD' at handover. When you return from your tea break, you find Kylie in tears. She says, 'Thank God you're back! You're the only one who has any time for me. That other old bag won't even let me have my things and she won't let me go to the kiosk! Can you make sure that you're always assigned to be my nurse?'. As a group, discuss the following questions.

♦ What should you do?
♦ How do you respond to the service user? State exactly the words you would use when speaking to the service user.
♦ Are the issues different for you depending on your own gender?

♦ Would you approach the staff member involved?
♦ How would you describe the behaviour exhibited here?
♦ Suggest ways in which this service user could be effectively managed:
   — as an inpatient service user,
   — as an outpatient service user.

Your brother has been seeing a new girlfriend for several weeks. One night, over the family dinner table, he says that he is finally going to 'meet the parents'. He's not too worried, he hasn't had any problems with his friends' parents before, and is actually curious because his girlfriend has not really told him much about them other than that her mother is a nurse who works part-time in a medical centre and her father is a senior bureaucrat of some kind in the government. Two nights later you get the report. He says, 'Her oldies are weird'. He goes on to describe the following: after each time the telephone is used, the mother cleans it with antibacterial spray; there was a whiteboard on the kitchen wall that was ruled into columns detailing a variety of schedules and rosters; the father, who only came out of his home office to eat and then returned, berated the mother for smearing the gravy on the side of his dinner plate; the dog wasn't allowed inside and they all had to say grace before eating. He says he has never seen anything like it. He asks for your opinion, as you have been working with 'loonies'. Discuss the following questions as a group.

♦ What does this story tell you about the girlfriend's family?
♦ What does it tell you about your brother?
♦ How might you explain his response to some of the things he observed?
♦ Do you agree with your brother's assessment of the family?
♦ What is the difference between a personality trait or traits and a personality disorder?

REFERENCES

Alford, B.A., Beck, A.T., 1997. The Integrative Power of Cognitive Therapy. Guilford Press, New York.

American Psychiatric Association (1994). Diagnostic and Statistical Manual of Mental Disorders, 4th ed. American Psychiatric Association, Washington DC.

American Psychiatric Association, 2000. Diagnostic and Statistical Manual of Mental Disorders, 4th ed., text rev. American Psychiatric Association, Washington DC.

Anderson, D.M., Keith, J., Novak, P.D., et al., 2002. Mosby's Medical, Nursing and Allied Health Dictionary, 6th ed. Mosby, St Louis.

Andrews, G., Hall W., Teeson M., et al. 1999. National Survey of Mental Health and Wellbeing, Report 2. The Mental Health of Australians. National Mental Health Strategy, Department of Health and Aged Care, Canberra.

Benjamin, L.S., 1974. Structural analysis of social behaviour. Psychol. Rev. 81, 392–425.

Blackburn, R., 2000. Treatment or incapacitation? Implications of research on personality disorders for the management of dangerous offenders. Legal Criminol. Psych. 5, 1–21.

Cleary, M., Siegfried, N., Walter, G., 2002. Experience, knowledge and attitudes of mental health staff regarding clients with a borderline personality disorder. Int. J. Ment. Health Nurs. 11 (3), 186–191.

Cloninger, R.C., 1986. A unified biosocial theory of personality theory and its role in development of anxiety states. Psychiatr. Dev. 3, 167–226.

Coid, J., Yang, M., Tyrer, P., et al., 2006. Prevalence and correlates of personality disorder in Great Britain. Br. J. Psychiatry 188, 423–431.

Dasgupta, P., Barber, J., 2004. Admission patterns of patients with personality disorder. Psychiatr. Bull. 28, 321–323.

Davison, G., Neale, J., 1998. Abnormal Psychology, seventh ed. John Wiley and Sons, New York.

Department of Health, 2003. Personality disorder: no longer a diagnosis of exclusion–policy implementation guidance for the development of services for people with personality disorder. <http://www.dh.gov.uk/en/Publicationsandstatistics/Publications/PublicationsPolicyAndGuidance/DH_4009546>.

Falconer, B., 2001. Personality disorders. In: Meadows, G., Singh, B. (Eds.), Mental Health in Australia: Collaborative Community Practice. Oxford University Press, Melbourne.

Farrell, G.A., 1997. Getting up to Speed with Evidence-Based Practice. Australian and New Zealand College of Mental Health Nurses, Sydney.

Freud, S., 1915. The instincts and their vicissitudes Collected Papers, 4. Hogarth Press, London.

Freud, S., 1931. Libidinal types. Collected Papers, vol 5. Hogarth Press, London.

Gallop, R., 2002. Trauma and personality: working with clients who have a diagnosis of borderline personality disorder. Seminar presentation, Rokeby Police Academy, Hobart, Tasmania.

Glod, C., 1998. Contemporary Psychiatric-Mental Health Nursing: The Brain–Behaviour Connection. F A Davis, Philadelphia.

Haywood, P., Bright, J.A., 1997. Stigma and mental illness: a review and critique. J. Ment. Illn. 6, 345–354.

Johnson, J., Cohen, P., Brown, J., et al., 1999. Childhood maltreatment increases risk for personality disorders during early adulthood. Arch. Gen. Psychiatry 56 (7), 600–606.

Lang, P.J., 1968. Fear reduction and fear behaviour: problems in treating a construct. In: Schlein, J.M. (Ed.), Research in Psychotherapy, III. American Psychological Association, Washington D C, pp. 90–102.

Leichsenring, F., Leibing, E., 2003. The effectiveness of psychodynamic therapy and cognitive behaviour therapy in the treatment of personality disorders: a meta-analysis. Am. J. Psychiatry 160 (7), 1223–1232.

Linehan, M.M., 1998. An illustration of dialectical behaviour therapy. In Session: Psychothe. Pract. 4 (2), 21–44.

Linehan, M.M., 2000. Commentary on innovation in dialectical behaviour therapy. Cogn. Behav. Ther. 7 (4), 478–481.

Livesly, W.J., 1986. Trait and behavioural prototypes of personality disorder. Am. J. Psychiatry 143, 728–732.

Livesly, W.J., 1991. Classifying personality disorders: ideal types, prototypes or dimensions? J. Personal. Disord. 5, 52–59.

Loranger, A., Sartorius, N., Andreoli, A., et al., 1994. The international personality disorder examination. The world health organization/alcohol, drug abuse and mental health administration international pilot study of personality disorders. Arch. Gen. Psychiatry 51 (3), 215–224.

Markham, D., 2003. Attitudes towards patients with a diagnosis of 'borderline personality disorder': social rejection and dangerousness. J. Ment. Health 12 (6), 595–612.

Marshall, S., Turnbull, J., 1996. Cognitive Behavioural Therapy: An Introduction to Theory and Practice. Baillière-Tindall, London.

Mattia, J.I., Zimmerman, M., 2001. Epidemiology. In: Livesley, W.J. (Ed.), Handbook of Personality Disorders: Theory, Research and Treatment. Guilford Press, New York.

Millon, T., Meagher, S.E., Grossman, S.D., 2001. Theoretical perspectives. In: Livesley, W.J. (Ed.), Handbook of Personality Disorders: Theory, Research and Treatment. Guilford Press, New York.

NICE (National Institute for Health and Clinical Excellence), 2009a.

Borderline personality disorder: treatment and management. <http://guidance.nice.org.uk/CG78/NICEGuidance/pdf/English>.

NICE (National Institute for Health and Clinical Excellence), 2009b. Antisocial personality disorder: treatment, management and prevention. <http://guidance.nice.org.uk/CG77/NICEGuidance/pdf/English>.

O'Brien, L., Flöte, J., 1997. Providing nursing care for a client with borderline personality disorder on an acute inpatient unit: a phenomenological study. Aust. N. Z. J. Ment. Health Nurs. 6 (4), 137–147.

Pap, A., 1953. Reduction—sentences and open concepts. Methods 5, 3–30.

Ryle, A., 1997. The structure and development of borderline personality disorder: a proposed model. Br. J. Psychiatry 170, 82–87.

Sadock, B.J., Sadock, V.A., 2003. Synopsis of Psychiatry: Behavioral Sciences/Clinical Psychiatry, 9th ed. Lippincott Williams, Philadelphia.

Samuels, J., Eaton, W., Bienvenu, J., 2002. Prevalence and correlates of personality disorders in a community sample. Br. J. Psychiatry 180, 536–542.

Sanislow, C., McGlashan, T., 1998. Treatment outcome of personality disorders. Can. J. Psychiatry 43, 237–250.

Smyth, E.E.M., 1989. Surviving Nursing. Addison-Wesley, Menlo Park, CA.

Tredget, J.E., 2001. The aetiology, presentation and treatment of personality disorders. J. Psychiatr. Ment. Health Nurs. 8 (4), 347–356.

Tyrer, P., Simonsen, E., 2003. Personality disorder in psychiatric practice. World Psychiatry 2 (10), 41–44.

Warren F., et al., 2003. Review of treatments for severe personality disorder. <http://www.personalitydisorder.org.uk/news/wp-content/uploads/Review_of_Treatments.pdf>.

Woods, P., Richards, D., 2002. The Effectiveness of Nursing Interventions with Personality Disorders: A Systematic Review of the Literature. School of Nursing, Midwifery and Health Visiting, University of Manchester, Manchester, UK.

World Health Organisation (WHO), 1992. The ICD-10 Classification of Mental and Behavioural Disorders. Available at: <http://www.who.int/classifications/icd/en/bluebook.pdf>.

Chapter | 17 |

Anxiety disorders

Sue Henderson and Stephen Elsom

CHAPTER POINTS

- Anxiety disorders are one of the most common mental health problems.
- People diagnosed with an anxiety disorder are less likely to seek treatment than people with a mood disorder.
- Every nurse should be able to recognize the different presentations of the various anxiety disorders and refer service users to appropriate services.
- All nurses should possess the skills to care for people experiencing a panic attack in any setting.
- Mobilizing appropriate coping skills and implementing stress-management techniques is a core nursing skill.
- The major psychotherapeutic methods of treating anxiety disorders include cognitive behavioural therapy and stress-management techniques such as progressive muscle relaxation.
- The most common drugs used in the treatment of anxiety disorders are antidepressants and anxiolytics.

DOI: http://dx.doi.org/10.1016/B978-0-7020-4493-9.00017-2

- acute stress disorder (ASD)
- adjustment-related disorders
- agoraphobia
- anxiety
- compulsions
- coping
- generalized anxiety disorder (GAD)
- obsessions
- obsessive–compulsive disorder (OCD)
- panic attack
- panic disorder
- phobic disorder
- post-traumatic stress disorder (PTSD)

LEARNING OUTCOMES

The material in this chapter will assist you to:

- define key terms related to anxiety disorders,
- distinguish between normal anxiety and the anxiety experienced in anxiety disorders,
- discuss the epidemiology, aetiology and treatment of anxiety disorders,
- explain the different types of anxiety disorders,
- describe the assessment of individuals diagnosed with anxiety disorders,
- discuss interventions appropriate to the care of individuals diagnosed with anxiety disorders,
- provide teaching to individuals and the community to facilitate early intervention for people diagnosed with anxiety disorders.

INTRODUCTION

Nurses frequently interact with anxious service users who are facing threats to their health and wellbeing. Experienced nurses become adept at reassuring and supporting service users in coping with the threat and crisis posed by ill health and trauma. Anxiety is a normal emotion experienced in varying degrees by everyone. Carpenito (2002, p. 113) defines anxiety as 'a state in which the individual/group experiences feelings of uneasiness (apprehension) and activation of the autonomic nervous system in response to a vague, non-specific threat'. Anxiety may manifest as:

- thought, for example excessive worry or an intrusive, unwanted idea,
- feeling, for example a feeling of impending doom,

- behaviours, for example performing repetitive actions or avoiding objects or situations,
- physical change, for example increased heart rate, trembling.

However, the presence of anxiety does not signify that the service user has an anxiety disorder. Anxiety disorders are specific diagnostic entities that are the primary problem.

Anxiety disorders are one of the most common mental health problems. They disrupt the individual's everyday life yet often go unrecognized by service users and health professionals alike. There is a tendency for service users, health professionals and others to dismiss the symptoms of anxiety disorders as nerves, worry or excessive shyness. As a result, anxiety disorders often go untreated, undertreated or inappropriately treated.

If this situation is to be reversed it is imperative that all nurses have an accurate understanding of anxiety and its relationship to anxiety disorders. A sound appreciation of the prevalence, causes, assessment, treatment and nursing management of anxiety will enable the nurse to provide evidence-based nursing care. In addition, a sound knowledge base will facilitate the accurate dissemination of information about anxiety disorders to service users, families and communities. Increased mental health literacy about anxiety disorders may facilitate early intervention for people with anxiety disorders, which could, with appropriate treatment, reduce the incidence of anxiety disorders.

CRITICAL THINKING CHALLENGE 17.1

Consider the following service user scenarios.

- Sharon organizes her clothes according to fabric type and colour.
- Michael continues to have nightmares 5 years after he was robbed at a petrol station.
- Seb has never liked spiders.
- Alicia stays at home all day every day.
- Glenda worries about everything and has done so for years.
- Nick avoids eating in public.

Now ask yourself these questions.

- Is this anxiety normal or does it constitute a disorder?
- How long must anxiety persist before it is classified as a disorder?
- What level of anxiety constitutes a disorder?
- What more needs to be known to be sure that the individual has met the diagnostic criteria for a specific anxiety disorder?

The common link in these presentations is excessive anxiety. In order to make this assessment we need to know how long the symptoms have been occurring. We also need to know how much time is devoted to the behaviours and to what degree they interfere with the individual's daily functioning.

For example, in examining Sharon's situation, if we found that Sharon organizes her clothes after cleaning the wardrobe, then this would not be regarded as a disorder. If Sharon rigidly arranged her clothes after completing the laundry but spent no more than a few minutes on the task, this behaviour may indicate a personality trait but not a disorder. However, if Sharon spends considerable time each day rearranging her clothes, feels distressed if she cannot complete the ritual and cannot leave the house until she has repeatedly checked that the clothes are in order, her behaviour may be considered a disorder.

EPIDEMIOLOGY

In the UK, 1 in 6 adults have a diagnosis of anxiety, depression and phobias while 1 in 14 people have a severe anxiety disorder likely to require specialist care and treatment (Office for National Statistics, 2001). Overall, men seem to have a lower rate of such disorders than women: 14% compared to 19% respectively (Office for National Statistics, 2001). However, there are no gender differences in diagnoses of panic disorder. These disorders are more likely to occur in middle age and symptoms are less likely to be reported by younger and older people.

People more likely to be diagnosed with an anxiety disorder tend to have an unskilled occupation, have no formal educational qualifications, rent accommodation and be economically inactive. They are more likely to be living alone, separated or divorced and single parents. As such, financial difficulties and a lack of social contacts may form the backdrop to anxiety disorders (Office for National Statistics, 2001). People with anxiety disorders are also more likely to have a comorbid physical health problem (Office for National Statistics, 2001). Sixty-seven per cent of people with two or more disorders also reported at least one physical complaint, compared to 38% of people with no disorder who reported a physical health issue (Office for National Statistics, 2001). Anxiety disorders have been reported to be higher among Irish males and Pakistani women, whereas they appear to be lower among Bangladeshi women, when compared to the general population (Nazroo and Sproston, 2002).

Comorbidity is the rule rather than the exception with mental disorders. Once again there are gender differences, with more males suffering from a substance use disorder in combination with an anxiety or mood disorder, while females are more likely to suffer from anxiety and have a concurrent mood or substance disorder. These gender differences have been simplistically referred to as 'women think, men drink'. In women, thinking is channelled into worry, while men may drink to cover their worries.

CRITICAL THINKING CHALLENGE 17.2

What do you think about the statement 'women think, men drink'? Is it a simplistic statement pandering to gender stereotypes? Would mental disorders be more evenly distributed between the sexes if males reduced their substance abuse? Without the cover of a substance, would more anxiety disorders emerge in males?

In 2006–2007 in the UK, £8.4 billion (12% of total spending by Primary Care Trusts) was spent on mental healthcare (Appleby and Gregory, 2008). While this is the single biggest spend area in health, it has been held to be disproportionate to the human and social costs of mental disorders (Royal College of Psychiatrists, 2008). However, there are significant regional variations in how this money is spent.

In an Australian study, Issakidis and Andrews (2002) examined the perceived need for care by people diagnosed with an anxiety disorder. Nearly 55% of respondents stated that they preferred to manage themselves. The reasons given by service users with an anxiety disorder for not accessing services were:

- 'I preferred to manage by myself,'
- 'I didn't think anything could help,'
- 'I didn't know where to get help,'
- 'I was afraid to ask for help or of what others would think of me' (stigma),
- 'I couldn't afford it,'
- 'I asked but didn't get help,'
- 'I got help from another source.'

Issakidis and Andrews (2002) concluded that attitudinal barriers were more significant than structural barriers in seeking help. This study revealed a pressing need for public and professional education about the recognition and treatment of anxiety disorders.

AETIOLOGY

There is no definitive cause of anxiety disorders. A number of theories have been postulated to explain why some people are more vulnerable than others to the development of an anxiety disorder. These theories represent the 'nature versus nurture' debate and include stress, biological, personality/temperament, psychodynamic, interpersonal and behavioural theories.

Stress theory

Stress theory was developed by Hans Selye (1956, 1974), an endocrinologist. Selye identified three stages of stress: alarm reaction, resistance and exhaustion. Alarm reaction is the physiological response to stress. In resistance the physiological response continues as the 'flight or fight' reaction. The person may adapt to this heightened state of arousal and begin to relax, or they may be unable to relax and deplete their physiological and emotional resources, leaving little in reserve. This last phase is exhaustion.

Biological theories

Biological theories include genetic and neurochemical theories.

Genetic theories

Diagnoses of anxiety disorders tend to run in families but families share both genes and environment. First-degree relatives share the greatest number of genes. Anxiety disorders have an increased incidence in first-degree relatives. Twin studies, which aim to separate the influence of genes and environment, indicate that specific anxiety disorders are not inherited but that a general tendency encompassing anxiety, mood and eating disorders is inherited (Kendler et al., 1995). Monozygotic twins have a concordance rate five times greater than that of dizygotic twins (APA, 2000). The development of a specific type of anxiety disorder then appears to be under the influence of the shared family environment (Crowe et al., 1983).

Neurochemical theories

Benzodiazepines reduce anxiety by facilitating the action of gamma-aminobutyric acid (GABA) (see Ch. 24). Because of this action it has been hypothesized that reduced GABA is associated with anxiety disorders. Increased noradrenaline is known to increase anxiety. Serotonin has been implicated in anxiety, aggression and mood disorders.

Personality/temperament theory

Both genes and environment influence personality type. Each human being is unique. We all have our own personalities and no two people are exactly alike. Having said this, it is also true that people can be grouped into broad categories such as introverted or extroverted, passive or aggressive and so on. This consistency of behaviour is referred to as personality. Young children are in the process of developing a personality. The cluster of traits they consistently display is referred to as temperament. Temperament is currently being studied in

Australia by the Australian Temperament Project (ATP). The study aims to:

> ...trace the pathways to psychosocial adjustment and maladjustment across the lifespan, and to investigate the contribution of personal, family and environmental factors to development and wellbeing. A major theme throughout has been the influence of an individual's temperament on his/her emotional and behavioural adjustment.

(Australian Institute of Family Studies, n.d.)

Analysis of data collected from the study indicates that a shy, inhibited temperament is associated with anxiety problems in adolescence (Prior et al., 2000). When the ATP study participants were in their late teens it was not possible to tell whether the presence of an anxiety disorder in adolescence would progress into adulthood. However, other researchers have found that the presence of an anxiety disorder in adolescence increased the risk of having an anxiety or depressive disorder in adulthood (Pine et al., 1998).

In reviewing the factors contributing to the development of anxiety disorders, Rapee (2002) concluded that a shy, inhibited temperament was the strongest predictor of the development of an anxiety disorder.

Psychoanalytic theory

Psychoanalytic theory postulates that anxiety occurs when the individual represses unacceptable thoughts and emotions. These unacceptable ideas and emotions then re-emerge in the form of anxiety. Freud (1936) believed that individuals mobilize defence mechanisms to control anxiety.

A psychoanalytic therapist would work with the individual to uncover the repressed material (the source of the anxiety) and bring it to a conscious level, so that it can then be dealt with and resolved. Resolution of the repressed material results in resolution of the anxiety.

Interpersonal theory

Sullivan (1952) believed that anxiety was generated by interpersonal problems; for example, insecure parents may transmit anxiety to their children, or anxiety may arise when people do not conform to social norms. Rapee (2002) found that an overprotective parenting style was associated with an inhibited temperament and anxiety disorders in offspring (Rapee, 2002).

Behavioural theory

Anxiety can be learned through experience and can be unlearned through new experiences. It makes sense that if a dog bites you, you can develop a fear of dogs. However, can people develop fears by watching others or by hearing about dangerous situations? Gerull and Rapee (2002) conducted a study to determine whether children learned to be fearful by watching others display fear. They showed toddlers a toy snake or spider paired with a picture of their mothers displaying either a positive, negative or neutral expression. Children were more likely to show fear of the toy when their mother displayed a negative expression. Mineka and Zinbarg (2006) argue that contemporary learning theory and research have the potential to explain the complex interplay between stressful learning events and contextual variables in the development and subsequent course of anxiety disorders.

ANXIETY AND STRESS-RELATED DISORDERS

Anxiety disorders may be classified as either primary or secondary anxiety disorders. *Primary* anxiety disorders are those in which the anxiety disorder is the principal disorder. *Secondary* anxiety disorders result from another cause; for example, anxiety secondary to a medical condition, or a substance-induced anxiety disorder.

The major presenting symptoms of anxiety disorders are panic, fear, stress, worry and ritualistic behaviours. These symptoms can be used to group the anxiety disorders:

- panic:
    - panic attack: can occur in any of the anxiety disorders,
    - panic disorder without agoraphobia,
    - panic disorder with agoraphobia;
- fear:
    - agoraphobia,
    - social phobia or social anxiety disorder,
    - specific phobia;
- stress:
    - adjustment disorder with anxiety,
    - acute stress disorder,
    - post-traumatic stress disorder;
- worry:
    - generalized anxiety disorder,
    - obsessions and rituals,
    - obsessive–compulsive disorder.

Panic attacks

A panic attack is not a discrete anxiety disorder. It can occur in any anxiety disorder and in many different mental disorders and medical conditions. A panic attack is defined as 'a discrete period of intense fear or discomfort in the absence of real danger' (APA, 2000, p. 430). Panic attacks have an abrupt onset and reach a peak

within 10 min or less. To qualify as having a panic attack the individual must experience at least four of the classic somatic or cognitive symptoms, namely palpitations, pounding heart or accelerated heart rate; sweating; trembling; sensations of shortness of breath; feelings of choking; chest pain; nausea or abdominal distress; feeling dizzy or lightheaded; derealization (feelings of unreality) or depersonalization (being detached from oneself); fear of dying, losing control or going mad; paraesthesia (numbness and tingling sensations); or chills/hot flushes (APA, 2000).

Panic-like symptoms are even more common than full-blown panic attacks. Panic-like symptoms are a subclinical condition consisting of a discrete period of intense fear accompanied by up to three of the classic symptoms of a panic attack.

There are three types of panic attack:

- unexpected: un-cued or 'out of the blue'; that is, there is no associated trigger,
- situationally bound: cued; that is, occurring on exposure to, or in anticipation of, a trigger,
- situationally predisposed: similar to situationally bound panic attacks, but the symptoms do not occur every time the individual is exposed to a trigger (APA, 2000).

Recurrent 'unexpected' attacks are required for a diagnosis of panic disorder. The unexpected nature of panic is illustrated in the case study of Danni.

CASE STUDY: DANNI

Danni [15] … was an outgoing, active teenager. 'Then one day I went to school and this overwhelming fear came over me: to this day I can't explain why… I started hyperventilating and my heart was racing. I felt sick and I had to go home.' She said that was the start of a downhill slide… Danni tried many treatments, and became addicted to oxazepam after being prescribed a series of medications (Mayer, 2001, p. 2).

Nursing interventions

A panic attack can occur in any setting, and therefore nurses must be prepared for a range of situations, from delivering first aid for a panic attack in a shopping centre, to managing the panicked service user in a fully equipped clinical environment.

The presenting symptoms of a panic attack may include palpitations, chest pain, sweating and shortness of breath. Consequently service users often present to the nearest accident and emergency department with their first panic attack. In this environment service users are assessed for physical problems and when none can be found they are frequently told that there is 'nothing' wrong and are discharged from the department without follow-up. A valuable opportunity to teach the service user about their condition and its management is missed. Early recognition and appropriate treatment can, at best, prevent the development of an anxiety disorder and, at the least, ensure that service users do not make continual visits to health professionals seeking a physical reason for their symptoms.

During a panic attack

Stay with the service user during the panic attack, as the panic may escalate if they are left on their own (Schultz and Videbeck, 2002). The presence of another individual has a calming effect on the panicking service user. An unattended service user in panic may try to escape their current situation, and in doing so put themselves in danger.

If the clinical environment in which the service user has presented with a panic attack is a high-stimulus area, take the service user to a calmer, more private setting. Avoid very small rooms or areas were the service user might feel trapped. Avoid public areas where the vulnerable service user can be observed by passers-by.

Some people lose control of their limbs or become dizzy during a panic attack and are unable to walk independently to another venue. In such a situation it is preferable to modify the environment (reduce noise, lighting, people moving and talking), rather than insist that the service user relocate. The panic attack will pass with time, whereas attempting to move a dizzy, fainting service user could result in injury, either to the service user should they fall or to the helper through muscle strain.

In treatment it may be beneficial to help the service user overcome the panic attack in the environment that triggered it. The service user's first response will be to flee the situation. In engaging in this behaviour they reinforce avoidance as a coping strategy.

The service user experiencing a panic attack may present with apparent cardiac symptoms. In a first-aid situation the nurse will not have access to monitoring equipment that can help exclude a cardiac cause for the symptoms. However, if the chest pain eases when the service user slows their breathing it is unlikely to be due to a heart attack. Nevertheless the nurse must be ready to activate an emergency plan, while at the same time remaining calm and presenting an image of confidence and control. An anxious service user can make a nurse anxious and in turn an anxious nurse can make an anxious service user more anxious. This ability to transmit anxiety from one person to another has been referred to as *infectious anxiety*. At its most extreme, infectious anxiety can cause mass hysteria.

Speak to the service user in short, simple and audible sentences. A service user at panic-level anxiety can only process one detail at a time and their sense of hearing can also be reduced (Stuart, 2005a). During the panic attack take a directive approach; instruct the service user to 'Please sit down' rather than asking, 'Would you like to sit down?' The service user experiencing panic will not be able to decide what to do when offered the choice of whether to sit or not, and needs direction at this time. When the service user has regained control they can resume responsibility for their own decisions. Continue with a calm, reassuring tone: 'You are having a panic attack' and 'I will stay with you'.

Instruct the service user to take a slow, medium breath (not a deep breath) through their nose and to hold it briefly before exhaling slowly through their nose. Aim to reduce the service user's respiration rate to 10 breaths per minute by using a 6 second cycle per respiration; for example, say 'in-2-3, out-2-3' (Andrews and Garrity, 2000). Instruct the service user to breathe using their diaphragm, not their chest. Continue coaching the service user until their anxiety subsides. Some service users are aware that they are hyperventilating and try to slow their breathing, whereas others are not aware and make no attempt to reduce their respiration rate. Shallow, increased breathing or deep breathing results in the service user exhaling too much carbon dioxide, which will manifest as dizziness and tingling or pins and needles in the extremities. To correct this you can ask the service user to breathe into a paper bag. They will then rebreathe the carbon dioxide and regain the correct balance. However, some people find the prospect of having a paper bag over their mouth and nose too smothering or embarrassing and will become more panicky. You must be prepared to modify any anxiety-reduction intervention to the individual concerned.

Continue to coach the service user in the slow-breathing technique because it is important for them to learn that the panic attack will pass and that reducing their breathing rate has helped them to regain control. As the service user's panic subsides, try and encourage them to stay and further reduce their anxiety rather than fleeing as soon as they can. This is an important step in proving to the service user that they can regain their composure, which is empowering, rather than reinforcing the idea that the current environment is a dangerous place. A service user who experiences a panic attack in a specific setting may come to associate that setting with danger and thus avoid it in future. This is how panic attacks can lead to agoraphobia, as the service user has another panic attack in another venue and adds this to the list of places to be avoided.

In a clinical setting, if the above techniques fail or the service user is experiencing disorganized thoughts, perceptual disturbances or agitation that could escalate to aggression, consider administering a prescribed anti-anxiety medication that can be given as necessary. Even in a clinical situation medication should only be used as a last resort because it communicates to the service user that they are incapable of regaining control and sets up a future expectation that anxiety can be eliminated by medication. Although benzodiazepines are very effective at reducing anxiety, they are associated with dependence and should only be used in the short term (preferably no longer than 2 weeks). Long-term use can result in withdrawal symptoms that mimic the anxiety symptoms that precipitated the service user taking them in the first place, thus convincing the service user that they cannot do without their 'pills'.

A small minority of service users experiencing very severe symptoms may require intravenous administration of a benzodiazepine by a medical practitioner.

After a panic attack

Once the panic attack has abated, tell the service user again that what they just experienced was a panic attack. Be aware that most of the information given to the service user during the panic attack will not have been retained. Continue to keep your explanations short and simple. Ask the service user if they have previously experienced a panic attack and, if so, when the last attack occurred, how many previous attacks they have had and whether there is anything in particular that triggers them.

Give the service user a list of the classic symptoms of a panic attack. Ask them to put a tick next to each symptom that they have experienced. Discuss the list with the service user to determine whether they agree that what they have experienced was a panic attack. Some service users may continue to believe that they have a physical problem that has yet to be diagnosed.

However, if this was the service user's first panic attack, and it has occurred in a community environment, it is important to refer the service user to a health professional for a thorough physical examination to exclude a physical cause for their symptoms. Once a physical cause for the service user's symptoms has been excluded and the diagnosis of panic attack has been confirmed, no further follow-up is warranted, as one panic attack does not constitute an anxiety disorder. However, the service user should be informed that if they have further panic attacks they should seek appropriate help early.

NURSE'S STORY: DEALING WITH PANIC ATTACK IN A&E

Kerryn Morgan is an accident and emergency nurse with many years of experience. Kerryn recounted an incident the previous weekend of a young mother who presented on a very busy night at the department. She was assessed and appointed a triage rating of T2 (urgent priority: to be seen within 2–4 h of presentation). The rationale for this rating was that the young mother had complained of chest pains and an irregular heart rate and although it looked as if she was having a panic attack, Kerryn was not willing to assume this without further investigation. The young woman was very flushed and kept fanning herself and dousing herself with water to cool down. She was very frightened and did not want to be left alone. Further questioning revealed that she had had a previous episode in her early teens and another during her pregnancy. Her pulse was regular but rapid.

Although Kerryn was unable to attend to her immediately, she responded to the young woman's distress by allowing the service user to remain near her while she attended to more urgent issues. Kerryn instructed the young woman to slow her breathing rate and explained that the tingling in her fingers was due to overbreathing and would abate once she was able to slow her breathing down. No further treatment other than empathy, respect and instruction on reducing the respiration rate was needed to resolve the panic attack.

Panic disorder

Panic disorder is defined as 'the presence of recurrent, unexpected panic attacks followed by at least one month of persistent concern about having another panic attack, or a significant behavioural change related to the attacks' (APA, 2000, p. 433). The individual must have experienced at least two unexpected panic attacks to be diagnosed with panic disorder. There are two types of panic disorder: panic disorder without agoraphobia and panic disorder with agoraphobia. The frequency and severity of panic disorder varies widely from one panic attack per week for months, to daily panic attacks, separated by weeks or months without an attack. The characteristics of panic disorder are:

- fear that attacks indicate the presence of an undiagnosed, life-threatening illness,
- remaining unconvinced by repeated negative medical tests and positive reassurance,
- fear that they are going crazy or have a weak character,
- development of avoidance behaviours,
- fear of having another attack.

The associated features of panic disorder include a constant or intermittent anxiety that is not focused on anything specific, apprehension about routine activities and anticipation of catastrophic consequences related to mild symptoms (for example, worrying that a headache is really an undiagnosed brain tumour). The service user may also be hypersensitive to medication side effects.

Panic disorder can lead to damage or loss of interpersonal relationships. The individual can be so disabled by the panic that they are no longer able to fulfill their usual roles.

Comorbid disorders to panic disorder include depression, with rates varying from 10 to 65%. In one-third of service users, depression precedes the panic disorder. In two-thirds of service users depression coincides with panic disorder. Service users will often self-medicate with alcohol or other medication and are at high risk of developing a substance use disorder. Other anxiety disorders and numerous general medical conditions are also common in panic disorder (APA, 2000). The case study of Ian illustrates role impairment and comorbidity associated with panic disorder.

CASE STUDY: IAN

Ian … 37, suffered a breakdown last year. He blamed work-related stress as the catalyst. 'About a year before the breakdown, I was having symptoms. I started getting tired, unable to deal with the stresses that I used to [deal with]. At that stage, it was a very physical thing that attacked my immune system. I got colds that lingered and IBS [irritable bowel syndrome]. I was always tired. Depressive tiredness is different: you wake up more tired than when you went to bed. Then I started having panic attacks. Getting to work became a nightmare: I couldn't get on the train. I felt run-down. I wasn't able to cope with even the basics. I became agoraphobic and more panicky. This is the stage where you should seek help, but I didn't.'

Eventually Ian … did go to his doctor, who told him to take a week off work. 'I took 2 weeks off and just lay in bed. After 2 weeks, I still felt bloody awful, but I went back to work and by Monday afternoon I knew it hadn't worked. I was completely unable to handle anything and I had very strange feelings of unreality. I was looking at the office as though I wasn't part of it. I was panicky, shaky and absolutely full of anxiety.'

Ian … stopped functioning after leaving his job and then – temporarily – his partner and son went to stay in a hotel. 'I still thought I could cure myself, it was all work-related and I just needed some peace. But … I realised how desperate I was. I went to bed and couldn't move because I was absolutely terrified. I felt physically paralysed. I lay like that for 2 days. I'd try to get out of bed but my breathing was all over the place. I'd been on edge for so long'.

Source: Kenny (2000), pp. 20–21.

Panic disorder occurs in 10% of service users in mental health settings, in 10–30% of general medical service users (especially in vestibular, respiratory and neurology settings) and in up to 60% of service users in cardiology settings (APA, 2000).

Panic disorder has a peak onset in adolescence and a smaller peak in the mid-thirties. It is rare in children and people over 45 years of age. Panic disorder has a chronic, fluctuating course. Agoraphobia usually develops within the first year of panic attacks.

Panic disorder is more common in families. A service user with a first-degree relative with panic disorder is eight times more likely to develop panic disorder than the general population. If the onset of symptoms occurs before the individual is 20 years old, then the likelihood is 20 times higher than in the general population.

The outcome of treatment in panic disorder is varied. In one study, 6 years after treatment 30% of service users were well, 40–50% had improved and 20–30% were the same or worse (APA, 2000).

Nursing interventions

Teaching plan: panic attacks

Select appropriate learning material about panic attacks and go through the main points with the service user. There are many pamphlets, self-help books, videos and internet resources to choose from. A list of suitable resources has been provided at the end of this chapter. It is important that you review all material before distributing it to a service user ensuring that it is evidence-based. Different service users will have different levels of understanding and it is important to pitch the material at the right level for maximum effect. The key activities that need to be undertaken are as follows.

- Inform the service user about the different levels of anxiety and encourage them to formulate a list of early warning signs of an impending panic attack.
- Support self-management and advise the service user to institute anxiety-reduction techniques early, to prevent a full-blown panic attack.
- Help the service user to identify stressors that exacerbate their anxiety.
- Inform the service user about the role of caffeine, nicotine and some prescribed medications, such as asthma medication, in increasing the heart rate, thus precipitating a panic attack in a predisposed person.
- Inform the service user that while vigorous exercise also increases the heart rate, a moderate to high level of fitness will reduce the heart rate and help the individual to cope with the stresses of daily life.
- Encourage the service user to practise anxiety-reduction techniques regularly, so that they can institute them when they need to.
- Provide the service user with a list of appropriate health professionals and self-help groups specializing in the management of panic attacks.
- After covering the above, schedule another session or refer the service user to an appropriate health professional to learn the slow-breathing technique.

Slow-breathing technique

Hyperventilation occurs during a panic attack, causing the service user to have symptoms such as shortness of breath, a lightheaded feeling, and tingling or a pins-and-needles sensation in the fingers, toes or lips. These sensations are uncomfortable and frightening, causing the service user to breathe even faster and thus induce even more unpleasant symptoms such as vertigo, chest pain and nausea. These symptoms increase the service user's fear that something is seriously wrong and their respiration rate continues to increase. To break this vicious cycle it is essential to help the service user reduce their respiration rate.

The aim is to teach the service user to reduce their respiration rate to 10 breaths per minute during rest. During a panic attack the nurse can act as a coach, talking the service user through the steps and offering encouragement. However, the aim is to teach the service user to regain control over their own hyperventilation so they can instigate slow breathing at the onset of escalating anxiety.

It is important that the service user uses their diaphragm to breathe, rather than their chest. Service users should also inhale and exhale through their nose. A stopwatch will be helpful initially so that the service user can practise the timing of their respirations into a regular, slow pattern. Ask the service user to breathe in for 3 s and then breathe out for 3 s. Have them use the stopwatch until they have developed a regular pattern. Encourage the service user to practise their slow-breathing technique regularly. They may wish to keep a record of their respiration rate for a while until they feel confident that they have reduced their respiration rate (Clinical Research Unit for Anxiety and Depression et al., 1999).

Putting the slow-breathing technique into practice

Because anxiety cannot be eliminated, it is important to learn how to cope with symptoms of anxiety. Service users can learn to tolerate symptoms of mild anxiety without anticipating that it will herald a panic attack. They can also practise reducing anxiety by implementing the slow-breathing techniques they have learned. There are several exercises, such as deliberately hyperventilating or shaking the head from side to side, that can induce panic symptoms (Clinical Research Unit for Anxiety and Depression et al., 1999). Service users should initially undertake these exercises in the presence of an experienced health professional specializing in anxiety management.

Agoraphobia

Agoraphobia is defined as 'anxiety about being in places or situations from which escape might be difficult (or embarrassing) or in which help may not be available in the event of having an unexpected or situationally predisposed panic attack or panic-like symptoms' (APA, 2000, p. 432). In addition to the typical symptoms of a panic attack, individuals may experience other symptoms that may be incapacitating or embarrassing, such as loss of bladder control, vomiting and headache. Typical agoraphobic situations include being outside the home alone, in a crowd or standing in a line, on a bridge and travelling in a bus, train or car. Individuals with agoraphobia avoid the situations they fear and as a result lead a severely restricted lifestyle. The extent of this restriction is illustrated in the case study below.

CASE STUDY: A DARK CLOUD

I wake each morning with this dark cloud hanging over me as I wonder how I will be able to cope with my household duties. Visiting friends used to be a pleasurable activity but I now begin to dread having to leave the house. If I have to walk any distance I find myself becoming breathless and agitated. My heart pounds and my vision is distorted.

Source: Neville (1986), p. 10.

Some people with agoraphobia will endure the feared situation, suffer intense distress and fear having another panic attack. To cope with their distress, people with agoraphobia will use a range of techniques, such as asking others to accompany them on outings, taking a mobile phone with them and checking for exits upon entering a building.

Types of agoraphobia

There are two main types of agoraphobia: panic disorder with agoraphobia, and agoraphobia without a history of panic disorder. Panic disorder with agoraphobia is the more prevalent of the two. People with panic disorder with agoraphobia are more likely to seek treatment (APA, 2000).

Social phobia (social anxiety disorder)

Social phobia is defined as a 'marked and persistent fear of one or more social or performance situations in which the person is exposed to unfamiliar people or to possible scrutiny by others. The individual fears that he or she will act in a way (or show anxiety symptoms) that will be humiliating or embarrassing' (APA, 2000, p. 456).

There are two types of social phobia: generalized social phobia and nongeneralized social phobia. *Generalized* social phobia includes fears related to most social situations such as initiating or maintaining conversations, participating in small groups, dating, speaking to authority figures, party attendance and public speaking. In *nongeneralized* social phobia, service users fear a single performance situation or several but not all social situations.

Examples of nongeneralized phobia performance situations include eating and drinking in public, writing in public and using a public toilet.

The features associated with social phobia include hypersensitivity to criticism, negative evaluation or rejection, difficulty in being assertive, low self-esteem, feelings of inferiority, poor social skills – avoiding eye contact when talking to a person, for example – and observable signs of anxiety such as a tremor or shaky voice. In addition, the socially phobic individual may experience underachievement at school and/or work and decreased social networks. In severe social phobia the individual is less likely to marry and may have suicidal ideation (APA, 2000).

Common conditions comorbid with social phobia include other anxiety, mood and substance-related disorders, anorexia nervosa and avoidant personality disorder.

In community samples the prevalence of social phobia is higher in females than in males, but in clinical samples the rate is similar for both males and females. Social phobia can occur across all age groups and has a lifetime prevalence of 3–13% (APA, 2000). Social phobia typically begins in the mid-teens and persists throughout a lifetime with a fluctuating course in response to stressors. Service users frequently describe a history of shyness. The social phobia may follow a humiliating event or new demand, such as a new job that requires public speaking. Social phobia tends to run in families. The generalized type is common in first-degree relatives.

Specific phobia

Specific phobia is defined as a 'marked and persistent fear that is excessive or unreasonable, cued by the presence or anticipation of a specific object or situation (e.g. flying, heights, animals, receiving an injection, seeing blood). Exposure to the phobic stimulus almost invariably provokes an immediate anxiety response … which may take the form of a panic attack' (APA, 2000, p. 449).

In specific phobia the person recognizes that the fear is excessive. They avoid the phobic stimulus or endure it with intense anxiety. The avoidance, anxious anticipation or distress interferes significantly with the individual's daily functioning. Individuals under 18 years of age must have symptoms for longer than 6 months to receive a diagnosis of specific phobia. This is in recognition that there are many fears related to a child's developmental level, such as fear of the dark or fear of strangers.

A useful mnemonic to remember the key elements necessary for a diagnosis of phobia is PHOBIA:

P: persistent
H: handicapping (restricted lifestyle)
O: object/situation
B: behaviour (avoidance)
I: irrational fears (recognized as such by service user)
A: anxiety response.

CASE STUDY: HEATHER

Heather is a 48-year-old woman whose husband of 18 years recently left her. Heather has always been shy and anxious, and recalls a particularly awkward adolescence. She remembers being 18, having few friends and being painfully shy with boys. She never went to school dances, rarely went out at night, tried to avoid looking people in the eye and hardly ever spoke to people unless she knew them well. Since these early days, Heather's confidence has grown a little as she matured, but she has always found it difficult to be in any social situation. Heather believes that she looks awkward and unattractive and whenever the conversation turns to her she immediately feels that people will think she is stupid. She avoids parties and dinners whenever she can and rarely starts conversations. She always tries to fit in with others and even avoids walking around in crowded places because she thinks everyone is watching her.

Source: Rapee (2001), p. xiii.

For a diagnosis of specific phobia, the individual's fear must result in significant interference with their functioning. Significant distress alone is not sufficient for a diagnosis of phobia.

There are five subtypes of specific phobia, depending on the type of trigger:

- animal: animals or insects,
- natural environment: storms, heights, water, etc. (generally childhood onset),
- blood/injection/injury: seeing blood or injury or receiving an injection or other procedure (vasovagal fainting response),
- situational: bridges, lifts, flying, etc.,
- other: choking, vomiting, contracting an illness.

Often more than one type will be present. Features associated with specific phobia include a restricted lifestyle. Comorbid conditions include other anxiety disorders, mood disorders and substance-related disorders.

Specific phobias are common in clinical settings but, with the exception of the blood/injection/injury type, are rarely the focus of attention. In contrast to other specific phobias, service users with the blood/injection/injury type experience an initial brief increase in heart rate and blood pressure, followed by a decreased heart rate and blood pressure. Three-quarters of service users will faint when their blood pressure drops. There is a risk to the service user's physical health if they avoid seeking treatment for a medical condition because of their phobia (APA, 2000). Some service users would rather die than have a needle. The case study below illustrates that this type of phobia is not confined to the 'weakling' stereotype.

CASE STUDY: FAINTING

A 32-year-old healthy male farmer told his physician during an examination that he always faints when stuck with a needle. The physician did not listen and assumed the service user was exaggerating, because the service user was otherwise very healthy, strong and able to deal with all the physical demands of farming, including delivering animals and giving them shots. The service user fainted before the needle was inserted for a blood sample, fell backward off the examination table and had to be lifted back onto the table while unconscious. Fortunately, except for some sore, stretched muscles, the service user was unhurt.

Source: Travis (1998), p. 57.

Less than a third of people diagnosed with a specific phobia seek professional treatment. Service users with a high level of impairment and those who are phobic about commonly encountered objects and situations are more likely to seek help.

Specific phobias develop in childhood and early adolescence. Females develop them at a younger age than males. Predisposing factors to the development of specific phobias include traumatic events such as being bitten by a dog, an unexpected panic attack in a specific situation, observation of others undergoing trauma and repeated warnings of danger by, for example, parents or the media.

Phobia rates are higher in individuals with other family members with a phobia. Blood/injection/injury phobias have strong familial patterns. Remission occurs in only 20% of service users with a phobia that persists into adulthood (APA, 2000).

Nursing and psychological interventions for phobias

Carpenito (2002, p. 380) defines fear as 'a state in which an individual or group experiences a feeling of physiological or emotional disruption related to an identifiable source that is perceived as dangerous'.

Exposure therapy is an effective nondrug therapy used in a range of anxiety disorders. Exposure therapy is defined as the gradual facing of feared situations to reduce associated anxiety and distress (Rogers and Gournay, 2001). *Systematic desensitization* is similar to exposure but pairs a conscious relaxation technique with exposure to decrease the anxiety response to an identified phobic trigger (Schultz and Videbeck, 2002). Exposure therapy relies on naturally occurring 'habituation' rather than a conscious induction of relaxation. Before commencing a course of exposure therapy the nurse must fully explain the procedure and provide support to the service user in the initial stages of therapy.

According to Rogers and Gournay (2001) there are several components of exposure: graded, prolonged, repeated, focused and practised.

Graded exposure

The service user develops a hierarchy of fears from most feared to least feared. These fears are written down in point form and discussed with the nurse. For example, the service user with social phobia may develop the following hierarchy:

- speaking to people in authority,
- initiating a conversation with a stranger at a party,
- eating in front of others.

The service user with agoraphobia would generate a different list of phobic triggers:

- visiting the shopping centre,
- walking to the end of the street,
- going to the letterbox,
- leaving the house and standing on the front step.

The same process would be followed by a service user with a specific phobia:

- patting a dog,
- standing next to a dog,
- standing within arm's reach of a dog,
- looking at pictures of dogs.

After the list has been generated and committed to paper, start with the least-fearful trigger and negotiate the manner and duration of exposure. Assist the service user to set goals for exposure. Ask the service user: 'What would you most like to be able to do if you didn't have this phobia?' Some examples elected by the service user with social phobia may include:

- looking people in the eye,
- speaking in a confident tone,
- inviting a friend over for a coffee,
- initiating a conversation with the boss,
- chatting up girls (or boys).

Prolonged exposure

The aim is for the service user to remain exposed to the phobic trigger for as long as it takes their anxiety to subside. This will vary from one service user to another. At least a 50% reduction from beginning-level anxiety is required for the exposure therapy to be effective.

Repeated exposure

The service user must face the phobic trigger at least daily for exposure therapy to be successful.

Focused exposure

The service user may revert to avoidance behaviours during the exposure. The service user has been using these maladaptive coping mechanisms for some time and it is difficult to break the habit. Examples include distraction techniques. Keep the service user focused on feeling the initial fear on exposure and then commenting on the natural reduction of anxiety that accompanies prolonged exposure.

Practised exposure

Practising exposure on a regular basis will maintain the gains. A family member can be enlisted to coach the service user to maintain a daily schedule of exposure (Rogers and Gournay, 2001).

CRITICAL THINKING CHALLENGE 17.3

Think of a person you know who has a phobia. What measures do they take to avoid coming in contact with the phobic stimulus? What effect does this avoidance behaviour have on their daily functioning?

Adjustment disorder

An adjustment disorder is an exaggerated emotional or behavioural response to a significant life change or stressor such as a relationship break-up, bereavement, divorce, business difficulties, illness, migration and so on. Adjustment disorders occupy a separate chapter from anxiety disorders in the *Diagnostic and Statistical Manual of Mental Disorders* (DSM-IV TR, APA, 2000). However, they are discussed here because adjustment disorders are characterized by the presence of a stressor.

The onset of adjustment disorder is within 3 months of exposure to the stressor. Acute adjustment disorder resolves within 6 months of the cessation of the stressor and its consequences. Chronic adjustment disorder occurs when a stressor, such as ill health, persists for longer than 6 months.

The symptoms experienced by the person are beyond what would normally be expected of a person in the given situation and significantly impair the individual's social, academic or occupational functioning. The decision of what is 'in excess of what would normally be expected' is subjective and thus prone to cultural and/or clinician bias.

People experiencing an adjustment disorder may have particular symptoms that dominate, such as depressed mood, anxiety or a disturbance of conduct (truancy, reckless driving, overspending, fighting). The diagnosis is only made when the person does not meet the diagnostic criteria for any other mental disorder. A normal grief reaction to the loss of a loved one would not be classified as an adjustment disorder; however, if the grief is excessive or prolonged, adjustment disorder may be diagnosed. Associated features include decreased performance at work or school, changed relationships, suicide attempts and suicide, substance abuse and somatic complaints.

Prevalence varies widely, from 2–8% of community samples to 12% of inpatients, up to a third of mental health outpatients and up to half of service users in specialist settings such as following cardiac surgery (APA, 2000).

Assessment consists of determining whether the person meets the criteria for another mental or personality disorder first, and exploring the nature of the stressor (duration, severity) and the individual's symptoms in relation to the stressor. Because the response is out of the norm, conducting a detailed assessment of the individual's personality traits and support structure would provide a sound base for a management plan.

As the disorder does not meet the diagnostic criteria of other DSM-IV TR disorders, first-line management consists of removal or modification of the stressor if possible, allowing the individual to ventilate feelings, crisis intervention, instituting problem-solving and stress management. Anti-anxiety medication or antidepressants are not appropriate in the initial stages but may be indicated at a later date. People experiencing ongoing stressors will need ongoing support, whereas those experiencing a response to an acute stressor may not require treatment or support after the initial crisis intervention. Most people experiencing an adjustment disorder recover fully.

Once the crisis has passed it can be helpful to teach service users a range of coping skills. Box 17.1 lists some common methods of coping with difficulties.

Box 17.1 **Common coping methods**

- Problem-solving: weighing up the pros and cons
- Tension reduction: play, exercise, hobbies
- Social skills: negotiation, humour, good communication
- Self-disclosure: sharing thoughts, experiences and feelings
- Structuring: organizing coping resources, planning ahead
- Seeking information: friends, self-help groups, health professionals, literature
- Stress monitoring: awareness of our own tension and events that increase it
- Assertive response: being able to request our needs and wants clearly, without infringing on others' rights
- Avoidance/withdrawal: getting away from things for a while. Not facing up to things at all is not adaptive.
- Self-medication: in the short term a glass of alcohol can help you relax. Self-medication becomes maladaptive when you rely on substances to relax.
- Social support network: friends can provide a great deal of support. The absence of friends and family or loneliness can be a precursor to mental illness.
- Beliefs/values: many service users say it is their belief in God or reliance on their values that has helped them through a crisis
- Wellness: keeping fit, eating nutritious meals and getting enough rest and sleep
- Self-esteem/confidence: prizing oneself

Stress-management techniques include progressive muscle relaxation, guided imagery and meditation.

CRITICAL THINKING CHALLENGE 17.4

Think of a time when you had a crisis in you life. How did you cope with the problem?

Acute stress disorder

Acute stress disorder (ASD) is a transient response to a severe trauma such as an accident, natural disaster, crime or combat. The characteristic symptoms of anxiety, dissociation and other intense autonomic arousal occur within 1 month after exposure to the stressor. The characteristic symptoms of ASD occur either while experiencing the trauma or within 1 month of the traumatic event. The diagnostic criteria require three or more of the following characteristic symptoms:

- numbing, detachment or no emotional response,
- being in a daze,
- derealization (feeling that the world is unreal or distorted),
- depersonalization (feeling of unreality, detachment or being outside one's body or mind, like an observer),
- dissociative amnesia (inability to recall significant aspects of the trauma).

The person persistently re-experiences the traumatic event in at least one of the following ways:

- recurrent images,
- recurrent thoughts or dreams,
- illusions,
- flashbacks,
- distress on reminders of the event.

The symptoms of ASD must last for at least 2 days and may persist for up to 4 weeks after the trauma. If the symptoms persist beyond 1 month after the trauma, ASD is reclassified as post-traumatic stress disorder (PTSD) (APA, 2000). Approximately 25–30% of people who experience a traumatic incident may subsequently develop PTSD (NICE, 2005a).

CASE STUDY: EMMA

Emma, a 23-year-old employed female, presents to her GP after an argument with her work colleague. Emma complains of feeling 'nervy' and on edge. She describes it as a feeling of tension that stops her from being able to relax. She lies awake until the early hours of the morning going over the argument. The feeling of tension has dulled her appetite and she does not enjoy her meals. Two days after the argument she is still thinking about it most of the time.

Nursing and psychological interventions

Debriefing

Debriefing is an interpersonal technique that assists people to mobilize adaptive coping strategies in order to overcome the effects of exposure to traumatic events. It is claimed that debriefing helps the individual gain a clear understanding of the trauma, come to terms with their thoughts and reactions to the trauma and identify any stress-related symptoms they may be experiencing. The debriefer provides information about the normal stress response to abnormal stressors, promotes problem-solving and supports the individual as they come to terms with the trauma. However, questions concerning the efficacy and safety of debriefing have been raised in recent literature (Wagner, 2005) and the National Institute for Health and Clinical Excellence (NICE) advises against brief or single-session debriefing as an initial response particularly when it focuses on the traumatic incident (NICE, 2005a). Where symptoms are mild and have persisted for less than 4 weeks it is recommended that 'watchful waiting' should be instigated (NICE, 2005a); that is, careful monitoring with the opportunity for increased support if symptoms worsen. If the person develops PTSD, trauma-focused psychological/cognitive behavioural therapy (CBT) should be offered as a first-line treatment (see below).

Progressive muscle relaxation

Progressive muscle relaxation is a useful technique to practise regularly to manage the stresses and strains of everyday life. It is not useful as a strategy to control panic in a person who has not previously mastered the technique, but it can be used in the early stages of anxiety. This is why it is so important for the service user to learn his or her own early warning signs of increased anxiety and institute anxiety-reduction techniques as soon as they emerge.

Progressive muscle relaxation follows a logical sequence, starting with the hands, then the arms, upward to the shoulders and neck, down the back and so on to the toes.

Start by instructing the service user to adopt a comfortable position in a chair with arm rests. Prepare the room so that there will be no interruptions for the duration of the session. Ask the service user to make a hard fist and hold it until you tell them to let their hands fall into their lap. Encourage the service user to notice the tension and then the feeling of relaxation. Continue throughout the body from the head to the toes.

All trainee health professionals have to start somewhere in developing their helping skills. The best way to master the technique of progressive muscle relaxation is to enrol in a class at the local community health centre and then practise the techniques regularly. Written scripts, setting out the exact wording in the correct sequence, can be used until you are skilled in the format. It is important to practise speaking in a calm, unhurried tone, which aids in relaxation. Relaxation CDs are available from retail outlets and can be useful, but it is advisable that the service user start with a personal instructor before moving to the pre-recorded method. Working with a health professional will increase motivation and adherence to the programme, whereas a CD can easily be turned off or ignored.

Guided imagery

Guided imagery can be used to deepen the relaxation response during progressive muscle relaxation. After achieving a state of relaxation the service user is asked to imagine a place that they find beautiful and relaxing (Fortinash and Holoday-Worret, 2008). Ask them to conjure up an image of the scenery and focus on specific aspects, such as the feeling of wind on their face, the sound of waves or the smell of the shore.

Meditation

Ask the service user to adopt a comfortable position in a quiet place. Every time they exhale they should say the word 'calm'. While guided imagery encourages the service user to use their imagination to conjure up pleasant images, meditation aims to still the mind. People who lead busy lives find this very difficult to do. The moment they have 5 min to spare they start thinking about the next three things they have to do. Tell the service user that as a thought comes into their head they should concentrate on their breathing and saying the word 'calm' as they exhale. They should practise meditation regularly.

Post-traumatic stress disorder

Post-traumatic stress disorder (PTSD) is defined as:

> ...development of characteristic symptoms following exposure to an extreme traumatic stressor involving direct personal experience of an event that involves actual or threatened death or serious injury, or other threat to one's integrity; or witnessing an event that involves death, injury, or a threat to the physical integrity of another person; or learning about unexpected or violent death, serious harm, or threat of death or injury experienced by a family member or other close associate.
>
> (APA, 2000, p. 463)

Traumatic events that may trigger PTSD include military combat, violent personal assault, disasters, a severe car accident, being diagnosed with a life-threatening illness and child sexual abuse. All these events are outside the realm of normal human experience.

The characteristic symptoms of PTSD include recurrent, intrusive recollections of the event; recurrent distressing dreams of the event; acting or feeling as if the traumatic event were recurring (flashbacks); intense distress at exposure to cues that resemble an aspect of the trauma; and physiological hyperarousal on exposure to the cues. Symptoms may develop immediately after the trauma but in some cases (approximately 15%) the onset of symptoms may be delayed by months or even years (NICE, 2005a).

The service user may adopt avoidance behaviours such as a persistent avoidance of the stimuli associated with the trauma, avoiding talking or thinking about the trauma, avoiding activities and places or people that remind the service user of the trauma. The service user may be unable to recall important aspects of the trauma, display decreased interest and participation in important activities, feel detached from others and have a restricted range of feelings towards loved ones. Service users may no longer expect to live a long life or have a career; they may suffer from increased arousal, difficulty falling asleep, irritability or outbursts of anger, difficulty concentrating, hypervigilance and an exaggerated startle reflex.

PTSD may be acute, with symptoms resolving within 3 months, or chronic, whereby symptoms persist for longer than 3 months. Some service users experience a delayed onset, with symptoms occurring at least 6 months after the trauma. Features associated with PTSD include survivor guilt, marital conflict, loss of employment and comorbid major depression, substance-related disorders or other anxiety disorders. The prevalence of PTSD varies with the group studied. Groups exposed to trauma, such as refugees or military personnel, can have rates of PTSD from a third to half of those exposed.

PTSD can occur at any age. Predisposing factors include the service user's premorbid personality, family background and the presence of a pre-existing mental health problem; however, PTSD can develop in individuals without any predisposing factors. Intriguingly, there is an increased vulnerability in service users with a first-degree relative with a history of PTSD or depression (APA, 2000).

Trauma-focused psychological therapy

Some people who experience symptoms of PTSD recover with little or no specialist treatment (NICE, 2005a). However, for others more specialist treatment is required, such as CBT which focuses specifically on coping with the traumatic experience. Eye movement desensitization and reprocessing (EMDR), based on the work of Dr Francine Shapiro, is another effective form of treatment (Coetzee and Regel, 2005; NICE, 2005a). It is based on the notion that the intensity of disturbing thoughts, and subsequent stress, can be reduced by eye movements. In therapy, as the person is asked to recall their traumatic episode, they are asked to focus on the therapist's moving finger (bilateral stimulation). By a mechanism which remains unknown, this appears to 'unfreeze' the traumatic memories allowing the person to focus on more positive thoughts.

However, it must be remembered that for some people it may be initially too overwhelming to discuss the traumatic incident. Here, it may take several sessions to build a trusting relationship prior to addressing the traumatic experiences.

Generalized anxiety disorder

Generalized anxiety disorder (GAD) is defined as 'excessive anxiety and worry (apprehensive expectation), occurring more days than not for a period of at least six months, about a number of events or activities. The individual finds it difficult to control the worry' (APA, 2000, p. 472). For a diagnosis of GAD to be made the anxiety and worry must be accompanied by at least three of the following symptoms: restlessness, being easily fatigued, difficulty concentrating, irritability, muscle tension and disturbed sleep. There may also be significant distress and an impairment in general functioning (NICE, 2011). The typical worries of the service user with GAD are about everyday routine events like job responsibilities, finances, health of family members and household tasks. The service user may shift from one worry to another.

Features not part of the diagnostic criteria but associated with GAD include muscle tension, trembling, twitching, feeling shaky, muscle aches and soreness. The service user may raise somatic complaints of sweating, nausea and diarrhoea. People with GAD are on edge and may have an exaggerated startle response. Hyperarousal, characterized by increased heart rate, shortness of breath and dizziness, is less prominent in GAD than in other anxiety disorders.

People with GAD are more likely to also have a mood disorder, other anxiety disorder, substance-related disorder, irritable bowel syndrome or headaches.

GAD is more common in females than males, and in families with relatives who have the disorder, and it runs a chronic, fluctuating course exacerbated by stress (Tyrer and Baldwin, 2006). Half of service users with GAD state that they have had the symptoms since childhood or adolescence (APA, 2000).

In general, NICE (2011) recommends a stepped approach to the care and treatment for GAD: from initial low-intensity psychological interventions (including guided, nonfacilitated self-help and psychoeducational programmes) through to CBT and applied relaxation to drug treatments (see Psychopharmacology, below). In complex cases, where there may be significant risk of harm or self-neglect, the person may receive additional input from crisis services or day hospitals, or may even require inpatient care (NICE, 2011). The needs of families and carers of the person who experiences GAD should also be assessed (NICE, 2011).

CASE STUDY: TAMARA

Tamara, a 25-year-old woman, presented with worries about her health, her career and her relationships. She said that she had always worried easily, but over the past several months she had felt more tense and agitated. The current increase in anxiety began following a dispute with a colleague who she believed had taken advantage of her, but since then she had been unable to assert herself with this colleague. She frequently worried about the quality of her work and worried that making a mistake would ultimately cause her to lose her job. Over this time she had developed a pattern of waking frequently during the night and being unable to get back to sleep for 2–3 h while thinking about all her worries. She had also come to see her GP for various somatic complaints over the years, which she worried were signs of a serious physical illness.

Source: Andrews and Hunt (1998), p. 28.

Nursing interventions

Problem-solving

Problem-solving may be a useful low-intensity intervention to help the person diagnosed with GAD to realize their own solutions to those issues which are causing them worry. The problem-solving technique should be familiar to nurses because the nursing process is based on a problem-solving framework. The first step is to describe the problem clearly and accurately. This is not as easy as it sounds, as people do not always identify the exact problem. For example, in the case study about Tamara, she states that she is worried that she will make a mistake and lose her job. Further probing reveals that Tamara had a dispute with a colleague and did not assert herself. Tamara's real problem is a lack of assertion skills.

The second step is to generate a list of possible solutions to the problem. Brainstorming is a process whereby any solution, no matter how far-fetched, is recorded. Tamara could ask an assertive cousin how she would deal with the situation, or she could watch other assertive people at her workplace to see how they go about asserting themselves, or she could hire an actor to take her place at the office to 'deal' with her colleague. While the third solution sounds outlandish, all solutions are listed because they may contain an element of usefulness in solving the problem. The last solution may indicate to Tamara that acting a part until she feels more confident may be more helpful than waiting until she feels confident to act.

Step three involves weighing the pros and cons of each generated solution and choosing the best or most practical solution.

The next step is to plan the best way to implement the chosen solution. What resources are needed and are they available? What does Tamara need to learn in order to implement the solution? A list is made in point form, detailing each step.

The plan is then implemented and evaluated. Did the solution work? What else needs to be done to solve the problem?

Although the problem-solving method looks easy, people with an anxiety disorder often have difficulty understanding their problems clearly and tend to choose solutions that reinforce the problem. Tamara may insist that she is in danger of losing her job and choose not to assert herself with her work colleague (avoidance behaviour) as a solution to her problem. It is for this reason that service users often need assistance in applying the problem-solving method in the early stages of therapy.

Obsessive–compulsive disorder

Between 1 and 3% of the UK population may have symptoms of obsessive–compulsive disorder (OCD) (NICE, 2005b). OCD consists of 'recurrent obsessions or compulsions that are severe enough to be time consuming (i.e. they take more than one hour a day) or cause marked distress or significant impairment' (APA, 2000, p. 456). To put it simplistically, *obsessions* are mental processes and *compulsions* are actions. There are some nuances, however, as the following definitions illustrate.

- Obsessions are 'recurrent persistent thoughts, impulses, or images that are experienced as intrusive and inappropriate and that cause marked anxiety or distress' (APA, 2000, p. 457). The most common obsessions are thoughts about contamination, repeated doubts (e.g. 'Did I turn the iron off?'), a need to have things in a particular order, aggressive or horrific impulses, and sexual imagery.
- Compulsions are 'repetitive behaviours (e.g. hand-washing, ordering, checking) or mental acts (e.g. praying, counting, repeating words silently), the goal of which is to prevent or reduce anxiety or distress, not to provide pleasure or gratification' (APA, 2000, p. 457). The most common compulsions are washing and cleaning, counting, checking, requesting or demanding assurances, repeating actions and arranging objects in order.

The case study below illustrates the link between obsessions and compulsions and how the service user does not gain any enjoyment from the ritual but relents in an effort to ward off uncomfortable anxiety.

Features associated with OCD include avoidance of situations that involve the content of the obsession, and hypochondriasis, with repeated visits to doctors for reassurance. The service user may feel guilty about the content of their thoughts or the time devoted to rituals; they may experience insomnia and abuse alcohol or drugs in

CASE STUDY: EXCESSIVE WASHING

A 26-year-old man is very concerned about cleanliness and hygiene. He spends a significant amount of time each day washing his hands and showering, especially after touching a toilet seat, doorknob or any other item he thinks may be dirty or contaminated. The service user explains that he is concerned about becoming infected or sick from touching these objects. He periodically acknowledges that the washing is excessive but explains that he becomes very anxious when he tries to avoid washing and eventually feels compelled to wash even more to make up for the omission.

Source: Fauman (2002), p. 223.

an effort to cope. Engaging in the 'rituals' is time-consuming and thus detracts from relationships, work and social activities.

Service users diagnosed with OCD have higher rates of major depression, experience other anxiety disorders and may also have an obsessive–compulsive personality disorder. Children diagnosed with OCD have an increased incidence of learning disorders and disruptive behaviours. One-third to half of people with Tourette's disorder also have OCD. Twenty to thirty per cent of service users with OCD display tics. Service users who engage in excessive washing may have concurrent dermatitis (APA, 2000).

In childhood, OCD is more common in males than females (APA, 2000). Controversially, it is thought by some that a small subset of children may develop OCD after an upper respiratory streptococcal infection ('strep throat') (Giedd et al., 2000). The acronym PANDAS, for paediatric autoimmune neuropsychiatric disorder associated with streptococcus, has been coined for this subgroup (Mell et al., 2005; Murphy et al., 2001).

The usual onset of OCD is gradual and occurs earlier in males (6–15 years) than females (20–29 years). It is common for the service user to experience exacerbations and remissions in response to stress. Only 5% of service users are free of symptoms between episodes. OCD has a higher concordance in monozygotic twins and first-degree relatives (APA, 2000).

Any assessment of OCD should take into consideration the person's cultural background and religious observances which may involve ritualistic behaviours (NICE, 2005b). Where the assessing nurse is unclear about the boundaries between symptoms of OCD and religious or cultural observances, advice and support should be sought from the appropriate community with the service user's consent (NICE, 2005b).

Nursing interventions

Any nurse who is offering psychological treatments to people with OCD must have undertaken aproropriate training and be in receipt of ongoing clinical supervision and support (NICE, 2005b).

Exposure and response prevention

The treatment of choice for OCD is a combination of exposure therapy and response prevention (ERP). Exposure has been described previously in the management of phobias. Service users with phobias cannot do things, whereas the service user with OCD cannot stop doing things. Therefore, it is important to add response prevention to the therapeutic regimen. Response prevention involves helping the service user to resist the urge to engage in compulsions and reducing the amount of time they spend engaging in rituals, with the ultimate aim of extinguishing the need to perform the rituals.

Start by determining the exact nature of the service user's obsessions and compulsions and how they interfere with the service user's everyday life. Ask the service user what might happen if they did not engage in the ritual. A written log of the amount of time spent on rituals can be a useful, accurate measurement of the problem and as a baseline against which response to future treatment can be measured.

Thorough education about the nature of OCD and information about exposure and response prevention is necessary before gaining the service user's informed consent to undertake the treatment plan. When the service user is exposed to the ritual trigger and asked not to perform the ritual they will experience significant discomfort and a strong urge to ritualize. If the service user gives in at this point and performs the ritual they will feel a flood of relief. It is this build-up of tension and then release of tension that reinforces the development of rituals in the first place. Exposure therapy involves exposing the service user to the stimuli that cue or trigger rituals. Response prevention during exposure ensures that the service user resists the urge to ritualize. The resulting tension from being unable to ritualize will build and build until it eventually peaks and then recedes. Repeated exposure and response prevention result in less initial tension and a quicker resolution of tension, until only a small amount of tension is felt when exposed to the ritual trigger (Treatment Protocol Project, 2004).

After a thorough explanation, the service user and nurse negotiate treatment goals. It is important that the service user agrees to commit to the treatment, as a therapeutic response requires a systematic, sustained approach. Giving in to the urge to ritualize before the tension peaks and falls naturally through habituation will not produce the desired treatment response. This does not mean that the service user is restrained or otherwise physically prevented from engaging in rituals, but rather that they make a strong commitment to stick with the treatment plan.

The nurse supports the service user during the exposure and coaches the service user not to respond to the urge to ritualize. Service users frequently believe that if they fail to engage in the ritual something dreadful will happen, and they may seek reassurance from the nurse that nothing bad will happen. The nurse must not reassure the service user because service users need to learn that this irrational fear has no basis in fact. By resisting the urge to ritualize, the service user will prove to himself or herself that their fear was groundless. This is more empowering than relying on external reassurance.

Exposure and response prevention require commitment and practice. Rituals have often built up over many years and will require a concerted effort to be eliminated. It will be necessary for the service user to repeatedly practise exposure and response prevention in a variety of settings. It may help to enlist the assistance of the service user's family in supervising them in the home setting. Family members must also understand the rationale for withholding reassurance and agree to reinforce the service user's adherence to the treatment plan.

THERAPIES WITH BROAD APPLICATIONS

CBT and psychopharmacology may be used in all the anxiety disorders as first- or second-line treatments (Ch. 23 also provides an overview of CBT and Ch. 24 discusses psychopharmacology). The next section explains these therapies.

Cognitive behavioural therapy

Cognitive behavioural therapy (CBT) was developed by Aaron Beck (1979) to challenge the service user's negative thought patterns. Cognition relates to our thoughts and the way we think. Service users with anxiety disorders often display distorted or irrational thinking. This does not mean they have lost touch with reality in the same way that a person with a psychosis has, but it does mean that their thoughts are not helpful in managing their condition. The efficacy of cognitive behavioural techniques in the treatment of anxiety disorders is well established (Furukawa et al., 2007, Hunot et al., 2007).

Rapee (2001) uses the phrase 'realistic thinking' to describe the thinking style promoted in CBT. This term is more neutral and service user-friendly than labelling a service user's thinking as distorted or irrational. The basic tenet of realistic thinking is that our feelings are directly caused by our beliefs, attitudes and thoughts about a

Table 17.1 Unrealistic thinking and rational responses		
Automatic thought	**Kind of cognitive distortion**	**Rational response**
Nothing will ever work out for me.	Overgeneralization	No one can look into the future. Concentrate on the present.
It will be awful if Jo turns me down.	Magnification	It might be upsetting, but it need not be awful unless I make it so.
Someone my age should be doing better than I am.	'Should' statements	Stop comparing yourself to others. All anyone can be expected to do is their best. What good does it do to compare myself to others? It only leads me to be down on myself, rather than get motivated.
I'm all alone in the world.	All-or-nothing thinking	It may feel like I'm all alone, but there are some people who care about me.
Everything is my fault.	Personalization	Stop playing this game of pointing blame at yourself. There's enough blame to go around. Better yet, forget placing blame and try to think through how to solve this problem.
I just don't have the brains for university.	Labelling and mislabelling	Stop calling yourself names like 'stupid'. I can accomplish a lot more than I give myself credit for.
Source: Nevid et al. (1994), pp. 270–271.		

situation, not the situation itself. For example, if you stood up in front of the class to present a case study from your last clinical rotation and several students burst into laughter, you might think they are laughing at your performance, when in reality a student had just told a joke. If you didn't know that the student had told a joke you might cling to your belief that you looked foolish. It is your interpretation of the situation, not the situation itself, that has produced your belief. Some examples of unrealistic thinking (automatic thoughts) are provided in Table 17.1.

The second important tenet of CBT is the understanding that extreme thoughts can lead to extreme emotions. The automatic thoughts in Table 17.1 are examples of extreme thoughts. Toning down these thoughts will lead to less extreme emotions, as can be seen in the 'Rational response' column. Anxious people tend to overestimate the likelihood of something bad happening. This kind of cognitive distortion has been referred to as 'catastrophizing' (Stuart, 2005b).

After the service user has learned to correctly identify their thoughts, they are ready to learn to think more realistically. This is referred to as cognitive restructuring and consists of:

- monitoring thoughts and feelings,
- questioning the evidence,
- examining alternatives,
- role reversal (Rapee, 2001).

Monitoring thoughts and feelings

The service user can use a realistic thinking record to monitor their thoughts and feelings. An illustration of the process of constructing a realistic thinking record, using the example of delivering a presentation to classmates, is set out in Table 17.2.

Questioning the evidence, examining alternatives and role reversal

In the second column of Table 17.2, the service user writes down what they think is going to happen. The 'Evidence' column relates to the types of evidence:

- past experience: how much has this happened before?
- general rules: is this something that generally happens?
- alternative explanations: what other explanations are there?
- role reversal: how would I feel if this was the other way around? (Rapee, 2001).

Probability

After listing all the evidence, the service user goes back and re-estimates the probability of an event happening. A rating of low, medium or high, or a percentage, can be used.

Table 17.2 Realistic thinking record

Event (what am I afraid of?)	Expectation (initial prediction)	Evidence (how do I know?)	Probability (how likely is it to happen?)	Degree of emotion (0–8)
Presentation of case study to classmates	I will say something stupid.	I have presented to my classmates before and I didn't say anything stupid. (past experience) Students usually listen to the presentation and then comment on their clinical experiences. (general rules)	15%	4
	My classmates will think I am stupid.	My classmates will realize that I am nervous talking in front of a group. (alternative explanations)	5%	2
	I will never become a registered nurse.	If I was listening to another student present their case study and they made a mistake I would not think they were stupid. (role reversal)	0%	1

Source: Rapee (2001).

Degree of emotion

The service user reviews the problem, the evidence and the likelihood of a catastrophe happening, and assigns a realistic emotional score. By working through the realistic thinking record, the service user can develop insight into the fact that it is the beliefs they attribute to a situation, not the situation itself, that is the problem. When the problem is written down and the fears are articulated, the evidence weighed, the probability estimated and the emotion re-evaluated, service users are helped to think more realistically. Garry McDonald, a well-known Australian actor, writes of CBT:

My progress came when I started cognitive behaviour therapy (CBT)... Meditation and CBT are the perfect partners. CBT is the Western version of mindfulness. You don't get the tremendous sense of wellbeing you get from meditation but you get the clarity much quicker. I just love CBT: you become a 'grown up', you make decisions, you live with mistakes, you get better. And better and better.

(McDonald, 1998, p. viii)

Cognitive restructuring can be combined with a range of behavioural techniques such as exposure, response prevention and progressive muscle relaxation. Other cognitive behavioural techniques that may be used in the treatment of anxiety disorders include thought stopping, distraction, reattribution, structured problem-solving and eye-movement desensitization (Barton et al., 2007).

Psychopharmacology

The two major groups of medications used in the treatment of anxiety disorders are antidepressants (such as selective serotonin-reuptake inhibitors, or SSRIs) and anti-anxiety drugs. Hypnotics may also be used for short term symptomatic relief when a person's sleep pattern is severely disturbed.

Antidepressants

Despite their name, antidepressants have many indications beyond their mood-elevating properties. Antidepressants are also indicated for anxiety and eating disorders and to manage chronic pain.

There is evidence that SSRIs are effective in the treatment of OCD (NICE, 2005b) and initial pharmacological treatment here could involve fluoxetine, fluvoxamine, paroxetine, sertraline or citalopram (NICE, 2005b). Clomipramine may be prescribed if there has been an unsuccessful trial of an SSRI, prior to which an electrocardiogram and blood pressure measurements should be undertaken if the person is at significant risk of cardiovascular disease (NICE, 2005b). For GAD, if a service user requests medication then sertraline is recommended in the first instance (NICE, 2011). For PTSD, paroxetine or mirtazapine may be used, and where these may not be effective then amitriptyline or phenelzine may be prescribed for those who are able to tolerate the side effects of such medication and, in the latter, dietary changes (NICE, 2005a). Drug treatment for PTSD may be commenced if a person does not consent to psychological treatment or when they are experiencing ongoing trauma (such as in domestic violence) (NICE, 2005a).

Further information on antidepressants can be found in Chapter 24.

Action

The different types of antidepressant work in different ways. They may:

- block neurotransmitter reuptake,
- inhibit neurotransmitter breakdown, or
- stimulate release of neurotransmitters.

There is a time lag of 1–2 weeks before the therapeutic effect occurs. Side effects, anti-anxiety and improved sleep effects occur earlier.

Selective serotonin-reuptake inhibitors

In the normal synapse, serotonin is released from a nerve cell and is then received by the next nerve cell. Some serotonin is then reabsorbed into the first nerve cell. Insufficient serotonin may be associated with depression and anxiety disorders. SSRIs block the reabsorption of serotonin into the first nerve cell. This blocking action results in an increased amount of serotonin being available at the next nerve cell (Keltner et al., 2001).

SSRIs have several advantages over the tricyclic antidepressants including minimal cardiac toxicity, safety in overdosage, mild side effects and being nonsedating. They are usually required in higher doses to treat anxiety disorders than for depressive disorders; however, service users with anxiety disorders are more likely to experience side effects, so the usual prescription regimen is to 'start low, go slow'.

Common side effects of SSRIs include nervousness and anxiety, insomnia (which can be counteracted by giving the dose in the morning), drowsiness or fatigue, gastrointestinal upsets such as nausea and diarrhoea, loss of appetite, weight loss and sexual dysfunction.

Less common side effects include dizziness, tremor, sweating and headache. Rare side effects include the potentially fatal serotonergic syndrome. To avoid serotonergic syndrome SSRIs should not be combined with monoamine oxidase inhibitors (MAOIs), reverse inhibitors of MAO-A (RIMA), tryptophan or St John's wort. A suitable drug-free interval is required when changing from one antidepressant to another. Serotonin syndrome presents with confusion, hypomania, restlessness, myoclonus, hyperreflexia, sweating, chills, tremor, diarrhoea, ataxia and headaches. While most cases of serotonin syndrome are mild (and can be treated by withdrawal of the SSRI), it can be potentially life-threatening, requiring emergency medical treatment in moderate or severe cases (Ables and Nagulli, 2010).

People who are under the age of 30 and prescribed an SSRI should be advised of the increased risk of suicidal thoughts and self-harm in a minority of people (NICE, 2011). This risk should be closely monitored during the early stages (over the first month) of this drug treatment (NICE, 2011).

The side effect profile of tricyclics, tetracyclics and MAOIs will not be discussed in this chapter, as they are not first-line treatment drugs for anxiety disorders.

Anti-anxiety medication

Anti-anxiety medications are also known as anxiolytics. There are two main groups of anti-anxiety medications: the benzodiazepines and the nonbenzodiazepines.

Benzodiazepines are prescribed more frequently in primary care than in mental health settings and include diazepam and oxazepam. They are often prescribed for problems that are more effectively managed with nondrug therapies. Benzodiazepines should not be the first-line therapy for anxiety disorders and must only be used for the short-term management during a crisis (NICE, 2011).

All benzodiazepines are equally effective but they differ in their metabolism, speed of onset and half-life. In addition to the relief of anxiety, benzodiazepines can be prescribed for sedation, premedication (to relieve anxiety and reduce memory of the procedure), as an anticonvulsant or to abort seizures, to ease alcohol withdrawal, to promote skeletal muscle relaxation and to induce sleep. Service users taking benzodiazepines are at increased risk of injury due to reduced alertness in driving or operating machinery. Long-term use of benzodiazepines can cause psychological and physical dependence. Service users with a history of alcohol abuse are at increased risk. Long-term use may lead to tolerance (a need to increase the dose to get the same effect) and rebound insomnia. Any central nervous system depressant drug will potentiate the effects of benzodiazepines. Potentiation may lead to increased sedation, unconsciousness and death. Common central nervous system (CNS) depressants include alcohol, antihistamines, analgesics, sedatives and tranquillizers. Service users over 60 years of age who take benzodiazepines have an increased vulnerability to confusion, memory impairment and oversedation, which could lead to falls (Hartikainen and Lönnroos, 2010).

Benzodiazepines may have an adverse effect on the individual's mood, leading to depression, emotional anaesthesia and aggression.

Withdrawal symptoms from benzodiazepines may occur between doses or during continuous use (interdose withdrawal). Service users may think these symptoms are due to the original problem. Withdrawal symptoms include increased anxiety, sleep disorder, aching limbs, nervousness and nausea. Forty-five per cent of service users discontinuing low-dose benzodiazepines experience withdrawal, as do up to 100% of service users on high doses. Short-half-life benzodiazepines are associated with more acute and intense withdrawal symptoms (NICE, 2011). Long-half-life benzodiazepines are associated with a milder, more delayed withdrawal.

Benzodiazepines should not be ceased abruptly. A safe, comfortable regimen is a dose reduction of 10–20% per week. Service users are allowed to stabilize between each reduction. Admission to hospital may be warranted for high-dose users or service users with a history of seizures or psychosis, or for more rapid withdrawal. More information on withdrawal can be obtained by contacting your local drug and alcohol services.

Benzodiazepine overdose is generally nonlethal unless combined with alcohol or other CNS depressants. The symptoms of overdose include hypotension, respiratory depression and coma. Overdose can be treated with flumazenil, with the lowest effective dose for the shortest amount of time (NICE, 2004). However, there is a high prevalence of contraindications with the use of flumazenil, which has led some to suggest that the drug should be used rarely and only then in consultation with the National Poisons Information Service (Thomson et al., 2006). If flumazenil is used, nurses will need to observe the service user carefully for several hours after a dose has been given for re-emergence of sedation as the drug wears off (NICE, 2004).

Nonbenzodiazepine anxiolytics

Buspirone can also be used to treat anxiety disorders. It has a different action from that of the benzodiazepines and is not a CNS depressant. It is a partial agonist (stimulant) of dopaminergic and serotoninergic receptors. Buspirone's action is primarily anxiolytic; it does not induce sedation and has no anticonvulsant or muscle-relaxant properties. The anxiolytic action is delayed, taking 1–2 weeks to take effect.

Hypnotics

Hypnotics are sedating medication used to promote sleep. They should only be used for the short-term management of an acute crisis where a person's sleep pattern has become disturbed, such as in PTSD (NICE, 2005a). Long-term use should be discouraged due to known problems with tolerance and dependence.

CONCLUSION

Anxiety disorders are one of the most common mental disorders. People who suffer from an anxiety disorder are less likely to seek treatment than people with a mood disorder. Nurses specializing in advanced anxiety management require additional, educational preparation. Core nursing skills include being able to recognize the symptoms of various anxiety disorders, refer service users with an anxiety disorder to appropriate services, manage panic in any setting, mobilize appropriate coping skills and implement stress-management techniques. The major psychotherapeutic methods of treating anxiety disorders include stress-management techniques such as progressive muscle relaxation. The major classes of drugs used in the treatment of anxiety disorders are antidepressants and anxiolytics.

The nurse's story earlier in this chapter highlights the fact that people diagnosed with anxiety disorders presenting to high-tech, physically orientated, clinical environments like an accident and emergency department believe they are physically ill and in grave danger. The triage system, set up to prioritize the emergency care of life-threatening conditions, rates panic attacks as a low priority; however, any hint of cardiac pathology is given a more urgent rating (as was the case in the nurse's story).

There is often a mismatch between the service user's perception of the urgency of the problem and the clinician's. Every area of healthcare has its 'core business'. The core business of an accident and emergency department is to deal with life-threatening conditions promptly. Pure panic attacks, no matter how distressing to the person having one, will never be given a high priority in such a setting. One way this problem has been tackled is to appoint psychiatric liaison nurses in accident and emergency departments. Such appropriately prepared nurses can triage mental health emergencies. The service user in panic is 'psychologically bleeding to death' and needs prompt intervention to manage their panic. However, the real tragedy of this story is not that accident and emergency departments are not set up to deal with psychiatric emergencies but that the mental health literacy of the public is so poor. This service user had had several previous panic attacks, her first when she was in her teens, yet she still did not know what was happening to her. There is an urgent need to inform the public about anxiety disorders and their management. Increased knowledge can translate into early recognition and intervention of anxiety disorders. Appropriate treatment can prevent further episodes and improve the service user's overall quality of life.

EXERCISES FOR CLASS ENGAGEMENT

Most members of the community have been exposed to at least one PTSD-level trauma in their lifetime, yet few develop PTSD (Breslau, 2002). Nurses are continually interacting with people exposed to a range of traumas. Working in groups, review the criteria for a PTSD-level trauma. Do you know someone who has been exposed to a PTSD-level trauma?

Did their response to the trauma meet the diagnostic criteria for ASD or PTSD?

With your group, discuss how to tell the difference between someone who worries about issues in their life and someone with GAD.

REFERENCES

Ables, A., Nagubilli, R., 2010. Prevention, recognition, and management of serotonin syndrome. Am. Fam. Physician 81 (9), 1139–1142.

Andrews, G., Garrity, A., 2000. Anxiety disorders: recognition and management. Aust. Fam. Physician 29 (4), 337–341.

Andrews, G., Hunt, C., 1998. Treatments that work in anxiety disorders. Med. J. Aust. 168 (12), 26–32.

APA (American Psychiatric Association), 2000. Diagnostic and Statistical Manual of Mental Disorders, fourth ed. text rev. American Psychiatric Association, Washington DC.

Appleby, J., Gregory, S., 2008. NHS spending: local variations in priorities: an update. <http://www.kingsfund.org.uk/publications/nhs_spending.html>.

Australian Institute of Family Studies, n.d. Australian temperament project. <http://www.aifs.org.au/atp/>.

Barton, D., Joubert, L., Alvarenga, M., et al., 2007. Anxiety disorders. In: Meadows, G. (Ed.), Mental Health in Australia: Collaborative Community Practice, second ed. Oxford University Press, Melbourne, pp. 493–508.

Beck, A.T., 1979. Cognitive Therapy and the Emotional Disorders. New American Library, New York.

Breslau, N., 2002. Epidemiologic studies of trauma, posttraumatic stress disorder, and other psychiatric disorders. Can. J. Psychiatry 47 (10), 923–929.

Carpenito, L.J., 2002. Nursing Diagnosis: Application to Clinical Practice, ninth ed. Lippincott, Philadelphia.

Clinical Research Unit for Anxiety and Depression, Lam-Po-Tang, J., Rosser, S., 1999. Panic: Patient Treatment Manual, Electronic Version. Clinical Research Unit for Anxiety Disorders, Melbourne.

Coetzee, R., Regel, S., 2005. Eye movement desensitization and reprocessing: an update. Adv. Psychiatr. Treat. 11, 347–354.

Crowe, R.R., Noyes, R., Pauls, D.L., et al., 1983. A family study of panic disorder. Arch. Gen. Psychiatry 40 (10), 1065–1069.

Fauman, M.A., 2002. Study Guide to DSM-IV TR. American Psychiatric Publications, Washington DC.

Fortinash, K.M., Holoday-Worret, P.A., 2008. Psychiatric Mental Health Nursing, fourth ed. Mosby, St Louis.

Freud, S., 1936. The Problem of Anxiety. W W Norton, New York.

Furukawa, T., Watanabe, N., Churchill, R., 2007. Combined psychotherapy plus antidepressants for panic disorder with or without agoraphobia. Cochrane Database Syst. Rev. 1, CD004364.

Gerull, F.C., Rapee, R.M., 2002. Mother knows best: the effects of maternal modelling on the acquisition of fear and avoidance behaviour in toddlers. Behav. Res. Ther. 40 (3), 279–287.

Giedd, J.N., Rapoport, J.L., Garvey, M.A., et al., 2000. MRI assessment of children with obsessive-compulsive disorder or tics associated with streptococcal infection. Am. J. Psychiatry 157 (2), 281–283.

Hartikainen, S., Lönnroos, E., 2010. Systematic review: use of sedatives and hypnotics, antidepressants and benzodiazepines in older people significantly increases their risk of falls. Evid. Based Med. 15, 59.

Hunot, V., Churchill, R., Teixeira, V., et al., 2007. Psychological therapies for generalised anxiety disorder. Cochrane Database Syst. Rev. 1, CD001848.

Issakidis, C., Andrews, G., 2002. Service utilisation for anxiety in an Australian community sample. Soc. Psychiatry Psychiatr. Epidemiol. 37 (4), 153–163.

Keltner, N.L., Hogan, B., Guy, D.M., 2001. Biological perspectives: dopaminergic and serotonergic receptor function in the CNS. Perspect. Psychiatr. Care 37 (2), 65–68.

Kendler, K.S., Walters, E.E., Neale, M.C., et al., 1995. The structure of the genetic and environmental risk factors for six major psychiatric

disorders in women: phobia, generalized anxiety disorder, panic disorder, bulimia, major depression, and alcoholism. Arch. Gen. Psychiatry 52 (5), 374–383.

Kenny, U., 2000. The anxiety epidemic. Herald Sun 8 October:20–21.

Mayer, P., 2001. Long torment of children's fears. Sunday Herald Sun 1 April:2–3.

McDonald, G., 1998. Foreword. In: Rapee, R.M. (Ed.), Overcoming Shyness and Social Phobia: A Step-By-Step Guide. Lifestyle Press, Killara, New South Wales, pp. vi–viii.

Mell, L.K., Davis, R.L., Owens, D., 2005. Association between streptococcal infection and obsessive-compulsive disorder, Tourette's syndrome, and tic disorder. Pediatrics 116 (1), 55–60.

Mineka, S., Zinbarg, R., 2006. A contemporary learning theory perspective on the etiology of anxiety disorders: it's not what you thought it was. Am. Psychol. 61 (1), 10–26.

Murphy, T.K., Petitto, J.M., Voeller, K.K., et al., 2001. Obsessive compulsive disorder: is there an association with childhood streptococcal infections and altered immune function? Semin. Clin. Neuropsychiatry 6 (4), 266–276.

Nazroo, J., Sproston, K. (Eds.), 2002. Ethnic Minority Psychiatric Illness Rates in the Community (EMPIRIC). <www.dh.gov.uk/assetRoot/04/02/40/34/04024034.pdf>.

Nevid, J.S., Rathus, S.A., Greene, B., 1994. Abnormal Psychology in a Changing World, second ed. Prentice Hall, Englewood Cliffs, NJ.

Neville, A., 1986. Who's Afraid of Agoraphobia? Facing up to Fear and Anxiety—a Self-help Guide. Arrow Books, London.

NICE (National Institute for Health and Clinical Excellence), 2004. Self-harm: the short-term physical and psychological management and secondary prevention of self-harm in primary and secondary care.

<http://www.nice.org.uk/nicemedia/live/10946/29421/29421.pdf>.

NICE (National Institute for Health and Clinical Excellence), 2005a. Post-traumatic stress disorder (PTSD): the management of PTSD in adults and children in primary and secondary care. <http://www.nice.org.uk/nicemedia/live/10966/29769/29769.pdf>.

NICE (National Institute for Health and Clinical Excellence), 2005b. Obsessive-compulsive disorder: core interventions in the treatment of obsessive-compulsive disorder and body dysmorphic disorder. <http://www.nice.org.uk/nicemedia/live/10976/29947/29947.pdf>.

NICE (National Institute for Health and Clinical Excellence), 2011. Generalised anxiety disorder and panic disorder (with or without agoraphobia) in adults. <http://www.nice.org.uk/nicemedia/live/13314/52599/52599.pdf>.

Office for National Statistics, 2001. Psychiatric morbidity among adults living in private households, 2000. <http://www.statistics.gov.uk/statbase/Product.asp?vlnk=8258&More=N>.

Pine, D.S., Cohen, P., Gurley, D., et al., 1998. The risk for early-adulthood anxiety and depressive disorders in adolescents with anxiety and depressive disorders. Arch. Gen. Psychiatry 55 (1), 56–64.

Prior, M., Smart, D., Sanson, A., et al., 2000. Does shy-inhibited temperament in childhood lead to anxiety problems in adolescence? J. Am. Acad. Child Adolesc. Psychiatry 39 (4), 461–468.

Rapee, R.M. (Ed.), 2001. Overcoming Shyness and Social Phobia: A Step-By-Step Guide, second ed. Lifestyle Press, Killara, New South Wales.

Rapee, R.M., 2002. The development and modification of temperamental risk for anxiety disorders: prevention of a lifetime of anxiety? Biol. Psychiatry 51 (9), 947–957.

Rogers, P., Gournay, K., 2001. Phobias: nature, assessment and treatment. Nurs. Stand. 15 (30), 37–45. (appeared previously in Mental Health Practice 2000, 3(8):30–35).

Royal College of Psychiatrists, 2008. Fair Deal for Mental Health. RCP, London.

Schultz, J.M., Videbeck, S.D., 2002. Lippincott's Manual of Psychiatric Nursing Care Plans, sixth ed. Lippincott Williams & Wilkins, Philadelphia.

Selye, H., 1956. The Stress of Life. McGraw-Hill, St Louis.

Selye, H., 1974. Stress without Distress. J B Lippincott, Philadelphia.

Stuart, G.W., 2005a. Anxiety responses and anxiety disorders. In: Stuart, G.W., Laraia, M.T. (Eds.), Principles and Practice of Psychiatric Nursing, eighth ed. Mosby, St Louis, pp. 260–284.

Stuart, G.W., 2005b. Cognitive behavioral treatment strategies. In: Stuart, G.W., Laraia, M.T. (Eds.), Principles and Practice of Psychiatric Nursing, eighth ed. Mosby, St Louis, pp. 654–667.

Sullivan, H.S., 1952. Interpersonal Theory of Psychiatry. WW Norton, New York.

Thomson, J., Donald, C., Lewin, K., 2006. Use of Flumazenil in benzodiazepine overdose. Emerg. Med. J. 23 (2), 162.

Travis, T.A., 1998. Solving Patient Problems: Psychiatry. Blackwell Science, Madison.

Treatment Protocol Project, 2004. Management of Mental Disorders. World Health Organization Collaborating Centre for Evidence in Mental Health Policy, Darlinghurst, NSW.

Tyrer, P., Baldwin, D., 2006. Generalised anxiety disorder. Lancet 368 (9553), 2156–2166.

Wagner, S.L., 2005. Emergency response service personnel and the critical incident stress debriefing debate. Int. J. Emerg. Ment. Health 7 (1), 33–41.

Chapter | 18 |

Eating disorders

Gail Anderson

DOI: http://dx.doi.org/10.1016/B978-0-7020-4493-9.00018-4

CHAPTER POINTS

- Eating disorders can have significant and potentially fatal medical consequences.
- A broad range of biological, psychological and social risk factors cause eating disorders.
- Disordered eating behaviours seen in anorexia nervosa and bulimia nervosa are driven by fear of weight gain.
- Eating disorders occur predominantly but not exclusively in Western societies.
- Eating disorders are on the rise among young men in Western societies.
- Eating-disordered behaviours include food avoidance, bingeing, vomiting, excessive exercise, use of appetite suppressants, and diuretic and laxative abuse.
- Eating disorders are usually chronic problems and remission and relapse of symptoms are common.
- Ambivalence and resistance to treatment are common.
- The major therapies used to treat eating disorders include cognitive behavioural therapy, interpersonal therapy, motivational enhancement therapy, family therapy and psychoeducation.
- Early detection and intervention improves treatment outcomes.
- Consistent therapeutic nursing care within a structured programme is the key to successful inpatient treatment of eating disorders.

KEY TERMS

- anorexia nervosa
- binge eating disorder
- bingeing
- body image disturbance
- bulimia nervosa
- cognitive behavioural therapy
- disordered eating
- family therapy
- interpersonal therapy
- motivational enhancement therapy
- nutritional rehabilitation
- psychoeducation
- purging
- refeeding syndrome
- weight loss
- weight restoration

LEARNING OUTCOMES

The material in this chapter will assist you to:

- develop an understanding of the major eating disorders within individual, family and social contexts,
- identify behaviours commonly associated with eating disorders,
- identify areas of health and wellbeing, including physical health, mental health, nutritional status and social and behavioural patterns, that are useful when assessing people suffering from eating disorders,
- recognize the potential medical complications associated with eating disorders,
- identify service users most at risk of refeeding syndrome,
- understand the ambivalence to treatment typically seen in eating-disordered service users,
- describe important aspects of nursing care for hospitalized service users diagnosed with anorexia nervosa,
- identify various approaches to the treatment of eating disorders, including cognitive behavioural therapy, interpersonal therapy, motivational enhancement therapy, family therapy, psychoeducation, supportive therapy and pharmacotherapy.

INTRODUCTION

The disorders discussed in this chapter are those classified by the *Diagnostic and Statistical Manual of Mental Disorders*, fourth edition (text revision; DSM-IV TR; APA, 2000), and *ICD-10 International Classification of Mental and Behavioural Disorders* (World Health Organisation (WHO) 1992) as eating disorders. They include anorexia nervosa, bulimia nervosa and other eating disorders not otherwise specified. This last category allows diagnosis of people whose disordered eating behaviours and symptoms are not entirely consistent with the criteria for anorexia nervosa or bulimia nervosa.

Eating disorders are characterized by one or more serious disturbances of eating behaviours such as food avoidance, self-induced vomiting, excessive exercising, recurrent episodes of uncontrolled eating and misuse of laxatives or diuretics in an effort to control weight. People with anorexia nervosa or bulimia nervosa are preoccupied with their weight, and judge their self-worth largely, or even exclusively, by their shape and weight and their ability to control them (Fairburn and Harrison, 2003). Although the DSM-IV TR and ICD-10 describes the criteria for diagnosis of specific eating disorders, symptoms have been known to occur on a continuum between these disorders (Tozzi et al., 2005). While service users cannot be diagnosed with anorexia nervosa, bulimia nervosa or unspecified eating disorders at the same time, their disordered eating behaviours can switch between these disorders over time. Body sculpting and cosmetic procedures to remove weight are also becoming more widely used in the twenty-first century.

Historically, descriptions of people diagnosed with eating disorders that might have been anorexia nervosa appear as early as the seventeenth century (Cartwright, 2004). Sometime during the late nineteenth and early twentieth centuries Western societies began to focus on thinness as a mark of beauty, and Russell (1995) argues that the incidence of anorexia nervosa has risen significantly since the 1950s. Bulimia nervosa was first documented in the 1900s and was identified in 1979 as a variant of anorexia nervosa (Russell, 1979).

CHARACTERISTICS OF EATING DISORDERS

Anorexia nervosa

Anorexia nervosa is a complex and usually chronic mental health problem with potentially fatal medical complications. It is characterized by determined efforts to lose weight or avoid weight gain (Box 18.1). If the onset of anorexia nervosa is prepubertal then the sequence of pubertal events is delayed or even arrested (growth

---

Box 18.1 Diagnostic criteria for anorexia nervosa

Anorexia nervosa is a disorder characterized by deliberate weight loss, induced and/or sustained by the patient. The disorder occurs most commonly in adolescent girls and young women, but adolescent boys and young men may be affected more rarely, as may children approaching puberty and older women up to the menopause. Anorexia nervosa constitutes an independent syndrome in the following sense:

a. the clinical features of the syndrome are easily recognized, so that diagnosis is reliable with a high level of agreement between clinicians;

b. follow-up studies have shown that, among patients who do not recover, a considerable number continue to show the same main features of anorexia nervosa in a chronic form.

Although the fundamental causes of anorexia nervosa remain elusive, there is growing evidence that interacting sociocultural and biological factors contribute to its causation, as do less specific psychological mechanisms and a vulnerability of personality. The disorder is associated with undernutrition of varying severity, with resulting secondary endocrine and metabolic changes and disturbances of bodily function. There remains some doubt as to whether the characteristic endocrine disorder is entirely due to the undernutrition and the direct effect of various behaviours that have brought it about (e.g. restricted dietary choice, excessive exercise and alterations in body composition, induced vomiting and purgation and the consequent electrolyte disturbances), or whether uncertain factors are also involved.

Diagnostic Guidelines

For a definite diagnosis, all the following are required.

a. Body weight is maintained at least 15% below that expected (either lost or never achieved), or body mass index (BMI) is 17.5 kg/m² or less. Prepubertal patients may show failure to make the expected weight gain during the period of growth.

b. The weight loss is self-induced by avoidance of 'fattening foods'. One or more of the following may also be present: self-induced vomiting, self-induced purging, excessive exercise and use of appetite suppressants and/ or diuretics.

c. There is body-image distortion in the form of a specific psychopathology whereby a dread of fatness persists as an intrusive, overvalued idea and the patient imposes a low-weight threshold on himself or herself.

d. A widespread endocrine disorder involving the hypothalamic–pituitary–gonadal axis is manifest in women as amenorrhoea and in men as a loss of sexual interest and potency. (An apparent exception is the persistence of vaginal bleeds in anorexic women who are receiving replacement hormonal therapy, most commonly taken as a contraceptive pill.) There may also be elevated levels of growth hormone, raised levels of cortisol, changes in the peripheral metabolism of the thyroid hormone and abnormalities of insulin secretion.

e. If onset is prepubertal the sequence of pubertal events is delayed or even arrested (growth ceases; in girls the breasts do not develop and there is a primary amenorrhoea; in boys the genitals remain juvenile). With recovery puberty is often completed normally, but the menarche is late.

Adapted from the World Health Organisation (1992) The ICD-10 Classification of Mental and Behavioural Disorders, pp. 138–139 with permission.

ceases: in girls the breasts do not develop and there is primary amenorrhoea, and in boys the genitals remain juvenile) (Royal Australian and New Zealand College of Psychiatrists, 2004).

The onset of anorexia nervosa typically begins with restricting food that is perceived to be fattening, and this dietary restriction becomes more rigid and severe as the disorder progresses. Other behaviours commonly used as a means of losing or controlling weight include excessive exercising, self-induced vomiting or purging and the use of appetite suppressants and/or diuretics. As weight loss progresses, service users feel a sense of identity, control and accomplishment that they didn't otherwise feel. They become preoccupied with thoughts of food and no matter how thin they become they see their bodies as fat and desire to lose more weight.

The essential diagnostic criteria defined in the ICD-10 (WHO, 1992) for anorexia nervosa are listed in Box 18.1.

Bulimia nervosa

Bulimia nervosa is characterized by overwhelming urges to over-eat (binge), followed by compensatory behaviour to avoid weight gain, such as self-induced vomiting, excessive exercise, food avoidance or laxative misuse. A cycle is often seen where self-induced nutritional restriction leads to an increased hunger for food, both physiologically and psychologically, which in turn encourages bingeing behaviour. For the person concerned with weight and body shape there then arises an overwhelming desire to prevent weight gain through behaviours such as vomiting, laxative abuse, over-exercising or restricting food intake again. The use of these compensatory behaviours leads to feelings of disgust and act to reinforce the person's sense of poor self-worth, and the bulimic cycle begins again.

The main feature that distinguishes bulimia nervosa from anorexia nervosa is that attempts to restrict food intake are punctuated by repeated binge eating, or episodes of eating during which there is an aversive sense of loss of control and an unusually large amount of food is eaten (Fairburn and Harrison, 2003). Service users diagnosed with bulimia nervosa are likely to have normal or near normal body weight.

The essential diagnostic criteria defined in the ICD-10 (WHO, 1992) for bulimia nervosa are listed in Box 18.2.

Unspecified eating disorder

The diagnosis of *unspecified* eating disorder is given when the disordered eating behaviour is not entirely consistent with the essential diagnostic criteria for either anorexia or bulimia nervosa. For example, a woman may have all the symptoms of anorexia nervosa except that she may still have a regular menstrual cycle. Binge eating disorder also fits into this category. Binge eating disorder is characterized

---

Box 18.2 Diagnostic criteria for bulimia nervosa

Bulimia nervosa is a syndrome characterized by repeated bouts of overeating and an excessive preoccupation with the control of body weight, leading the patient to adopt extreme measures so as to mitigate the 'fattening' effects of ingested food. The term should be restricted to the form of the disorder that is related to anorexia nervosa by virtue of sharing the same psychopathology. The age and sex distribution is similar to that of anorexia nervosa, but the age of presentation tends to be slightly later. The disorder may be viewed as a sequel to persistent anorexia nervosa (although the reverse sequence may also occur). A previously anorexic patient may first appear to improve as a result of weight gain and possibly a return of menstruation, but a pernicious pattern of overeating and vomiting then becomes established. Repeated vomiting is likely to give rise to disturbances of body electrolytes, physical complications (tetany, epileptic seizures, cardiac arrhythmias, muscular weakness) and further severe loss of weight.

Diagnostic guidelines

For a definite diagnosis, all the following are required.

a. There is a persistent preoccupation with eating, and an irresistible craving for food; the patient succumbs to episodes of overeating in which large amounts of food are consumed in short periods of time.

b. The patient attempts to counteract the 'fattening' effects of food by one or more of the following: self-induced vomiting, purgative abuse, alternating periods of starvation and use of drugs such as appetite suppressants, thyroid preparations or diuretics. When bulimia occurs in diabetic patients they may choose to neglect their insulin treatment.

c. The psychopathology consists of a morbid dread of fatness and the patient sets herself or himself a sharply defined weight threshold, well below the premorbid weight that constitutes the optimum or healthy weight in the opinion of the physician. There is often, but not always, a history of an earlier episode of anorexia nervosa, the interval between the two disorders ranging from a few months to several years. This earlier episode may have been fully expressed, or may have assumed a minor cryptic form with a moderate loss of weight and/or a transient phase of amenorrhoea.

Adapted from the World Health Organisation (1992) The ICD-10 Classification of Mental and Behavioural Disorders, pp. 139–140 with permission.

---

by recurrent episodes of binge eating without compensatory behaviours to avoid weight gain, a lack of self-control during the binge eating and marked distress after a binge. As binge eating disorder does not involve avoidance of weight gain, it has a strong association with obesity.

Eating disorders in children and adolescents

Special medical consideration, including early and more aggressive refeeding to a healthy weight range, is required for children and adolescents with eating disorders as they can more rapidly become medically compromised and permanently lose growth potential (Hamilton, 2007). Emaciation occurs more rapidly as younger service users have lower energy stores than adults, and children also dehydrate more quickly than adults do (RCP, 2005).

In order to prevent potentially irreversible physical growth and developmental complications, paediatricians, child psychiatrists and nurses who are aware of the physiological differences and psychosocial developmental needs of these younger service users should treat children and adolescents with eating disorders. Unlike adults, children should continue to grow in height during the course of their treatment. Therefore their height measurements and healthy target weights need to be revised every 3 months. When nursing adolescents with eating disorders, the philosophy should be consistent with nursing care aimed at promoting the achievement of adolescent developmental tasks as well as management of the eating disorder (Anderson, 1996). Bulimia nervosa is rarely seen in children.

Eating disorders in males

Behaviours such as excessive exercise to increase bulk, bingeing and purging and steroid use are not uncommon among young males and there is concern that eating disorders are increasing among men. There is an increased prevalence in certain subgroups of males who are vulnerable to weight and shape concerns, such as wrestlers and homosexual men (Clarke-Stone and Joyce, 2003) and athletes (Muise et al., 2003). The clinical features of eating disorders specific to males include loss of libido, decrease in spontaneous early morning erections, nocturnal emissions and desire to masturbate associated with malnutrition and lower testosterone levels and higher rates of comorbid depression and substance use.

The increased incidence of eating disorders in men may be due to an increasing obsession among men in Western societies with their appearance. In contrast to the popular thin ideal of feminine beauty, young men experience two conflicting social pressures. One is the pressure to 'bulk up' or become more muscular. A condition termed *muscle dysmorphia* that is most prevalent in males has been described (see Ch. 20). In contrast to people with eating disorders who see themselves as fat when they are thin, people with muscle dysmorphia feel ashamed of looking small when they are actually well built (Grieve, 2007; Pope et al., 2000). The other recent social pressure on young men is highlighted by the current popularity of some male role models in the media spotlight, such as musicians and singers, who have been diagnosed with anorexia nervosa or look particularly underweight. The impact of these underweight role models on the prevalence of disordered eating among men is yet to be studied.

INCIDENCE AND PREVALENCE

The eating disorders are encountered predominantly in Western industrialized countries but appear to be increasing in non-Western countries. Incidence and prevalence rates are difficult to report accurately as many people with eating disorders go undetected. For example, one Australian study (O'Dea and Abraham, 2002) investigated eating, weight, shape and exercise behaviours in young men, and found that one in five men worried about their weight and shape, followed rules about eating and limited their food intake, and while 9% reported disordered eating, none of the population studied had sought treatment.

Incidence rates refer to the number of new cases in the population over a specified time. Incidence rates for anorexia nervosa have been estimated to be 8 per 100 000 people per year, and 13 per 100 000 people per year for bulimia nervosa (Hoek, 2006). The incidence rate for anorexia nervosa in males has been reported to be below 1 per 100 000 people per year (Hoek, 2006).

Prevalence rates refer to the actual number of cases in the population at a particular point in time. Eating disorders are more common among adolescent girls and young women, with a 0.3% average prevalence rate reported for anorexia nervosa and 1% for bulimia nervosa (Hoek, 2006). Studies of lifetime prevalence have reported various rates, from 0.3 to 3.7% for anorexia nervosa and 1 to 4.2% for bulimia nervosa (APA, 2006). Machado et al. (2007) reported a 2.7% prevalence rate for unspecified eating disorder. One Australian study (Hay, 1998) reported a 1% prevalence of binge eating disorder using DSM-IV TR criteria and a 2.5% prevalence using a broader definition. Binge eating disorder has been described as almost as common among men as women, with approximately 40% of sufferers being male (Pope et al., 2000).

AETIOLOGY AND RISK FACTORS

There is no single cause for eating disorders, although genetic, biological, psychological, family, social and cultural factors have all been implicated in their development.

Gender

Being female in a culture where thinness is equated with beauty and popularity is a risk factor for developing an eating disorder. Paxton (2000) argues that evolutionary factors that predispose women to being more conscious of their appearance may be involved. Ninety per cent of service users with anorexia nervosa are female. Patton et al. (1999) argue that dieting is the most important predictor of new eating disorders, and that differences in the incidence of eating disorders between the sexes can be largely accounted for by the higher rates of dieting and mental disorders in females.

Age

Onset of anorexia nervosa generally occurs during adolescence, although eating disorders are occurring more frequently in children aged from 6 to 12 years (Hamilton, 2007). Bulimia nervosa and binge eating disorder are more likely to first occur in late adolescence or early adulthood, although service users with these disorders may not present for treatment until much later in life.

History of dieting

Most eating disorders start with dieting behaviours. One study of adolescent girls found that severe dieters were 18 times more likely to develop an eating disorder than non-dieters, and that moderate dieters were five times more likely to develop these symptoms (Patton et al., 1999). Service users seeking treatment for binge eating disorder, however, have been reported to have weight problems prior to dieting and binge eating behaviour (Reas and Grilo, 2007).

Social factors

Low self-esteem and concerns about appearance and body image are exacerbated for many young people by social and cultural pressures to conform to a particular thin ideal of beauty. The media and associated influences such as the fashion industry have been criticized for many years for promoting unrealistically thin images of women. In addition, the ideal bodies presented in the media have become thinner over time. Body comparison, or the process of comparing one's body with others, such as friends or models and film stars, is recognized as a factor contributing to body dissatisfaction, dieting and symptoms of disordered eating (Paxton et al., 1999, Stormer and Thompson, 1996). Recent pressure is being placed on the fashion, media, marketing and advertising industries to encourage a greater diversity of more realistic weight and body shapes. It will be interesting to see if this pressure has an impact on lowering future incidence and prevalence rates of eating disorders. However, it must be remembered that while all young people are exposed to media and marketing industries, they do not all develop eating disorders. Low self-esteem is a common factor in those who do develop eating disorders, and interventions aimed at improving the self-esteem of children and adolescents may also help to decrease the number of people affected by eating disorders. Furthermore, the onset of anorexia nervosa can also be associated with other stressful life events such as loss and grief, child abuse or neglect, bullying or other developmental traumas. Urban living has also been identified as a risk factor for bulimia nervosa but not for anorexia nervosa (Van Son et al., 2006).

CRITICAL THINKING CHALLENGE 18.1

How would you describe a 'normal' interest in body image and dieting versus an obsessional interest?
   Is your answer different for males and females?
   Does age affect what is considered 'normal'?
   Given the high incidence of dieting behaviour in the community, do you think eating-disordered behaviour is deviant?

Psychological factors

Common personality traits found in service users with anorexia nervosa include low self-esteem, perfectionism, obsessionality, alexithymia (difficulty identifying and expressing feelings verbally) and intimacy concerns along with a sense of not feeling in control of one's life. Young people with bulimia nervosa tend to be more impulsive and self-critical, and demonstrate labile moods in response to environmental events (Sigman, 2003).

Cognitive behavioural theories have been proposed to account for the development and maintenance of eating disorders. Fairburn and Harrison (2003) describe two main origins of the restriction of food intake characterizing the onset of eating disorders as a need to feel in control of life, which gets displaced onto controlling eating, and over-evaluation of shape and weight in those who have been sensitized to their appearance.

In the psychodynamic literature, service users diagnosed with anorexia nervosa have been described as having difficulties with separation and autonomy (often manifested as overly close or enmeshed relationships with parents), affect regulation (including the direct expression of anger and aggression) and negotiation of psychosexual development (APA, 2006).

Service users diagnosed with bulimia nervosa have been understood in a number of ways, ranging from viewing symptoms as manifestations of impulsivity or problems with emotion regulation and dissociative states to viewing them along a spectrum of self-harming behaviours commonly seen in borderline personality organization (Westen and Harnden-Fischer, 2001).

Familial factors

Despite its limitations, research indicates that family functioning can play a part in the development and maintenance of weight concerns and eating disorders (May et al., 2006). Negative paternal comments and dieting have been known to influence self-esteem, body image and the eating behaviours of children (Cartwright, 2004). Freeman (2002) suggests that families with a child diagnosed with anorexia nervosa often have one parent who is over-involved while the other is passive. Anorexia nervosa can also develop in over-controlled and rigid families that have difficulty expressing and resolving conflict, while bulimia nervosa is more likely to develop when family systems are chaotic (Hamilton, 2007).

McIntosh et al. (2000) suggest that the families of individuals diagnosed with restricting anorexia nervosa are more positive than the families of individuals diagnosed with bulimia nervosa or binge eating/purging anorexia nervosa. In a discussion of bulimia nervosa, Zerbe (1993) identified family discord, lack of consistency, lack of warmth and emotional connection to the child, and failure to protect the child from sexual and physical abuse or perpetuating such abuse as influential. Families of service users diagnosed with bulimia nervosa have also been shown to have higher rates of substance abuse, affective disorders and certain personality traits such as perfectionism (Lilenfeld et al., 2000).

Genetic and biological factors

Biological factors known to predispose people to developing eating disorders include genetics and gene–environment interactions (Strober et al., 2000). Women who have been diagnosed anorexia nervosa often have daughters with similar problems and the risk of a first-degree relative of an affected person developing an eating disorder is ten times that of the general population (Beumont, 2000, p. 81). Molecular genetic studies are currently attempting to identify specific genes that contribute to this vulnerability for eating disorders.

Alterations of central nervous system serotonin activity may also directly affect eating behaviours as well as other symptoms of mental health problems such as depression and obsessive–compulsive symptoms. Low levels of serotonin activity are associated with impulsivity and may predispose to bulimia nervosa, whereas high levels are associated with rigidity and constraint and may predispose to anorexia nervosa. Furthermore, the neurotransmitters serotonin and noradrenaline are regulated by leptin, which acts on the hypothalamus to regulate appetite and weight. It may be that individuals diagnosed

with bulimia have a normal response to leptin but as they try to reduce their weight past their body's 'set-point' for weight they fail because of the body's overwhelming drive to maintain this set point (Abraham and Llewellyn-Jones, 2001).

The risk of developing anorexia nervosa has also been shown to increase with the number of perinatal complications (Favaro et al., 2006).

MEDICAL COMPLICATIONS

The protein–calorie malnutrition seen in anorexia nervosa affects every organ in the body, and nurses must be aware of the potential medical complications as these can be life-threatening and require urgent resuscitation. Acute complications of anorexia nervosa include bradycardia and cardiac compromise, hypothermia, dehydration, electrolyte disturbance (with purging), gastrointestinal motility disturbances, renal problems, infertility and perinatal complications (Miller et al., 2005).

The abnormalities seen in service users with bulimia nervosa, particularly electrolyte disturbances, are usually related to frequent vomiting or laxative and diuretic misuse. Binge eating disorder carries similar medical risks and long-term consequences to those seen in obesity, such as hypertension, high blood cholesterol, heart disease and increased risk of diabetes and stroke.

Most of the medical complications of anorexia nervosa, with the exception of potentially irreversible osteoporosis, can be reversed with restoration of adequate nutrition and healthy weight range. However, the long-term effect of anorexia nervosa and protein–calorie malnutrition on cognition and brain functioning requires further research.

Cardiovascular effects

Fainting and collapse are common reasons for presentation at accident and emergency departments and often indicate serious cardiovascular complications (Cartwright, 2004). Cardiac irregularities caused by protein–calorie malnutrition include bradycardia (heart rate less than 50 beats per minute), hypotension (blood pressure less than 80/50 mmHg) and cardiac arrhythmias. electrocardiogram (ECG) abnormalities, including a prolonged QTc interval and non-specific ST-segment depression or T-wave changes, can be associated with electrolyte disturbances as well as malnutrition. The abuse of the emetic *ipecacuanha* can lead to cardiomyopathy. As cardiac arrest can result from arrhythmias, cardiac monitoring is recommended for service users with acute medical compromise such as bradycardia or a prolonged QTc interval on ECG.

Electrolyte abnormalities

Electrolyte abnormalities, including low potassium, chloride and sodium levels, are common in the purging subtype of anorexia nervosa and bulimia nervosa. Frequent vomiting can result in metabolic alkalosis and hypokalaemia, whereas laxative misuse can lead to metabolic acidosis, hyponatraemia and hypokalaemia.

Renal dysfunction

Reduced glomerular filtration rate, elevated serum urea nitrogen and hypovolaemia can occur in both anorexia and bulimia nervosa. Reduced urine production can indicate severe dehydration or progressive renal insufficiency. Associated renal failure is sometimes seen in older adolescents and adults.

Gastrointestinal effects

Service users who severely restrict their dietary intake describe feeling bloated or full even after eating small amounts of food, which can indicate shrinking of the stomach, or delayed gastric emptying. Binge eating, on the other hand, can lead to gastric dilation and, in rare cases, stomach rupture or death. In assessing bowel activity, diarrhoea can be a sign of laxative abuse, while constipation may result from inadequate food intake including lack of fibre bulk, dehydration or decrease in gastric motility. It should be noted that laxatives used by service users can include those found in common household food items, such as artificial sweeteners, chewing gum and diet drinks.

Recurrent vomiting can lead to enlarged parotid and salivary glands, and oesophagitis or oesophageal or gastric tears. Abdominal pain or involuntary regurgitation of food is associated with both the trauma and frequency of vomiting.

Endocrine effects

One of the diagnostic criteria for anorexia nervosa in postmenarcheal females is amenorrhoea. Amenorrhoea in anorexia nervosa is due to the effects of protein–calorie malnutrition on central regulatory structures such as the pituitary gland and the hypothalamus. Gonadotropins and oestradiol (hormones responsible for reproduction and sexual development) levels are generally low in females diagnosed with anorexia nervosa. Decreased serum testosterone levels and accompanying loss of libido are commonly found in underweight males. Service users diagnosed with bulimia may have irregular menses or 'periods' (oligomenorrhoea). Thyroid function (in particular triiodothyronine (T_3) levels) may be depressed in low-weight service users diagnosed with anorexia nervosa and is consistent with clinical findings such as dry skin and brittle hair, fatigue and cold intolerance.

Musculoskeletal effects

Osteopenia (low bone mineral density), osteoporosis and associated risk of fractures are common in longstanding and severe cases of anorexia nervosa (Grinspoon et al., 2000). Irreversible decreased bone mineral density is associated with prolonged malnutrition, low oestrogen levels and amenorrhoea for longer than 6 months, and decreased muscle mass. A dual-energy X-ray absorbtiometry (DEXA) scan is generally ordered to assess bone mineral density when service users diagnosed with an eating disorder have experienced amenorrhoea for longer than 6 consecutive months. Growth retardation can occur in children when the onset of the disorder occurs before closure of the epiphyses.

Dental and oral effects

Dental erosion and caries can occur with recurrent self-induced vomiting. Riboflavin deficiency may cause fissures of the lips, especially in the corners of the mouth, and iron and zinc deficiencies cause glossitis and loss of taste sensation (RCP, 2005).

Skin/integument effects

Protein–calorie malnutrition leads to loss of subcutaneous fat, and lanugo, a fine, downy hair that grows on the face and body, is often seen. Lanugo is believed to be an adaptation to loss of body fat, and functions to help preserve body temperature. Cool hands and feet with bluish discolouration (peripheral cyanosis), callous on the dorsum of the dominant hand due to repeated self-induced vomiting, brittle nails and dry skin are commonly seen. Carotenaemia, a yellow/orange discolouration of the skin caused by vitamin A overload, usually from eating carrots, is occasionally seen (seen best on the hands or soles of the feet).

Neurological effects

Structural changes in the brain including loss of brain volume, cerebral atrophy and ventricular dilatation have been reported (Fairburn and Harrison, 2003; Rome and Ammerman, 2003) and there are concerns that some of these changes persist even after refeeding. Severe electrolyte imbalances can lead to abnormal electrical discharges in the brain and seizures.

Cognitive changes

Cognitive changes associated with the biological impact of protein–calorie malnutrition include impaired concentration and comprehension, and a pervasive obsession with food-related issues (which can be assessed by asking how much of the service user's time is taken up with thinking about food). In children and adolescents, poor concentration can lead to difficulties keeping up with schoolwork.

The cognitive effects of starvation can also impair a service user's ability to engage in psychological interventions and underscore the need for nutritional rehabilitation in order to enhance effective use of psychotherapeutic interventions and ultimate emotional and psychological recovery.

The competence of the service user to make an informed decision is a very important consideration in assessment and treatment. Legal intervention including involuntary hospitalization under the Mental Health Act 1983, amended 2007, or Children Act 1989 are considered when service users with life-threatening symptoms refuse treatment.

COMORBIDITY

Many service users with eating disorders have additional comorbidity with other mental health problems that increases the complexity of treatment. The most common comorbidities are Axis I mental disorders including depression, anxiety and obsessive–compulsive disorder, body dysmorphic disorder and chemical dependency, and Axis II personality disorders such as borderline personality disorder.

Symptoms of depression such as low mood, irritability and social withdrawal can be seen in very underweight people due to the effects of malnutrition. These symptoms do not necessarily warrant a diagnosis of major depressive disorder as they often reverse with nutritional rehabilitation.

Anxiety disorders may precede eating disorders and anxiety may also develop or worsen as weight is restored and treatment progresses. Obsessive–compulsive behaviours (see Ch. 17) are observed in service users diagnosed with eating disorders, particularly anorexia, and usually take the form of repetitive counting and ritualistic eating patterns such as chewing food a certain number of times. In most cases the obsessive–compulsive symptoms tend to resolve as the starvation resolves, unless the condition was premorbid. As well as obsessive–compulsive disorder, social phobia and panic disorders have been identified (Godart et al., 2006). Service users diagnosed with anorexia nervosa and comorbid body dysmorphic disorder have been shown to have a high rate of attempted suicide (Grant et al., 2002).

Substance misuse occurs particularly in service users diagnosed with bulimia nervosa, and includes the use of legal and illicit drugs, such as alcohol, tobacco and amphetamines and the typical drugs used for weight loss, such as caffeine, emetics, diuretics and laxatives. Children

and adolescents diagnosed with anorexia nervosa are less likely to substance abuse although some young people with bulimia nervosa consume alcohol. Some studies support a familial relationship between substance use disorders and eating disorders, and monitoring for substance misuse throughout treatment has been recommended (Herzog et al., 2006; Piran and Gadalla, 2007).

ASSESSMENT

A comprehensive multidisciplinary assessment determines whether a diagnosis for a specific eating disorder is met and identifies symptoms and behaviours that need to be addressed in the service user's treatment programme.

Physical assessment

A full medical examination includes weight and height measures, vital signs, cardiovascular and peripheral vascular function, metabolic status, dermatological manifestations and evidence of self-harm (APA, 2006). The physical assessment, including blood chemistry, urinalysis and ECG, will detect any of the medical complications previously described.

Medical complications develop at higher weights in those who lose weight rapidly. Recording the history of highest and lowest weights since the onset of the disorder helps assess the rapidity of weight loss. It is also useful to note any significant relationships between life events and weight loss as this gives insight into causal factors that can be addressed in treatment.

In adults, height and weight are used to calculate the body mass index (or BMI) (see Box 18.3), which helps

---

Box 18.3 Calculation of body mass index

To calculate body mass index (BMI), divide weight in kilograms by height squared in metres. For example, a person who is 163 cm tall and weighs 55 kg would have a body mass index of 20.75. To calculate:

1.63 squared equals 2.65
55 divided by 2.65 equals a BMI of 20.75 kg/m^2

Range:

BMI<16 kg/m^2	requires specialist management
BMI<18.5 kg/m^2	underweight
BMI 19–25 kg/m^2	normal weight
BMI>25 kg/m^2	overweight
BMI>30 kg/m^2	obese

Note: These ranges relate to white populations. Norms for Asian populations may be lower.

---

determine the degree of starvation. Children and adolescents are assessed on percentage of ideal body weight or gender-specific standardized growth charts. Plotting the child's previous growth patterns helps to identify any crossing over of centiles above or below that expected on the child's growth curve trajectories.

Rather than undressing the child or adolescent, sexual or pubertal development can be assessed by asking them to point to the diagrammatic picture most closely matching their own body development on the five-stage Tanner rating scales for pubertal changes, that accompany most standardized child growth charts.

Mental state examination

A mental state examination will confirm the specific diagnosis, identify any comorbid mental health problems and exclude other primary diagnosis such as depression, which can present as loss of appetite without the body image disturbance and fear of weight gain. Other aspects of the service user's mental state that greatly influence clinical course and outcome include mood, anxiety and substance use disorders, as well as motivational status, personality traits and personality disorders (APA, 2006). Denial and minimization are common in adolescents diagnosed with anorexia nervosa and can complicate the assessment process (Couturier and Lock, 2006). Parents or carers of young service users are interviewed to help validate assessment findings.

Body image assessment

Body image attitudes develop during childhood and dissatisfaction tends to increase during adolescence and young adulthood. It is useful therefore to understand the service user's perception of their weight during childhood and identify any significant events that might have triggered negative responses to body image, such as teasing or bullying and criticism about weight or body shape.

Assessing the degree and nature of body image disturbance assists in diagnosis, in understanding the severity of the disorder and in guiding treatment programmes. According to Crowther and Sherwood (1997), assessment of body image considers three components: body image distortion (a disturbance of perception in which service users describe their body or parts of it as large or fat despite concrete evidence to the contrary), body image dissatisfaction (a disturbance of cognition and affect that leads to a negative evaluation of physical appearance) and body image avoidance (a disturbance of behaviour that leads to repetitive body checking and avoidance of social situations that provoke anxiety about the body).

Simple questions that can give insight into the service user's body image include 'When I look at you I see you as very thin. How do you see yourself?', 'How do you feel when you look at yourself in the mirror?' and 'What weight would you like to be?'

CRITICAL THINKING CHALLENGE 18.2

Outline the things that have influenced your personal body image.

Do you believe that your personal body image has been affected more by your individual temperament or by family, cultural and social issues?

To what extent has the mass media affected your personal body image?

Nutritional assessment

A dietitian on the multidisciplinary team usually performs a nutritional assessment. The dietary history is used to identify specific deficiencies and should include information on fluid intake, consumption of alcohol and caffeine, smoking, use of vitamin supplements and measurement of weight and height (RCP, 2005). Energy input, including the amount and types of food eaten and avoided, are assessed. It is not unusual for service users diagnosed with anorexia nervosa and sometimes service users diagnosed with bulimia nervosa to avoid whole food groups such as meat, dairy products and carbohydrates. Some foods are so feared because of a service user's beliefs about uncontrollable weight gain that they become labelled as 'fear foods'.

It is also important to ascertain the amount of energy output or weight-controlling behaviours including exercise and sports participation, and the frequency, amount and type of any bingeing and purging behaviours.

Disordered eating behaviours and rituals

Disordered eating behaviours commonly seen in people diagnosed with anorexia nervosa develop in order to avoid weight gain. The extent of the service user's struggle with food can be assessed by observing mealtime behaviours. Box 18.4 provides examples of some frequently observed eating abnormalities.

Service users sometimes eat excessive amounts of some foods because of their perceived benefits in promoting weight loss. For example, a common addition to meals is chilli sauce, which is believed, in the absence of concrete evidence, to increase metabolic rate. It is also not unusual for service users to drink large quantities of diet caffeinated soft drinks, coffee or water if they perceive that this as helpful in avoiding weight gain. For example, caffeine in soft drinks and coffee is mistakenly believed to increase metabolic rate, and the sweetener in diet drinks can have a laxative effect when taken in large doses. Large quantities of fluid can also help to suppress hunger pains, and increased water consumption (water loading)

Box 18.4 **Examples of eating abnormalities**

- Refusal to eat
- Cutting up food into tiny pieces and then eating pieces individually, or by colour, or in groups of numbers (e.g. two peas followed by two pieces of carrot)
- Attempting to remove any oil from food, e.g. by pressing food into absorbent serviettes, scraping margarine from sandwiches
- Restricting foods so as to eat the same thing every day
- Fear of touching food
- Adding large amounts of condiment to food or concocting strange mixtures
- Eating so slowly that the time to eat a meal is extended sometimes by up to several hours, which can then often lead into the next mealtime
- Constant fidgeting at the table
- Obsessive calorie counting or measuring of all food quantities
- Leaving the table during or immediately after the meal, usually to vomit or throw away food hidden during the meal
- Excessive use of diet foods or diet products
- Excessive preoccupation with the preparation and serving of food to others
- Avoidance of eating with others

is often used by service users prior to weighing to give a false impression of weight gain.

Bingeing can be spontaneous or planned and after a time can occur in a ritualistic manner; for example, choosing the same time and place every evening or certain nights of the week. Bingeing that is planned can cause great anxiety if the person is prevented from carrying out the ritual by events outside their control. Some service users diagnosed with bulimia will, over time, choose food that is easily regurgitated or food that is economical if they cannot finance their binges. A binge episode is usually terminated in response to one or more of the following: abdominal fullness, distension and pain, running out of food, the need to sleep or social interruptions.

Self-induced vomiting usually but not always follows a binge, and techniques used to induce vomiting include *ipecacuanha*, putting fingers down the throat or vomiting on demand. Signs that vomiting may be occurring include weight loss or no weight gain despite apparent adherence to a prescribed nutritional programme, leaving the meal table immediately after a meal to go to the shower or toilet, or the smell or presence of vomit in the toilet, sink or shower.

Diuretic and laxative abuse tends to be ineffective in achieving real weight loss. Diuretics only cause fluid loss and laxatives work on the large bowel, in which

only approximately 12% of the nutrition from food is absorbed and so most nutrition has entered the bloodstream before the laxatives act. Excessive exercise is also a common strategy used by people with an eating disorder to lose or avoid gaining weight. They tend to engage in fat-burning exercise rather than muscle-building or muscle-strengthening exercise.

Family assessment

A family history is used to identify factors that may have contributed to the development of the eating disorder, and family stressors that can be addressed to facilitate the service user's recovery. Any family history of eating disorder, affective disorder, anxiety, substance use or other mental health problems has implications for treatment. It is also important to assess the quality of relationships, the level of support available within the family, the way family members communicate with each other, family attitudes towards eating and appearance, and the effect the eating disorder has on family and social relationships. Treasure et al. (2003) argue that the carer's response to the unwell family member is an important mediator of service user outcome in mental health problems.

During the assessment, one is mindful that many families and carers are often emotionally exhausted by their own struggle to help their family member manage the disordered eating. Feelings of guilt, failure, anger, blame and fear are common in families. As no direct evidence exists to prove that families cause eating disorders, blaming family members is harmful and would impair their desire, willingness and capacity to participate actively and constructively in treatment and recovery (APA, 2006).

While family involvement is strongly encouraged, confidentiality issues must be taken into account for both adolescents and adults. The decision to involve families, spouses and/or partners of adult service users should be made in consultation with the service user.

TREATMENT

People diagnosed with eating disorders are challenging to treat and the recovery process is likely to take an average of 5–7 years, with remission and relapse of symptoms occurring during this time. Treatment can range from less than 1 year for mild cases to a lifetime in chronic cases. Service users who do not recover within 7 years of initial diagnosis are considered to have chronic eating disorders and are known to be very treatment-resistant. Early detection and intervention generally improves treatment outcome.

Several studies have explored the treatment experience of eating disorders from the perspectives of both service user and family (Malson et al., 2004; McMaster et al., 2004) and nursing staff (King and Turner, 2000; Ramjan,

2004; Ryan et al., 2006). These studies highlight the complexity of treatment and some of the frustrations experienced by both consumers and healthcare professionals during treatment.

Services available for treating people diagnosed with eating disorders include outpatient programmes, day patient programmes and inpatient care in both medical and mental healthcare settings. Typically the age and the medical and mental state of the service user and the availability and expertise of local healthcare providers determine the most appropriate treatment service. A multidisciplinary team approach is needed as medical and nursing care, nutritional rehabilitation, psychotherapy and, particularly in children and adolescents, family therapy are all integral parts of treatment.

The aims of treating people diagnosed with anorexia nervosa have been described by the American Psychiatric Association (APA, 2006) as:

- to restore service users to a healthy weight (associated with the return of menses and normal ovulation in female service users, normal sexual drive and hormone levels in male service users and normal physical and sexual growth and development in children and adolescents),
- to treat physical complications,
- to enhance motivation to cooperate in the restoration of healthy eating patterns and participate in treatment,
- to provide education regarding healthy nutrition and eating patterns,
- to help service users reassess and change core dysfunctional cognitions, attitudes, motives, conflicts and feelings related to the eating disorder,
- to treat associated mental health problems, including deficits in mood and impulse regulation and self-esteem and behavioural problems,
- to enlist family support and provide family counselling and therapy where appropriate,
- to prevent relapse.

Service users rarely seek treatment, especially those with anorexia nervosa, and when they do ambivalence about complying with treatment is always present. Ambivalence and resistance to treatment occur largely because the eating disorder functions to give the service user a sense of identity, control and accomplishment that they may not otherwise feel.

The majority of service users diagnosed with bulimia nervosa should be treated in an outpatient basis (NICE, 2004). The aims of treating bulimia nervosa have been described by the American Psychiatric Association (APA, 2006) as:

- to reduce and, where possible, eliminate binge eating and purging behaviour,
- to treat physical complications,

- to enhance motivation to cooperate in the restoration of healthy eating patterns and participate in treatment,
- to provide education regarding healthy nutrition and eating patterns,
- to help service users assess and change core dysfunctional thoughts, attitudes, motives, conflicts and feelings related to the eating disorder,
- to treat associated mental health problems including deficits in mood and impulse regulation, self-esteem and behaviour,
- to enlist family support and provide family counselling and therapy where appropriate,
- to prevent relapse.

Binge eating disorder is generally treated on an outpatient basis. The aims of treating binge eating disorder include normalized eating patterns, reduction or elimination of binge episodes, stabilization of weight within a healthy weight range, effective treatment of any underlying psychopathology and prevention of relapse.

Hospitalization

Service users diagnosed with eating disorders are admitted to hospital when they require the safety and containment provided by nursing care. Those diagnosed with anorexia nervosa are more likely to require hospitalization than service users diagnosed with bulimia nervosa. Box 18.5 lists some of the medical indications for hospitalisation. Other indications for admission include significant risk of self-harm, comorbid mental disorders requiring hospitalization, severe family dysfunction or abusive relationships and a resistance to outpatient treatment in very malnourished service users.

Box 18.5 Medical indications for hospitalization

Heart rate <50 beats per minute
Blood pressure <80 mmHg systolic and 50 mmHg diastolic
Postural systolic blood pressure drop >10 mmHg
Temperature <35.6°C
Cardiac rhythm or conduction disturbance, e.g. prolonged QTc interval (>0.44 s) on ECG
Severe electrolyte abnormalities
Acute dehydration
Weight <75% of predicted ideal body weight
Rapid weight loss in the presence of medical complications
Arrested growth and development in children and adolescents
Medical complications in service users with insulin-dependent diabetes or at-risk pregnancy
Uncontrollable bingeing and purging
Suicide or self-harm risk

The discharge weight range and/or other goals of the admission are made clear to the service user prior to or early in their admission. Inpatient programmes generally consist of either a short-term admission for medical stabilization or a longer admission for weight restoration. Psychological treatment should focus not only on eating behaviour and attitudes to an individual's weight and shape, but also wider issues affecting the person's life with the expectation that the person will achieve weight gain (NICE, 2004). Strict behavioural programmes should not be used in the care and treatment of anorexia nervosa (NICE, 2004). When the service user is medically stable, increasing levels of supervised physiotherapy assist the service user to gain weight as muscle rather than fat as well as promoting bone health.

It is essential for service users, families and staff to have realistic expectations and clear goals for the admission. Service users do not leave hospital 'cured' of their eating disorder but will be medically stable, more weight restored and therefore more cognitively able to engage in ongoing individual psychotherapy or family therapy after discharge. As eating disorders are usually chronic problems, relapse of symptoms and two or more admissions to hospital are not uncommon.

CASE STUDY: LUCY

Lucy, aged 15 years, achieves well at school and wants to be a chef or dietitian. She lives in the inner city with her parents, who are both 'busy' doctors. Her older brother, who is outgoing and popular, is studying to become a lawyer. Lucy's mother says, 'She's always been a good girl but more recently she has distanced herself from us and spends a lot of time alone in her bedroom'.

The family describe themselves as very close and loving despite both parents working long hours. Lucy used to discuss things with her mother 'like a best friend' and describes her father as 'He's okay but he's not around that much'. Lucy started preparing meals for the family 12 months ago, but now refuses to eat with her family. Her weight has dropped from 55 kg to 36 kg in the past year. During the same period she has grown from 160 cm to 162 cm tall.

Lucy was admitted to hospital after the family's efforts to encourage her to eat failed and she fainted on the way to school. Her parents held firm about the admission despite Lucy screaming, 'I'll know you don't love me if you make me stay here!' Lucy required cardiac monitoring in a high-dependency ward before being transferred to the adolescent ward. Her eating-disordered behaviours included severe food restriction and excessive exercise. There was no evidence of vomiting or laxative abuse. She sees herself as fat and believes the hospital bed should be occupied by someone who is sick, not by her.

Lucy was commenced on overnight nasogastric supplemental feeds and encouraged to eat her meals during the day. She gradually progressed to an oral diet, which was supplemented with Ensure Plus when she didn't complete all the food on her plate. Lucy finally reached and maintained her goal weight by eating food prior to discharge. Lucy's mood improved as her weight gain progressed. She actively participated in individual and group therapy sessions on the ward, focusing mainly on self-esteem, coping strategies and the expression of feelings in more healthy ways. Lucy's family engaged well in family therapy and Lucy was able to use these sessions to talk with her parents and brother about how she was feeling. Lucy went home at her discharge goal weight of 52 kg. Her discharge plan included continuing monitoring of her physical and mental health through the hospital's adolescent eating disorders clinic, gradual weight increase according to height/weight requirements for her age and ongoing family therapy sessions. Lucy started menstruating again 4 months after discharge. Lucy is well engaged with the staff and has agreed to seek help early if she experiences any relapse in eating-disordered thoughts or behaviours.

Nutritional rehabilitation

Refeeding is indicated when there is evidence of protein–calorie malnutrition. The cornerstones of nutritional treatment are nutritional education, meal planning, establishment of regular eating patterns and discouragement of dieting (American Dietetic Association, 2006). The service user will be fearful of excessive weight gain in the early stages of eating normally, so the nurse can provide reassurance that the aim is to increase weight slowly. The service user is encouraged to eat a wide variety of foods and 'fear foods' are introduced slowly. An experienced dietitian works with the service user to develop an appropriate meal plan and an intake of 2200–2500 kcal daily will generally achieve a weekly weight gain of 0.5–1 kg in most service users on an inpatient basis and 0.5 kg if the person is an outpatient (NICE, 2004; RCP, 2005). Nutritional support and the regular monitoring of a service user's physical state should be accompanied by supportive therapy and psychological interventions, such as cognitive behavioural therapy (CBT) (NICE, 2004).

Liquid nutritional supplements are given to malnourished service users if they are unable to eat sufficient food to achieve the necessary weight gain. Nasogastric (or enteral) feeding is not usually considered unless the service user is medically compromised and cannot achieve adequate weight gain without assistance and only then for the minimum amout of time possible (RCP, 2005). Nocturnal nasogastric feeding has been shown to be more effective than oral refeeding in weight restoration during hospitalization in girls (Robb et al., 2002) and boys (Silber et al., 2004). Service users' reactions to nasogastric feeds are varied. Some express relief that they do not have to eat what they perceive as the enormous amounts required for weight gain and view positively the fact that the responsibility for weight gain has been taken away from them (Abraham and Llewellyn-Jones, 2001). Others find it very distressing and, for those service users with a history of abuse, it may even reactivate feelings associated with sexual abuse (RCP, 2005). Liquid nutritional supplements are given for the shortest possible time as service users need to relearn how to eat normally.

ETHICAL DILEMMA

Kathy is a 28-year-old woman with a 12-year history of anorexia nervosa who is admitted with severe medical complications resulting from starvation. This is her fifth admission in the past 18 months, during which time she has spent only 4 months in total in the community. All her admissions have aimed at weight gain but the last two were considered successful and she was discharged at a low body mass index because the team felt they should work on improving her quality of life. Weight gain distressed Kathy so much that she had immediately starved herself on discharge. Her mother has given up work to look after her and feels very depressed about Kathy's last two admissions. Kathy is refusing nasogastric tube feeds and has requested that she be allowed to go home to die.

Questions

1 What rights do health professionals have to enforce nasogastric feeding?
2 Is it ethical to enforce treatment when the service user clearly doesn't want to endure any more pain?
3 Is it fair to refuse treatment when the parents want to continue trying for recovery?

The following principles might help guide your discussion.

♦ The Mental Health Act 1983, amended 2007, and the Children Act 1989 provide the legal context for the feeding of a person against their will (NICE, 2004).
♦ The potential risk of the condition: assess the degree to which failure to deliver treatment will result in premature death from the physical or psychological complications of the disorder.
♦ Beneficence: estimate the likely benefit of imposed treatment. Short-term results from refeeding are considered beneficial and can lead to an improved quality of life. In an acute crisis the intervention of refeeding can be life-saving.

♦ Non-maleficence: evaluate the intent to avoid harm. Goldner et al. (1997, p. 453) stress that 'it is important to evaluate the physical risks of all interventions, and the negative psychological effects of imposing treatment against the person's wishes' when considering the enforcement of treatment. It is also important to ask who will carry the burden of care for the person and whether it can be rightfully expected that they will do so. This might be particularly important in cases where service users have endured numerous refeeding episodes and the family has cared for the service user only to watch their loved one go through the agonizing fall back into starvation (from Goldner et al., 1997).

Nursing care

Initially, medical resuscitation and stabilization take priority if life-threatening complications are present. Vital signs such as fourth-hourly heart rate, temperature and blood pressure (until normal readings are sustained for a minimum of 72 h) provide insight into the body's ability to maintain homeostasis. Nurses are responsible for:

• monitoring vital signs and acting appropriately when vital signs indicate medical instability,
• ensuring the service user's physical safety and containment,
• monitoring emotional status, and providing support to contain the anxiety and distress of both service users and their families,
• initiating and encouraging the refeeding process,
• monitoring weight gain by regularly weighing service users,
• administering prescribed medication,
• supervising a programme designed to achieve nutritional rehabilitation, normalized eating behaviours and reduction in compensatory behaviours.

Hospitalization usually produces distress in service users diagnosed with eating disorders who are resistant to treatment and driven by a desire to lose weight. Promoting a milieu of emotional nurturance and containing the anxiety and distress felt by service users diagnosed with eating disorders and their families is a constant challenge for nurses. Supportive individual therapy, group counselling and psychoeducation for service users and their families are therapies commonly used by nursing staff working in specialist eating disorder services to contain anxiety and distress.

Ryan et al. (2006) identified three constructs of inpatient nursing care for service users diagnosed with eating disorders as (1) 'loving' or empathetic support, (2) discipline, surveillance and authoritative containment and (3) constant and ever-present care. Ramjan (2004) studied nurses working in two medical wards and identified three major themes for specific difficulties that nurses need to overcome: struggling for understanding, struggling for control and struggling to develop therapeutic relationships. Similarly, King and Turner (2000) found that nurses experience difficulty developing therapeutic alliances with service users when their core nursing values of trust, privacy, being non-judgemental, maintaining confidentiality and assuring service user's rights and advocacy were challenged by the behaviours of service users diagnosed with eating disorders. All three of these Australian studies reflect the complexity of nursing care for this group and the need for constant awareness of counter-transference issues (see Ch. 23).

The keys to effective nursing care of inpatients diagnosed with anorexia nervosa include:

- identifying and acting to reverse signs and symptoms indicating medical instability,
- understanding that eating-disordered behaviours are driven by fear and anxiety regarding change,
- finding a balance between, on the one hand, setting firm limits and encouraging the necessary nutritional rehabilitation and behavioural programme, while on the other hand simultaneously developing a therapeutic relationship with the service user,
- containing the service user's and their family's anxiety and distress through supportive therapy and psychoeducation,
- facilitating and motivating the service user to change, rather than trying to impose or enforce a particular behavioural change,
- consistently adhering to the plan of care and appropriate limit-setting,
- maintaining clear professional boundaries,
- developing, 'owning' and regularly reviewing a behavioural programme with service users, if appropriate,
- having realistic expectations regarding what can be achieved during a hospital admission given the complexity and chronicity of the problem,
- awareness of counter-transference issues and adequate professional supervision and support,
- enjoying the challenge of caring for individual service users and assisting them to know and care for themselves in more healthy ways through change,
- maintaining a positive regard for service users in the face of resistance to treatment and chronicity of the disorder.

NURSE'S STORY: WORKING WITH ADOLESCENTS WHO HAVE BEEN DIAGNOSED WITH ANOREXIA

When I first started working with adolescents who had anorexia nervosa I was scared that I would say or do the wrong thing. I didn't understand why it was so difficult for them to eat. Boy was I on a steep learning curve! I was used to trying to meet my patient's needs and advocate for them, but I could see that if I went along with what these patients wanted to do, they would lose more weight. But when I first tried to confront them about their behaviour they would lie to me or get angry with me, and I found this really hard to take.

Luckily, I work in a great team and was able to learn 'on the job'. My senior nursing colleagues taught me much about the illness and about how the behaviours I was seeing were not directed at me personally, but reflected the patient's overwhelming fear of change. I discovered that I wasn't responsible for making them gain weight, but that my job was to try and get to know what it was like for them to have their illness. Then I could encourage them to better manage their fears and start taking responsibility for positively changing their own thoughts and behaviours. Now that I understand just how hard it is for these patients to change, I am better able to support them. Along with a sense of confidence in my nursing care came a feeling of job satisfaction. I enjoy my work with these young people and now feel that I am making a positive difference in their lives.

Therapeutic relationship

Effective nursing management incorporates a therapeutic alliance *with* the service user and *against* the disorder. This alliance is enhanced by empathetic comments and behaviours and constant positive regard, reassurance and support for change. Positive regard for the person can be displayed by externalizing the eating-disordered thoughts and behaviours as separate from the intrinsic regard held for the person; for example 'Is "the anorexia" making it really difficult for you to eat today?' and 'I know it's hard for you to eat when "the anorexia" is telling you not to. How can I best help you to fight "the anorexic thoughts"?'

Unless a particular situation is life-threatening, stand-over enforcement tactics and invasion of privacy (e.g. observing service users in the bathroom) are unnecessary and destructive for both the development of therapeutic relationships and the promotion of the service user's self-responsibility and motivation for change. Food avoidance and the use of compensatory behaviours will be reflected to a great extent in the service user's pattern of weight gain and in their blood and urine test results. Generally, if they fail to gain the expected amount of weight each week in hospital, they have either restricted their oral intake or participated in compensatory behaviours. Invading privacy or engaging in confrontation will result in an angry eating-disordered response rather than encouraging positive growth and motivation for change. Taking control of eating and ceasing compensatory behaviours are ultimately the responsibility of the service user. The goal for nurses is not to enforce change but to gradually encourage the service user's motivation for change by exploring and challenging their individual perspective on, and experience of, their eating disorder. Younger children, however, may need a more directive approach than adolescents and adults.

Normalization of eating patterns

Meal times are usually very stressful for service users, and the nurse can help by providing support and encouragement, by acting as a role model for healthy eating behaviour, by encouraging the discussion of non-food-related subjects and by promoting normal socialization at meal times. When service users engage in ritualistic behaviours (see Box 18.4) the nurse notes these behaviours and discusses them in private with the service user after the meal is finished, validating their difficulty with eating, praising positive efforts and offering encouragement to eat normally during the next meal. Adequate after-meal support and praise for effort encourages the continued development of normal eating behaviours.

Service users are encouraged to eat breakfast, lunch, dinner and three snacks each day. Main meals should be eaten within 30 min and snacks within 15–20 min. Nurses generally record the amount of food eaten and document the service user's eating behaviours and any other observations in the progress notes. This information is particularly helpful in planning strategies for ongoing care.

Caring for service users in a specialist eating disorders setting enables the development of a supportive dining room milieu where eating-disordered service users can also encourage each other. Taking the service users to a café for coffee and eating out in public can provide the service user with further exposure to and experience in coping with social eating.

Binge eating and purging behaviours

Service users diagnosed with bulimia nervosa and binge eating disorder may find that eating three normal-sized meals and snacks each day helps reduce the desire for binge eating episodes. Nurses can explore triggers or patterns of events that precede bingeing and compensatory behaviours, and support service users to develop strategies to prevent purging, such as expressing their feelings

and seeking support from others, distraction, relaxation activities, and avoiding going into the bathroom for 1 hour after meals.

Monitoring weight gain

It is common practice to set a minimum healthy target weight range for service users with anorexia nervosa at the beginning of treatment. Ultimately, the return of a normal menstrual cycle reflects a healthy minimum weight for young adult females. However, service users are generally discharged from hospital at lower weights, with the expectation of continuing weight gain until their healthy target is reached, while participating in ongoing supportive outpatient treatment.

Most treatment facilities aim for an average weekly weight gain of 1 kg in inpatient settings and 0.5 kg in outpatient settings, requiring an extra 3500–7000 calories per week (NICE, 2004). The frequency of weighing, or monitoring of expected weight gain, varies between treatment settings, but twice a week is sufficient to monitor and reward progress.

In an outpatient setting any team member can undertake monitoring of weight gain, but in the hospital environment it is generally the responsibility of the nurse. Service users are usually weighed in the morning before food or drink consumption, wearing only a hospital gown. Techniques commonly used by service users to project a false increase in weight include drinking large amounts of water just prior to weighing, or hiding weights on their person. Therefore they are usually asked to void just prior to weighing and a urinalysis is attended to. Low specific gravity (<1.010) suggests water loading and high pH (8–9) suggests purging. A sudden increase in weight or an increase that is not consistent with the service user's current eating behaviour should alert the nurse to discuss with the service user and the treating team possible reasons for weight gain outside that expected. A random (unexpected) weight measurement can be undertaken outside the normal weighing time if the service user is suspected of manipulating their real weight.

Refeeding syndrome

Nurses need to be aware of refeeding syndrome, which is a rare but potentially fatal complication of initial intensive refeeding in severely malnourished service users. Refeeding syndrome refers to an imbalance of electrolytes and fluid shifts that can occur when a severely anorexic service user commences nutritional rehabilitation. On refeeding, there is an exceptionally high demand for phosphate to make adenosine triphosphate (ATP), phospholipids, glycogen and the synthesis of protein to rebuild lean body mass (Rome and Ammerman, 2003). Phosphate levels can drop significantly, especially during the first week of refeeding, giving rise to potential cardiac and respiratory failure. Supplemental phosphate is usually given prophylactically for at least the first 1–2 weeks of refeeding and the dose is adjusted according to serial serum phosphate levels. Vitamin and mineral supplements are also prescribed. Electrolyte abnormalities should be corrected prior to refeeding, then monitored daily until they have stabilized within normal ranges. Service users most at risk of developing refeeding syndrome include those with a very low body mass index, a history of severe dietary restraint, vomiting, laxative misuse or bingeing, and those with concurrent medical conditions such as diabetes, infection or major organ failure (RCP, 2005). During refeeding, nurses monitor for clinical signs of refeeding syndrome, such as delirium, arrhythmias, fluid retention and oedema, and ensure that prophylactic phosphate and vitamin and mineral supplements are ingested. If signs of refeeding syndrome become evident, urgent medical consultation is sought in order to normalize electrolyte levels and prevent cardiovascular and other organ systems failure, seizures and death. The prescribed rate of refeeding, with gradually increasing increments, should minimize the risk of refeeding syndrome.

Psychotherapeutic techniques and treatments

While the complications of anorexia nervosa are well documented, there is limited evidence of the most appropriate treatment (Fairburn, 2005). Discussed below are examples of psychotherapeutic techniques and treatments often used in the care and treatment of service users diagnosed with eating disorders. In clinical practice, a combination of some of these therapies or other psychotherapies not described below, such as psychodynamic psychotherapy, dialectical behaviour therapy and narrative therapy, have been used. Systematic reviews of treatment options for anorexia nervosa (Bulik et al., 2007), bulimia nervosa (Shapiro et al., 2007) and binge eating disorder (Brownley et al., 2007) are available. The cognitive capacity of the service user needs to be taken into account and, as a general rule, the more malnourished the service user is, the more directive the psychotherapy needs to be.

Supportive therapy

Bloch (2006) argues that supportive therapy is a skill that should be utilized by every mental health professional. Components of supportive therapy described by Bloch (2006) include:

- reassurance (by removing doubts and misconceptions and highlighting strengths),
- explanation (clarification of day-to-day practical questions and external reality),
- guidance (direct advice and teaching of coping skills),
- suggestion (aiming to induce change and influence adherence),
- encouragement (in specific contexts to promote self-esteem and endorse behaviours about which the service user is hesitant or anxious),
- effecting changes in the service user's environment (to remove or alter detrimental social elements and, conversely, to maximize potentially beneficial ones),
- permission for catharsis (sharing with the therapist pent-up feelings such as fear, grief, sorrow, concern, frustration and envy).

A supportive psychotherapy specifically for use with adults who have a diagnosis of anorexia nervosa has been described by McIntosh et al. (2006). This therapy aims to maintain a therapeutic relationship that facilitates the return to normal eating and to enable other life issues that have an impact on the eating disorder to be addressed.

Goal setting

Working with service users to set achievable goals aims at a collaborative approach to increase the service user's awareness, enhance change and provide a positive experience of achievement (outside that of weight loss) when the goal is reached. Goals need to be achievable. For example, it may be possible for a service user diagnosed with bulimia to reduce bingeing in the short term and later aim for cessation of bingeing. Specific goals are best, specifying how much and how often. For example, a service user diagnosed with anorexia might initially aim to eat one new 'fear food' a day. Service users can enlist their family's help in achieving goals, and when each goal is achieved, the service user is encouraged to aim for a higher goal. For example, a service user might aim to go out for coffee once a week with her family and friends, and when this is achieved she may increase the goal to twice a week or progress to having a meal at a restaurant.

Keeping a journal can help service users to identify obstacles that prevent the achievement of their goals, as well as encouraging the identification and expression of feelings. When goals are not met, the service user is encouraged to explore the barriers to achieving the goal and evaluate what lessons may still have been learned, or gains achieved, by aiming for the goal. For example, a service user who could not reduce their bingeing may have increased their understanding of the reasons for the binge and gained valuable insight into what maintains the behaviour. This insight can then be used to develop a new approach to binge reduction.

Socratic questioning

One of the most common techniques for encouraging motivation is the use of Socratic questioning, which is basically teaching by questioning rather than telling. This technique helps the service user to recognize problems, clarify meanings, feelings and consequences, and promotes new insights and beliefs, which can lead to change. The basis of Socratic questioning is to highlight the adaptive function that the person's belief plays in their life and to help them explore that belief in light of other evidence. For example, if the person believes they will be happier if their weight is lower, one could ask them if their happiness is increasing as they lose weight. The aim is to break the cycle of negative thinking and behaviours.

Cognitive behavioural therapy

In the treatment of eating disorders, cognitive behavioural therapy (CBT) is tailored to focus on cognitively restructuring the dysfunctional thoughts and behaviours that maintain eating-disordered pathology. Under this model, eating disorders are viewed as being maintained by the overvalued idea that self-worth is contingent on appearance, and weight and shape are seen as the primary or exclusive construct in self-esteem (Surgenor and Thornton, 2000). Generally the treatment is delivered in three stages, the first stage being the most intense, with six sessions over 3 weeks. The first phase involves self-monitoring, weighing, prescribing regular patterns of eating and developing self-control strategies. Phase two focuses on eliminating dieting, problem-solving and modifying thoughts that link body and weight with self-esteem. The final phase focuses on relapse prevention and developing skills to manage stressors (Surgenor and Thornton, 2000).

CBT is now the leading evidence-based treatment for adults diagnosed with bulimia nervosa (Agras et al., 2000; Cooper, 2005). It has also been developmentally adapted for adolescents with binge eating disorder (Fairburn et al., 1993; Schapman-Williams et al., 2006) and bulimia nervosa (Fairburn et al., 1993; Lock, 2005). The course of treatment for CBT for bulimia nervosa should be for 16–20 sessions over 4–5 months (NICE, 2004).

Interpersonal therapy

Interpersonal therapy is a brief, time-limited psychotherapy that encourages service users to make changes in their relationships, thereby improving self-esteem and problem-solving skills. Interpersonal therapy has been defined as a:

> ... time limited (up to 20 sessions) non-interpretive, individual psychotherapy with a focus on linking current interpersonal functioning to eating problems, although the eating disorder symptoms per se are explicitly never directly the focus of sessions.

(Surgenor and Thornton, 2000, p. 108)

Interpersonal therapy focuses on how relationships are initiated and maintained and addresses issues of social isolation, role transitions and interpersonal role disputes. To date, research into the effectiveness of interpersonal therapy is inconclusive for service users diagnosed with anorexia but shows some promise for service users diagnosed with bulimia nervosa (Surgenor and Thornton, 2000).

Motivational enhancement therapy

Motivational enhancement therapy targets denial, ambivalence and resistance to change and can be helpful, particularly in chronic eating disorders. Motivational enhancement therapy recognizes that the service user's perception of their health problems and their motivation to change must be considered during treatment as change is a wilful choice and cannot be imposed in a lasting way. Prochaska and Di Clemente (1992) proposed a stages-of-change model that incorporates pre-contemplation (not perceiving a problem), contemplation (reviewing the possibility of change), preparation (preparing for change), action (change), maintenance and relapse. George et al. (2004) argue that psychological treatment needs to match the service user's stage of change if it is to be successful.

Motivational interviewing is basically an adaptation of the Socratic style and proceeds from the assumption that change is produced collaboratively and cannot be imposed from outside (Bemis-Vitousek, 2000). The skill in motivational interviewing is to raise doubts for the service user about their beliefs regarding the goal of thinness and to help them to 'make discoveries on their own and say it in their own words' (Bemis-Vitousek, 2000, p. 99). Interventions initially seek to ascertain the service user's current level of motivation, engage them in treatment at that level, and work towards increasing stages of motivation.

Psychoeducation

Psychoeducation is a technique that all nurses use, often without thinking to call it such. It involves providing information about the eating disorder that enables the service user to better understand their health problems and its effects, and to develop more effective coping strategies to overcome difficulties they are experiencing. The service user is considered responsible for change and change is believed to be more likely if they have information about the mechanisms that cause and maintain their disorder. Rome and Ammerman (2003) suggest that improved compliance with nutritional rehabilitation may be achieved when service users are provided with explanations of why and how their physical symptoms occur. Some examples of psychoeducation provided by nurses include providing information about:

- the biological factors that regulate weight: this can include discussion of how dieting largely works against the body's weight regulators, causing stress to both physical and psychological functioning,

- the psychological and physical effects of starvation: education on the effects of starvation also provides some hope for service users that their intrusive thoughts about food will resolve and that any physical discomfort associated with eating will reduce, as the stomach returns to normal size and emptying is no longer delayed,
- techniques for coping with stress and anxiety (e.g. relaxation techniques),
- the physical side effects of vomiting, laxative and diuretic abuse,
- the binge/purge cycle and how it affects self-esteem: nurses can help service users to reduce and even eliminate vomiting through supportive counselling before or after meals and by using distracting tactics or teaching relaxation techniques to manage the urge to vomit immediately after meals. Equally, bingeing can be dealt with in similar ways, with emphasis on identifying and managing the cues to bingeing. Service users can also be informed of the benefits of eating regularly, thereby reducing the physical and psychological drive to binge,
- how exercise can be beneficial to a healthy lifestyle if taken appropriately, and the importance of establishing a healthy pattern of exercise based on muscle strengthening and stress relief rather than fat burning,
- healthy weight ranges: this is important to assist the service user to aim for a normal weight. It also challenges the service user's beliefs about what is healthy for them personally, as they can firmly believe that they are immune from normal nutritional and weight guidelines and are healthy at a much lower weight than others,
- the short- and long-term medical consequences of eating disorders,
- relapse prevention.

Psychoeducation can also be extremely useful for parents, family members and friends to increase their understanding of, and facilitate strategies to cope with, the disorder. The more information families have, the less they will blame themselves and the more open they will be to positive changes that can improve outcomes.

Family therapy and support

Family therapy has shown promise as an effective treatment for younger service users with anorexia nervosa (Lock et al., 2006a,b; Robin et al., 1999) and may produce better results than individual therapy in children (Rosen, 2003). A family-based approach is essential in the management of this younger population and families need to be involved and engaged as an important resource by the treating team. There is often a tendency

for carers to inadvertently reinforce the behaviours of anorexia nervosa, particularly as the distress about eating is so intense that they can give in to the anorexic behaviours (Treasure et al., 2003). If families of children and adolescents are not engaged with and committed to the treatment programme, or are unable to work together to provide clear, firm boundaries regarding food and anorexic behaviours, relapse can almost be predicted. To facilitate change, families need to develop effective coping strategies for dealing with the anorexic behaviours as well as changing their interactional patterns to accommodate for the young person's growth and development.

Understanding the complexity of the mental health problem and having realistic expectations of its chronicity can often assist families in containing their anxiety. Although confidentiality about specific details of the treatment plan may be necessary for the service user's benefit, it is important that the nurse supports the family and provides education to help them understand the factors that drive and maintain eating disorders as well as the current treatment plan. It can be helpful to focus on developing coping strategies for stressful situations such as meal times and eating out, or for dealing with eating-disordered behaviours such as bingeing and vomiting. Education and support also aim to help readjust family interactional patterns that may support the maintenance of the disorder. Finally, it is important to involve the family in discharge planning, particularly if the service user will be living with them or relying on them for emotional and practical support.

Self-help programmes

Service users diagnosed with bulimia nervosa and binge eating disorder may benefit from an evidence-based guided self-help programme as a first or additional treatment (Carter and Fairburn, 1998; NICE, 2004). An excellent self-help guide on eating disorders has been developed by Northumberland, Tyne and Wear NHS Foundation Trust (http://www.ntw.nhs.uk/pic/selfhelp#).

Pharmacotherapy

Pharmacotherapy is not used as a first-line treatment for service users diagnosed with anorexia nervosa but has been shown to be helpful when used in combination with CBT for service users diagnosed with bulimia nervosa (NICE, 2004; Zhu and Walsh, 2002). Antidepressants, specifically fluoxetine which is a selective serotonin-reuptake inhibitor (SSRI), can be beneficial for reducing bingeing and purging in the treatment of bulimia nervosa and for reducing binges in binge eating disorder. The effective dose of fluoxetine for people diagnosed with bulimia nervosa is higher than for depression (60 mg per day) (NICE, 2004). The long-term effects of SSRIs for people diagnosed with binge eating disorders are unknown (NICE, 2004). However, the role of antidepressants is best assessed after nutritional rehabilitation in low-weight service users diagnosed with anorexia nervosa, as food can be the best 'medicine' in improving mood.

The atypical antipsychotic olanzapine has been used judiciously to treat the symptoms of anxiety, body image distortions and severe obsessions, and has shown promising results in diminishing thought intrusion and distorted body image (Brambilla et al., 2007; Mondraty et al., 2005). Its use is also associated with weight gain.

Monoamine oxidase inhibitors and tricyclic antidepressants are rarely used for treatment of eating disorders because of their side effects.

A mental state examination will determine whether pharmacotherapy is warranted to treat specific comorbid symptoms of depression, anxiety or OCD in both underweight and weight-restored service users.

CASE STUDY: MARY

Mary is a 32-year-old single unemployed white female with a 12-year-old son. Mary and her son live with her parents in a small rural community. Mary's only source of income is a government sickness benefit.

At the age of 14, Mary was diagnosed with anorexia nervosa. She experienced some resolution of her eating disorder between the ages of 18 and 24, and during this time gave birth to her son. Mary moved in with her parents when the child was 2 years old. She has been admitted to hospital 19 times in the past 14 years for problems including severe electrolyte imbalance, dehydration, suicidal depression, a drug overdose and anorexia nervosa.

WEIGHT/HEIGHT

Mary is 160 cm tall. Her lowest weight has been 24 kg and highest 55 kg. Currently she weighs 30 kg but does not wish to weigh more than 38 kg.

MARY'S SON

Her son is 12 years old and in year 7 at school. He is a sensitive child, and is Mary's reason to keep going. They have little close time together as his grandfather has taken over much of the parenting role. Mary asks her son to lie to her parents about the amount of food she is eating. Mary met the child's father through friends, but the relationship was violent and broke up after a year while Mary was pregnant. They no longer have any contact.

MARY'S BEST FRIEND

Mary's only good friend is a busy single mother with four children who lives in a regional town about 3 h drive from Mary. The distance makes it difficult for Mary to see her very often.

MARY'S MOTHER

The main person in Mary's life is her mother and Mary has always felt she could not cope without her approval. She is a very dominating and controlling person, especially about Mary's eating behaviour, and does not listen to Mary. She works as the receptionist at Mary's general practitioner's surgery. This means she has access to Mary's file, which raises considerable privacy and confidentiality issues.

MARY'S FATHER

Mary has occasional arguments with her father, who she finds impersonal and not prepared to listen to her. He is the father figure for the child, but has a tendency to 'take over', insisting on picking the child up from school is an example.

MARY'S SIBLING

Mary has a sister who is 3 years younger than her and is married with one child. Mary believes her sister was the favourite child, as she was a straight-A student at school. She has been losing weight recently and Mary believes that she has an eating disorder. They are only just on speaking terms but Mary has not seen her lately because of conflict between her sister and her parents.

CURRENT SITUATION

Mary is having psychotic delusions that restrict her ability to shop for food. Mary believes that if she goes into the supermarket calories will leap from the fruit and vegetables onto her body. Mary is becoming obsessive about her son's weight. Currently she is unable to manage the video conferencing counselling sessions through the district health service because she cannot concentrate for long periods. Her weight has dropped to 28 kg and she has not been able to manage any other involvement with her community mental health nurse because of fatigue. At present there is no form of communication between the psychiatrist and the community mental health nurse. She reports that she now uses between 40 and 80 laxatives daily. She is vomiting once or twice a day, can no longer work for long periods and has to rely on public transport. Mary recognizes that she is unable to manage activities that she had been able to complete 6 months ago, due to fatigue. Mary is preparing for her death. She refuses to spend any money on herself as she wishes to leave her son some money. She was admitted to the local hospital a week ago and is due to be discharged today at a weight of 30 kg.

In the case study, Mary's community mental health nurse is on extended leave and you are acting as her interim community mental health nurse.

What care plans would you, as her community mental health nurse, develop with this young woman in your community setting?

Consider the role of the team and yourself as a community mental health nurse in relation to the following areas:

- goal setting,
- addressing eating-disordered thoughts and behaviours,
- medical monitoring,
- nutritional monitoring and rehabilitation,
- family support,
- monitoring of mental state.

OUTCOME

Mortality rates in anorexia nervosa are among the highest of the mental disorders (APA, 2006; Birmingham et al., 2005; Hoek, 2006). Crude mortality rates are generally reported as 5–10%, with suicide and electrolyte imbalances leading to cardiac arrest being the most common causes of death.

The general consensus is that 50% of service users with a diagnosis of anorexia nervosa have good outcomes, 30% have intermediate outcomes and 20% have poor outcomes. Recovery rates among adolescents have been reported as slightly better, with approximately 50–70% recovering, 20% improved and 10–20% developing chronic anorexia nervosa (Steinhausen, 2002). However, Halvorsen et al. (2004) reported that 41% of service users in their adolescent study who no longer had an eating disorder did, however, have an Axis I diagnosis, most commonly depression or anxiety disorders. Factors associated with worse outcomes include other psychological symptoms such as depression, mood and anxiety disorders, social functioning, longer duration of disorder and substance abuse (Berkman et al., 2007).

Considerable variability occurs in the course of bulimia nervosa but persistence of symptoms has been shown, with approximately 30% of service users continuing to engage in recurrent binge eating and purging behaviours at long-term follow-up (Keel et al., 1999). Remission and relapse of symptoms is common and one recent study concluded that the probability of remission at 60 months was 74% for bulimia nervosa and 83% for unspecified eating disorders, and the probability for relapse among those with remission was 47% for bulimia nervosa and 42% for unspecified eating disorders (Grilo et al., 2007). Factors clearly associated with worse outcomes include depression, substance use and poor impulse control (Berkman et al., 2007). More research is needed to better understand the course of service users with unspecified eating disorders and binge eating disorder.

The following is an extract from a letter written by a recovering, now young adult, service user:

It's now been 6 years since I was first diagnosed with anorexia nervosa. I know I still have many years ahead to learn about life and to learn from my mistakes and experiences, but this recovery process has taught me so much about confronting myself, challenging myself and training my mind to think positively and it does work. Thank you for firmly confronting my disorder when I couldn't and for hanging in with me, keeping me alive and supporting me long enough for me to finally get to the point where I feel strong enough as a person to not need or want this illness any more.

CONCLUSION

This chapter has provided an introduction to the major eating disorders encountered in nursing practice and has included a focus on the medical complications, assessment and treatment of eating disorders. The eating disorders are multidimensional, encompassing a range of psychological and physical health issues. Although they are chronic disorders with a relatively low incidence, the severity of their impact in terms of mortality and morbidity is high. Many sufferers encounter difficulties in accessing appropriate services and this difficulty, coupled with the shame, denial and ambivalence to treatment commonly associated with these disorders, results in delayed treatment for many. This is of particular concern because of the known effectiveness of early treatment in preventing or reducing progression to severe and chronic disorder.

What of the future? In modern Western societies there seems to be an ever-increasing concern with body image, weight, shape and appearance for both women and men. For some this leads to severe disruption and diagnosis with one of a growing list of disorders including the eating disorders. A greater emphasis on primary prevention strategies, particularly targeting the self-esteem, body image and resilience of the very young, both males and females, may prove helpful.

A multidisciplinary approach to treatment of eating disorders is crucial and nurses committed to caring for service users have much to contribute in both inpatient and community treatment settings. Service users are admitted to hospital when they require 24-hour nursing care. In order that optimal care is provided, it is essential that nurses receive adequate education and supervision when managing these very complex service users.

More evidence-based research is needed to better understand the relative importance of biological and psychosocial risk and protective factors, and to continue developing more effective treatment therapies to facilitate better outcomes. One needs only to look at the outcome data of current treatments to see that more research is needed to enhance outcomes. Nurses are in a key position to undertake research designed to better understand eating disorders and promote evidence-based effective nursing strategies that enhance care and outcomes.

EXERCISES FOR CLASS ENGAGEMENT

In a group, discuss the influence of the media, marketing and advertising industry on the development of eating disorders among young women and men.

Discuss the reasons that body image dissatisfaction tends to increase during adolescence.

ACKNOWLEDGEMENT

Elaine Painter and Fran Sanders are acknowledged for their contribution to this chapter.

REFERENCES

Abraham, S., Llewellyn-Jones, D., 2001. Eating Disorders: The Facts. Oxford Medical Publications, Sydney.

Agras, W., Walsh, T., Fairburn, C.G., et al., 2000. A multicentre comparison of cognitive behavioural therapy and interpersonal psychotherapy for bulimia nervosa. Arch. Gen. Psychiatry 57 (5), 459–466.

American Dietetic Association, 2006. Position of the American Dietetic Association: nutritional intervention in the treatment of anorexia nervosa, bulimia nervosa and other eating disorders. J. Am. Diet. Assoc. 106 (12), 2073–2082.

Anderson, G., 1996. Nursing care of the adolescent with special needs: anorexia nervosa. In: Adams, A., McQuellin, C., Nagy, S. (Eds.), Nursing the Infant, Child and Adolescent, Interactions and Care. McLennan & Petty, Sydney.

APA (American Psychiatric Association), 2000. Diagnostic and Statistical Manual of Mental Disorders, fourth ed., text rev. American Psychiatric Association, Washington DC.

APA (American Psychiatric Association), 2006. Practice Guideline for the Treatment of Patients with Eating Disorders, third ed. American Psychiatric Association, Washington DC.

Bemis-Vitousek, K., 2000. Developing motivation for change in individuals with eating disorders. In: Gaskill, D.,

Sanders, F. (Eds.), The Encultured Body: Policy Implications for Healthy Body Image and Disordered Eating Behaviours. QUT, Kelvin Grove, Queensland, pp. 95–105.

Berkman, N.D., Lohr, K.N., Bulik, C.M., 2007. Outcomes of eating disorders: a systematic review of the literature. Int. J. Eat. Disord. 40 (4), 293–309.

Beumont, P., 2000. Anorexia nervosa as a mental and physical illness: the medical perspective. In: Gaskill, D., Sanders, F. (Eds.), The Encultured Body: Policy Implications for Healthy Body Image and Disordered Eating Behaviours. QUT, Kelvin Grove, Queensland, pp. 80–94.

Birmingham, C.L., Su, J., Hlynsky, J.A., et al., 2005. The mortality rate from anorexia nervosa. Int. J. Eat. Disord. 38 (2), 143–146.

Bloch, S., 2006. Supportive psychotherapy. In: Bloch, S. (Ed.), An Introduction to the Psychotherapies, fourth ed. Oxford University Press, Oxford, pp. 215–235.

Brambilla, F., Garcia, C.S., Fassino, S., et al., 2007. Olanzapine therapy effects in anorexia nervosa: psychobiological effects. Int. Clin. Pharmacol. 22 (4), 197–204.

Brownley, K.A., Berkman, N.D., Sedway, J.A., et al., 2007. Binge eating disorder treatment: a systematic review of randomised controlled trials. Int. J. Eat. Disord. 40 (4), 337–348.

Bulik, C.M., Berkman, N.D., Brownley, K.A., et al., 2007. Anorexia nervosa treatment: a systematic review of randomised controlled trials. Int. J. Eat. Disord. 40 (4), 310–320.

Carter, J., Fairburn, C., 1998. Cognitive—behavioral self-help for binge eating disorder: a controlled effectiveness study. J. Consult. Clin. Psychol. 66, 616–623.

Cartwright, M.M., 2004. Eating disorder emergencies: understanding the medical complexities of the hospitalized eating disordered patient. Crit. Care Nurs. Clin. North Am. 16 (4), 515–530.

Clarke-Stone, S., Joyce, H., 2003. Understanding eating disorders. Nurs. Times 99 (44), 20–23.

Cooper, M., 2005. Cognitive theory in anorexia nervosa and bulimia nervosa: progress, development and future directions. Clin. Psychol. Rev. 25, 511–531.

Couturier, J.L., Lock, J., 2006. Denial and minimization in adolescents with anorexia nervosa. Int. J. Eat. Disord. 39 (3), 212–216.

Crowther, J., Sherwood, N., 1997. Assessment. In: Garner, D., Garfinkel, P. (Eds.), Handbook of Treatment for Eating Disorders, second ed. Guilford Press, New York, pp. 34–49.

Fairburn, C., 2005. Evidence-based treatment of anorexia nervosa. Int. J. Eat. Disord. 37 (Suppl.), S26–S30.

Fairburn, C., Harrison, P.J., 2003. Eating disorders. Lancet 361 (9355), 407–416.

Fairburn, C., Marcus, M.D., Wilson, G.T., 1993. Cognitive behavioural therapy for binge eating and bulimia nervosa: a comprehensive treatment manual. In: Fairburn, C.G., Wilson, G.T. (Eds.), Binge Eating: Nature, Assessment and Treatment. Guilford Press, New York, pp. 361–404.

Favaro, A., Tenconi, E., Santonastaso, P., 2006. Perinatal factors and the risk of developing anorexia nervosa and bulimia nervosa. Arch. Gen. Psychiatry 63 (1), 82–88.

Freeman, C., 2002. What Causes Anorexia Nervosa? Overcoming Anorexia Nervosa. University Press, New York.

George, L., Thornton, C., Touyz, S., et al., 2004. Motivational enhancement and schema-focused cognitive behavioural therapy in the treatment of chronic eating disorders. Clin. Psychol. 8 (2), 81–85.

Godart, N., Berthoz, S., Rein, Z., et al., 2006. Does the frequency of anxiety and depressive disorders differ between diagnostic subtypes of anorexia nervosa and bulimia? Int. J. Eat. Disord. 39 (8), 772–778.

Goldner, E.M., Birmingham, C.L., Smye, V., 1997. Addressing treatment refusal in anorexia nervosa: clinical, ethical and legal considerations. In: Garner, D., Garfinkel, P. (Eds.), Handbook of Treatment for Eating Disorders, second ed. Guilford Press, New York, pp. 450–461.

Grant, J.E., Won Kim, S., Eckert, E.D., 2002. Body dysmorphic disorder in patients with anorexia nervosa: prevalence, clinical features and delusionality of body image. Int. J. Eat. Disord. 32 (3), 291–300.

Grieve, F.G., 2007. A conceptual model of factors contributing to the development of muscle dysmorphia. Eat. Disord. 15 (1), 63–80.

Grilo, C.M., Pagano, M.E., Skodol, A.E., et al., 2007. Natural course of bulimia nervosa and of eating disorder not otherwise specified: 5-year prospective study of remissions, relapses, and the effects of personality disorder psychopathology (CME). J. Clin. Psychiatry 68 (5), 738–746.

Grinspoon, S., Thomas, E., Pitts, S., et al., 2000. Prevalence and predictive factors for regional osteopenia in women with anorexia nervosa. Ann. Intern. Med. 133 (10), 790–794.

Halvorsen, I., Andersen, A., Heyerdahl, S., 2004. Good outcome of adolescent onset anorexia nervosa after systematic treatment: intermediate to long-term follow up of a representative country sample. Eur. Child Adolesc. Psychiatry 13 (5), 295–306.

Hamilton, J., 2007. Eating disorders in preadolescent children. Nurse Pract. 32 (3), 44–48.

Hay, P., 1998. The epidemiology of eating disorder behaviours: an Australian community-based survey. Int. J. Eat. Disord. 23 (4), 371–382.

Herzog, D.B., Franko, D.L., Dorer, D.J., et al., 2006. Drug abuse in women with eating disorders. Int. J. Eat. Disord. 39 (5), 364–368.

Hoek, H.W., 2006. Incidence, prevalence and mortality of anorexia nervosa and other eating disorders. Clin. Opin. Psychiatry 19 (4), 389–394.

Keel, P.K., Mitchell, J.E., Miller, K.B., et al., 1999. Long-term outcome of bulimia nervosa. Arch. Gen. Psychiatry 56 (1), 63–69.

King, S., Turner, de S., 2000. Caring for adolescent females with anorexia nervosa: registered nurses' perspective. J. Adv. Nurs. 32 (1), 139–147.

Lilenfeld, L.R., Stein, D., Bulik, C.M., et al., 2000. Personality traits among currently eating disordered, recovered and never ill first degree relatives of bulimic and control women. Psychol. Med. 30 (6), 1399–1410.

Lock, J., 2005. Adjusting cognitive behaviour therapy for adolescents with bulimia nervosa: results of case series. Am. J. Psychother. 59 (3), 267–281.

Lock, J., Couturier, J., Agras, W., et al., 2006a. Comparison of long-term outcomes in adolescents with anorexia nervosa treated with family therapy. J. Am. Acad. Child Adolesc. Psychiatry 45 (6), 666–672.

Lock, J., le Grange, D., Forsberg, S., et al., 2006b. Is family therapy useful for treating children with anorexia nervosa? Results of a case series. J. Am. Acad. Child Adolesc. Psychiatry 45 (11), 1323–1328.

Machado, P.P., Machado, B.C., Goncalves, S., et al., 2007. The prevalence of eating disorders not otherwise specified. Int. J. Eat. Disord. 40 (3), 212–217.

Malson, H., Finn, D.M., Treasure, J., et al., 2004. Constructing 'the eating disordered patient': a discourse analysis of accounts of treatment experiences. J. Commun. Appl. Soc. Psychol. 14 (6), 473–489.

May, A.L., Kim, J., McHale, S.M., et al., 2006. Parent–adolescent relationships and the development of weight concerns from early to late adolescence. Int. J. Eat. Disord. 39 (8), 729–740.

McIntosh, V., Bulik, C., McKenzie, J., et al., 2000. Interpersonal psychotherapy for anorexia nervosa. Int. J. Eat. Disord. 27 (2), 125–139.

McIntosh, V.V., Jordan, J., Luty, S.E., et al., 2006. Specialist supportive clinical management for anorexia nervosa. Int. J. Eat. Disord. 39 (8), 625–632.

McMaster, R., Beale, B., Hillege, S., et al., 2004. The parent experience of eating disorders: interactions with professionals. Int. J. Ment. Health Nurs. 13 (1), 67–73.

Miller, K.K., Grinspoon, S.K., Ciampa, J., et al., 2005. Medical findings in outpatients with anorexia nervosa. Arch. Intern. Med. 165 (5), 561–566.

Mondraty, N., Birmingham, C.L., Touyz, S., et al., 2005. Randomised controlled trial of olanzapine in the treatment of cognitions in anorexia nervosa. Australas. Psychiatry 13 (1), 72–75.

Muise, A.M., Stein, D.G., Arbess, G., 2003. Eating disorders in adolescent boys: a review of the adolescent and young adult literature. J. Adolesc. Health 33 (6), 427–435.

NICE (National Institute for Health and Clinical Excellence), 2004. Eating Disorders: Core Interventions in the Treatment and Management of Anorexia Nervosa, Bulimia Nervosa and Related Eating Disorders. <http://guidance.nice.org.uk/CG9>.

O'Dea, J.A., Abraham, S., 2002. Eating and exercise disorders in young college men. J. Am. Coll. Health 50 (6), 273–278.

Patton, G., Selzer, R., Coffey, C., et al., 1999. Onset of adolescent eating disorders: a population-based cohort study over three years. Br. Med. J. 318 (7186), 765–768.

Paxton, S., 2000. Individual risk factors and socio-cultural contexts for disordered eating. In: Gaskill, D., Sanders, F. (Eds.), The Encultured Body: Policy Implications for Healthy Body Image and Disordered Eating Behaviours QUT, Kelvin Grove, Queensland, pp. 24–33.

Paxton, S., Schutz, H., Wertheim, E., et al., 1999. Friendship clique and peer influences on body image attitudes, dietary restraint, extreme weight loss behaviours and binge eating in adolescent girls. J. Abnorm. Psychol. 108 (2), 255–266.

Piran, N., Gadalla, T., 2007. Eating disorders and substance abuse in Canadian women: a national study. Addiction 102 (1), 105–113.

Pope, H., Phillips, K., Olivardia, R., 2000. The Adonis Complex. How to Identify, Treat, and Prevent Body Obsession in Men and Boys. Touchstone, Simon & Schuster, New York.

Prochaska, J.O., Di Clemente, C.C., 1992. The transtheorectical model of change. In: Norcross, J.C., Goldfried, M.R. (Eds.), Handbook of Psychotherapy. Integration Basic Books, New York, pp. 300–334.

Ramjan, L.M., 2004. Nurses and the 'therapeutic relationship': caring for adolescents with anorexia nervosa. J. Adv. Nurs. 45 (5), 495–503.

RCP (Royal College of Psychiatrists), 2005. Guidelines for Nutritional Management of Anorexia Nervosa. Council Report CR130.

Reas, D.L., Grilo, C.M., 2007. Timing and sequence of the onset of overweight, dieting and binge eating in overweight patients with binge eating disorder. Int. J. Eat. Disord. 40 (2), 165–170.

Robb, A.S., Silber, T.J., Orrell-Valente, J.K., et al., 2002. Supplemental nocturnal nasogastric re-feeding for better short-term outcome in hospitalised adolescent girls with anorexia nervosa. Am. J. Psychiatry 159 (8), 1347–1353.

Robin, A., Siegel, P., Moye, A., et al., 1999. A controlled comparison of family therapy versus individual therapy for adolescents with anorexia nervosa. J. Am. Acad. Child Adolesc. Psychiatry 38 (12), 1482–1489.

Rome, E.S., Ammerman, S., 2003. Medical complications of eating disorders: an update. J. Adolesc. Health 33 (6), 418–426.

Rosen, D.S., 2003. Eating disorders in children and young adolescents: etiology, classification, clinical features and treatment. Adolesc. Med. State Art Rev. 14 (1), 49–59.

Royal Australian and New Zealand College of Psychiatrists, 2004. Australian and New Zealand clinical practice guidelines for the treatment of anorexia nervosa. Aust. N. Z. J. Psychiatry 38 (9), 659–670.

Russell, G., 1979. Bulimia nervosa: an ominous variant of anorexia nervosa. Psychol. Med. 9 (3), 429–448.

Russell, G., 1995. Anorexia nervosa through time. In: Szmukler, G., Dare, C., Treasure, J. (Eds.), Handbook of Eating Disorders: Theory, Treatment and Research. Wiley, Chichester, pp. 5–17.

Ryan, V., Malson, H., Clarke, S., et al., 2006. Discursive constructions of 'eating disorders nursing': an analysis of nurses' accounts of nursing eating disorder patients. Eur. Eat. Disord. Rev. 14 (2), 125–135.

Schapman-Williams, A.M., Lock, J., Couturier, J., 2006. Cognitive-behavioural therapy for adolescents with binge eating syndromes: a case series. Int. J. Eat. Disord. 39 (3), 252–255.

Shapiro, J.R., Berkman, N.D., Brownley, K.A., et al., 2007. Bulimia nervosa treatment: a systematic review of randomised controlled trials. Int. J. Eat. Disord. 40 (4), 321–336.

Sigman, G.S., 2003. Eating disorders in children and adolescents. Pediatr. Clin. North Am. 50 (5), 1139–1177.

Silber, T.J., Robb, A.S., Orrell-Valente, J.K., et al., 2004. J. Dev. Behav. Pediatr. 25 (6), 415–418.

Steinhausen, H.-C., 2002. The outcome of anorexia nervosa in the 20th century. Am. J. Psychiatry 159 (8), 1284–1293.

Stormer, S., Thompson, J., 1996. Explanations of body image disturbance: a test of maturational status, negative verbal commentary, social comparison, and sociocultural hypotheses. Int. J. Eat. Disord. 19 (2), 193–202.

Strober, M., Freeman, R., Lampert, C., et al., 2000. Controlled family study of anorexia nervosa and bulimia nervosa: evidence of shared liability and transmission of partial syndromes. Am. J. Psychiatry 157 (3), 393–401.

Surgenor, L., Thornton, C., 2000. Eating disorders and disturbed body image: a view from psychology. In: Gaskill, D., Sanders, F. (Eds.), The Encultured Body: Policy Implications for Healthy Body Image and Disordered Eating Behaviours. QUT, Kelvin Grove, Queensland, pp. 106–118.

Tozzi, F., Thornton, L.M., Klump, K.L., et al., 2005. Symptom fluctuation in eating disorders: correlates of diagnostic crossover. Am. J. Psychiatry 162 (4), 732–740.

Treasure, J., Gavan, K., Todd, G., et al., 2003. Changing the environment in eating disorders: working with carers/families to improve motivation and facilitate change. Eur. Eat. Disord. Rev. 11 (1), 25–37.

Van Son, G., Van Hoeken, D., Bartelds, A., et al., 2006. Urbanisation and the incidence of eating disorders. Br. J. Psychiatry 189 (6), 562–563.

World Health Organisation (WHO), 1992. The ICD-10 Classification of Mental and Behavioural Disorders. Available at: <http://www.who.int/classifications/icd/en/bluebook.pdf>.

Westen, D., Harnden-Fischer, J., 2001. Personality profiles in eating disorders: rethinking the distinction between Axis 1 and Axis 11. Am. J. Psychiatry 158 (4), 547–562.

Zerbe, K.J., 1993. Whose body is it anyway? Understanding psychosomatic aspects of eating disorders. Bull. Menninger Clin. 57 (2), 161–177.

Zhu, A., Walsh, T., 2002. Pharmacological treatment of eating disorders. Can. J. Psychiatry 47 (3), 227–234.

Chapter | **19** |

Substance-related disorders and dual diagnosis

Janette Curtis

CHAPTER POINTS

- It is estimated that 24% of the UK population consume alcohol or other drugs at levels that are hazardous or harmful (NICE, 2010a).
- Alcohol consumption is the third-highest risk factor for disease burden in developed countries.
- Alcohol-related harm is estimated to cost £20 billion and the problem appears to be escalating (Prime Minister's Strategy Unit, 2004).
- There are over 30 000 hospital admissions in the UK for alcohol-dependence syndrome (Prime Minister's Strategy Unit, 2004).
- Around half of all violent crime is associated with alcohol misuse, and at peak times around 70% of all admissions to casualty departments are alcohol-related (Prime Minister's Strategy Unit, 2004).
- Alcohol is also associated with liver disease, pancreatitis, some cancers, diabetes, epilepsy, motor vehicle accidents and a range of injuries and social problems such as neglect and abuse. Alcohol misuse accounts for 22 000 premature deaths every year.

DOI: http://dx.doi.org/10.1016/B978-0-7020-4493-9.00019-6

- There is a considerable degree of coexistence between substance use disorder (particularly alcohol) and other mental health disorders.
- Psychoactive drugs can cause harm through intoxication or dependence. They are classified as depressants, stimulants or hallucinogens.
- Specific assessment tools and criteria are used for a service user who presents with a substance misuse or who has a dual diagnosis.
- Interventions include harm reduction, management of the intoxicated service user, withdrawal, and early and brief interventions.
- Accurate assessment and appropriate care and treatment of service users with a dual diagnosis is essential.
- Treatment for dual diagnosis service users can include pharmacological treatment and psychological interventions to reduce substance use.

KEY TERMS

- abstinence
- affective disorders
- alcohol use disorders
- anxiety disorders
- assessment
- coexisting disorder
- comorbidity
- dependence
- detoxification
- drug use disorders
- dual diagnosis
- harm reduction
- harmful use
- hazardous use
- illicit
- injecting drug use
- intoxication
- medically assisted alcohol withdrawal
- pharmacodynamics
- pharmacokinetics
- physical dependence
- psychoactive drugs
- psychological dependence
- psychosis
- risk
- substance misuse
- substance-related disorders
- therapeutic use

- tolerance
- toxicity
- withdrawal

LEARNING OUTCOMES

The material in this chapter will assist you to:
- discuss the incidence and significance of substance-related disorders and dual diagnosis,
- differentiate between and describe the pharmacokinetics and pharmacodynamics of psychoactive drugs,
- identify the importance of undertaking an alcohol and other drug assessment for all mental health service users,
- describe a range of interventions that can be used for service users with a coexisting substance use disorder and a mental health problem,
- apply your knowledge of the nursing process to the service user who is dependent on alcohol and/or other drugs,
- critically analyse the range of treatment services available for service users with a dual diagnosis.

INTRODUCTION

Wherever nurses work they will come across people who have problems with substance use or misuse, whether the substances are licit or illicit. The same can be said of people who have problems with their mental health: they will be found in all areas in which nurses work. Nurses and other health professionals may also have times in their lives when they experience difficulty with their own mental health or substance use. Problems with the use of substances and with mental health might occur separately or concurrently. It is important that all nurses understand the concerns associated with these issues in order to offer the best care possible.

This chapter explores issues of substance use, substance-related disorders and dual diagnosis. It begins by outlining the use of alcohol and other drugs, and highlights the costs of substance misuse to the individual, family and community. The pharmacological dimension of psychoactive drugs is explored, terms are defined and the diagnostic criteria for substance misuse are presented. The skills needed to ask questions which will elicit information and undertake a comprehensive assessment are detailed, and specific interventions such as early and brief interventions and harm reduction are explored. Interventions for assessing and working with service users who are intoxicated or withdrawing from substances are described.

The final section of the chapter discusses dual diagnosis (a diagnosed mental disorder and substance use disorder), including the clinical significance of dual diagnosis, an exploration of why people with a mental disorder may use alcohol and other drugs, as well as treatment models and interventions. The emphasis throughout this chapter is on the misuse of alcohol and other drugs. You will find additional information and specific nursing interventions for dual diagnosis in other relevant chapters. The interventions described are applicable to any service user with a substance use disorder, including the service user who is dually diagnosed.

SUBSTANCE USE AND MISUSE

> *Globally, alcohol consumption causes 3.2% of deaths (1.8 million) and 4.0% of the disability-adjusted life years lost (58.3 million). Overall, there are causal relationships between alcohol consumption and more than 60 types of disease and injury. Alcohol consumption is the leading risk factor for disease burden in low-mortality developing countries, and the third-largest risk factor in developed countries.*

(WHO, 2004a)

Alcohol and illicit drug use contribute to major stress on families, the economy, workplace injuries and violence. The Prime Minister's Strategy Unit estimated that alcohol misuse costs £20 billion per year (Prime Minister's Strategy Unit, 2004). Furthermore, 1.2 million violent incidents (and 360 000 incidents of domestic violence) are alcohol-related. Up to 17 million working days a year are lost through alcohol-related absence, and alcohol is thought to be implicated in 1000 suicides and 22 000 premature deaths per year (Prime Minister's Strategy Unit, 2004). Cigarette smoking kills 120 000 in the UK each year and is implicated in a third of all cancers. People who smoke regularly lose on average 16 years from their life expectancy compared to nonsmokers (Department of Health, 1998).

Excluding tobacco, alcohol is the most used drug in the UK. It is present on most social and celebratory occasions, from diplomatic banquets to informal meetings with friends. Social drinking is a rule-laden activity. Drunkenness may be considered appropriate during certain rites of passage, such as stag nights, but there is a clear line between this form of social interaction and continuous, excessive drinking, which has a strong impact on the individual, the community and the economy. Negative effects can follow heavy or excessive regular (chronic) alcohol consumption or single (acute) episodes of alcohol misuse.

Illicit drug use (illegal drugs and the illicit use of drugs and volatile substances, including the nonmedical use of prescription drugs) can also be acute or chronic, and have negative effects on individuals, their families and the community.

EPIDEMIOLOGY

The UK and Ireland have the highest rates of alcohol consumption in the English-speaking world; followed by Australia and New Zealand. Conditions associated with hazardous and harmful alcohol use include some cancers, liver disease, pancreatitis, diabetes and epilepsy. Alcohol is also a significant factor in motor vehicle fatalities and injuries, falls, drowning, burns, suicide and occupational injuries. In addition, the social costs associated with the excessive use of alcohol include such factors as neglect, and physical and verbal abuse

Chronic, excessive alcohol consumption can result in thiamine deficiency, which affects the central nervous system and can lead to what is termed Wernicke's encephalopathy (Anderson et al., 2002; Kolb and Whishaw, 2003; Lopatko et al., 2002). *Wernicke's encephalopathy* is the acute phase of the syndrome, which results in damage to the sixth nerve, causing nystagmus (involuntary, rhythmic movement of the eyes), ataxia (staggering gait) and confusion. This is reversible with thiamine therapy. *Korsakoff's syndrome* is the chronic phase of the syndrome, resulting in short-term memory loss and confabulation (Kolb and Whishaw, 2003). Recovery from this syndrome is usually incomplete. Irreversible alcohol-related dementia may also occur (Ambrose et al., 2001).

In 2009–2010, of the 206 889 people aged over 18 years who received treatment for a drug-related problem, most (84%) were using opiates and/or crack cocaine. Seven per cent were using cannabis, while 5% were using powder cocaine as a primary drug (Roxburgh et al., 2010). Most (73%) were male, white (88%) with a median age of 33 years. Some 46% of this group reported that they had previously injected, whereas 20% were injecting at the start of the treatment period, presenting additional health hazards such as drug overdose and the acquiring of blood-borne infections such as hepatitis C virus (HCV) or HIV (Roxburgh et al., 2010).

Pregnant and/or breastfeeding women

There is evidence that high levels of alcohol consumption during pregnancy can contribute to a variety of adverse outcomes in the newborn child. However, the evidence of the effects on the fetus of drinking lower levels is less clear. Overall, the most consistent evidence to date identifies an average of one standard drink per day as the level below which no discernible evidence has been found of harm to the unborn child (Royal Women's Hospital, 2005).

357

However, the National Institute for Health and Clinical Excellence (NICE) recommends that pregnant women or women trying to conceive should avoid drinking alcohol (NICE, 2008). There is particular risk of miscarriage during the first 3 months of pregnancy. However, if the woman does wish to drink alcohol they should be advised to drink no more than 1 to 2 UK units once or twice a week in order to minimize any potential risk to the baby (1 unit equates to half a pint of ordinary-strength lager or beer, or a single shot (25 ml) of spirits. One small (125 ml) glass of wine (12% alcohol by volume) is roughly equal to 1.5 UK units) (NICE, 2008). Likewise, pregnant women should be informed of the risks of smoking, such as an increased risk of having a low birth weight baby and preterm birth (NICE, 2008). There is no specific evidence of a risk associated with cannabis use during pregnancy, other than the associated known harmful risks of smoking (NICE, 2008).

PHARMACOLOGY OF PSYCHOACTIVE DRUGS

The World Health Organization (WHO) uses the term 'drug' to describe a chemical entity used nonmedically and self-administered for its psychoactive effect. The psychoactive effect is an essential component of the description and usually includes a change in mood, arousal and/or perception, cognition (thinking) and/or behaviour (WHO, 2004b).

All psychoactive drugs have the capacity to produce drug dependence. These drugs may be produced in a laboratory (e.g. amphetamines or ecstasy) or extracted from plants (e.g. heroin or cocaine). They can also be legal (such as alcohol) or illicit (e.g. cannabis). Psychoactive drugs can cause harm either through intoxication or through dependence (Whelan, 1999). They can be classified in many ways. One of the most common methods is to classify them as depressants, stimulants or hallucinogens. Some drugs have multiple actions and therefore can be placed in more than one category (Teesson and Hall, 2001).

Depressants are drugs that slow down the activity of the brain. When used in small doses they produce relaxation or drowsiness; in larger doses they produce a loss of consciousness similar to a deep sleep. Some can produce impaired coordination, depression and, in large quantities, coma and death. Depressant drugs include ethanol (alcohol), benzodiazepines (e.g. diazepam), sleeping tablets (e.g. zopiclone), opioids and painkillers (e.g. codeine, morphine, heroin), and solvents and inhalants (e.g. petrol, nitrous oxide, amyl nitrate) (Teesson and Hall, 2001).

Stimulant drugs accelerate activity in the nervous system and increase the body's sense of arousal. In small doses they increase awareness and concentration and decrease fatigue. Irritability, activity, nervousness and insomnia increase as the amount taken increases, and some individuals experience delusions and hallucinations. Excessive doses can lead to convulsions and death. Stimulants include amphetamines (commonly known as speed), methamphetamines (commonly known as crystal meth, ice), d-amphetamine (dexamphetamine) and methylphenidate (Ritalin). Other stimulant drugs include cocaine, nicotine, caffeine and 3,4-methylenedioxymethamphetamine (MDMA, commonly known as ecstasy) (Teesson and Hall, 2001).

Hallucinogens (also called psychedelics or psychotomimetics) share properties with both of the previous categories. However, their specific function is to distort perception and consequently induce hallucinations (auditory, tactile and/or visual). In small doses some hallucinogens such as cannabis reduce inhibitions and cause the user to become more relaxed and feel more sociable. Hallucinogens include lysergic acid diethylamide (LSD), psilocybin (magic mushrooms) and mescaline (part of the Mexican cactus, peyote). Some amphetamine derivatives such as MDMA (ecstasy) are chemically related to mescaline and have both stimulant and hallucinatory properties and may be placed in both categories for classification purposes (Teesson and Hall, 2001).

Although cannabis is commonly placed with the hallucinogenic group of drugs, it is often difficult to classify in pharmacological terms as it has a mixture of mood, cognitive, motor and perceptual effects and does not clearly belong with any one drug class (Ashton, 2001).

HOW DO DRUGS WORK?

The effects of drugs on the body can be understood through two concepts: pharmacokinetics and pharmacodynamics.

Pharmacokinetics is the study of the action of drugs within the body, including the mechanisms of absorption, distribution, metabolism and excretion (Anderson et al., 2002). The pharmacokinetics of each drug differs; for example, the oral administration of amphetamines produces peak cardiovascular effects after approximately 1 hour, while central nervous system (CNS) effects peak about 2 h after administration. The effects last for 4–6 h. However, if the drug is administered intranasally (snorting), the effects are felt within a few minutes. Intravenous injection produces even faster results. Amphetamines are eliminated by metabolism in the liver and excreted by the kidneys, and much is excreted as unchanged amphetamine (Latt et al., 2002).

In comparison, smoking cannabis delivers the active ingredient tetrahydrocannabinol (THC) rapidly to the blood and brain. Plasma THC peaks at the end of smoking (approximately 14 min) and falls to low values within 2 h. If cannabis is consumed orally, its absorption is lower and its effects are more variable and also often less pronounced. THC is fat-soluble, which results in a slow elimination of metabolites, and it can be detected in the urine several days after administration and well after the acute effects of THC have disappeared (Todd et al., 2002).

Pharmacodynamics is the study of how a drug acts on a living organism, including the pharmacological response and the duration and magnitude of response observed relative to the concentration of the drug at an active site in the organism (Anderson et al., 2002). As with pharmacokinetics, each drug action is different: for example, amphetamines activate the CNS and have peripheral sympathomimetic actions. The CNS stimulation results in euphoria, an increased feeling of wellbeing, increased energy and confidence, improved cognitive and psychomotor performance, insomnia and suppression of appetite. Sympathomimetic effects include elevated blood pressure and tachycardia (Latt et al., 2002).

In contrast, the effects of cannabis are mediated by the actions of THC at CB1 receptors in the brain and peripheral tissues (e.g. endothelial cells and testes). Cannabis taken in low doses produces a mixture of stimulatory and depressant effects; at high doses the effects are mainly depressant. The effects of cannabis include euphoria, relaxation and a feeling of wellbeing. In addition, there are perceptual distortions such as altered time sense. Memory, cognition and skilled task performance are impaired, although many users may feel confident and highly creative. Peripheral effects include tachycardia, vasodilatation and hypotension. Cannabis stimulates the appetite and is also an antiemetic, and people who have taken cannabis often experience 'the munchies' when they feel hungry and crave certain foods (Todd et al., 2002). As with all psychoactive drugs, the effects vary between individuals depending on the amount taken, the manner of administration, the frequency of use, concurrent use with other drugs, past exposure and the environment in which the drug is used.

CORE DIAGNOSES FOR SUBSTANCE USE

Substance use exists on a continuum that extends from abstinence through intermittent nonhazardous (and sometimes beneficial) use, hazardous use and harmful use, to dependence (Saunders and Young, 2002). In general, the greater the frequency of use and the greater the amount of substances consumed per occasion, the more severe the consequences for the user's health, the psychosocial consequences and the risk of dependence. However, problems may occur due to occasional, high-level (binge) use, and/or repeated harmful but not dependent use. The terms *substance abuse* and *dependence* can be difficult to define precisely, as there are extraneous factors that must be taken into account, such as culture

and ideology. For example, in some cultures the use of psychoactive drugs for religious or spiritual ceremonies is accepted but in other cultures is prohibited. The term substance abuse is often associated with addiction and dependence. It is considered value-laden, and has limited use in contemporary addiction literature in the UK (Hussein Rassool, 2002).

The *Diagnostic and Statistical Manual of Mental Disorders*, fourth edition (text revision; DSM-IV TR; APA, 2000) is often used to diagnose substance dependence. It focuses on social and interpersonal consequences of substance 'abuse', such as failure in role obligations, and recurrent legal, social or interpersonal problems. Substance 'abuse' can therefore be defined as the use of drugs or alcohol in a way that disrupts prevailing social norms, remembering that these norms vary with culture, gender and generation (Saunders and Young, 2002).

The descriptive terms that are most often used are:

- intoxication,
- hazardous use,
- harmful use,
- episodic heavy drinking or 'binge' drinking,
- dependence.

These are discussed on the following pages.

Intoxication

Intoxication occurs when a person's intake of a substance exceeds their tolerance and produces behavioural and/or physical changes. There is no formally agreed definition, although it is usually taken to refer to an elevated blood alcohol concentration such that a person cannot function within their normal range of physical/cognitive abilities. Susbtance intoxication leads to reversible behavioural or psychological changes due to ingestion of (or other exposure to) a substance acting on the CNS (e.g. belligerence, mood lability, cognitive impairment, impaired judgement, impaired social or occupational functioning) and develops during or shortly after use of the substance (APA, 2000).

Women become intoxicated after drinking smaller amounts of alcohol than men, because their smaller body weight, smaller liver size and smaller blood volume give a higher concentration of alcohol in their vital organs for a given dose. It is important for nurses to manage intoxication correctly because it complicates assessment and service user care, even when it is not life-threatening. Intoxication can be dangerous because it can mimic or mask serious illness or injury (infections, hypoxia, head injury, hypoglycaemia, temporal lobe epilepsy, drug toxicity, meningitis, cerebral vascular accidents and transient ischaemic accidents).

Psychoactive drugs affect mood, cognition, behaviour and physiological functioning. Intoxication can be life-threatening because it can cause altered physical functioning (for example, depressed respiration, alterations in temperature regulation and altered mental function such as panic or paranoia, which can result in accidental injuries). The essential feature of substance intoxication is that it is reversible and is due to the recent ingestion of, or exposure to, a substance. The maladaptive behavioural or psychological changes associated with intoxication are due to the direct physiological effects of the substance on the CNS and develop during or shortly after the use of the substance. The symptoms are not due to a general medical condition or are not better accounted for by another mental disorder. Intoxication is often associated with substance use or dependence, but this category does not apply to nicotine (APA, 2000).

With regards to alcohol, the Department of Health recommends that adult men should not regularly drink more than four units of alcohol per day and women no more than three units (Department of Health, 1995). One UK unit of alcohol is defined as 8 g (or 10 ml) of alcohol which is the amount contained in half a pint of ordinary strength beer, cider or lager (3–4% alcohol by volume), or a standard measure of spirits. After an episode of heavy drinking it is advisable to have 2 days alcohol-free to allow the body to recover. Medical advice is to drink no more than 21 units of alcohol per week in men and 14 units in women (Royal College of Psychiatrists, 1988). Those people who drink above these levels do so *hazardously*: that is, this level of alcohol use increases the risk of future harm.

Hazardous use

Hazardous use is defined as a repetitive pattern of use that poses a risk of harmful physical and psychological consequences (potential problem). Hazardous substance use is defined in terms of at-risk behaviours such as sharing intravenous needles, bingeing and using substances in unsafe settings, such as when using machinery (Saunders and Young, 2002).

Harmful use

The term *harmful use* is used when the pattern of substance use is actually causing harm (NICE, 2011). Men who drink above 50 units of alcohol per day and women who drink 35 units per day or more are drinking at levels which are 'definitely harmful' (NICE, 2011). It is estimated that 24% of adults drink hazardous or harmful amounts of alcohol (NICE, 2010b) and 6.4 million people may be said to be moderate to heavy drinkers; that is, they drink above the maximum recommended weekly levels (Prime Minister's Strategy Unit, 2004).

Episodic heavy drinking or 'binge' drinking

'Binge' drinkers are described as people who drink to get drunk (Prime Minister's Strategy Unit, 2004) where large quantities of alcohol may be consumed in a short period of time. Men who drink more than eight units per day and women who drink more than six units can be classified as 'binge drinkers', and it is estimated that 5.9 million people in the UK drink double the maximum daily recommended amount at least once a week (Prime Minister's Strategy Unit, 2004). Such people are more likely to do this under the age of 25 years, and although this is more likely to be among males, over the past 15 years women's binge drinking has increased. Such patterns of alcohol use increase the risk of accidents, violence, sexual assault and alcohol poisoning.

Dependence

The term *alcohol dependence* is now considered a more precise term diagnostically when compared to the previous term *alcoholism* (NICE, 2011).

Saunders and Young (2002) describe one paradox of substance use, which is the persistent use of a substance despite negative consequences. Often these negative consequences contradict the original motive for substance use in the early stages. For example, a person who is alcohol-dependent may have initially used alcohol as a way of coping with anxiety, yet now maintains dependent use despite increased financial, relationship, physical and employment worries. The individual may consider that the reinforcing effects of alcohol use outweigh the negative consequences of its use. Dependence can be both physical and psychological. It is often referred to as a psychobiological syndrome (Saunders et al., 2001), which exists along a continuum. It consists of a number of behavioural, emotional, cognitive and physiological disturbances that cluster together at the same time. There may be evidence of tolerance and/or withdrawal. The substance may often be taken in larger amounts or over a longer period than was intended. There may be a persistent desire or unsuccessful efforts to cut down or control substance use. A great deal of time may be spent in activities necessary to obtain the substance (e.g. visiting multiple doctors or driving long distances), use of the substance (e.g. chain smoking) or recovering from its effects. The person may give up or reduce important social, occupational or recreational activities because of substance use (APA, 2000).

ASSESSMENT AND DIAGNOSIS

The use of alcohol and other drugs is very common in the UK (as well as other countries) and substance misuse must be considered as a possibility with every service user that a nurse sees in any setting. Specific assessment tools and criteria are used for a service user who presents with a substance disorder or who has a dual diagnosis.

Because of the wide variety of substances available and the range of possible uses, it is important to carefully elicit a substance use history from the service user. The purpose of eliciting information about substance use is to assist in making a diagnosis so that an appropriate management strategy can be developed and implemented (DeCrespigny and Cusack, 2003). A study undertaken by Carta et al. (2002) of 173 mental health professionals, of whom 134 were nurses, found a knowledge and skill gap in assessment and management of substance misuse problems, such as basic knowledge like the number of grams of alcohol contained in a standard drink and the recommended number of alcohol-free days per week.

Presentation, setting and history

The process of assessment will be influenced by the nature of the presentation and the setting. For example, people who present to an emergency department are likely to be distressed due to recent trauma or pain or because family members or friends have been admitted with illness or trauma (Saunders et al., 2001). In this setting, the emphasis should be on obtaining key information about the service user's substance use for their immediate management. The recent substance use history is important in order to assess the type of substance used, and also the level and frequency of use, to identify whether a withdrawal state could occur (Gowing et al., 2000). It is also important in gauging a service user's requirements for analgesia and any potential risk of infection if the person is an injecting drug user.

Information regarding the service user's past substance use history is also important as this assists in the planning of interventions that may be useful in identifying triggers for using and to prevent relapse. A developmental and family history should be documented as well as identifying the age of first use of each substance used and how its/their use has developed over time. Following on from this, the nurse needs to work with the service user to identify when he or she thinks the substance use became problematic, as well as identifying any periods of abstinence or any change in the use of substances.

Substance use history

A service user's substance use (prescribed and nonprescribed) must be measured to determine whether the level of use may cause harm or whether withdrawal is imminent (Anderson et al., 2002). For alcohol there is an agreed low level of consumption, but alcohol interacts with many medications including some herbal preparations. There are too many medications with the potential to interact with alcohol to be listed here, but comprehensive and up-to-date information on alcohol and medication interactions can be found in the *British National Formulary* and associated website.

NURSE'S STORY: WORKING IN SUBSTANCE MISUSE SERVICES

The ultimate challenge and 'high' of working in substance misuse services is the experience of assisting a service user and seeing them creating a happier life out of what is sometimes chaos. My part in providing the information and the skills that help that process of recovery gives me a sense of wellbeing and achievement about what I do. I am only talking about small steps here. Every small step no matter how hesitant is a cause for celebration and joy. You cannot do the service user's work for them but you can provide assistance to them on the journey they must make. That is where skill is needed. The skill is assessing where the service user is on the motivational cycle and being able to provide assistance that helps them towards their recovery, yet recognizing that everybody has different recovery goals and that each person's needs are unique. So, the passion for me is in feeling that I am doing something to help people out of this mess. Even if it is only by offering my respect, recognition, skills and time. The downside is that you cannot do it for them, and the struggle with addiction and dependence is a hard and lonely one. At those times when people give up on their goals I remind myself that these problems were a long time developing and will be a long time in being resolved, and that a step back is just that, not the end of the game.

Maureen (20 years working in substance misuse services)

Taking a substance use history

When asking about substance use, it is important to approach the topic in an open manner and substance use as an accepted behaviour. Asking questions about alcohol and tobacco before asking about illicit drug use is less confronting. It will also help to legitimize subsequent questioning and make the person more comfortable.

In a substance use assessment it is essential to clarify the elements listed below. Health services may have a standard substance use assessment form, which will cover each of these elements.

For alcohol use, it is important to establish the:

- quantity and frequency of consumption,
- beverage(s) type.

With tobacco use, two important questions are:

- 'How many cigarettes do you smoke each day?'
- 'Do you smoke within half an hour of waking up in the morning?'

With other drug use you will need to establish:

- the type of drug used,
- how it is administered (injected, inhaled),
- how often the drug is used,

- how much is used,
- how long the person has been using the drug,
- the time and amount of the last dose (where possible clarify in exact terms, e.g. grams of alcohol, standard drink units, grams of cannabis, milligrams of methadone) in order to predict and manage withdrawal.

It can often be difficult to discuss personal issues with people we do not know. However, the following hints can help make a substance misuse assessment flow more smoothly.

- Ensure that the environment is as quiet and private as possible.
- If it is not possible to be completely private, speak quietly so that others do not hear all the personal details.
- When you are interviewing the service user, note any inconsistencies in what you are being told.
- If the service user becomes angry, leave the question and rephrase it later.
- A substance use history can also be elicited from the service user's friends or family.
- If there is a discrepancy between what the service user tells you and what significant others tell you, record this and clarify details when possible.
- How you ask the questions is important. It is important to remain nonthreatening and nonjudgemental (remember that many of the substances used are illegal and service users may well be guarded about revealing the full extent of their use unless or until they feel that you can be trusted).
- Although many service users may drink at levels higher than those recommended, do not assume that they see this as problematic. The service user may lead a very different lifestyle to yours and might not conform to what you consider to be acceptable behaviour.
- Such considerations must not affect the therapeutic process. Remember that substance use is a health issue, not a moral one (Curtis and Harrison, 2001). Although illicit drugs may be involved, it is the service user's health and not the legal aspect that nurses are concerned about.
- It is always important to check with senior nursing staff about any legal issues of confidentiality and duty of care. Respective legal and policy requirements must be observed and enforced in given clinical situations, and failure by a nurse to abide by such procedural guidelines may place a nurse in jeopardy (Staunton and Chiarella, 2003).
- Introduce drinking/substance use as a normal everyday occurrence. For example, ask: 'What is your favourite drink?' or 'What do you like to drink?' Phrase questions in a way that assumes the service user does drink alcohol or use other drugs. By asking questions in this way, it gives them permission to talk about their substance use. For example, ask the service user: 'When did you last drink enough to make you merry or even drunk?' rather than 'Have you ever been drunk?', which is more likely to elicit a yes/no answer.
- When asking about the number of drinks consumed or the frequency of other drug use, suggest a quantity towards the extreme range of the scale. For example, 'How many drinks would you normally consume in an evening? Five cans?' or 'How many sleeping tablets do you take at a time? Five or six?'. A person is more likely to admit to a high level if you imply that such a number is not out of the question. However, you must also be careful that you do not encourage the service user to overestimate their alcohol and other drug use (Allen, 2003).

Observations

An assessment of a person's physical and mental state may reveal evidence of recent substance use, such as the smell of alcohol on a person or signs of withdrawal. A person who has misused substances for some time may have a decline in global functioning, which may be seen by a decline in health status and poor hygiene. Signs of current drug use are outlined in Box 19.1. An assessment should include:

- general appearance: look for evidence of malnutrition, in which the person can look gaunt, and for signs of agitation, which may indicate stimulant use or withdrawal from a substance. People who regularly inject drugs will often wear long sleeves and long trousers even in hot weather in an attempt to cover up injection marks,
- signs of intoxication: such as ataxia, confused thinking, being argumentative or the smell of alcohol on the person's breath,
- signs of withdrawal: such as tremor and sweating, particularly of the hands and face,
- stigmata: such as abscesses at injection sites, inflammation of the nasal septum from snorting cocaine, bruising and scars unrelated to surgery, which might indicate accidents while under the influence of substances,
- pulse rate, blood pressure and evidence of head injury.

CRITICAL THINKING CHALLENGE 19.1

When assessing a service user for possible substance use, which of the following would alert the nurse to possible opiate use?

A. pupillary constriction
B. liver disease
C. reddened eyes
D. tactile hallucination

During an initial interview, the nurse asks the service user if he has ever experienced blackouts. Blackouts are:

A. an inability to perform work requiring concentration.
B. amnesia for events that occurred while intoxicated.
C. a state of unconsciousness from an overdose of alcohol.
D. denial of the unpleasant effects of drinking.

Box 19.1 Signs of current drug use

Puncture marks
Cellulitis
Phlebitis
Skin abscesses
Erosion or irritation around nostrils/septum
Irritation around mouth or nose
Tenderness or liver pain

Tests

Mental status examination

A mental status examination is essential (see Ch. 10), paying particular attention to:

- clouding of consciousness,
- perceptual abnormalities, especially visual and auditory hallucinations,
- thought abnormalities, especially paranoid ideation,
- suicidal ideation,
- altered cognition.

Laboratory tests

Laboratory tests may provide evidence of substance misuse. Physiological markers of consumption are most widely used to verify a diagnosis of substance use. For example, blood alcohol concentration (BAC) is one physiological marker: the average blood alcohol that is removed from the body being approximately 15 mg per 100/ml of blood per hour (Edwards et al., 2003). The mean corpuscular volume (MCV) of red blood cells, serum gamma-glutamyl transferase (GGT), serum aspartate aminotransferase (AST) and especially carbohydrate-deficient transferrin (CDT), considered to be a more sensitive measure of excessive alcohol consumption, can also give an indication of recent alcohol consumption (Dawe et al., 2002).

Screening tests

Screening tests may also be used. These instruments usually take the form of self-reported questionnaires and are used for diagnostic purposes. One of the most widely used screening instruments is the Alcohol Use Disorders Identification Test (AUDIT), which is designed to screen for a range of drinking problems, particularly harmful and hazardous use. It is especially suitable for primary healthcare settings and has reliability across cultural groups and a range of specific populations including women, mental health service users, university students and the unemployed.

The AUDIT is a self-report measure comprising 10 items, which are scored by adding each of the items. Items 1–8 are scored on a 0–4 scale, and items 9 and 10 are scored 0, 2 or 4. A score of 8 or above has frequently been used to indicate the presence of alcohol problems. While studies have found this cut-off point to have adequate sensitivity and specificity for adult men, a lower cut-off point of 4 may be more useful for women and adolescents (Saunders et al., 1993).

The AUDIT is in the public domain and is reproduced in Box 19.2. It may be used without cost. (A copy of the AUDIT and guidelines are available free of charge from the WHO website [http://www.who.int/]: follow the menu options.)

INTERVENTIONS

Many different types of intervention can be used when working with people with substance use issues. Interventions presented in this chapter can be offered in a mental health unit. For more specialized substance misuse interventions, contact your local drug and alcohol service.

Early and brief interventions

Studies have shown that early intervention (talking to people at an early stage in their substance use) is an effective way to prevent later possible complications (Chang, 2002; Dale and Marsh, 2000a, 2000b; Denis et al., 2007). Brief interventions for substance use involve sessions of 5–15 min and often include the provision of self-help materials such as pamphlets or substance use diaries. This may extend to a brief assessment, providing advice (in a one-off session) as well as assessing the service user's readiness to change (motivational interview), harm reduction and follow-up (Fielden and Marsh, 2007). The components of brief interventions include providing feedback to the service user on risk or impairments due to drug use, listening to the service user's concerns, advising the service user about the consequence of continued drug

Box 19.2 Alcohol use disorders identification test (AUDIT) screening instrument

Please circle the answer that is correct for you.

1. How often do you have a drink containing alcohol?
    Never
    Monthly or less
    2–4 times a month
    2–3 times a week
    4 or more times a week

2. How many drinks containing alcohol do you have on a typical day when you are drinking?
    1 or 2
    or 4
    or 6
    7 to 9
    10 or more

3. How often do you have six or more drinks on one occasion?
    Never
    Less than monthly
    Monthly
    Weekly
    Daily or almost daily

4. How often have you found that you were not able to stop drinking once you had started?
    Never
    Less than monthly
    Monthly
    Weekly
    Daily or almost daily

5. How often during the last year have you failed to do what was normally expected of you because of drinking?
    Never
    Less than monthly
    Monthly
    Weekly
    Daily or almost daily

6. How often during the last year have you needed a first drink in the morning to get yourself going after a heavy drinking session?
    Never
    Less than monthly
    Monthly
    Weekly
    Daily or almost daily

7. How often during the last year have you had a feeling of guilt or remorse after drinking?
    Never
    Less than monthly

Monthly
Weekly
Daily or almost daily

8. How often during the last year have you been unable to remember what happened the night before because you had been drinking?
    Never
    Less than monthly
    Monthly
    Weekly
    Daily or almost daily

9. Have you or someone else been injured as a result of your drinking?
    No
    Yes, but not in the last year
    Yes, during the last year

10. Has a relative or friend or a doctor or other health worker been concerned about your drinking or suggested you cut down?
    No
    Yes, but not in the last year
    Yes, during the last year

From the World Health Organisation (1992) The ICD-10 Classification of Mental and Behavioural Disorders with permission.

use, defining treatment goals such as reducing or ceasing drug use and discussing and implementing strategies for treatment (for example, identifying triggers for drug use and strategies to overcome these, and offering a follow-up session; Hulse et al., 2002a) (see Ch. 23 for more information on therapeutic interventions).

CASE STUDY: HELEN

Helen has been a service user of community health services for approximately 6 months receiving care for a leg ulcer, which is exacerbated by Type II diabetes. She is 63 years old and lives by herself. Her husband died approximately 12 months ago. She has one married daughter and three grandchildren, who live in New Zealand. On previous visits Helen was well groomed, her house was clean and she seemed pleased to see the community nurse, offering her cups of tea and cakes that she had cooked. Recently, though, Helen seemed to have lost interest in caring for herself. On the last visit she appeared unkempt, her clothes were wrinkled and had food stains on them. Her hygiene was poor and the smell of urine and body odour was quite strong. The community nurse had noticed two empty bottles of sherry on the table and a half-full sherry bottle. Helen was irritable and her words were slurred. She stated that she felt lonely and bored without her daughter and husband, and that 'the sherry helps me to forget'. Helen denied any previous problems with alcohol or other substances, but she did say that sherry had helped her to cope with the death of her husband, and that the doctor had then given her some pills and gradually they had made her feel better. Helen 'thinks' that she 'mostly remembers' to take her diabetes medication, but she doesn't know what all the fuss is about, as there is nothing wrong with her.

Questions

How would you assess Helen?
  Physical assessment?
  Mental health assessment?
  Substance use assessment?
What are the issues involved in caring for Helen?
What are the priorities in providing care for Helen?
  Short term?
  Longer term?
What services need to be included in Helen's care?
If you were Helen's community nurse, what management plan would you develop in consultation with Helen?

CRITICAL THINKING CHALLENGE 19.2

In the case study above, you are working in a community mental health centre and have arranged to visit Helen. The community nurse has given you Helen's history in her referral letter.

♦ How will you prioritize this situation?
♦ What types of assessment will you initiate?
♦ What questions might you ask?
♦ Who will you discuss Helen's situation with?
♦ What follow-up plan might you implement?

Brief interventions are recommended for service users experiencing relatively few problems related to their substance use and who have low levels of dependence (Dunn et al., 2001; Fielden and Marsh, 2007). Brief interventions are recommended for service users with a dependence on nicotine, low to moderate dependence on alcohol or low to moderate dependence on cannabis. It is not recommended for service users with severe dependence. If brief interventions consist of only one session, it should include advice on how to reduce drug use or drinking to a safer level, provision of harm-reduction information, and discussion of harm-reduction strategies (Dale and Marsh, 2000b).

NURSE'S STORY: WHY I WORK AS A NURSE IN SUBSTANCE MISUSE SERVICES

A question I get asked regularly, not only in the workplace but also at dinner parties, is: 'Why do you want to work with drug addicts?' To be honest I have never really been able to come up with a clear answer but I will give it a go. I have nursed in drug and alcohol for 15 years. I enjoy the job.

A skill learned early in my career was to engage service users honestly and openly with the expectation that this would be reciprocated. I find it a great privilege to be allowed into the complex layers of drug and alcohol dependency, allowing me the opportunity to offer solutions to health and social needs. There is great scope in working with service users holistically and not merely with their first presenting issue.

I have a very strong belief that as nurses we are not in a position to judge who is worthy of healthcare. Some of my colleagues treat drug-dependent service users with little respect and understanding. Part of my job is to challenge those beliefs, address fears, educate and assist service users in receiving nondiscriminatory healthcare.

One rare gem that comes with drug and alcohol nursing is that of working with a team of people who know how to look after each other. Having a black sense of humour and being able to share a bottle of wine and many laughs keeps balance in your life and the ability to enjoy a fantastic career.

Inga Heyman

Motivational interviewing

Motivational interviewing (MI) is based on the transtheoretical model developed by Prochaska and DiClemente (1983) and is one of the most widely used and easily available interventions. The basic idea is to ascertain which stage of 'readiness to change' the person is at and then to provide information or targeted support to move the person onto the next stage. A detailed explanation is given in Chapter 23.

The nurse's story below, by Isabella, is an illustration of the way in which a practising nurse, who works in a substance misuse service, uses the technique. Motivational interviewing can be used in clinical work with service users in any setting.

NURSE'S STORY: USING MOTIVATIONAL INTERVIEWING

When we talk about motivational interviewing, we very often fall into the trap of thinking it is very formal, done in the office, with the nurse and service user sitting down and talking about things, but in actual fact it is very different from that. Take Thursday afternoon, for example. Thursday is very often the day that service users receive benefits and payments into their accounts and you find that suddenly service users become quite agitated and edgy and that they come up to staff and say that they have to go out and pay a water bill or a phone bill or something and that it can't possibly wait. It becomes their major focus for that day, when in fact we know that they are going out to use. So we really need to be on our toes about motivational interviewing.

Some of the techniques that we use might be to develop discrepancy in their thinking because they are very focused on wanting to go, so what we might do is to bring them back to their initial goals. You might say, 'One of your goals was to stay here. What if you just wait a bit longer?'. We often use techniques aimed at delaying the decision, so we might try distracting them. For example, if it's around meal time we might say, 'Why don't you go and have lunch and think about this for a while and then come back and make that decision then?' That sort of thing. This type of conversation can happen walking down the corridor, outside or even when the service user is at the door with their bags packed.

Also, if they do leave, it triggers everyone else in the place and they start to think that they need to go as well. So what we try to do, what we have to do, is to put those strategies in place really early about what the potential triggers are for that person, and look at some of the strategies that we can use on the Thursday because they may not realize when they first come in that it is going to be an issue. But we know that similar patterns will take over, so we need to anticipate that.

I don't think it is a difficult technique to use, but in saying that, I instinctively did it for years without actually putting a name to it. It just seemed that a lot of my interactions involved negotiation; negotiating with service users about what their goals were if they seemed to be a bit off track and going back to their original goals. It is all about negotiation. Personally, I was working with it for years and it was not until I started further study that I thought, 'Oh, that's what it is called'. You can put it in words then and think, 'Oh, that is what we are doing'. Once you learn more about it you can add to your skills and enhance them.

Motivational interviewing could even be used by a student nurse on placement if they have a general understanding, not just about drug and alcohol, but an understanding of some of the issues with addiction or misuse, just knowing what the national standards or national guidelines are. If they have a service user in any setting, whether it is medical surgical, maternity or on a paediatric ward and they detect that that person may have an issue with alcohol or any other sort of drug, just a brief intervention is the starting block for any sort of motivational interviewing. It may be that in a general conversation when they are washing the service user that they find out that the service user might drink a lot. The

student could ask a few more questions and say, 'Have you ever thought about cutting back or stopping, or has it ever caused you any concerns or harm?' If the service user says yes, the student could contact their mentor or they might already be aware of what services are available. It would be good if the students did know what services are available, and get them in contact. That's a start.

Motivational interviewing is all about developing dissonance and that is what you can do in a brief intervention. The service user might be precontemplative if they are sitting in hospital after an accident or they might have moved over to the contemplative mode, but to get them to move over to the action stage might be where the student nurse is the key and can play a pivotal part in bringing it to someone's attention. Generally you find that the student nurse is the one who spends more time with the service users and gets into general conversations with them. I think that is really good.

Getting someone to think about their drinking or substance use and putting some strategies in place to help them seems to be a technique that can be used with all people, not just people who are heavy alcohol or drug users. A person doesn't have to be at 'rock bottom' before you can use this technique; it can be used with anyone at all. I was teaching brief interventions with alcohol to students this morning and they started talking about the ways in which they could use it. It just came up in a general conversation. I think that the student needs to know just the basics. If we stick with alcohol, then what you need to know are the stages of change and also some of the national guidelines put out for drinking: what is acceptable and what can be seen as hazardous drinking. Helping might be as simple as handing that person a brochure. If the service user turns around and says, 'No, I don't want this,' the nurse could still say, 'Here is a brochure for the future'. That's it. It's that easy.

Isabella

Harm reduction

Harm reduction is described as 'the guiding principle used to identify a range of strategies that target the consequences of drug use rather than focusing on the drug itself' (Roche and Evans, 2000, p. 151). Harm reduction represents a new way of conceptualizing and responding to illegal (and legal) drug problems and related harm. The major advantage is that it allows individuals, agencies and policy makers to consider a whole range of interventions and responses to drug use (Marlatt and Witkiewitz, 2002). The principle of harm reduction has been particularly successful in its contribution to the containment of the spread of HIV/AIDS (Bedell, 2007). Harm-reduction strategies aim to reduce problems associated with the continuing use of alcohol and other drugs.

Typical harm-reduction strategies include:

- needle- and syringe-availability programmes,
- methadone maintenance or other pharmacotherapies to reduce the harm associated with injecting drug use, such as the spread of infection through sharing needles,
- suggestions for alternative routes of administration for drugs, such as inhaling or oral use rather than intravenous use, and information on where not to inject, such as into arteries or close to nerves and tendons. Service users should be encouraged to avoid injecting into the neck, breasts, groin or veins below the waist,
- Narcan (naloxone) for ambulance crews. This is an opioid antagonist (it reverses the effect of opioids) that is effective in the treatment of opioid overdose,
- training in safe injecting practices such as using clean needles,
- information on using a reduced quantity of the drug if the person has not used it for an extended period of time,
- supervised injecting rooms,
- provision of information on low-risk using practices such as not mixing drugs or using alone.

Harm-reduction strategies may be appropriate for service users who continue to use alcohol or other drugs or who are likely to relapse.

Managing an intoxicated service user

Service users who are aggressive or disruptive because they are intoxicated can risk their own safety and the safety of others. Intoxicated service users can be frightened and frightening, disruptive and/or upset. They can be difficult to manage and may become loud and aggressive to staff and other service users, and so how they are approached and treated is an important part of managing intoxication. When dealing with an intoxicated person always approach them in a friendly and respectful manner, because authoritarian or patronizing attitudes can provoke anger and aggression. If other intoxicated people accompany the service user, ask them to wait outside, as they may exacerbate the situation and distract the service user. When talking to the service user use the service user's name and use slow, distinct speech with short, simple sentences; however, do not talk down to them. Maintain eye contact, but without being intrusive. Most importantly, make other staff aware of the situation for your own safety and the safety of others. (See Ch. 22 for useful skills such as anger management, aggression management and techniques for preventing violence.)

All intoxicated service users must be kept under observation. A thorough physical and mental status examination will reveal the extent of intoxication. If the intoxication does not diminish with falling serum levels, the service user must be assessed for other possible causes of their condition. Maintenance of airway and breathing is of utmost importance in the comatose service user because vomiting is likely to occur in grossly intoxicated people (Townsend, 2002).

Any service user presenting with seizures should be assessed for alcohol withdrawal, benzodiazepine withdrawal or stimulant intoxication as well as other possible causes. Information about substance use can be obtained from the service user or from friends and family (Townsend, 2002). The seizures must be treated according to policy and the service user should be observed for at least 4 h post-seizure using the Glasgow Coma Scale (GCS). The GCS is a standardized system for assessing the degree of conscious impairment in the critically ill and for predicting the duration and ultimate outcome of coma, primarily in service users with head injuries. It assesses three determinants: eye opening, verbal responses and motor responses (Anderson et al., 2002).

Substance withdrawal

Withdrawal is usually but not always associated with substance dependence. Most individuals going through withdrawal have a craving to readminister the substance to reduce the symptoms. The diagnosis of withdrawal is recognized for the following groups of substances: alcohol, amphetamine, cocaine, nicotine, opioids and sedatives, hypnotics or anxiolytics (APA, 2000). The signs and symptoms of withdrawal vary, but most of the symptoms are the opposite of what is observed during intoxication (Box 19.3). The dose and duration of drug use affects the withdrawal process.

'Detoxification' is most often defined as the process by which alcohol- or drug-dependent persons recover from intoxication in a supervised manner so that withdrawal symptoms are minimized (Heather and Tebbutt,

---

> ### Box 19.3 **Indications of intoxication**
>
> - Alcohol: loss of control of voluntary movements, slurred speech, disinhibition, low blood pressure, smells of alcohol
> - Benzodiazepines: slurred speech, loss of control of voluntary movements, sedation, nystagmus (repetitive eye movement), low blood pressure, drooling, disinhibition
> - Opioids: pinpoint pupils (pupillary constriction), sedation, low blood pressure, slowed pulse, itching and scratching
>
> Reprinted from Hulse G, White J, Cape G 2002 Management of alcohol and drug problems. Oxford University Press, Melbourne, with permission.

1989, p. 47). However, for alcohol the term *medically assisted alcohol withdrawal* is more current (NICE, 2010a) (see below). Withdrawal from a substance can take place in an inpatient unit or in the person's own home. The service user might be medicated or nonmedicated, depending on the severity of the withdrawal and the service user's wishes. Symptoms of withdrawal range in severity from mildly uncomfortable to life-threatening; however, careful assessment and management can alleviate many of the symptoms (Gowing et al., 2000). The onset and length of withdrawal syndrome depends on the half-life of the drug taken. Nursing management of withdrawal focuses on five main areas:

- minimizing progression to severe withdrawal,
- decreasing risk of injury to self/others,
- eliminating risk of dehydration, electrolyte and nutritional imbalance,
- reducing risk of seizures,
- identifying presence of concurrent illness that masks/mimics withdrawal (Checiniski, 2002).

A Cochrane review found that no available treatment (biological and psychological) has been demonstrated to be effective in the treatment of amphetamine withdrawal (Srisurapont et al., 2001) and that evidence about the treatment for amphetamine psychosis or amphetamine dependence is very limited (Shoptaw et al., 2009a, 2009b). A review of cognitive behavioural therapy (CBT) for cannabis users suggest that although there is not enough evidence to draw clear conclusions, counselling, including CBT, may have beneficial effects (Denis et al., 2007).

Alcohol withdrawal

Severe alcohol withdrawal is potentially life-threatening and it is important to anticipate when it might occur. Minor (mild or moderate) withdrawal usually occurs within 24 h after the person has had their last drink and begins to experience 'the shakes'. Often the tremor is associated with hypertension, restlessness, sweating, diarrhoea, headache, difficulty sleeping, decreased appetite and anxiety. Most service users do not experience all symptoms, and symptoms usually subside after 2 or 3 days of abstinence (Anderson et al., 2002). For some individuals the symptoms are more severe; 15% of chronic alcohol users will experience seizures 2 or 3 days after their last drink (Saunders and Young, 2002).

In the UK, benzodiazepines are often used in the treatment for alcohol withdrawal (NICE, 2010a). The dose is titrated depending on the severity of the withdrawal according to the symptoms and, in most cases, medication will be decreased after a few days and discontinued after 1 week. NICE (2010a) also recommend prophylactic thiamine for people who have consumed amounts of alcohol at harmful levels or who are dependent before

and during a planned medically assisted alcohol withdrawal and where they:

- are malnourished or at risk of malnourishment, or
- have decompensated liver disease, or
- are in acute withdrawal.

Identifying persons at risk of alcohol withdrawal, and monitoring the withdrawal state using a standardized assessment tool, has contributed to a substantial reduction in complications of alcohol withdrawal. Rating scales available include the Alcohol Withdrawal Scale (AWS), the Clinical Institute Withdrawal Assessment for Alcohol (Revised) Scale (CIWA-AR) (NICE, 2010a) and the Short Alcohol Withdrawal Scale (SAWS) (Sullivan et al., 1989). However, a substance misuse service may have its own standard scale to use. Benzodiazepines are used widely to treat anxiety and insomnia, and it is important to recognize the potential for addiction and misuse that these drugs have for people with a predisposition to alcohol and/or drug use. Some service users who use benzodiazepines as well as alcohol on a regular basis will need to be withdrawn more slowly; however, the use of these drugs for short periods in a controlled unit such as an inpatient unit is probably safe and warranted for most service users (Todd, 2002).

Fewer than 5% of people with chronic alcohol use who withdraw from alcohol may experience a major withdrawal syndrome known as *delirium tremens* (Saunders and Young, 2002). This syndrome occurs 3–10 days after the person has had their last drink. The service user may present with agitation, disorientation, high fever, paranoia and visual hallucinations (Townsend, 2002). A medical practitioner must see service users who present with a major withdrawal syndrome.

Nursing attention for a service user experiencing delirium tremens must be vigilant. The service user must be nursed in a separate room. Intravenous fluid replacement may be required if there is severe dehydration and excessive sweating. In addition, specific electrolyte replacement (calcium, phosphate, magnesium and/or potassium) may be required. It is essential to reduce any agitation and the service user must be kept calm, to reduce exhaustion. Intravenous diazepam may be prescribed to relieve withdrawal symptoms, and antipsychotic medication such as haloperidol may also be prescribed (Ntais et al., 2007).

There are some factors that predict the likely severity of the alcohol withdrawal syndrome. One factor is whether the service user has a long history of regular heavy alcohol use that meets the criteria of hazardous or dependent, as detailed earlier in this chapter (Saunders and Young, 2002). Another factor is the use of other psychotropic drugs, particularly CNS depressants (Dale and Marsh, 2000a). Furthermore, if the person has a past history of withdrawal syndrome, particularly delirium tremens, this places them at greater risk of withdrawal.

The Index for Suspicion of Alcohol Withdrawal (see Box 19.4) is a useful tool for nurses to use as a guide to questions to ask a service user regarding their alcohol use and to alert them to the possibility of withdrawal.

Other interventions

Evidence supports the need to offer a wide spectrum of treatment approaches, although no experimental studies have unequivocally demonstrated the effectiveness of 12-step programmes (Ferri et al., 2007). Nonresidential rehabilitation services include self-help groups, of which the most common are Alcoholics Anonymous (AA) and Narcotics Anonymous (NA), which are self-help groups based on an abstinence philosophy. Community drug and alcohol services provide a range of interventions including individual and group counselling, pharmacotherapies such as methadone maintenance for opiate-dependent service users, CBT, which teaches service users to moderate their responses to their environment by improving social coping and problem-solving skills, and motivational interviewing (Hulse et al., 2002b). (All these therapeutic interventions are described more fully in Ch. 23.) The goal of motivational interviewing is to encourage the service user to recognize both the problems and the benefits associated with drug use and to determine whether the consequences outweigh the benefits (Rubak et al., 2005). Other approaches include residential treatment services and a therapeutic communities,

which offer rehabilitation to a person after they have completed their withdrawal programme.

Integrating different treatment philosophies that meet the needs of service users has been shown to be problematic (MacDonald et al., 2004; Torrey et al., 2002), but the most important aspect of treatment interventions is to match the service user to the counsellor and to the treatment (Dale and Marsh, 2000b).

CRITICAL THINKING CHALLENGE 19.3

A 36-year-old man is admitted to the unit on which you are working, with the following symptoms: temperature 38.1 °C, pulse rate 106 beats per minute, respirations 28 per minute, blood pressure 189/93 mmHg, profuse perspiration and tremulousness. He appears highly agitated.

A mental status examination reveals confusion, disorientation and visual and tactile hallucinations. His partner informs you that he has been a heavy drinker of alcohol, but he stopped 2 days ago. What substance-induced disorder is the service user experiencing?

A. Substance-induced psychosis
B. Alcohol-withdrawal syndrome
C. Delirium tremens
D. Substance-induced anxiety disorder

When the nurse does an initial admission interview on a service user being admitted for withdrawal, which of the following areas is it critical to assess?

A. Type(s) of drug used
B. Family history
C. Reason for admission
D. Physical history

DUAL DIAGNOSIS

Several terms are used to describe someone who has more than one disorder concurrently. Mental health and substance misuse professionals use the terms *dual diagnosis, comorbidity* and *coexisting disorder* interchangeably. There is no universal acceptance of any one term. There are many issues which underpin dual diagnosis, including:

- a primary mental health problem which precipitates or leads to substance misuse,
- substance misuse which worsens or alters the course of mental health problems,
- intoxication and/or substance dependence leading to psychological symptoms,
- substance misuse and/or withdrawal leading to mental disorder (Department of Health, 2002).

There is a considerable degree of coexistence between substance use disorders and other mental health disorders.

The prevalence of dual diagnosis is between 30 and 70% of those presenting to health and social care settings (Crome et al., 2009). Laudet et al. (2000) report that the rate of co-occurring substance use and mental health disorders in the USA ranges between 29 and 59%. Drake et al. (2001) state that substance misuse is the most common and clinically significant dual diagnosis among individuals with mental disorders. Studies tend to show that:

- increased rates of substance misuse are found among those with mental health problems affecting around a third to a half of people with severe mental health problems,
- alcohol misuse is the most common form of substance misuse,
- where drug misuse occurs it often coexists with alcohol misuse,
- homelessness is often associated with substance misuse problems,
- community mental health teams generally report that 8–15% of their clients have dual diagnosis problems, although higher rates of dual diagnosis may be found in inner cities,
- prisoners have a high prevalence of drug dependency and dual diagnosis (Department of Health, 2002, p. 7).

Alcohol and other drugs, even at low levels of consumption, can interact adversely with most of the medications commonly prescribed for the treatment of mental health problems.

There are many theories about dual diagnosis, but most fit into three categories. The first is that there is a direct causal relationship between the two disorders whereby the presence of one disorder makes the other more likely to develop; for example, a dependant cannabis user may become more likely to suffer from the symptoms of psychosis. The second explanation highlights an indirect causal relationship between the two disorders whereby one disorder makes the other more likely to develop, and the third is that there are common factors that increase the risk of both disorders. For example, a severely depressed person may be having psychotic episodes and turning to cannabis for self-medication. There is growing evidence that simple causal hypotheses are not sufficient to explain the association (Teesson and Proudfoot, 2004). Prevalence rates of dual diagnosis vary significantly, depending on the definitions used and the populations studied. Most studies exclude tobacco use from their data; however, McEvoy and Allen (2003) estimate that 70–80% of people with schizophrenia and 65–78% of people with a mood disorder smoke, while Ziedonis and Williams (2003) state that people with mental health problems smoke nearly half of all cigarettes consumed in the USA, and that their risk of developing tobacco-related medical illnesses is two to three times that of the rest of the population.

Patterns of dual diagnosis are dependent on the drug and the type of mental disorder (Kandel et al., 2001).

For example, the highest rates of substance misuse were seen among people diagnosed with antisocial personality disorders, and greater dependence on substance use was seen in individuals who used illicit drugs. Patterns of comorbidity also appear to be age dependent (Prigerson et al., 2001). Younger people with dual diagnosis were more likely to use illicit substances; older people were more likely to use legal substances such as alcohol (Kandel et al., 2001). Although the studies vary a little in their results, they all demonstrate that the prevalence rates for service users with a dual diagnosis are considerable and that nurses and other health professionals must find ways to address the problem.

Clinical significance of dual diagnosis

There is considerable evidence to suggest that service users with a dual diagnosis do less well than those with either a mental health problem or a substance use problem. They are more difficult to manage due to their complex health and social needs, have higher rates of nonadherence with treatment, and are more likely to be violent and to be exposed to violence (Drake et al., 2001; Teesson and Hall, 2001). Service users with a dual diagnosis are more likely to have a chronic disability and consequently result in more service utilization (MacDonald et al., 2004). They have less access to treatment services (Holmwood, 2002) and a greater chance of experiencing difficulties in relationships, employment prospects, social isolation, poor health and chronic financial difficulties (Teesson and Proudfoot, 2004). These service users often have a number of surrounding issues that combine and add to the complexity of treatment goals and outcomes. 'Such issues may include impending legal action from illegal activity, having a child placed in care due to parental alcohol and/or other drug use, lack of accommodation and psychological problems' (Dale and Marsh, 2000b, p. 45).

Why do people with a mental disorder use nonprescribed drugs?

A number of reasons have been proposed for the increase in numbers of people with mental health problems using nonprescribed drugs. Since deinstitutionalization, the number of people with a chronic mental disorder living in the community has increased and this exposes them to a substance-using culture that they may not have been exposed to when separated from mainstream society and living in institutions. Furthermore, an increase in the social acceptability and prevalence of substance use may contribute to higher levels of disorders. There may also be increased awareness of and interest in dual diagnosis, with more clinicians actively assessing their service users, or it may be that substance use can precipitate or perpetuate a mental health problem.

In a frequently cited work, Smith and Hucker (1994) suggest that people with a mental health problem use psychoactive drugs for the following reasons:

- to self-medicate symptoms of mental disorder,
- to reduce the side effects of prescribed medication,
- to facilitate social interaction,
- to participate in certain subcultures,
- to develop an identity more acceptable than that of a person with a mental health problem,
- to help cope with the disabilities of mental health problems such as isolation, poverty, lack of affordable housing and social drift.

Williams and Cohen (2000) suggest that the availability of illicit drugs in mental health facilities may be a contributory factor, and that some individuals are introduced to drug use when they are inpatients for treatment of mental health problems. However, it is becoming clear that simple causal hypotheses are not sufficient to explain the association between mental health problems and substance use (Teesson and Proudfoot, 2004).

It has been identified that nicotine may improve the poor attention to and processing of sensory stimulation of individuals diagnosed with schizophrenia. Nicotine improves eye acceleration and integration of visual information into motor commands for people diagnosed with schizophrenia (McEvoy and Allen, 2003). Management of the side effects of medication may be another reason for tobacco dependence: medications are metabolized more quickly and blood levels are lower in people who smoke. Smokers with mental health problems report that smoking reduces their symptoms and improves their cognitive functioning. Cigarettes were rated as a core need by all subjects in the study and rated as more important than food (Ziedonis and Williams, 2003). However, evidence from recent clinical trials shows that continued smoking adversely affects treatment for marijuana dependence and that smoking cessation is recommended for substance-dependent people. Cessation could actually protect against relapse in the illicit drug user (Cantwell, 2003).

Assessing substance misuse in a mental health unit

Due to the possible high prevalence of dual diagnosis, people presenting to a mental health unit should undergo a substance misuse assessment (Alverson et al., 2000; Drake et al., 2001; Prigerson et al., 2001; Crome et al., 2009). For example, mental disorders (particularly schizophrenia and depression) are commonly associated with alcohol use or dependence (Lopatko et al., 2002). In addition, anxiety disorders and substance use are also commonly dually diagnosed (McKeehan and Martin, 2002). It may sometimes be difficult to discern whether depression is the result or the cause of an alcohol-use disorder (Libby et al., 2005). With repeated use of large doses of stimulants a psychotic state resembling acute schizophrenia can develop and is characterized by agitation, paranoid delusions and visual hallucinations. It is sometimes difficult to differentiate stimulant-induced psychosis from acute paranoid schizophrenia, although psychotic symptoms usually subside as the drug concentration declines (Latt et al., 2002). Drug use can mask a mental health problem, exacerbate the symptoms and prolong the episode (McKeehan and Martin, 2002; White, 2001). Depression, anxiety disorders and bulimia are all more common in women with alcohol problems than in men with alcohol problems (Royal Women's Hospital, 2005).

Guidelines for differentiating between a primary psychotic disorder and a substance-misuse disorder are provided in Box 19.5.

Box 19.5 Guidelines for differentiating between a primary psychotic and a substance-induced disorder

Substance-induced psychotic symptoms can result from intoxication, chronic use or withdrawal.

- Intoxication with cannabis can induce a transient, self-limiting psychotic disorder characterized by hallucinations and agitation.
- Prolonged heavy use of psychostimulants (e.g. amphetamines) can produce a psychotic picture similar to schizophrenia.
- Hallucinogen-induced psychosis is usually transient, but may persist if use is sustained.
- Heavy alcohol use has been associated with alcoholic hallucinosis and morbid jealousy.
- Psychotic symptoms can also occur during withdrawal (e.g. delirium tremens) and delirious states.

A *nonsubstance-induced* psychotic disorder should be considered when:

- psychosis preceded the onset of substance use,
- psychosis persists for longer than 1 month after acute withdrawal or severe intoxication,
- psychotic symptoms are not consistent with the substance used,
- there is a history of psychotic symptoms during periods (>1 month) of abstinence,
- there is a personal or family history of a nonsubstance-induced psychotic disorder.

Lubman DI, Sundram S. Substance misuse in patients with schizophrenia: a primary care guide. Med J Aust 2003; 178 Suppl May 5:S71–S75 © Copyright 2003 *The Medical Journal of Australia* – reproduced with permission.

Caring for service users with a dual diagnosis

Service users with dual diagnoses can be very complex and difficult to treat and care for. Nursing staff are usually not trained or educated in both areas (substance misuse and mental health) and, as noted earlier in this chapter, nurses may hold negative attitudes towards service users who use alcohol and other drugs. Dually diagnosed service users often evoke powerful, unpleasant feelings in health professionals, and nurses may feel unskilled in working with them and overwhelmed by the multiplicity of their problems (Lubman and Sundram, 2003). Many nurses are pessimistic regarding outcomes and believe that intensive time spent with these service users will produce minimal gains. In addition, dually diagnosed service users may feel stigmatized by mental health nurses' attitudes when these are related to an abstinence model that is in direct contrast to the harm-minimization model supported by the substance misuse sector.

This group of service users offers many challenges to nursing staff, as most dually diagnosed service users have a range of personal and social problems and have difficulty maintaining a concurrent level of wellness in both areas. Continued drug use (e.g. of cannabis) may exacerbate positive symptoms of schizophrenia and lead to decompensation and admission or readmission to hospital.

The key principles of history taking and assessment have been detailed under the section on assessment in this chapter. Developing a collaborative therapeutic alliance is essential and the nurse needs to adopt an empathetic and nonjudgemental approach. It is important to accurately assess service users and to screen them for substance use, as many service users with schizophrenia or other mental disorders may often deny or understate their substance use. Once a diagnosis has been made, appropriate management combines pharmacological treatment of the psychotic episode and psychosocial interventions to reduce substance use. Ideally, a service user's mental state should be relatively stable before attempting withdrawal, although this is not always possible. Early and brief interventions can be used in both outpatient and inpatient settings.

Management principles for service users diagnosed with schizophrenia and substance use are outlined in Box 19.6.

As with all aspects of nursing care, safety is the main concern. If a service user has been admitted to a mental health facility in a psychotic state, it is essential that the psychosis be managed, and when the service user's mental state is more settled the nurse can engage in psychosocial interventions to assist the service user with their problematic substance use. These interventions will need to be continued once the service user has been discharged from hospital. If the service user is at risk of withdrawal from one or more substances, withdrawal strategies as outlined earlier in this chapter need to be implemented immediately. The service user will need to be monitored closely and medically

Box 19.6 Management principles for service users diagnosed with schizophrenia and substance misuse

Assessment
- Screen service users with psychosis for substance misuse.
- Determine severity of use and associated risk-taking behaviours (e.g. injecting practices, unsafe sex).
- Exclude organic illness or physical complications of substance misuse.
- Seek collateral history: families or close supports should be involved where possible.

Treatment
- First engage the service user using a nonjudgemental attitude.
- Inform the service user:
  - give general advice about harmful effects of substance misuse,
  - advise about safe and responsible levels of substance use (NH&MRC, 1999),
  - make individual links between substance misuse and service user's problems (e.g. cannabis use and worsening paranoia),
  - inform the service user about safer practices (e.g. safe sexual practices).
- Treat psychotic symptoms and monitor the service user for side effects.
- Help the service user establish advantages and disadvantages of current use and motivate service user to change.
- With medical staff, evaluate the need for concurrent substance use medications (e.g. methadone, acamprosate, nicotine-replacement therapy).
- Refer the service user to appropriate community services as appropriate.
- Devise relapse–prevention strategies that address both psychosis and substance misuse.
- Identify triggers for relapse (e.g. meeting other drug users, family conflict) and explore alternative coping strategies.

Lubman DI, Sundram S. Substance misuse in patients with schizophrenia: a primary care guide. Med J Aust 2003; 178 Suppl May 5:S71–S75 © Copyright 2003 The Medical Journal of Australia – reproduced with permission.

examined and appropriate medication prescribed. When the service user is more settled, the nurse can begin to explore reasons for the service user's substance use, including the relationship of the substance to the service user's mental health problems, treatment, and feelings of social isolation related to negative symptoms.

The service user's readiness to change and their degree of commitment to treatment of both mental disorder and substance use needs to be explored (Lubman and Sundram, 2003). (Refer to Ch. 23 for motivational interviewing and other interventions.) Remember: service users may be at different stages of readiness in their problematic drug use and mental disorder, and interventions need to reflect this. For example, a service user may be at a pre-contemplation stage for their substance use and at an action stage for their mental health problem.

Adopt a concrete problem-solving approach with the service user whenever possible. For example, set tasks that are readily achievable, such as keeping a daily diary of substance use or psychotic symptoms. During the sessions, focus on specific skills to deal with high-risk situations. This may involve assertion training, useful for learning to say 'no' to a dealer. The nurse could consider the use of role play to assist the service user. Remember that a long-term perspective with ongoing intervention is required.

NURSE'S STORY: BEST PRACTICE ADVICE

I have found, from 25 years' experience working in a mental health unit, that almost every person admitted to a mental health unit has a dual diagnosis or at least a problem with alcohol and/or drugs. My advice is: 'Don't be concerned: expect it as the norm'. Stop expecting to deal only with your bit. You need to be able to deal with the whole person. The mental health nurse has a responsibility to find out more about substance misuse, even if it is only how to recognize symptoms and how and when to refer to other services.

Sue, Unit Manager

Service delivery models for dual diagnosis service users

Todd et al. (2002) found that most of the barriers to treatment related to the structure and organization of services within which treatment was delivered. Outcomes and effectiveness of the treatments offered were limited by poor communication between the agencies involved. Effective cooperation between mental health and substance misuse services is essential to ensure that the service user receives treatment that best manages their condition. There are differences in philosophy and opinions regarding the best way to treat service users with a dual diagnosis and, like all treatment options, there are advantages and disadvantages in each model (of separate services or integrated services). Differences in dual disorder combinations, symptom severity and degree of impairment affect the extent to which one treatment model can suit all individuals (Jeffery et al., 2007).

Several models have been proposed for approaching addiction treatment in the mental health setting:

- the sequential model, which posits that individuals should be kept in the mental health facility until they are mentally stable and then transferred to a separate drug-treatment programme,
- the parallel model, in which service users are concurrently treated for their mental health and substance use problems but in separate settings,
- the integrated model, where both substance misuse and mental health problems are treated under the one setting by specially trained professionals.

Research shows that there is no clear evidence supporting an advantage of any one model of service delivery. 'The current momentum for integrated programmes is not based on good evidence. Implementation of new specialist substance misuse services for those with serious mental illness should be within the context of simple, well designed clinical trials' (Jeffery et al., 2007, p. 10).

CONCLUSION

Alcohol and drug use are commonplace in the UK. Many people do not experience problems with their use; however, it is estimated that about 10% of the population at any one time consume substances at levels that are hazardous or harmful. People who have a coexisting substance misuse and mental health problem are at greater risk. Research demonstrates that this group of people experiences more social problems and has less positive treatment outcomes.

As nurses it is important to assess every service user for substance use and to offer timely and effective treatment. Thorough assessment is the key to offering appropriate and timely management of dually diagnosed service users and to identifying those service users who are at risk of harm associated with substance use, but have not been previously diagnosed. Treatment may take the form of brief interventions that can be offered in the mental health setting, or drug and alcohol and mental health services may need to find ways of working together to offer appropriate and timely services to these service users.

Rates of tobacco use are high among service users with a dual diagnosis, and interventions must be made available to assist service users in reducing or ceasing their tobacco use. Alcohol is still the most used substance and it is important to undertake an accurate history and to follow area health service protocols to minimize the risk of withdrawal.

Despite the high prevalence of dual diagnosis, there is little evidence on the nature of best practice for this service user group. However, recommendations from the research literature suggest that a programme which treats both disorders concurrently, with preference given to an integrated model of treatment, is most beneficial. In addition, service users need to be matched with counsellors and to treatment philosophies, and services need to work together to offer a holistic approach.

Service users who have a mental health problem do not necessarily have a substance use problem and, conversely, service users of substance misuse services do not necessarily have a mental health problem. However, many service users who use treatment services do have a dual diagnosis. Before any intervention is offered, it is imperative that all service users undergo an adequate substance use assessment and a mental status examination.

EXERCISES FOR CLASS ENGAGEMENT

Discuss the following questions with your group.

♦ Your partner's brother is admitted to a mental health unit where you are a student. You know that he is quite a heavy user of cannabis, but he does not tell the admitting nurse this and he whispers to you, 'Please don't tell them, they will never let me out'. What will you do?

♦ How would you feel if you observed another student drinking vodka during a lunch break when you are both working together in a clinical practicum? What would you do?

♦ Are you aware of negative attitudes and feelings that might impede your interactions and therapeutic response to a service user with a substance-related disorder? How do you deal with your negative feelings and attitudes in order to establish a therapeutic relationship with the service user?

♦ What role does the Nursing and Midwifery Council (NMC) have in responding to a complaint about a nurse using substances when on duty?

REFERENCES

Allen, J.P., 2003. Assessment of alcoholic patients: advances and future challenges. In: Galanter, M., Begleiter, H., Lagressa, D. (Eds.), Recent Developments in Alcoholism, Vol. 16. Research on Alcohol Treatment. Kluwer Academic, New York, pp. 13–24.

Alverson, H., Alverson, M., Drake, E., 2000. Addictions services: an ethnographic study of the longitudinal course of substance abuse among people with severe mental illness. Community Ment. Health J. 36 (6), 557–569.

Ambrose, M.L., Bowden, S.C., Whelan, G., 2001. Working memory impairments in alcohol-dependent participants without clinical amnesia. Alcohol. Clin. Exp. Res. 25 (2), 185–191.

Anderson, D.M., Keith, J., Novak, M.A., et al., 2002. Mosby's Medical, Nursing and Allied Health Dictionary. Mosby, St Louis.

APA (American Psychiatric Association), 2000. Diagnostic and Statistical Manual of Mental Disorders, fourth ed. text rev. American Psychiatric Association, Washington DC.

Ashton, C.H., 2001. Pharmacology and effects of cannabis: a brief review. Br. J. Psychiatry 178, 101–106.

Bedell, R., 2007. The art and science of scaling up needle and syringe programmes. Addiction 102 (8), 1179–1180.

Cantwell, R., 2003. Substance use and schizophrenia: effects on symptoms, social functioning and service use. Br. J. Psychiatry 15 (3), 324–329.

Carta, B., Happell, B., Pinikahana, J., 2002. Mental health professionals' knowledge and perceptions of problematic alcohol and substance use: a questionnaire survey. Aust. J. Prim. Health 8 (3), 67–74.

Chang, G., 2002. Brief interventions for problem drinking and women. J. Subst. Abuse Treat. 23 (1), 1–7.

Checiniski, K., 2002. Treatment strategies and interventions. In: Hussein Rassool, G. (Ed.), Dual Diagnosis: Substance Misuse and Psychiatric Disorders. Blackwell Science, Oxford.

Crome, I., Chambers, P., with Frisher, M., Bloor, R., Roberts, D., 2009. The relationship between dual diagnosis: substance misuse and dealing with mental health issues. <http://www.scie.org.uk/publications/briefings/files/briefing30.pdf>.

Curtis, J., Harrison, L., 2001. Beneath the surface: collaboration in alcohol and other drug treatment. An analysis using Foucault's three modes of objectification. J. Adv. Nurs. 34 (6), 737–744.

Dale, A., Marsh, A., 2000a. Evidence-based Practice Indicators for Alcohol and Other Drug Interventions: Literature Review. Best Practice in Alcohol and Other Drug Interventions Working Group, Perth.

Dale, A., Marsh, A., 2000b. A Guide for Counsellors Working with Alcohol and other Drug Users: Core Counselling Skills. Best Practice in Alcohol and Other Drug Interventions Working Group, Perth.

Dawe, S., Loxton, N., Hides, L., et al., 2002. Review of Diagnostic Screening Instruments for Alcohol and other Drug Use and other Psychiatric Disorders, second ed. Publications Department, Commonwealth Department of Health Ageing, Brisbane, Queensland.

DeCrespigny, C., Cusack, L., 2003. Alcohol, Tobacco and Other Drugs: Guidelines for Nurses and Midwives. Clinical Guidelines. Flinders University, Adelaide.

Denis, C., Lavie, E., Fatseas, M., et al., 2007. Psychotherapeutic interventions for cannabis abuse and/or dependence in outpatient settings. Cochrane Database Syst. Rev. 3, CD005336.

Department of Health, 1995. Sensible drinking: report of an inter-departmental working group. <http://www.dh.gov.uk/en/Publicationsandstatistics/Publications/PublicationsPolicyAndGuidance/DH_4084701>.

Department of Health, 1998. Smoking kills: a white paper on tobacco. <http://webarchive.nationalarchives.gov.uk/+/www.dh.gov.uk/en/Publicationsandstatistics/Publications/PublicationsPolicyAndGuidance/DH_4006684>.

Department of Health, 2002. Mental health policy implementation guide: dual diagnosis good practice guide. <http://www.dh.gov.uk/en/Publicationsandstatistics/Publications/PublicationsPolicyAndGuidance/DH_4009058>.

Drake, R.E., Essock, S.M., Shaner, A., et al., 2001. Implementing dual diagnosis services for clients with severe mental illness. Psychiatr. Serv. 52 (4), 469–475.

Dunn, C., De Roo, L., Rivara, F., 2001. The use of brief interventions adapted from motivational interviewing across behavioural domains: a systematic review. Addiction 96 (12), 1179–1180.

Edwards, G., Marshall, J., Cook, C., 2003. The Treatment of Drinking Problems. A Guide for the Helping Professions, fourth ed. Cambridge University Press, Cambridge.

Ferri, M., Amato, L., Davoli, M., 2007. Alcoholics Anonymous and other 12-step programmes for alcohol dependence. Cochrane Database Syst. Rev. 3, CD005032.

Fielden, S., Marsh, D., 2007. It's time for Canadian community early warning systems for illicit drug overdoses. Harm Reduct. J. 4 (10) <http://www.harmreductionjournal.com/content/4/1/10/>.

Gowing, L.J., Ali, R.L., White, J.M., 2000. The management of opioid withdrawal. Drug Alcohol. Rev. 19 (3), 309–318.

Heather, N., Tebbutt, J., 1989. The Effectiveness of Treatment Services for Drug and Alcohol Problems. AGPS, Canberra.

Holmwood, C., 2002. Comorbidity of mental disorders and substance use: a brief guide for the primary care clinician. <http://www.parc.

net.au/comorbidityresource2.pdf> (13.06.07.).

Hulse, G., White, J., Cape, G., 2002a. Management of Alcohol and Drug Problems. Oxford University Press, Melbourne.

Hulse, G., White, J., Conigrave, K., 2002b. Identifying treatment options. In: Hulse, G., White, J., Cape, G. (Eds.), Management of Alcohol and Drug Problems. Oxford University Press, Melbourne.

Hussein Rassool, G., 2002. Dual Diagnosis, Substance Misuse and Psychiatric Disorders. Blackwell Science, Oxford.

Jeffery, D.P., Ley, A., McLaren, S., et al., 2007. Psychosocial treatment programmes for people with both severe mental illness and substance misuse (review). Cochrane Collab. 1, 1–37.

Kandel, D.B., Huang, F., Davies, M., 2001. Comorbidity between patterns of substance use dependence and psychiatric syndromes. Drug Alcohol. Depend. 64, 233–241.

Kolb, A., Whishaw, S., 2003. Fundamentals of human neuropsychology. <http://en.wikipedia.org/wiki/korsakoffs_syndrome>.

Latt, N., White, J., McLean, S., et al., 2002. Central nervous stimulants. In: Hulse, G., White, J., Cape, G. (Eds.), Management of Alcohol and Drug Problems. Oxford University Press, Melbourne.

Laudet, A.B., Magura, S., Vogel, H.S., et al., 2000. Addictions services: support, mutual aid and recovery from dual diagnosis. Community Ment. Health J. 36 (5), 457–476.

Libby, A.M., Orton, H.D., Stover, S.K., et al., 2005. What came first, major depression or substance use disorder? Clinical characteristics and substance use comparing teens in a treatment cohort. Addict. Behav. 30 (9), 1649–1662.

Lopatko, O., McLean, S., Saunders, J.B., et al., 2002. Alcohol. In: Hulse, G., White, J., Cape, G. (Eds.), Management of Alcohol and Drug Problems. Oxford University Press, Melbourne.

Lubman, D., Sundram, S., 2003. Substance misuse in patients with schizophrenia: a primary care guide. Med. J. Aust. 178 (9), 571–575.

MacDonald, E., Luxmoore, M., Pica, S., et al., 2004. Social networks of people with dual diagnosis: the quantity and quality of relationships at different stages of substance use treatment. Community Ment. Health J. 40 (5), 451–464.

McEvoy, J., Allen, T., 2003. Substance abuse (including nicotine) in schizophrenic patients. Curr. Opin. Psychiatry 16 (2), 199–205.

McKeehan, M.B., Martin, D., 2002. Assessment and treatment of anxiety disorders and co-morbid alcohol/other drug dependency. Alcohol. Treat. Q. 20 (1), 45–59.

Marlatt, G.A., Witkiewitz, K., 2002. Harm reduction approaches to alcohol use: health promotion, prevention, and treatment. Addict. Behav. 27 (6), 867–886.

National Health and Medical Research Council, 1999. A Guide to the Development, Implementation and Evaluation of Clinical Practice Guidelines. NHMRC, Canberra.

NICE (National Institute for Health and Clinical Excellence), 2008. Antenatal care. <http://guidance.nice.org.uk/CG62/NICEGuidance/pdf/English>.

NICE (National Institute for Health and Clinical Excellence), 2010a. Alcohol-use disorders: diagnosis and clinical management of alcohol-related physical complications. <http://guidance.nice.org.uk/nicemedia/live/12995/48991/48991.pdf>.

NICE (National Institute for Health and Clinical Excellence), 2010b. Alcohol-use disorders - preventing the development of hazardous and harmful drinking. <http://guidance.nice.org.uk/PH24>.

NICE (National Institute for Health and Clinical Excellence), 2011. Alcohol-use disorders: diagnosis, assessment and management of harmful drinking and alcohol dependence. <http://guidance.nice.org.uk/CG115>.

NSW Department of Health, 2000. Alcohol and Other Drugs Policy for Nursing Practice. NSW Department of Health, Sydney.

Ntais, C., Pakos, E., Kyzas, P., et al., 2007. Benzodiazepines for alcohol withdrawal. Cochrane Database Syst. Rev. 3, CD005063.

Prigerson, H.G., Desai, R.A., Rosenheck, R.A., 2001. Older adult patients with both psychiatric and substance abuse disorders: prevalence and health service use. Psychiatr. Q. 79 (1), 1–18.

Prime Minister's Strategy Unit, 2004. Alcohol harm reduction strategy for England. <http://www. newcastle-staffs.gov.uk/documents/ community%20and%20living/ community%20safety/caboffce%20 alcoholhar%20pdf.pdf>.

Prochaska, J.O., DiClemente, C.C., 1983. Stages and processes of self-change of smoking: toward an integrative model of change. J. Consult. Clin. Psychol. 51 (3), 390–395.

Roche, A., Evans, K., 2000. Harm reduction. In: Stokes, G., Chalk, P., Gillen, K. (Eds.), Drugs and Democracy: In Search of New Directions. Melbourne University Press, Melbourne.

Roxburgh, M., Donmall, M., White, M., Jones, A., 2010. Statistics from the National Drug Treatment Monitoring System (NDTMS). 1 April 2009 – 31 March 2010. <http://www.nta.nhs.uk/uploads/ ndtmsannualreport2009- 10finalversion.pdf>.

Royal College of Psychiatrists, 1988. A consensus statement on a better response to alcohol related problems prepared at a meeting held on 6 November 1987, at the Royal College of Psychiatrists. Psychiatr. Bull. 12, 33–34.

Royal Women's Hospital, 2005. Women's alcohol and drug service. <http://www.rwh.org.au/wads/ health-info.cfm?doc_id=3820> (27.06.07.).

Rubak, S., Sandbaek, A., Lauritzen, T., et al., 2005. Motivational interviewing: a systematic review and meta analysis. Br. J. Gen. Pract. 55 (513), 305–312.

Saunders, J., Young, R., 2002. Assessment and diagnosis. In: Hulse, G., White, J., Cape, G. (Eds.), Management of Alcohol and Drug Problems. Oxford University Press, Melbourne.

Saunders, J., Aasland, O.G., Babor, T.F., et al., 1993. Development of the alcohol use disorders identification test (AUDIT). WHO collaborative project on early detection of persons with harmful alcohol consumption II. Addiction 88, 791–804.

Saunders, J., Young, R., Dore, B., 2001. Substance misuse. In: Bloch, S., Singh, B. (Eds.), Clinical Foundations in Psychiatry. Melbourne University Press, Melbourne.

Shoptaw, S.J., Kao, U., Heinzerling, K., Ling, W., 2009a. Treatment for amphetamine withdrawal. Cochrane Database Syst. Rev. 2, CD003021.

Shoptaw, S.J., Kao, U., Ling, W., 2009b. Treatment for amphetamine psychosis. Cochrane Database Syst. Rev. 1, CD003026.

Smith, J., Hucker, S., 1994. Schizophrenia and substance abuse. Br. J. Psychiatry 165, 13–21.

Srisurapont, M., Jarusuraisin, N., Kittirattanapaiboon, P., 2001. Treatment for amphetamine dependence and abuse. Cochrane Database Syst. Rev. 4, CD003022.

Staunton, P.J., Chiarella, M., 2003. Nursing and the Law. Elsevier, Sydney.

Sullivan, J., Sykora, K., Schneiderman, J., et al., 1989. Assessment of alcohol withdrawal: the revised clinical institute withdrawal assessment for alcohol scale (CIWA-AR). Br. J. Addict. 84, 1353–1357.

Teesson, M., Hall, W., 2001. Substance-related disorders. In: Meadows, G., Singh, B. (Eds.), Mental Health in Australia: Collaborative Community Practice. Oxford University Press, Melbourne.

Teesson, M., Proudfoot, H., 2004. Comorbid mental disorders and substance use disorders: epidemiology, prevention and treatment. <http://www.vrb.gov.au/ pubs/comorbid.pdf>.

Todd, F., 2002. Coexisting alcohol and drug use and mental health disorders. In: Hulse, G., White, A., Cape, G. (Eds.), Management of Alcohol and Drug Problems. Oxford University Press, Melbourne.

Todd, F., McLean, S., Krum, H., et al., 2002. Cannabis. In: Hulse, G., White, A., Cape, G. (Eds.), Management of Alcohol and Drug Problems. Oxford University Press, Melbourne.

Torrey, W.C., Drake, R.E., Cohen, M., et al., 2002. The challenge of implementing and sustaining integrated dual disorders treatment programs. Community Ment. Health J. 38, 507–521.

Townsend, M.C., 2002. Essentials of Psychiatric Mental Health Nursing. FA Davis, Philadelphia.

Whelan, G., 1999. The pharmacological dimension of psychoactive drugs. In: Hamilton, M., Kellehear, A. (Eds.), Drug Use in Australia: A Harm Minimisation Approach. Oxford University Press, Melbourne.

White, A., 2001. Links between cannabis and psychosis. In: Barrows, G. (Ed.), Directions in Psychiatry. Forum 8 Conference. 13–14 July 2001, Orietta Press, Tasmania, pp. 12–14.

Williams, R., Cohen, J., 2000. Substance use and misuse in psychiatric wards: a model task for clinical governance? Psychiatr. Bull. 24, 43–46.

WHO (World Health Organization), 1992. AUDIT: The Alcohol Use Disorders Identification Test. Guidelines for use in primary health care. <http://www.who.int>.

WHO (World Health Organization), 2004a. Global status report on alcohol. Department of Mental Health and Substance Abuse, WHO. <http://search.live.com/results.aspx? srch=106&FORM=AS6&q=WHO+al cohol+policy> (25.06.07.).

WHO (World Health Organization), 2004b. Alcohol Policy. Global Status Report. 25 June 2007, WHO, Geneva.

Ziedonis, D., Williams, J., 2003. Management of smoking in people with psychiatric disorders. Curr. Opin. Psychiatry 16 (3), 305–315.

Chapter | 20 |

Somatoform and dissociative disorders

Ruth Elder

CHAPTER POINTS

- The somatoform disorders are mental health problems that present as physical disorders.
- The somatoform disorders are not to be confused with malingering, which is the intentional production of symptoms to avoid some responsibility or duty.
- Somatization is a method of expressing anxiety and distress and is found in all cultural groups.
- The distress and suffering experienced by service users diagnosed with a somatoform disorder are real, although the medical basis for their symptoms is not.
- Service users diagnosed with a somatoform disorder are most frequently encountered in primary healthcare settings.
- The dissociative disorders are marked by an abrupt, temporary change in consciousness, cognition, memory, identity or behaviour.

DOI: http://dx.doi.org/10.1016/B978-0-7020-4493-9.00020-2

KEY TERMS

- amnesia
- conversion
- depersonalization
- derealization
- dissociation
- fugue
- hypochondriasis
- hysteria
- **la belle indifference**
- malingering
- medically unexplained symptoms
- neurosis
- primary gain
- reassurance
- secondary gain
- somatization

LEARNING OUTCOMES

The material in this chapter will assist you to:

- define somatoform and dissociative disorders,
- define key terms related to somatoform and dissociative disorders,
- distinguish disorders that present as physical disorders from malingering,
- describe the major conditions categorized as somatoform or dissociative disorders,
- describe the assessment of people diagnosed with somatoform and dissociative disorders,
- discuss interventions appropriate to people diagnosed with somatoform and dissociative disorders.

INTRODUCTION

The disorders discussed in this chapter are the somatoform disorders and dissociative disorders. In both groups of disorders, sufferers present complaining of physical symptoms, although no medical condition is found to exist. All these disorders as well as the anxiety disorders, phobias, compulsions and obsessions (see Ch. 17) and disorders of sexual functioning were once classified as 'neurotic reactions' or 'neurotic disorders'. The term *neurosis* is not widely used in *The ICD-10 Classification of Mental and Behavioural Disorders*, and is mainly of historical interest and can be found in a number of seminal texts on psychiatry. The concept of neurosis was developed in

1769 by William Cullen at Edinburgh University, who believed that madness was the result of excessive irritation of the nerves (Porter, 2002) and used the term to refer to nervous system disease. Since the time of Freud its meaning has changed to refer to a nonpsychotic disorder characterized mainly by anxiety. The disorders that fall under the label of neurosis are *ego-dystonic*; that is, the symptoms are experienced as distressing to the individual.

SOMATOFORM DISORDERS

The somatoform disorders (see Box 20.1) are a heterogeneous group of disorders the distinguishing characteristic of which is the presence of physical symptoms in the absence of a readily apparent medical condition. In order for the service user to be diagnosed as suffering from a somatoform disorder the symptoms cannot be fully accounted for by a physical disease or another mental disorder, or the effects of drugs or medication. There is usually no evidence of injury. However, these disorders are often confused with actual physical disorders and the service user suffering from them truly believes they are physically ill. The symptoms cause the afflicted person significant distress and can interfere with their normal functioning. Although no medical condition exists, hospitalization can occur, and numerous diagnostic tests and even surgery are performed (Clarke and Smith, 2001). These disorders well illustrate how 'suffering and illness are only indirectly related to the presence or absence of disease' (Epstein et al., 1999, p. 221).

The somatoform disorders should be distinguished from *malingering*. The physical symptoms are not fabricated intentionally, whereas in malingering there is the intentional production of symptoms in order to avoid some specific duty or responsibility. In malingering, the incentive for the person to become sick is clearly identifiable. For example, the person might be required to stand trial, or wants to evade the police, or is simply looking for a bed for the night.

The symptoms that accompany the disorders are referred to as either *somatization* or, more commonly now, *medically unexplained symptoms* (MUS). In general health settings they are referred to as functional, which means they have no organic basis. The syndromes (see Box 20.2) derived from the symptoms tend to be chronic, although the common symptoms that characterize them are highly prevalent in the population at large (such as fatigue, weakness, sleeping difficulties, headache, muscle and joint aches/pains, problems with memory, attention and concentration, anxiety and depression, nausea, shortness of breath and dizziness; Barsky and Borus, 1999). In the various syndromes, the symptoms tend to accrue over time rather than clustering simultaneously (Escobar, 1996).

Box 20.1 Diagnostic criteria for the somatisation/somatoform disorders

The main features are multiple, recurrent and frequently changing physical symptoms, which have usually been present for several years before the patient is referred to a psychiatrist. Most patients have a long and complicated history of contact with both primary and specialist medical services, during which many negative investigations or fruitless operations may have been carried out. Symptoms may be referred to any part or system of the body, but gastrointestinal sensations (pain, belching, regurgitation, vomiting, nausea, etc.), and abnormal skin sensations (itching, burning, tingling, numbness, soreness, etc.) and blotchiness are among the commonest. Sexual and menstrual complaints are also common. Marked depression and anxiety are frequently present and may justify specific treatment.

The course of the disorder is chronic and fluctuating, and is often associated with long-standing disruption of social, interpersonal and family behaviour. The disorder is far more common in women than in men, and usually starts in early adult life. Dependence upon or abuse of medication (usually sedatives and analgesics) often results from the frequent courses of medication.

Diagnostic guidelines

A definite diagnosis requires the presence of all of the following:

a. at least 2 years of multiple and variable physical symptoms for which no adequate physical explanation has been found;
b. persistent refusal to accept the advice or reassurance of several doctors that there is no physical explanation for the symptoms;
c. some degree of impairment of social and family functioning attributable to the nature of the symptoms and resulting behaviour.

Differential diagnosis

In diagnosis, differentiation from the following disorders is essential.

Physical disorders

Patients with long-standing somatization disorder have the same chance of developing independent physical disorders as any other person of their age, and further investigations or consultations should be considered if there is a shift in the emphasis or stability of the physical complaints which suggests possible physical disease.

Affective (depressive) and anxiety disorders

Varying degrees of depression and anxiety commonly accompany somatization disorders, but need not be specified separately unless they are sufficiently marked and persistent as to justify a diagnosis in their own right. The onset of multiple somatic symptoms after the age of 40 years may be an early manifestation of a primarily depressive disorder.

Hypochondriacal disorder

In somatization disorders the emphasis is on the symptoms themselves and their individual effects, whereas in hypochondriacal disorder attention is directed more to the presence of an underlying progressive and serious disease process and its disabling consequences. In hypochondriacal disorder the patient tends to ask for investigations to determine or confirm the nature of the underlying disease, whereas the patient with somatization disorder asks for treatment to remove the symptoms. In somatization disorder there is usually excessive drug use, together with noncompliance over long periods, whereas patients with hypochondriacal disorder fear drugs and their side effects, and seek for reassurance by frequent visits to different physicians.

Delusional disorders

This covers schizophrenia with somatic delusions, and depressive disorders with hypochondriacal delusions. The bizarre qualities of the beliefs, together with fewer physical symptoms of more constant nature, are most typical of the delusional disorders.

Adapted from the World Health Organisation (1992) The ICD-10 Classification of Mental and Behavioural Disorders, pp. 129–130 with permission.

The word *somatoform*, which means 'having bodily form', has both Greek and Latin roots (Escobar et al., 2002). *Soma* is the Greek word for 'body', while *form* derives from the Latin *forma* meaning 'form' or 'shape'. The word is intended to convey the idea that a mental disorder or psychological problem can appear in the guise of somatic symptoms. This idea that a disease can take bodily form but actually reside in the mind derives, philosophically, from Western medicine's foundation in Cartesian dualism, which assumes a division between mind and body (Kirmayer, 1996). This framework also assumes that symptoms are psychological and/or physical

Allergy: multiple chemical sensitivity
Cardiology: atypical or noncardiac chest pain, mitral valve prolapse
Dentistry: temporomandibular joint dysfunction, atypical facial pain
Ear, nose and throat: tinnitus, dizziness, globus syndrome
Gastroenterology: irritable bowel syndrome, non-ulcer dyspepsia
Gynaecology: premenstrual syndrome, chronic pelvic pain
Infectious diseases: chronic (postviral) fatigue syndrome (CFS)
Internal medicine: CFS, chronic Lyme disease, hypoglycaemia, chronic candidiasis
Military medicine: Gulf (Persian) War syndrome
Occupational medicine: multiple chemical sensitivity, sick building syndrome
Orthopaedics: carpal tunnel syndrome, low back pain, herniated disc
Neurology: tension headache
Plastic surgery: silicone-associated connective tissue disease
Rehabilitation medicine: repetitive strain injury, chronic whiplash
Respiratory medicine: hyperventilation syndrome, dyspnoea, habit cough, laryngeal dysfunction
Rheumatology: fibromyalgia, fibrositis

Sources: Adapted from Escobar et al. (2002) and Wessely et al. (1999).

defects that reside within the service user, and the possibility that they may be situationally caused is not generally entertained. This division of mental disorders into either physical or emotional means that it is very common for service users diagnosed with a somatoform disorder to be diagnosed with a comorbid anxiety and/or mood disorder. For example, somatization disorder commonly coexists with anxiety disorders (34%), depression (55%), personality disorders (61%) and panic disorders (26%) (Bass and Tyrer, 2000; Clarke and Smith, 2001; Holloway and Zerbe, 2000; Kipen and Fiedler, 2002). Hypochondriasis often occurs in conjunction with panic disorder (Hardy et al., 2001). Mood, anxiety and personality disorders are common in service users diagnosed with body dysmorphic disorder (BDD; Veale et al., 1996). Castillo (1997, p. 190) argues that the diagnostic practice of distinguishing between physical and mental disorders is an outcome of a disease-centred paradigm 'which assumes that each symptom cluster has a separate biological cause that can best be treated with separate medications'.

Unlike many of the other major mental disorders, the somatoform group are not linked by shared aetiologies, family histories or other factors, but through their

manifestation as an organic problem (Morrison, 1995). Although the ICD-10 (World Health Organisation (WHO) 1992) classifies the somatoform disorders separately from the anxiety disorders, service users with a somatoform disorder are also, as noted above, often anxious or depressed (Clarke and Smith, 2001). Clinically, therefore, the disorders can be very hard to distinguish from one another. At one time all the somatoform disorders fell under the heading of 'hysteria' (Kirmayer and Robbins, 1991 cited in McWhinney et al., 1997) (see Ch. 2 for a discussion of the origins of the term hysteria). Throughout the eighteenth century hysteria was generally believed to be a malady that affected mainly women (Shorter, 1994). During the second half of the nineteenth century, hysteria was one of the most commonly diagnosed mental disorders (Castillo, 1997).

The original conception of hysteria allowed for the presence of emotional symptoms. Not only did it encompass the common somatic symptoms of paralyses and anaesthesias, generalized aches and pains, and visual disturbances, but it was also characterized by anxiety and panic, depressive and dissociative symptoms and perceptual disturbances such as hallucinations.

The somatoform disorders, and somatization disorder in particular, need to be distinguished from somatization as a process which nearly everyone engages in from time to time. This process is the topic of the next section.

The process of somatization

Somatization was first introduced into the lexicon of psychiatry by the German psychoanalyst Wilhelm Stekel in the early 1900s (Lipsitt, 2001). He used the term to refer to symptoms similar to those of conversion disorder. Over time it has come to characterize the psychological process whereby anxiety or psychological conflict is translated into physical complaints, although no mechanism has been found. These complaints might be pain, such as a headache, or reflect a concern with bodily functions such as elimination.

Somatization is extremely common, so common in fact as to be a part of normal experience (Singh, 1998). Cross-cultural studies indicate that somatization is the most common means of expressing anxiety (Kirmayer 1984, cited in Castillo, 1997). Somatic symptoms are experienced by 80% of people in any 1 week (Merskey, 2000). For many people, somatization is a form of coping and is one of the characteristic responses of people who have suffered trauma (Punamaki et al., 2002). Somatoform symptoms are also common in refugees who have experienced severe trauma either in their countries of origin or during or after their flight (Waitzkin and Magaña, 1997). From a cross-cultural perspective also, there appears to be little reason for distinguishing among anxiety, somatoform and mood disorders (Castillo, 1998). In many cultures, illness is experienced holistically and no distinction is made between mental and physical illnesses. Finally, the expression of emotions in the form of bodily symptoms can occur when it is either difficult to put the feelings into words or when there are not the words with which to express psychological and emotional states (Singh, 1998).

Epidemiology

It has generally been thought that the somatoform disorders were relatively rare in the community as a whole. This belief was largely based on a US survey, the Epidemiological Catchment Area (ECA) Study, which found the lifetime prevalence of somatization disorder to be about 0.13% (Singh, 1998). However, a recent study by Baumeister and Härter (2007) suggests that at a 12-month prevalence rate of 11% in the general population, they occur frequently, and are the third-highest occurring disorders. Women outnumber men at a 5:1 ratio and the lifetime prevalence rate among women is 1–2% (Sadock and Sadock, 2005). In an Italian community sample, BDD was found to have a 1-year prevalence of 0.7% (Otto et al., 2001) and a point prevalence of 0.7% in a community sample of women aged 36–44 years (Otto et al., 2001). In a sample of female Turkish students, 4.8% were diagnosed with BDD (Cansever et al., 2003).

The somatoform disorders are usually encountered in primary healthcare settings, rarely mental health ones, which may go some way to explaining why they appear to have been of little interest to mental health nurses. In primary care settings no medical explanation can be given for the symptoms of about a third of service users (Escobar et al., 2002), which is not to say that all these service users may be diagnosed with a somatoform disorder, rather that unexplained somatic symptoms are exceedingly common. Between 5 and 9% of primary care patients exhibit hypochondriacal symptoms (Hardy et al., 2001).

The somatoform disorders can also assume great importance in certain clinical settings. For example, it has been estimated that as many as 50% of patients presenting with gastrointestinal symptoms have a functional disorder (Ringel and Drossman, 1999). In the UK as many as 4% of people attending neurology clinics suffer from a conversion disorder (Perkin 1989, cited in Halligan et al., 2000). In the USA 12% of patients in dermatological settings and 15% seeking cosmetic surgery were found to have BDD (Phillips et al., 2001).

Most of the somatoform disorders are more common in women than men (Sadock and Sadock, 2005), although hypochondriasis and BDD are roughly equally distributed between the sexes (Phillips and Castle, 2001). This distribution, for somatization disorder at least, might be an artefact of the diagnostic criteria. Kihlstrom and Kihlstrom (2001) argue that the DSM-IV TR effectively redefined somatization as a female disorder by requiring that there be one sexual or reproductive symptom. Somatization disorder and conversion disorder tend to be more common among the less educated and those on low incomes (Singh, 1998), although it has not always been so (Shorter, 1994). In the late nineteenth century, Morel, a French psychiatrist, and in the early twentieth century, Thomas Saville, a London neurologist, found hysteria and hypochondria to be equally distributed among the rich and the poor (Shorter, 1994).

Somatization disorder and BDD usually begin in adolescence (Patterson et al., 2001). Conversion disorder usually appears first in adolescence or early adulthood, but might occur at any time.

Aetiology

The causes of the somatoform disorders are unknown. However, somatization has been recognized since the ancient Egyptians (Sadock and Sadock, 2003), and BDD has been recognized for centuries. References to it can be found in Greek mythology, and European, Russian and Japanese literature (Biby, 1998). Theories about their possible origins can be divided roughly into two: those that consider the disorders to originate in organic structures and processes (*neurogenesis*) and those that believe they originate in mental phenomena (*psychogenesis*) (Shorter, 1994). The latter position reached its apotheosis in psychoanalytic doctrine in the first half of the twentieth century, but can be traced to the seventeenth-century physician Thomas Sydenham, who believed somatization to be a disease of the mind (Sharpe and Carson, 2001). The former position is much older, but was out of favour while psychoanalytic doctrine was dominant. The term hysteria itself, by focusing on a particular bodily function, namely the uterus, suggested a belief in its organic basis. However, Thomas Willis, a seventeenth-century neurologist, believed the symptoms derived from the head (Sharpe and Carson, 2001). Briquet, a nineteenth-century French physician, was convinced that hysteria had a genetic component (Shorter, 1994). He was among the first to believe that patients inherited psychosomatic illnesses. Pierre Janet (1903) also thought that the condition he termed *psychasthenia* was biological in origin (Shorter, 1994).

Psychodynamic theory

Psychodynamic theory explains somatization as an outcome of early life experiences and as a defence against psychological conflict (see Ch. 7). Emotions are expressed physically when they cannot be expressed verbally through either guilt or fear (Hardy et al., 2001).

Used as a defence mechanism, the service user stands to accrue a number of short-term advantages, which are referred to as primary and secondary gains. The *primary gain* is the decrease in anxiety which results from psychological pain and conflict. A physical symptom gives legitimacy to 'feeling bad'. Rather than changing the 'self', the problem is a body part. The *secondary gain* is the attention and support provided by others for a physical illness. Through physical conditions and symptoms the person might be able to avoid their obligations, such as going to work or doing the housework. For example, in conversion disorder the person who witnesses a fatal accident might develop blindness, as might a person who feels guilty about looking at erotic material. Keeping the upsetting material out of consciousness and thus helping reduce anxiety is the primary gain. Secondary gain is achieved when the symptom helps the person avoid a particular duty, for example in the case of a soldier who develops a paralysis of the hand and therefore cannot fire a gun.

The concepts of primary and secondary gains are not intended to imply that the symptoms are simulated or figments of the imagination: the symptoms are not 'all in the mind'. Service users really do experience the symptoms in the body.

Amplification

Amplification theory proposes that in some people normal bodily sensations are amplified or heightened. Some people simply may be hypersensitive to normal bodily stimuli and attribute pathological meaning to normal somatic sensations and functions (Hardy et al., 2001). Others, however, may become susceptible to media influence, public health campaigns or simple word of mouth, so symptoms that were previously ignored or dismissed are brought into awareness and assume new meaning (Barsky and Borus, 1999).

Interpersonal theory

Interpersonal theory has been used as an explanation for hypochondriasis. This theory suggests that children diagnosed with hypochondriasis model their behaviour on the responses to pain and illness they have observed in another family member or other adults who are ill. From an interpersonal perspective the antecedents of hypochondriasis are believed to be found in childhood adversity where early attachments have been marked by insecurity, which, in turn, produces persistent separation anxiety (Noyes Jr et al., 2002).

Developmental theory

Developmental theory suggests that translating psychological distress into physical symptoms is a learned response. The child may not have learnt adequate verbal and cognitive skills to express their psychological distress (Kirmayer and Looper, 2006). Parents may also model somatic behaviour, thus teaching it to their children.

Personality

Personality factors appear to be important in the genesis of the somatoform disorders. For example, the personality characteristics of anxiousness and fearfulness are commonly associated with these disorders (Bass and Tyrer, 2000). Furthermore, high numbers of service users with diagnoses of anxiety disorders or major depression suffer from the somatoform disorders.

Biological theories

There is as yet no strong evidence for any biological basis for the somatoform disorders, although a number of interesting hypotheses are being pursued. Sharpe and Carson (2001) suggest that new evidence supports the idea that the functional disorders are disturbances of the nervous system.

Behavioural theory

Both respondent and operant conditioning have been used to explain the somatoform disorders (Tazaki and Landlaw, 2006). In respondent conditioning, if a service user experienced a traumatic event (unconditioned stimulus) which led to their experiencing negative emotions such as fear or anger and these negative emotions were accompanied by physiological changes such as tachycardia and hyperventilation (conditioned response), then the future experience of the emotions alone may lead to the physiological changes. In operant conditioning, service users diagnosed with a somatoform disorder may have experienced positive consequences of their complaints of physical symptoms, such as attention and sympathy; or, through their complaints they may have avoided unpleasant consequences. Either experience could result in a conditioned response.

Familial factors

BDD has been found to be four times as prevalent in those who have first-degree relatives with the condition. For hypochondriasis, studies have indicated high rates of concordance for twins (Hardy et al., 2001).

Culture

According to Shorter (1994), culture is important in shaping perceptions of illness. In this theory, culture shapes illness behaviour by conferring legitimacy and, hence, respectability, to certain forms of behaviour. In Western cultures greater legitimacy is accorded somatic complaints, and both service users and doctors act to interpret symptoms as indicative of bodily, rather than psychological, processes.

Assessment

Service users diagnosed with a somatoform disorder are likely to present with somatic or physical symptoms, not emotional or psychological ones.

The first step in assessment is taking a comprehensive history. The point to keep in mind here is that it is the service user's concerns that are paramount, rather than the health professional's need to diagnose. Fischhoff and Wessely (2003, pp. 595–596) provide some questions that can help focus on the areas of concern to the service user, rather than the health professional.

- What decisions face them?
- What concerns weigh on them, including nonmedical issues (e.g. insurance, family)?
- What conflicting claims, beliefs and observations confuse them?
- What information, and misinformation, do they have already?
- Which knowledge gaps and misconceptions provide the greatest barrier to understanding?

It is useful to enquire as to any stresses in the service user's life at the time the symptom(s) first appeared. Depression and anxiety frequently accompany the somatoform disorders and somatic symptoms are often features of these disorders.

Service users with multiple somatic complaints are also likely to be severely functionally impaired (Hiller et al., 1997), so enquiries should be made about their activities of daily living, and their occupational and social functioning.

Somatization disorder

Somatization disorder is characterized predominantly by multiple physical complaints, and usually runs a chronic course (Bass and Tyrer, 2000; Escobar et al., 2002). People with unexplained somatic symptoms have usually sought medical treatment many times over many years (Maynard, 2003). The symptoms they present with tend to be multiple and recurring. They will often present in a dramatic way, providing vivid descriptions of the effect of the symptoms on their lives, but are vague about the details of the symptoms themselves. The most common symptoms service users complain about are headaches, abdominal distress, dizziness, palpitations, anxiety, consitipation or diarrhoea, depression or anxiety (Treatment Protocol Project, 2000).

Service users are often described as appearing anxious and/or angry. The distress service users experience should be treated as real, as should the experience of the symptoms. They are not lying or imagining their symptoms. The service user should be asked what they think has caused the symptoms, how the symptoms interfere with their everyday activities and how they handle them. Examples of helpful questions the nurse could ask the service user are listed in Box 20.3.

Communication is often impaired because there are sometimes gaps in the service user's history, and they are often inclined to overdramatize, to make false generalizations about what is happening to them from limited

---

Box 20.3 Helpful questions

Why do you think you are having this problem?
At what age did you start having this problem?
How do you feel about it?
How many healthcare providers have you seen over the past 5 years?
What do you consider to be the major stressors in your life now?
How does your body usually respond to stress?
Is there something that you fear is wrong with you?
What do you think would help your problem most right now?
How is this problem affecting your life?
If the problem cannot be cured, what would you consider to be reasonable goals?

Reprinted from Maynard C, 2003, Assess and manage somatization, Nurse Practitioner 28(4), with permission from Lippincott, Williams and Wilkins, http://www.lww.com

---

evidence and to oversimplify. They are also said to be very demanding of health professionals' time and attention, because despite the numerous negative tests they will not be reassured that there is nothing physically wrong with them. They may also express feelings of helplessness in the face of perceived failures on the part of health professionals to cure them and at the same time will usually refuse to see a psychiatrist or will simply ignore the referral. In contrast to service users diagnosed with other chronic disorders, such as rheumatoid arthritis or diabetes, Holloway and Zerbe (2000) report that service users diagnosed with somatization disorder tend to be passive with respect to finding a cure.

Most physicians (see, for example, Singh, 1998 and Barsky and Borus, 1999) advocate ruling out a physical cause for the service user's complaints before contemplating the possibility of a psychological cause for the symptoms. However, Epstein et al. (1999) argue that such a strategy simply prioritizes organic disease, and perpetuates the idea that there is a division between mental and physical phenomena.

It is often useful, if possible, to interview the service user's family and friends. They frequently report that they are tired of the service user's demands. They might describe the service user as so self-absorbed in their symptoms that they neglect important relationships and are no longer emotionally available.

Hypochondriasis

People diagnosed with hypochondriasis are intensely preoccupied with their bodily functions and report a wide range of symptoms. Whereas the service user diagnosed with somatization disorder is focused on the symptoms, the service user diagnosed with hypochondriasis is focused on what the symptoms might signify (Singh, 1998). They often misinterpret ordinary bodily functions such as gastric noises and sensations, or are intensely aware of their heartbeats and breathing and attribute them to a serious physical illness. They either fear or are convinced they have a serious illness, despite medical assurances to the contrary. While a type of somatoform disorder, hypochondriasis is also a frequent symptom in many mental health problems. Although most people diagnosed with hypochondriasis fear a physical illness, a very small number fear insanity. The symptoms experienced are not imaginary or simply 'all in their mind'.

People diagnosed with this disorder persistently try to elicit caring responses from their families and doctors. Unfortunately, their attempts are frequently met with withdrawal or withholding of care.

It is important to exclude symptoms of depression, anxiety and psychosis amongst people presenting with hypochondriacal symptoms. Physical disease also needs to be excluded. The service user often has a sound understanding of symptoms and medical terminology as a result of previous medical consultations. They frequently become upset when told that there is nothing wrong and reject outright psychological explanations of their problem. Careful assessment will often uncover a stressful event, such as the death of a close relative, which coincides with the onset of hypochondriacal behaviour.

Hypochondriacal behaviour often leads to a number of other behaviours designed to avoid or check for disease and which can interfere with normal functioning. For example, the service user may avoid exercise, develop rigid patterns of eating and drinking, and repeatedly inspect their body. Disturbances in sleeping patterns and increased feelings of anxiety because of worry about health are also experienced. There are often impairments in social and occupational functioning because work, university or important dates are frequently missed because of imaginary ills.

Pain disorder

Service users diagnosed with this disorder experience pain that either cannot be explained by any physiological findings or is described as grossly out of proportion to the condition of which the service user complains. Examples of some of the pain syndromes are listed in Box 20.4.

Box 20.4 Chronic pain syndromes

Trigeminal neuralgia
Burning mouth syndrome
Chronic pelvic pain
Fibromyalgia
Headaches
Cancer pain

A truly traumatic event such as a car accident can sometimes precipitate the disorder. For others, however, pain appears as a gradually increasing and entrenched facet of their lifestyle. Since the beginning of the twentieth century, psychogenic pain disorders have been on the increase, which, according to Meyer (1999), may be because it is far more difficult to attribute vague, diffuse pain symptoms to psychological causes.

A full physical assessment for pain disorder is needed, with particular attention paid to previous injuries or trauma. The service user's body should be examined for any physical abnormalities or changes. As with all the somatoform disorders it is useful to consider recent stresses in the service user's life and their usual ways of coping with them. The ways in which the pain has interfered with the service user's everyday functioning should also be considered.

Conversion disorder

Like most of the somatoform disorders, conversion disorder is typically diagnosed after organic pathology and malingering have been excluded and possible psychological stressors identified. The ICD-10 diagnostic criteria for conversion disorders are listed in Box 20.5. The service user may deny that they are consciously responsible for their symptoms. It is important to try to uncover recent stresses in the person's life that might have precipitated the symptoms. Examining what a symptom might represent can enhance understanding of their behaviour. For example, if the service user is 'blind' then it can be useful to consider what it might be that the service user does not wish to see. If the symptom is itchiness, then is there someone or something that the service user finds intensely irritating? If the service user complains of numbness, then there may be an event or person that has hurt them deeply. If the service user is seeking attention and asking to be taken care of, then consider whether there are responsibilities they wish to avoid.

CASE STUDY: PAULINE

Pauline is 19 years old. She has been diagnosed with chronic fatigue syndrome. About 2 years ago, while she was travelling home from school one afternoon, she felt overcome with nausea. When she got home she was weak and feverish; she had a sore throat, a headache, her joints ached and she had muscle tenderness. She went to see her local doctor, who confirmed a low-grade fever but was unable to find anything else wrong. Blood counts, X-rays and viral studies all proved negative. Over the next year, Pauline's condition did not improve. Her doctor referred her to a number of specialist physicians, none of whom were able to find anything wrong.

Box 20.5 Diagnostic criteria for the dissociative (conversion) disorders

The common theme shared by dissociative (or conversion) disorders is a partial or complete loss of the normal integration between memories of the past, awareness of identity, immediate sensations and control of bodily movements. There is normally a considerable degree of conscious control over the memories and sensations that can be selected for immediate attention, and the movements that are to be carried out. In the dissociative disorders it is presumed that this ability to exercise a conscious and selective control is impaired, to a degree that can vary from day to day or even from hour to hour. It is usually very difficult to assess the extent to which some of the loss of functions might be under voluntary control. These disorders have previously been classified as various types of 'conversion hysteria', but it now seems best to avoid the term 'hysteria' as far as possible, in view of its many and varied meanings.

Dissociative disorders are presumed to be 'psychogenic' in origin, being associated closely in time with traumatic events, insoluble and intolerable problems, or disturbed relationships. It is therefore often possible to make interpretations and presumptions about the individual's means of dealing within intolerable stress, but concepts derived from any one particular theory, such as 'unconscious motivation' and 'secondary gain', are not included among the guidelines or criteria for diagnosis. The term 'conversion' is widely applied to some of these disorders, and implies that the unpleasant affect, engendered by the problems and conflicts that the individual cannot solve, is somehow transformed into the symptoms. The onset and termination of dissociative states are often reported as being sudden, but they are rarely observed except during contrived interactions or procedures such as hypnosis or abreaction.

Change in or disappearance of a dissociative state may be limited to the duration of such procedures. All types of dissociative state tend to remit after a few weeks or months, particularly if their onset was associated with a traumatic life event. More chronic states, particularly paralyses and anaesthesias, may develop (sometimes more slowly) if they are associated with insoluble problems or interpersonal difficulties. Dissociative states that have endured for more than 1–2 years before coming to psychiatric attention are often resistant to therapy.

Individuals with dissociative disorders often show a striking denial of problems or difficulties that may be obvious to others. Any problems that they themselves recognize may be attributed by patients to the dissociative symptoms. Depersonalization and derealization are not included here, since in these syndromes only limited aspects of personal identity are usually affected, and there is no associated loss of performance in terms of sensations, memories or movements.

Diagnostic guidelines

For a definite diagnosis the following should be present:

a. the clinical features as specified for the individual disorders (such as amnesia, either partial or complete, for recent events that are of a traumatic or stressful nature, stupor, loss of ability to move the whole or a part of a limb or limbs and so forth);

b. no evidence of a physical disorder that might explain the symptoms;

c. evidence for psychological causation, in the form of clear association in time with stressful events and problems or disturbed relationships (even if denied by the individual).

Convincing evidence of psychological causation may be difficult to find, even though strongly suspected. In the presence of known disorders of the central or peripheral nervous system, the diagnosis of dissociative disorder should be made with great caution. In the absence of evidence for psychological causation the diagnosis should remain provisional, and enquiry into both physical and psychological aspects should continue.

Adapted from the World Health Organisation (1992) The ICD-10 Classification of Mental and Behavioural Disorders, pp. 122–123 with permission.

NURSE'S STORY: LISTENING TO A SERVICE USER'S PHYSICAL COMPLAINTS

We get quite a few patients in here (an orthopaedic ward) who often express their depression in physical complaints. For example, Mrs Taylor, who is 84 years old, broke her left hip about a month after the death of her husband. She's been in here 14 days now and we asked the doctor to see her because we were concerned about her lack of progress. She's really reluctant to get out of bed, always very anxious about falling again and tearful a lot of the time. She complains constantly about the pain and whimpers whenever we touch her. Her face screws up and she starts breathing really fast. We know she has some pain, but her complaints about it are out of proportion to what we would expect her to be experiencing at this time. She is also overly focused on her bowels. The problem here in part is that she is not eating very much and her fluid intake is also poor.

The way we manage her is to try and make sure that we listen to her before asking her to do anything. So in the morning, for example, when we want her to get up to go to the shower, we listen patiently to her for about 5 min and acknowledge what she says, before making the request. We let her make all her complaints. We don't say that she can't talk about her bowels or whatever, or that we won't listen to her if she starts complaining again, but we don't dwell on them. We find, then, that although she still pulls faces and makes exaggerated noises, she'll gather her toiletries, her clean clothes and go to the shower. We also ask if she wants some pain relief about half an hour before we want her to get out of bed. We are trying to let her know that we are listening to her, not just ignoring her, and that we will meet her need for pain relief as necessary.

In conversion disorder, which is characterized mainly by neurological symptoms, service users report a loss of or change in their motor or sensory function, such as weakness, paralysis, anaesthesia or memory loss, in the absence of a neurological or physical condition or positive findings. The paralyses or anaesthesias reported rarely follow known anatomical pathways and a paralysed limb often will be moved inadvertently. The conversion anaesthesia usually follows what is known as a stocking–glove distribution; the individual might complain that they are unable, for example, to feel pinpricks to their wrist or above the ankle. Some of the most common symptoms, apart from paralyses and anaesthesias, include blindness, seizures and uncoordinated walking. They may also complain of speech impairments or being unable to speak above a whisper, choking or difficulty swallowing, and tremors. The symptoms usually interfere with normal activities and can cause major disability. If the symptoms are prolonged and interfere with normal bodily functions, they can sometimes cause physiological damage. The service user might complain bitterly about the symptoms and yet display a remarkable degree of indifference to their symptoms, even if the symptom is blindness or paralysis. This lack of concern is known as *la belle indifference*, which means 'beautiful indifference'. Symptoms usually arise in response to particular, severe stressors.

CASE STUDY: JIM

Whenever Jim spent time with his fiancée he developed a headache. The headache left as soon as he was no longer in her presence. The headaches vanished altogether when he broke off the engagement.

Body dysmorphic disorder

Of all the somatoform disorders, body dysmorphic disorder (BDD), which is characterized by a distressing preoccupation with an imagined or slight defect in physical appearance, appears to have captured the most interest from nurses. It is often the case in service users diagnosed with BDD that the defect they complain about would not have been noticed unless they had drawn your attention to it. If there is a real defect, then the overwhelming distress experienced by the service user is out of proportion to the actual defect. The service user believes they are ugly or deformed. They cannot be reassured by others that there is nothing wrong or that the defect is slight or unnoticeable. People diagnosed with this disorder usually complain about defects to the face. These defects are either entirely imagined or highly exaggerated. Sometimes a real defect exists, but the person's concern about it is excessive. This preoccupation may have a delusional quality. Some authors have argued that BDD is related to, or a variant of, one of the nonsomatoform disorders, including psychosis, mood disorder, social phobia and obsessive–compulsive disorder.

Many service users diagnosed with BDD have a history of cosmetic surgery and, because the skin is the most common area of preoccupation, of having visited dermatologists in particular. The most common areas of preoccupation are skin (>60%), hair (>50%) and nose (approximately 40%) (Phillips 1991, cited in Patterson et al., 2001). The concerns most frequently identified are skin elasticity, skin colouring and perceived imperfections such as acne, moles, scarring and cellulite. Men diagnosed with the disorder usually become preoccupied with dermatological problems such as acne or scarring, hair loss or the dimensions of their nose or genitals (Phillips and Castle, 2001). When assessing a service user for this disorder, Hill (2006) suggests that the nurse ask the service user about whether they have undergone previous cosmetic procedures and enquire as to their thoughts and feelings about the outcomes. She also advises that it is important to ask the service user how long they spend worrying about their appearance.

CASE STUDY: MARIAN

Marian, a 32-year-old woman diagnosed with major depression, has been in an inpatient on a mental health ward for 4 days. She states that when she woke this morning she was unable to move her right arm. While relating this story to the nurse, she displays little concern for the symptom and states that she would be happy to see the doctor after she has had breakfast. Her arm hangs limply by her side. Marian had lost her job about 6 weeks before her admission and her ex-husband, who is overseas and used to beat her, is behind in providing monetary support for their two children, aged 4 and 6. Marian's parents, who visited Marian the previous evening, and who have been supporting Marian and her children, angrily demanded that she write to him to send money urgently.

Many service users will avoid social situations because they feel embarrassed and very self-conscious about their appearance. Consequently they can become house-bound and isolated. They have a poor self-image and are inclined to believe that a change in their appearance would markedly improve their lives.

Similarly to people diagnosed with obsessive–compulsive disorder (see Ch. 17), some service users can spend many hours a day performing repetitive activities such as checking themselves in the mirror, comparing themselves to others, grooming themselves, attempting to camouflage the imagined defect, picking their skin or seeking reassurance. These activities, like the imagined defect that led to their performance, can also lead to social isolation and occupational impairment.

This is not a trivial disorder, because large numbers of service users are hospitalized. Many service users diagnosed with BDD have suicidal ideation and some will attempt suicide; as many as 24% are successful (Veale et al., 1996).

There are a number of different types of BDD. One of these is *muscle dysmorphia*, a problem that occurs mainly in men who perceive themselves as small, or smaller than their true size, despite working out for many hours per day, and despite being very muscular. This disorder used to be referred to as 'reverse anorexia' or 'bigorexia'. The disorder is similar to anorexia (see Ch. 18) in that the person becomes obsessed with their body image and suffers from an actual perceptual distortion when they look in the mirror: they see themselves as much smaller than others do. This disorder affects a large number of men, but apparently only a small number of weightlifters (Olivardia, 2001).

Another variant of BDD is *apotemnophilia*, where the service user wishes to be an amputee. In 2000, two cases were reported in the UK where a surgeon had performed single-leg amputations on two service users who felt 'incomplete' with four limbs. Although the service users were reported to be very happy with the results, the hospital that employed the surgeon was not (Ramsay, 2000).

Interventions

Health professionals find service users suffering from any of the somatoform disorders among the most challenging to treat (Servan-Schreiber et al., 2000; Starcevic, 2002). Among the challenges is finding an acceptable treatment. Not surprisingly, people with one of the somatoform disorders are usually reluctant to undergo psychotherapeutic treatments when they believe their problems to be physiological. However, those treatments that have been shown to be effective for the management of anxiety and mood disorders are also often effective in the somatoform disorders (Simon, 2002). The next challenge is finding out whether the treatment really works. Most service users do not visit mental health professionals, and neither do they want to. The third challenge is resisting providing services the service user might want and that could harm them. The service user might want and demand a physical treatment such as surgery, that if provided will prove ineffective, not just at the physical level (the service user has no organic illness for which the treatment could be effective) but also at the psychological level: the treatment will neither improve the quality of their life nor change their behaviour. Hence a practical model for effectively working with service users is a biopsychosocial one (Epstein et al., 1999; Lyles et al., 2003).

The behaviours associated with these disorders tend to elicit negative responses from healthcare providers, who are inclined to be pessimistic about treatment outcomes, and whose distaste for and frustration with these service users has not always been well hidden. The unhelpful labels of 'demanding', 'manipulative', 'difficult' and 'uncooperative' are applied by some although, as Kihlstrom and Kihlstrom (2001) point out, frustration can arise from the health professional's inability to confirm the symptoms. Equally, however, service users are often dissatisfied with healthcare professionals, whom they resent and mistrust and whom, they often feel, have rejected them. This apparent stand-off between professionals and service users has resulted in an apparent mismatch between treatment strategies: those that benefit the professionals and the system, versus those that assist the service user. Because service users truly believe they have a physical illness, they are frequently dissatisfied with what they perceive to be their healthcare providers' failure to treat them properly. Compounding this perception is the fact that the treatments offered often will not have helped, so they are likely to present with a history of numerous medical attendances, and many are more likely to receive physical treatments. For example, service users diagnosed with BDD may receive dermatological and surgical treatment, even though the outcomes from dermatological and plastic surgery treatments are generally poor with this group of service users (Phillips et al., 2001). A service user-focused strategy would be one wherein symptoms are relieved, the service users are less concerned that they are ill, can engage in their usual activities of daily living, and enjoy a high quality of life.

While most of the interventions discussed in this section are directed towards service users, it is important that nurses also take care of themselves. In caring for these service users it is not uncommon for the nurse to feel useless, threatened, uncertain and fed-up. This care is important to ensure that the nurse can remain helpful to the service user. Nurses can care for themselves by ensuring balance in their lives but also by receiving ongoing supervision and informal support from colleagues for the care of these service users. Principles for intervening in somatization are outlined in Box 20.6.

The therapeutic relationship

The therapeutic relationship established between the nurse and the service user is the foundation of all interventions with service users diagnosed with a somatoform disorder (Epstein et al., 1999; Lyles et al., 2003). This relationship is often a long-term one, because service user progress tends to be slow and they are often resistant. However, the evidence points directly to the importance of the relationship in improving service user outcomes (Lyles et al., 2003), even though establishing the relationship can be difficult. The difficulty is in finding a common language with which to work (Clarke and Smith, 2001). The nurse needs to listen to the service user and try to understand the experiences from the service user's perspective. The nurse needs to understand the service user's explanatory model of their illness and their beliefs about health and disease. In order to do this effectively it is necessary to understand the service user's language. Service users may need to be asked what they mean by certain phrases such as 'chemical imbalance' (Epstein et al., 1999). It is also unhelpful to describe the service user's symptoms as somatization; it is more useful to be more concrete: for example, 'pounding in the chest'.

If possible, the relationship needs to shift its focus from the physical to the psychosocial (Singh, 1998), but this can take time and requires careful attention to cues from the service user that they are ready to talk about these issues. Acknowledging that the physical symptom is real to the service user but reducing the amount of time discussing physical complaints can help this process. It is also helpful to see the service user regularly for a set time, so the service user does not have to produce symptoms in order to receive attention (Servan-Schreiber et al., 2000). Scheduling more frequent visits initially – for example, weekly for 4–6 weeks and tapering off to monthly as the service user improves – can help build the relationship. In between visits, weekly telephone contact initiated by the nurse and independently of any symptoms the service user might be experiencing, can help avert potential problems. The nurse's initiative has been shown to help service users with medically unexplained symptoms 'shift their thinking toward managing symptoms rather than reacting to them' (Lyles et al., 2003, p. 67). These visits are also important in reassuring the service user that continued follow-up by the nurse will be sufficient to detect any organic illnesses should they arise. Nurses should accept and legitimize the service user's suffering, while exploring symptoms, pathological findings, life context and emotions (Epstein et al., 1999). Enhancing the service user's verbal communication skills can also develop the relationship. The service user can be helped to be clear and straightforward in their communication. Therapeutic groups, where service users receive feedback from their peers, can also be helpful.

The focus of the therapeutic relationship needs to be on the specific personal and social difficulties experienced by the service user, and working through possible solutions. The service user also needs to be encouraged to verbalize their fears and anxieties.

Reassurance

Great care needs to be taken in offering reassurance to service users. For service users diagnosed with BDD, reassurance is rarely helpful, although they seek it constantly (Patterson et al., 2001). Reassurance appears to be effective with service users who experience hypochondriacal symptoms and sometimes with some service users who have medically unexplained symptoms (MUS) (Holloway and Zerbe, 2000; Page and Wessely, 2003). Barsky and Borus (1999) argue that for service users with MUS reassurance should be limited and cautious. Service users can be told that they do not have a life-threatening illness but do have a serious health problem that can cause significant impairment (Servan-Schreiber et al., 2000). They can be told that although the cause of the symptoms is unknown the factors that help perpetuate them can be addressed (Treatment Protocol Project, 2000). These factors include stress, depression, insomnia and inactivity.

While most service users are reassured by negative results, if these are presented to service users with MUS in a way that suggests their 'illness' is in their head, then they may feel rejected. Negative results are not an explanation of why the service user feels as they do. It is important that the service user be given an explanation that fits their frame of reference. Empowering explanations are marked by 'a tangible, usually physical, causal mechanism [chemicals or neurones in the brain]; they exculpate the service user by attributing symptoms to causes for which the service user could not be blamed; and they involve the service user by invoking internal adjustment or suggesting external factor(s) that the service user could influence' (Salmon et al., 1999, p. 375).

Relief of symptoms

There is little agreement among authors about whether to focus on symptoms. Some argue that to focus on symptoms leads to their amplification and perpetuation (Barsky and Borus, 1999) or reinforcement (Servan-Schreiber et al., 2000). Others believe that such a focus shows compassion (Fischhoff and Wessely, 2003). Overall, it seems that a balance needs to be achieved and a distinction made between people diagnosed with a somatoform disorder and those who have somatic symptoms. The reality of the symptoms for the service user needs to be acknowledged: they can be told that the symptoms are not 'all in their head'. The focus, over the long term, should be on the service user, their beliefs and expectations, their everyday functioning, and how the symptoms interfere with their functioning rather than the symptoms themselves (Epstein et al., 1999; Escobar, 1996; Maynard 2003; Servan-Schreiber et al., 2000). In this way, unwittingly reinforcing the symptoms by challenging them and thus making them the centre of the therapeutic encounter can be avoided. Simon (2002) argues for a rehabilitative rather than biomedical approach that focuses on how best to live with symptoms.

However, it is important to focus on relieving the symptoms as much as possible. Such relief may be provided through carefully listening to the service user's history and acknowledging uncertainty. Naming the condition (Fischhoff and Wessely, 2003; Starcevic, 2002) has also proved helpful. Service users generally do not want to be told, 'There is nothing wrong with you' or 'You have no illness'. These statements serve only to heighten the service user's concerns. Instead, a concrete rendering of their symptoms is needed, which might involve saying, 'Your headaches are a result of the stress you've been experiencing at work leading you to tense your muscles'.

Cognitive behavioural therapy

For service users who attend mental health professionals, cognitive behavioural therapy (CBT) has proved effective (Sharpe and Carson, 2001). Cognitive behavioural interventions have been found to reduce the intensity and frequency of somatic complaints (Servan-Schreiber et al., 2000). CBT aims to help the service user modify the thoughts that reinforce their symptoms (see Ch. 23 for a discussion of CBT). A basic premise is that the service user's beliefs are false. There are numerous techniques that aim to overcome false beliefs. For example, the service user can be taught about the relationship between cognitive beliefs and physiological responses. For example, simply believing that one is in danger can stimulate the sympathetic responses that raise blood pressure and heart rate (Hardy et al., 2001). Service users also can be encouraged to formulate alternative explanations for their experience of bodily symptoms. They can be encouraged

to write a list for and against the chances of having a particular disease (Hardy et al., 2001). There is often a physiological explanation for a service user's symptoms that the service user can be educated about. For example, the service user may be unaware of how stress can lead to muscular tension in their neck and shoulders that, in turn, can give rise to headaches. These types of explanation can also be used to help overcome the service user's belief that the mind and body are separate; for example, a preoccupation with bodily functions can lead to anxiety, which can lead to hyperventilation, which can produce a tingling in the fingers.

Some service users with a diagnosis of hypochondriasis may be helped by insight therapy or explanatory therapy (Hardy et al., 2001). This therapy seeks to help service users understand the origin of their symptoms, which might be an earlier traumatic event that led to an intense focus on bodily symptoms.

Therapies that focus on the body, such as relaxation, exercise, physiotherapy and massage, are often well accepted by service users (Epstein et al., 1999). These therapies are also useful in helping reduce anxiety. Sometimes training the service user in assertiveness and general social skills, so they learn to ask for what they want clearly and directly, can help the service user cope better. The service user's new abilities with these skills also provide opportunities to reward them with praise and support, helping undermine their previous dependence on gaining support from physical symptoms.

Behaviour therapy has a place especially in the treatment of those service users who achieve secondary gains from their symptoms. However, it is also useful when the service user agrees that whatever they have been doing about the symptoms has not been successful so far. The service user's beliefs can be challenged gently.

CBT is also useful in helping service user's diagnosed with BDD develop a more realistic picture of themselves. It can also help the service user resist the urge to engage in compulsive behaviours such as checking their appearance in the mirror, and face social situations that were previously avoided (Patterson et al., 2001).

Psychopharmacology

Medications have a place in the treatment of coexisting mental health problems such as depression and anxiety. Careful education about side effects is necessary so that the service user does not discontinue the medication through misattribution of symptoms to side effects of the medication (Holloway and Zerbe, 2000). They also have a role in the treatment of real physical illnesses, but care needs to be taken with those medications that somatizing service users are apt to over-use, such as anti-anxiety agents, analgesics and hypnotics (Clarke and Smith, 2001), which also have the potential to be addictive. If they are prescribed, then they are administered for a specific time over a specific period: for example, an analgesic might be prescribed for the first 2 days of the menstrual period. In pain disorder, the medications used for pain tend to be limited to aspirin and nonsteroidal anti-inflammatory agents.

Antidepressants have been shown to be beneficial in the MUS syndromes, even in the absence of a depressive disorder (Kroenke and Swindle, 2000; Simon, 2002). They have also proved efficacious in the treatment of the various functional pain syndromes (Singh, 1998).

Successful treatment of BDD with the tricyclic antidepressant imipramine has been reported (Fontenelle et al., 2002). The selective serotonin-reuptake inhibitor (SSRI) antidepressants are also used. Clomipramine, fluoxetine and fluvoxamine have all been used effectively (Phillips, 1995). These medications appear to help by reducing the distressing preoccupation with the body and its associated depression and anxiety. They are especially helpful in cases where the person has attempted suicide. Patterson et al. (2001) suggest that service users diagnosed with BDD can be helped to accept medication by telling them that it will help with their feelings of distress and demoralization about their appearance.

Support

Many of the somatoform disorders are chronic; therefore it is unlikely that the service user will be cured. In these cases a number of mental health professionals suggest that care, rather than cure, is the appropriate intervention model (Holloway and Zerbe, 2000; Singh, 1998). Kroenke and Swindle (2000, p. 206) have termed this the 'hand-holding' approach; that is, 'regularly scheduled visits with a primary care provider, limited subspecialty referrals or diagnostic testing, legitimation of the service user's complaints and sustained reassurance'. Nurses especially can play an important role by visiting or phoning service users regularly and spending time listening to the service user's concerns. This routine can help minimize the service user's need to develop new symptoms in order to get the support and attention they crave. The goal is to help the service user express their emotional conflicts verbally and to reduce, if not eliminate entirely, their reliance on expressing them in physical complaints.

Supportive therapies are usually the treatment of choice for people diagnosed with hypochondriasis. Communication needs to be simple, straightforward and clear. The results of all laboratory tests and screening procedures need to be told to the service user. The condition needs to be fully explained. The service user should be told they have a fear of disease, and what this means should be discussed with them. Service users will often vacillate between accepting and rejecting the diagnosis. This vacillation means they will need to be seen supportively for some time. Some service users may never fully accept the diagnosis, so long-term education will be in order.

Family involvement

It is also useful to involve the family in treatment if possible. The family can be educated about the disorder, especially with a view to helping them understand what their contribution to the realization of secondary gains might be. They can also be enlisted in helping the service user avoid unnecessary treatments and surgery, and to respond supportively without recourse to talking about disease. They can be taught to help get the service user to exercise and avoid inactivity. They can learn to respond supportively without encouraging 'pain' or 'disease' (Katon 1993, cited in Meyer, 1999, pp. 81–82).

Validation

Validation has been found to be a useful strategy with service users with a diagnosis of hypochondriasis. There is no point in telling service users that their symptoms are imaginary and that they must give them up. As Starcevic (2002) argues, service users with a diagnosis of hypochondriasis need to feel accepted. He suggests that we can convey acceptance by validating the service user's experience. He provides the following examples of validating statements:

- 'It is reasonable to concentrate so much on your body when it keeps sending you signals,'
- 'I understand why you're listening to your body, as the body seems to be trying to tell you something, and perhaps only you can make some sense of it, despite what the doctors tell you,'
- 'You seem to be expressing something through symptoms that are difficult to understand, but the language of symptoms is yours and the one with which you are now trying to communicate as best as you can' (Starcevic, 2002, p. 172).

Rather than telling the service user, 'You are a hypochondriac', it can be helpful to reframe the diagnosis as 'excessive worry about health' or 'fear of illness' (Hardy et al., 2001). This reframing can also help overcome potential service user resistance to understanding their behaviour as hypochondriacal. If an alternative rational explanation is available for a service user's symptoms, then it should be given. For example, a 'pounding heart' is a normal response to exertion, not a sign of heart disease.

Reality therapy

Reality therapy or confrontation–insight therapy has had some limited success with service users diagnosed with pain disorder. The therapy involves confronting the service user with the fact that there is no plausible reason for their pain, but there are 'rewards'. This type of confrontation is not intended to be conflictual, or to drive the service user away from therapy.

Lifestyle interventions

Servan-Schreiber et al. (2000) recommend physical exercise for 20 min three times a week for service users who believe they are physically impaired. The service user should be encouraged to get moving psychologically and physically (Katon 1993, cited in Meyer 1999, pp. 81–82). Inactivity and rest tend to be counterproductive in that the service user might then ruminate on their symptoms.

CRITICAL THINKING CHALLENGE 20.1

How do you think you might react to service users who seem to be always complaining about physical symptoms that you know are not real? If you think you might feel angry or frustrated, can you identify why you might feel that way?

DISSOCIATIVE DISORDERS

The dissociative disorders are functional disorders in that they are not caused by direct damage to the brain, whether through disease or injury or other physical insult. They are generally considered to occur very rarely, although there is little in the way of strong data about incidence and prevalence rates. It might simply be, as Simeon (2004) suggests, that they are rarely diagnosed, because they are poorly recognized. Simeon (2004) cites one study which rates the prevalence of depersonalization disorder at 2.4%, which is similar to the prevalence of schizophrenia, and states the ratio of males to females as 1:1 and the age of onset as 16 years. Dissociative identity disorder was once considered exceedingly rare, although during the late 1970s and 1980s it was more frequently diagnosed, especially in North America.

Previously, the dissociative disorders were known as hysterical neuroses of the dissociative type. They are marked by an abrupt, temporary change in consciousness, cognition, memory, identity or behaviour. Service users suffering from one of these disorders frequently report that they suddenly cannot remember important events or aspects of their own identity such as who they are or how old they are. Many studies demonstrate

a relationship between traumatic events, whether in childhood or more recently, and dissociative phenomena. Such events include physical and sexual abuse or assault, childhood neglect and death of family members. Dissociation as a response to trauma is considered a coping mechanism; that is, it provides a means for the person to physically, emotionally or cognitively absent themselves from the traumatic situation. However, the link between trauma and dissociation is not clear cut, because trauma in itself does not necessarily lead to dissociation (Kihlstrom, 2005).

Pierre Janet (1889, cited in Witztum and van der Hart, 1998), in the early part of the twentieth century, first conceptualized the dissociative disorders as forms of 'splitting off' or dissociating parts of consciousness. Certain parts of the personality were considered to separate from the habitual personality and slip outside the control of conscious awareness. These personality parts could then assume a life of their own. However, it was Freud who developed the idea of a dynamic unconscious, where emotions and ideas unacceptable to the person were kept out of awareness or repressed. The person is thus protected from the anxiety and emotional pain associated with psychological conflicts or other disturbing circumstances by compartmentalizing and 'forgetting' the unpleasant material.

Amnesia is a feature of dissociative amnesia, dissociative fugue and dissociative identity disorder. To the outside observer, who is not aware of the presence of a disorder, the person might appear to be functioning entirely normally. Unlike service users with amnesia related to dementia or other organic processes, there is rarely confusion or disorganized behaviour.

Similarly to the somatoform disorders and the process of somatization, the dissociative disorders and the process of dissociation need to be distinguished. The experience of mild dissociation is very common, occurring in more than 95% of the world's cultures, and is most often considered normal (Kleinman, 1996, p. 23). Nearly everyone experiences dissociation at some time or another. For example, a person might be driving somewhere and, while focused on their own internal thoughts, might be unaware of what is happening around them. They then suddenly realize that they can't remember driving during the previous few minutes, or they might find themselves driving to work instead of to a friend's house. Daydreaming is a very mild form of dissociation. Another form of dissociation is when we are surprised at how quickly time has gone by when we 'get lost' in a book or some other enjoyable activity. Hypnosis is an example of a dissociative state produced in normal people.

Two particular types of dissociation are depersonalization and derealization. *Depersonalization* involves a 'disrupted integration of self-perceptions with the sense of self' (Simeon, 2004). Subjectively, the person feels estranged, detached or disconnected from their own being. Depersonalization is often a symptom in numerous other mental health problems and physical illnesses, such as panic attacks and schizophrenia. Many people without such problems also experience depersonalization during periods of anxiety or stress (Clarke and Smith, 2001), and sometimes when intoxicated, but they usually continue to function and do not feel overwhelmed by it. This conception of depersonalization needs to be distinguished from that used to describe the behaviours of distancing oneself from others or from one's work, or of treating others as objects, that some healthcare workers, particularly nurses, adopt as a means of coping with the high level of work-based stress known as burnout.

Depersonalization is often accompanied by the experience of *derealization*, which is another, related, phenomenon whereby the person's sense of the object world is altered. The person might perceive objects to be bigger or smaller than they really are, or once-familiar objects might now seem strange.

Dissociative amnesia

This disorder is sometimes referred to as *psychogenic amnesia*. Service users diagnosed with dissociative amnesia are suddenly aware that they are unable to remember autobiographical, past events, which are usually of a particularly stressful or traumatic nature, during a particular period. It has been extensively documented among soldiers who have been in combat (Witztum and Maragalit, 2002). The most common form is *localized amnesia*, where the person forgets the events of a few hours to a few days. This type of amnesia can occur in people who might have survived a car crash in which another family member has been killed (APA, 2000). *Selective amnesia* is the failure to recall some, but not all, events during a short period of time; for example, an abused child might remember only some of the events connected to abusive episodes. *Generalized amnesia* is the loss of a whole lifetime's memories. *Systematized amnesia* is the loss of memory for a specific category of information: for example, all memories relating to a particular person.

Primary and secondary gains can also be associated with amnesia. The soldier who forgets the horrors witnessed during combat protects himself from painful emotions, as does the mother who forgets the car accident in which her children were killed.

Dissociative fugue

Dissociative fugue is a very rare disorder and is most likely to occur after a critical event. The amnesia associated with this disorder encompasses the whole or a very large part of the person's life. A service user diagnosed with this disorder suddenly and unexpectedly travels far away, often thousands of miles from home. The journey can last from a few hours to many days, and sometimes several months, at a time. The dissociated part of the personality appears to take control of the person's life. The person is unable to remember their past. They may also be confused about their identity, unable to remember their name or their occupation. A very small number adopt a new identity.

Other types of trauma might also be seen, such as war experiences. Families may also report that there have been times when the service user has mysteriously disappeared for varying periods of time and/or been found in places some distance from their homes. Families may also be able to provide information about trauma or stressful situations previously experienced by the service user. Family and friendship relations in general may have become highly disrupted because of the service user's apparent abrupt withdrawal.

Dissociative identity disorder

Dissociative identity disorder (or DID), a rare disorder that is often severe and chronic, is most popularly known by its former name of multiple personality disorder. It has sometimes been confused in the popular imagination with schizophrenia, to which it is not related. Service users diagnosed with this disorder have at least two distinct personalities. Neither or none of the personalities should be confused with having imaginary playmates. The development of autonomous personalities appears to resolve deep-seated conflicting beliefs and desires, because the alternate personalities often have characteristics quite different to those of the core or host personality. The transition or switching from one personality to another is rapid and the core personality usually forgets or is unaware of the existence of the others, although the host is often aware that they have lost time or that there are periods of blackout. The alternate personalities, however, are usually aware of the core personality. The alternate personalities are relatively self-contained, having their own set of roles and relationships distinct from those of the core personality, and are in control at different times or situations. The alternate personalities allow the person to cope in situations or with events that the core personality finds overwhelming.

The classic story of split personality is Robert Louis Stevenson's *Dr Jekyll and Mr Hyde* (Stevenson, 1925). *Sybil* (Schreiber, 1975) and *The Three Faces of Eve* (Thigpen, 1960) were two best-selling books about this disorder that were also made into films, which helped further popularize this condition. Despite this popularity, however, little is known about the incidence of this disorder. It is overwhelmingly a disorder of females, with 90% of cases occurring in women and most of these in the USA (Meyer, 1999). People diagnosed with this disorder

CASE STUDY: MARLA

Marla was a 23-year-old doctor's receptionist who failed to return to work from lunch one day. She had been working for the doctor for 6 months and there had been no indication that anything was wrong. Ten days later she was found in a small town 600 miles away. She had been taken in by a woman who had been unable to find out her name, but was concerned because 'she seemed so confused'. Marla's true identity became known when she suddenly 'came to'. She was unable to account for how she had come to the town. In therapy it emerged that Marla had suffered physical abuse by her stepfather from the age of 8 until 14, when he died.

rarely seek treatment. If they become known to mental health professionals, it is usually because they may have attempted suicide or are suffering from another disorder, usually major depression or schizophrenia.

This condition is also most likely the one that service users suffer from when they are believed to be 'possessed' or, in some cultures such as India, where there is an expectation of possession. In some other cultures, such as Indonesia, Malaysia and Latin America, as well as India, dissociative disorders are associated with trance states, which are usually induced and which are not usually associated with distress or dysfunction.

A history of childhood physical or sexual abuse or neglect is common in service users' backgrounds who have been diagnosed with dissociative identity disorder. Common symptoms of dissociation include headaches, switching, mood swings, time lapses, auditory hallucinations, intrusive memories and anxiety (McAllister, 2000). Seemingly innocuous triggers such as certain fruits, sounds or colours can start the dissociative process. The person will usually have experienced a loss of time and be unable to recall events from when the alternate personality dominated. Some service users diagnosed with dissociative identity disorder also suffer from an eating disorder or are dependent on substances.

Depersonalization disorder

When a service user experiences one or more episodes of feelings of unreality or their feelings of depersonalization become persistent or recurrent, then the person may be suffering from *depersonalization disorder*. The service user's sense of their personal reality is lost or altered, such that they feel estranged from themselves, as if they are in a dream, or feel 'spaced out', or that their actions are mechanical, or that they are otherwise detached from their body or mind. The core symptoms of the disorder are emotional numbing, visual derealization and altered body experience (Simeon 2004, p. 346). People

diagnosed with this disorder often report that they feel they are 'going crazy' and are often highly anxious. Time and space can feel distorted. Their symptoms may have arisen in response to severe stress and there may be a history of strenuous attempts to adjust. Service users might be reluctant to reveal their symptoms for fear that they will be thought crazy or will not be understood, or they may lack the words to describe their experiences (Simeon, 2004). Many will be highly distressed. In order to be diagnosed with this disorder the feelings must not have been induced by drugs, although marijuana, hallucinogens, ecstasy and ketamine have all been implicated in precipitating the disorder (Simeon, 2004).

Assessment

As with the somatoform disorders, underlying organic pathology, such as brain tumour or temporal lobe epilepsy, must be ruled out. The focus of assessment will be identity, memory and consciousness. Although the symptoms appear abruptly, often in response to severe stress, sometimes a history of emotional and/or physical abuse and trauma can be uncovered. These disorders have the potential to interfere with social and occupational functioning, so these aspects are worth exploring. Like the somatoform disorders, the dissociative disorders need to be distinguished from malingering.

Interventions

Currently available information about the treatment of the dissociative disorders is largely reliant on case reports and the experiences of clinicians (Maldonado et al., 2002). The dissociative disorders are difficult to manage, and interventions tend to be targeted at troublesome symptoms. The interventions in this section will usually be applicable to all the dissociative disorders, although exceptions and particular cases will be identified. First and foremost among the interventions is the development of a sound therapeutic relationship. Such a relationship is crucial, as progress is often slow and long-term, and because these disorders are often poorly recognized the relationship is necessary to forming a diagnosis. The significance of a diagnosis is that it can bring profound relief by helping the service user realize that they are not suffering alone. In some cases, psychodynamically orientated psychotherapy might be offered (see Ch. 23). However, this form of treatment is usually outside the expertise of most nurses. Hypnotic techniques are still used with DID and are most likely to be provided by hypnotherapists (see below). Drugs may be used to treat any coexisting disorders, especially depression and anxiety, but there are none specific to the dissociative disorders. Nursing interventions will be psychotherapeutically orientated and will target social and environmental supports, advocating and teaching stress-reduction strategies and skill-acquisition strategies where necessary (see Ch. 23). For the highly anxious service user, techniques such as relaxation training, breathing exercises and meditation, which can ease their level of arousal, can be helpful; for the service user with lower levels of arousal, more intensely stimulating techniques such as exercise can prove helpful.

If there is a history of childhood abuse, then the service user can benefit from being able to disclose the abuse and their feelings about the abuse in a nonjudgemental, safe environment. Sometimes their lost memories can be recovered through hypnosis (Degun-Mather, 2002), deep relaxation techniques (see Ch. 23) or free association (McAllister, 2000). Hypnosis involves inducing a trance in the service user. In the trance, service users can recall to consciousness memories that were once lost and some can regress to earlier stages of development (Sadock and Sadock, 2003). Free association was a technique developed by Freud. The fundamental rule guiding the technique is that the service user tells the analyst whatever comes into their mind. Inevitably, however, the service user censors the material, usually unconsciously through the defence mechanism of repression, sometimes consciously, as when the service user feels embarrassed. This censoring is known as 'resistance' and becomes the focus of the therapeutic encounter.

Some service users are receptive to explanations that their dissociative disorder is psychogenic in origin. For example, a service user can be told that they have blocked out events that would be too stressful or traumatic to bear consciously (Degun-Mather, 2002). They can also be told that this is a natural defence against pain.

The family is often included in therapy where possible. Such therapy can help the family learn new ways of interacting with the service user, so they no longer reinforce any secondary gains the service user is achieving.

CRITICAL THINKING CHALLENGE 20.2

Do you believe that simply listening to a service user diagnosed with one of the somatoform or dissociative disorders can be helpful to the service user? Why or why not?

In what way can dissociation serve to protect a service user from overwhelming anxiety?

CONCLUSION

In this chapter the somatoform and dissociative disorders have been discussed. The somatoform disorders are mental health problems that present as physical disorders. Service users diagnosed with these disorders often prove difficult to treat because they perceive their problems as physical, not psychological. Somatization is an extremely common means of communicating anxiety and some members of all cultural groups express their distress in this way. The dissociative disorders are marked by an abrupt, temporary change in consciousness, cognition, memory, identity or behaviour.

EXERCISES FOR CLASS ENGAGEMENT

In a group, discuss how you might respond to a service user who insists that the dyspepsia she experiences is cancer and not related to the problems she is experiencing in her marriage and at work.

Discuss the advantages and disadvantages of excluding physical causes for a service user's symptoms before considering possible psychological reasons.

REFERENCES

APA (American Psychiatric Association), 2000. Diagnostic and Statistical Manual of Mental Disorders, fourth ed. text rev. American Psychiatric Association, Washington DC.

Barsky, A.J., Borus, J.F., 1999. Functional somatic syndromes. Ann. Intern. Med. 130 (11), 910–921.

Bass, C., Tyrer, P., 2000. The somatoform conundrum: a question of nosological values. Gen. Hosp. Psychiatry 22 (1), 49–50.

Baumeister, H., Härter, M., 2007. Prevalence of mental disorders based on general population surveys. Soc. Psychiatry Psychiatr. Epidemiol. 42 (7), 537–546.

Biby, E.L., 1998. The relationship between body dysmorphic disorder and depression, self-esteem, somatisation, and obsessive-compulsive disorder. J. Clin. Psychol. 54 (4), 489–499.

Cansever, A., Uzun, O., Dönmez, E., et al., 2003. The prevalence and clinical features of body dysmorphic disorder in college students: a study in a Turkish sample. Compr. Psychiatry 44 (1), 60–64.

Castillo, R.J., 1997. Culture and Mental Illness: A Client-Centered Approach. Brooks/Cole, Pacific Grove, CA.

Castillo, R.J. (Ed.), 1998. Meanings of Madness. Brooks/Cole, Pacific Grove, CA.

Clarke, D., Smith, G., 2001. Somatoform disorders. In: Meadows, G., Singh, B. (Eds.), Mental Health in Australia: Collaborative Community

Practice. Oxford University Press, Melbourne, pp. 375–386.

Degun-Mather, M., 2002. Hypnosis in the treatment of a case of dissociative amnesia for a 12-year period. Contemp. Hypn. 19 (1), 33–41.

Epstein, R.M., Quill, T.E., McWhinney, I.R., 1999. Somatization reconsidered: incorporating the patient's experiences of illness. Arch. Intern. Med. 159 (3), 215–222.

Escobar, J., 1996. Overview of somatisation: diagnosis, epidemiology, and management. Psychopharmacol. Bull. 32 (4), 589–596.

Escobar, J.I., Hoyos-Nervi, I., Gara, M., 2002. Medically unexplained physical symptoms in medical practice: a psychiatric perspective. Environ. Health Perspect. 110 (Suppl. 4), 631–636.

Fischhoff, B., Wessely, S., 2003. Managing patients with inexplicable health problems. Br. Med. J. 326 (7389), 595–597.

Fontenelle, L.F., Mendlowicz, M.V., Mussi, T.C., et al., 2002. The man with the purple nostrils: a case of rhinotrichotillomania secondary to body dysmorphic disorder. Acta Psychiatr. Scand. 106 (6), 464–467.

Halligan, P.W., Bass, C., Wade, D.T., 2000. New approaches to conversion hysteria. Br. Med. J. 320 (7248), 1488–1490.

Hardy, E.R., Warmbrodt, L., Chrisman, S.K., 2001. Recognizing hypochondria in primary care. Nurse Pract. 26 (6), 26–35.

Hill, M.J., 2006. Body dysmorphic disorder: implications for practice. Dermatol. Nurs. 18 (1), 13.

Hiller, W., Rief, W., Fichter, M., 1997. How disabled are patients with somatoform disorders? Gen. Hosp. Psychiatry 19 (6), 432–438.

Holloway, K.L., Zerbe, K.J., 2000. Simplified approach to somatisation disorder: when less may prove to be more. Postgrad. Med. 108 (6), 89.

Janet, P., 1889. L'automatisme Psychologique. Félix Alcan, Paris.

Janet, P., 1903. Les Obsessions et la Psychasthénie, vols. 1–2. Félix Alcan, Paris.

Kihlstrom, J.F., 2005. Dissociative disorders. Annu. Rev. Clin. Psychol. 1, 227–253.

Kihlstrom, J.F., Kihlstrom, L.C., 2001. Somatisation as illness behavior. Adv. Mind Body Med. 17 (4), 240–243.

Kipen, H.M., Fiedler, N., 2002. Environmental factors in medically unexplained symptoms and related syndromes: the evidence and the challenge. Environ. Health Perspect. 110 (Suppl. 4), 597–599.

Kirmayer, L.J., 1996. Cultural notes and somatoform and dissociative disorders 1. In: Mezzich, J.E., Kleinman, A., Fabrega Jr, H. (Eds.), Culture and Psychiatric Diagnosis: A DSM-IV TR Perspective. American Psychiatric Press, Washington, pp. 151–158.

Kirmayer, L.J., Looper, K.J., 2006. Abnormal illness behaviour: physiological, psychological and social dimensions of coping with distress. Curr. Opin. Psychiatry 19 (1), 54–60.

Kleinman, A., 1996. How is culture important for DSM-IV TR?. In: Mezzich, J.E., Kleinman, A., Fabrega Jr, H. (Eds.), Culture and Psychiatric Diagnosis: A DSM-IV TR Perspective. American Psychiatric Press, Washington, pp. 15–26.

Kroenke, K., Swindle, R., 2000. Cognitive-behavioral therapy for somatisation and symptom syndromes: a critical review of controlled clinical trials. Psychother. Psychosom. 69 (4), 205–215.

Lipsitt, D.R., 2001. The time has come to speak of many things. Adv. Mind Body Med. 17 (4), 249–256.

Lyles, J.S., Hodges, A., Collins, C., et al., 2003. Using nurse practitioners to implement an intervention in primary care for high-utilizing patients with medically unexplained symptoms. Gen. Hosp. Psychiatry 25 (2), 63–73.

McAllister, M.M., 2000. Dissociative identity disorder: a literature review. J. Psychiatr. Ment. Health Nurs. 7 (1), 25–33.

McWhinney, I.R., Epstein, R.M., Freeman, T.R., 1997. Rethinking somatization. Ann. Intern. Med. 126 (9), 747–750.

Maldonado, J.R., Butler, L.D., Spiegel, D., 2002. Treatments for dissociative disorders. In: Nathan, P.E., Gorman, J.M. (Eds.), A Guide to Treatments that Work, second ed. Oxford University Press, New York, pp. 463–496.

Maynard, C.K., 2003. Assess and manage somatization. Nurse Pract. 28 (4), 20–29.

Merskey, H., 2000. Pain, psychogenesis, and psychiatric diagnosis. Int. Rev. Psychiatry 12 (2), 99–102.

Meyer, R.G., 1999. Case Studies in Abnormal Behaviour. Allyn & Bacon, Boston.

Morrison, J., 1995. DSM-IV TR Made Easy: The Clinician's Guide to Diagnosis. Guilford Press, New York.

Noyes Jr, R., Stuart, S., Langbehn, D.R., et al., 2002. Childhood antecedents of hypochondriasis. Psychosomatics 43 (4), 282–289.

Olivardia, R., 2001. Mirror, mirror on the wall, who's the largest of them all? The features and phenomenology of muscle dysmorphia. Harv. Rev. Psychiatry 9 (5), 254–259.

Otto, M.W., Wilhelm, S., Cohen, L.S., et al., 2001. Prevalence of body dysmorphic disorder in a community sample of women. Am. J. Psychiatry 158 (12), 2061–2063.

Page, L.A., Wessely, S., 2003. Medically unexplained symptoms: exacerbating factors in the doctor–patient encounter. J. R. Soc. Med. 96 (5), 223–227.

Patterson, W.M., Bienvenu, O.J., Chodynicki, M.P., et al., 2001. Body dysmorphic disorder. Int. J. Dermatol. 40, 688–690.

Phillips, K.A., 1995. Body dysmorphic disorder: clinical features and drug treatment. CNS Drugs 3, 30–40.

Phillips, K.A., Castle, D.J., 2001. Body dysmorphic disorder in men. Br. Med. J. 323 (7320), 1015–1017.

Phillips, K.A., Grant, J., Siniscalchi, J., et al., 2001. Surgical and nonpsychiatric treatment of patients with body dysmorphic disorder. Psychosomatics 42 (6), 504–510.

Porter, R., 2002. Madness: A Brief History. Oxford University Press, Oxford.

Punamaki, R.-L., Kanninen, K., Qouta, S., et al., 2002. The role of psychological defences in moderating trauma and post-traumatic symptoms among Palestinian men. Int. J. Psychol. 37 (5), 286–297.

Ramsay, S., 2000. Controversy over UK surgeon who amputated healthy limbs. Lancet 355 (9202), 476.

Ringel, Y., Drossman, D.A., 1999. From gut to brain and back—a new perspective into functional gastrointestinal disorders. J. Psychosom. Res. 47 (3), 205–210.

Sadock, B.J., Sadock, V.A., 2003. Somatoform disorders. In: Sadock, B.J., Sadock, V.A. (Eds.), Kaplan and Sadock's Synopsis of Psychiatry: Behavioral Sciences/Clinical Psychiatry, ninth ed. Lippincott Williams & Wilkins, Philadelphia, pp. 643–660.

Sadock, B.J., Sadock, V.A., 2005. Kaplan and Sadock's Pocket Handbook of Clinical Psychiatry, fourth ed. Lippincott Williams & Wilkins, New York.

Salmon, P., Peters, S., Stanley, I., 1999. Patients' perceptions of medical explanations for somatisation disorders: qualitative analysis. Br. Med. J. 318 (7180), 372–376.

Schreiber, F.R., 1975. Sybil: The True Story of a Woman Possessed by Sixteen Different Personalities. Penguin, Harmondsworth.

Servan-Schreiber, D., Tabas, G., Kolb, N., 2000. Somatizing patients: part II, practical management. Am. Fam. Physician 61, 1423–1428. 1431–1432.

Sharpe, M., Carson, A., 2001. 'Unexplained' somatic symptoms, functional syndromes, and somatization: do we need a paradigm shift? Ann. Intern. Med. 134 (9/2), 926–930.

Shorter, E., 1994. From the Mind into the Body: The Cultural Origins of Psychosomatic Symptoms. Free Press, New York.

Simeon, D., 2004. Depersonalisation disorder: a contemporary overview. CNS Drugs 18 (5), 343–354.

Simon, G.E., 2002. Management of somatoform and factitious disorders. In: Nathan, P.E., Gorman, J.M. (Eds.), A Guide to Treatments that Work, second ed. Oxford University Press, New York, pp. 447–462.

Singh, B., 1998. Managing somatoform disorders. Med. J. Aust. 168, 572–577.

Starcevic, V., 2002. Overcoming therapeutic pessimism in hypochondriasis. Am. J. Psychother. 56 (2), 167–178.

Stevenson, R.L., 1925. Dr Jekyll and Mr Hyde. Dent, London.

Tazaki, M., Landlaw, K., 2006. Behavioural mechanisms and cognitive-behavioural interventions in somatoform disorders. Int. Rev. Psychiatry 18 (1), 67–73.

Thigpen, C.H., 1960. The Three Faces of Eve. Pan, London.

Treatment Protocol Project, 2000. Management of Mental Disorders. World Health Organization Collaborating Centre for Mental Health and Substance Abuse, Sydney.

Veale, D., Boocock, A., Gourna, K., et al., 1996. Body dysmorphic disorder: a survey of fifty cases. Br. J. Psychiatry 169 (2), 196–201.

Waitzkin, H., Magaña, H., 1997. The black box in somatisation: unexplained physical symptoms, culture, and narratives of trauma. Soc. Sci. Med. 45 (6), 811–825.

Wessely, S., Nimnuan, C., Sharpe, M., 1999. Functional somatic syndromes: one or many? Lancet 354 (9182), 936–939.

Witztum, E., Maragalit, H., 2002. Combat-induced dissociative amnesia: review and case example of generalized dissociative amnesia. J. Trauma Dissociation 32 (2), 35–55.

Witztum, E., van der Hart, O., 1998. Possession and persecution by demons: Janet's use of hypnotic techniques in treating hysterical psychosis. In: Castillo, R.J. (Ed.), Meanings of Madness. Brooks/Cole, Pacific Grove, CA.

World Health Organisation (WHO), 1992. The ICD-10 Classification of Mental and Behavioural Disorders. Available at: <http://www.who.int/classifications/icd/en/bluebook.pdf>.

Part | 4 |

Developing skills for mental health nursing

Chapter | **21** |

Settings for mental healthcare

Ruth Elder and Alicia Powell

CHAPTER POINTS

- The quality of the environment is important to service user recovery and rehabilitation.
- The preferred environment for the care of people with mental health problems is in the home.
- Environmental strategies in the care of people with a mental health problem became more important in the eighteenth century, when it was noticed that patients were more 'manageable' in a pleasant environment.

DOI: http://dx.doi.org/10.1016/B978-0-7020-4493-9.00021-4

- Confinement of people with mental health problems in large public asylums was largely an innovation of the nineteenth century.
- The therapeutic milieu is a consciously organized environment.
- Maxwell Jones in the USA and Thomas Main in the UK pioneered the concept of the hospital and environment as treatment tools.
- The goals of the therapeutic milieu are containment, structure, support, involvement, validation, symptom management and maintaining links with family and the community.
- The principles on which the therapeutic milieu is based include open communication, democratization, reality confrontation, permissiveness, group cohesion and the multidisciplinary team.
- The principle guiding the care of service users in the community is that of the least-restrictive alternative.
- The therapeutic community residence is an environment that encourages the development of the service user as a person in interaction with others, rather than as someone suffering from a health problem or disability.
- The preferred contemporary setting for the provision of mental healthcare is the community.
- There are a variety of community-based mental health services for service users with varying needs. These include Community Mental Health Teams, Assertive Outreach Teams, Early Intervention Services, Child and Adolescent Services, Older Persons Services and Home Treatment Teams.
- The main model underpinning mental health service provision in the UK is the Care Programme Approach.
- The principles of caring in the community are recovery-based and include self-determination, normalization and a focus on service user strengths and the community as a resource.
- There is a current move to reconfigure mental health service provision in the UK, with the aim of enhancing efficiency, personalization of care and cost-effectiveness.

KEY TERMS

- care coordination
- community care
- community integration
- community meeting
- continuity of care
- custodial care
- deinstitutionalization

- democratization
- empowerment
- group cohesion
- least-restrictive alternative
- milieu
- milieu therapy
- moral treatment
- multidisciplinary team
- normalization
- observation
- open communication
- partnership
- permissiveness
- reality confrontation
- revolving door
- therapeutic community

LEARNING OUTCOMES

The material in this chapter will assist you to:
- define and describe the therapeutic milieu,
- discuss the contribution of a therapeutic milieu to service user recovery,
- discuss the role of the nurse in the therapeutic milieu,
- describe the components and functions of the multidisciplinary team,
- examine principles of caring in the community.

INTRODUCTION

The biomedical model, which is focused on alleviating symptoms through the use of biological treatments such as psychotropic drugs and electroconvulsive therapy, has tended to underplay the usefulness of the environment as an aid to the care of people with mental health problems. However, far from being an outmoded concept or form of treatment, the setting in which care takes place is an important and necessary component of service user recovery and is a means of assessing and supporting people with mental health problems. People who are acutely mentally unwell to such a degree that they may pose a risk to themselves or others may need the protection afforded by a well-structured inpatient ward. On discharge, many will also need ongoing assistance in the form of supported accommodation in order to regain lost functioning, and will need assistance with integration into the community to ensure their continued wellbeing.

This chapter is concerned with the environment as a therapeutic tool. *Milieu, therapeutic milieu, milieu therapy* and *therapeutic community* are terms that have been used in psychiatry to refer to the qualities of the environment believed to be beneficial to people with mental health problems. These terms can refer to a wide variety of programmes and contexts, from whole institutions, to mental health inpatient wards located in general hospitals, to community residences. Despite a number of attempts to differentiate them, the terms lack precise definitions and are often used interchangeably. For the purposes of this chapter, however, the terms milieu and milieu therapy are used to refer to inpatient mental healthcare settings, whereas *therapeutic community* is be used to refer to environments where the emphasis is on normal functioning rather than a disorder or disability.

This chapter begins by providing the historical context and development of ideas about the therapeutic potential of the environment in which care occurs. A discussion of the history of the terms should aid clarity and understanding and the appraisal of their usefulness in modern mental healthcare. The brief history will then be followed by an examination of the application of the concepts in a variety of settings.

HISTORICAL OVERVIEW

Ideas about what is considered a suitable environment for the care of people with mental health problems have varied little over time or across cultures. On the whole, people diagnosed with mental disorders have been considered a domestic responsibility (Porter, 2002), irrespective of beliefs about the nature of mental disorder. However, these beliefs have at times been highly influential, even if the conclusions drawn from them have been contradictory. For example, throughout most of history it has been believed that people with mental health problems were possessed by supernatural forces. This belief usually led to their being feared and avoided. However, one exception to this rule is the Belgian colony of Gheel (sometimes spelt Geel), whose role as a haven for people with mental health problems was founded on familial/community support and has existed since the thirteenth century. At Gheel is the church of St Dymphna, the patron saint of the 'mentally ill', to which those with mental health problems seeking to exorcize their affliction have made pilgrimages (Sedgwick, 1982). Many of them settled there. The inhabitants of this farming town made their homes available for shelter and care, and their fields for work, to severely disturbed people diagnosed with mental disorders. This township thus became one of the precursors of the idea of a community-based, therapeutic environment. Seven hundred years later, Gheel continues to serve as an example for the successful integration of modern treatments (Goldstein and Godemont, 2007).

However, the acceptance of people with mental health problems by the townspeople of Gheel has proved

exceptional during much of the period it has been in existence. In the seventeenth century, when it was more generally believed that people with mental health problems were 'insane' – that is, they were believed to be without reason and akin to wild beasts rather than possessed – small, private and public asylums were developed, where they could be segregated from the sane. The asylums varied markedly in the quality of care they provided, and many meted out brutal treatments. Two infamous asylums of the time were St Mary of Bethlehem in London, from whence the word *bedlam* is derived, and the Hôpital Générale in Paris. The inmates at both were chained and tortured, and at Bedlam the inmates were put on display for the amusement and edification of Sunday visitors.

The eighteenth-century Enlightenment brought a general reforming zeal as well as new ideas about what was referred to as 'madness' as a mental condition which could be best treated by mental means. Furthermore, greater experience caring for people diagnosed with mental disorders gave rise to the idea that the asylum could be used as a therapeutic tool, as opposed to being solely a means of confinement. One of the foremost advocates of this progressive thinking was Philippe Pinel (1745–1826). Pinel, who is considered the founder of modern psychiatry, freed the inmates of the Bicêtre and Salpêtrière asylums in Paris from their chains (Shorter, 1997). He also provided them with nourishing food, warm baths and useful activity, abolished whips and other instruments of torture and treated them with kindness. An important outcome of these acts was that many inmates improved dramatically, and others were less violent when allowed to move around. Pinel coined the term *'le traitement moral'* which translated as 'moral treatment', a phrase later popularized by the Englishman and Quaker tea merchant, William Tuke (1732–1822) (Shorter, 1997). Tuke's humanitarian philosophy, which was in stark contrast to the bleedings, purges, chains and denial of basic necessities of life that had marked other treatment approaches, was that mental disorder was best treated by beautiful scenery, pleasant distractions and physical comfort. He put his policies of care and kindness into practice at the York Retreat, which he established for the care of members of the local Quaker community suffering from mental disorders.

An important assumption on which moral treatment rested was that a closed environment was most conducive to the reanimation of reason by psychiatry (Porter, 2002). Consequently, purpose-built and -designed institutions for confining people with mental health problems were constructed during the nineteenth century (Porter, 2002). Unfortunately, the humanitarian aspirations of the eighteenth century eventually collapsed under the weight of the huge numbers of patients increasingly housed within them. These large, public institutions were rarely intended to be therapeutic, but were custodial. The patients were housed and fed, but little occurred in the way of treatment. By the time of World War I they were little more than vast warehouses (Shorter, 1997).

In the twentieth century, the changes and ideas that led to the development of modern therapeutic communities took two different courses. One led to changes within asylums themselves, while the other led to the development of structures outside the currently existing institutions. In both cases, though, their development was partly a reaction to the institutions developed in the nineteenth century.

THERAPEUTIC COMMUNITIES

The therapeutic community has been described as 'one of the most significant innovations in the history of psychiatry' (Mills and Harrison, 2007). Overturning earlier ideas about the nature of social control, its essence was the flattening of professional hierarchies and the institution of democratic as opposed to authoritarian processes.

Two of the most important early contributors to the development of therapeutic community during the twentieth century were Thomas Main (1946) in the UK and Maxwell Jones (1953) in the USA (Tuck and Keels, 1992). They were among the first modern psychiatrists to recognize the role of the social environment in affecting change in both staff and patients. The foundations for Main's therapeutic aims were laid at Northfield Military Hospital in the UK, where two psychiatrists, John Rickman and Wilfred Bion, had experimented with group treatments (Mills and Harrison, 2007). Jones built his ideas on the observations made by him and other psychiatrists during World War II, that some army units created pathology among soldiers. Jones, however, pioneered the idea that 'a hospital might become therapeutic as a social organization' (Main, 1980, p. 53). Jones believed that all human social organization comprised a setting for social and interpersonal relations that could either enhance or limit human potential for health and wellbeing.

Jones used the concept of therapeutic community to describe his innovations in the wards of large asylums during the 1940s and 1950s, although the term *therapeutic community* can be traced to an earlier lecture given by the American psychiatrist Harry Stack Sullivan in 1939 (Mills and Harrison, 2007). For Jones, the essence of the concept of therapeutic community was a change to the organizational ethos of large mental institutions. He started this change in 1940 when he altered the structure of a psychiatric unit at the Maudsley Hospital in London from a punitive, authoritarian one to one where the patients, 100 soldiers with 'effort syndrome', a psychosomatic disorder marked by fatigue, were encouraged to become actively involved in their treatment, educated about their symptoms and given a work programme

(Watson, 1992). The outcomes of these changes were staff who behaved less like custodians and more like facilitators, and a more democratic ward culture. Following the war, Jones tested his theories about therapeutic communities on a group of men with severe antisocial personality disorders. His aim was to reduce 'acting-out behaviours' and to focus on developing social skills. Prior to his experiment the men had failed to respond to any of the currently available therapies; in the therapeutic community, nearly half of them improved.

One of the most important tenets to be derived from Jones's work is that, in order to be therapeutic, a setting has to be engineered that way. In the inpatient care setting, a therapeutic milieu is a consciously organized environment demanding deliberate decision making (Tuck and Keels, 1992) and experienced staff who understand inpatient mental healthcare (Delaney, 1992). The concept of milieu means more than just the physical environment. It includes the social, emotional, interpersonal, professional and managerial elements that comprise a particular setting. In a therapeutic milieu these elements are not considered simply part of the usual background to treatment but critical influences on therapy. The principal components of the therapeutic milieu are outlined in Box 21.1.

In its original conception, the milieu was intended not only to meet a service user's need for psychiatric, medical and nursing care, but also their need for recreation, occupation and social interaction. These needs were to be met through open communication, democratization, reality confrontation, permissiveness, group cohesion and the multidisciplinary team (MDT; see Box 21.2). Democratization, reality confrontation, permissiveness

---

Box 21.1 Components of the therapeutic milieu

A belief that the environment is the treatment agent
The participation of the patients and the staff in decision making
The use of a multidisciplinary treatment team
Open communication
Individualized goal-setting with patients

Box 21.2 Principles governing the inpatient therapeutic milieu

Open communication
Democratization
Reality confrontation
Permissiveness
Group cohesion
Multidisciplinary team

and communalism were identified by Rapoport (1960, cited in Watson, 1992) as the four fundamental themes characterizing the therapeutic community. Each of these components is considered in the next section.

PRINCIPLES GOVERNING THE INPATIENT THERAPEUTIC MILIEU

Open communication

In the therapeutic milieu, great value is placed on communication. In the conventional medical model, the process of communication tends to follow hierarchical lines: information flows upwards to the doctor, and prescriptions are ordered downwards to the service and nursing staff. In the therapeutic milieu, however, staff and service users are considered team members, each of whom has a valuable contribution to make to the service user's recovery. However, in order to be able to contribute effectively it is necessary that everyone, including the service user, has all the information necessary to make informed decisions. Effective decisions rely on everyone knowing and working towards the same goals.

Open communication helps build morale and is considered to have a therapeutic effect on staff as well as service users. Staff need to be clear about what behaviour is expected and acceptable, and staff and service users are expected to be candid about their feelings, perceptions and needs. Open communication can be facilitated through warmth and the formation of trusting, one-to-one relationships. Thomas et al. (2002) found that one of the most valued aspects of hospitalization for service users was socialization with staff and other service users (Thomas et al., 2002). An important assumption underlying the therapeutic milieu is that normal functioning results from the social interaction and peer pressure attending activities designed to facilitate open communication. Interaction with others promotes a capacity for self-acceptance and self-realization, and can be facilitated by regular group and community meetings.

In a short-stay environment, the community meeting might be held at best once a week, but is more often an ad hoc affair used to address unit crises (Munich, 2000). Kahn (1994, p. 23) argues that the contemporary emphasis on short inpatient stays has led to mental healthcare facilities 'characterized by disorganization, dysphoria and fear'. He suggests that the service user–staff community meeting is one of the major means of restoring the therapeutic potential of inpatient units. The typical community meeting is held in a large room where all the staff and service users can be seated comfortably in a circle. Kahn (1994) has outlined six techniques, based on Yalom's (1983) standard principles of group therapy, for ensuring the effectiveness of community meetings in short-stay inpatient units (see Box 21.3).

CRITICAL THINKING CHALLENGE 21.1

A therapeutic milieu is based on open communication. However, open communication can be in conflict with a service users's right to privacy. Do you think these two principles can be reconciled?

Box 21.3 The six principles of effective community meetings

1. Plan ahead. Choose staff members to lead, deputize and plan the community meeting beforehand.
2. Establish the rules and norms for the conduct of the meeting at the start.
   a. Get everyone involved by giving advance notice of the meeting, encouraging all to attend, seeking out stragglers and reminding them that the community meeting is about to start.
   b. At the meeting, ask all attendees to introduce themselves; address everyone by name.
3. Infuse energy by using humour and empathy to help group members deal with difficult issues and appear eager to participate.
4. Choose relevant topics and issues of concern to patients such as maintaining safety and order, controlling impulses, expressing strong feelings, reducing isolation, establishing supports, taking advantage of the treatment programme, and developing plans for the future.
5. Address unit processes by discussing the needs of the unit using the framework of containment, structure, support, involvement, validation and symptom management.

Reprinted from Kahn EM (1994). The patient-staff community meeting: Old tools, new rules. *Journal of Psychosocial Nursing and Mental Health Services*, 32(8), 22–26, with permission from SLACK Incorporated.

Democratization

Democratization is a core element of a therapeutic community. The aim is to create an environment in which staff and service users feel free to express themselves without fear of rejection and to participate in decision making to the extent of their abilities. In a therapeutic community, service users have opportunities to take an active part in ward affairs. They can participate in setting some rules and can be encouraged to solve problems through enquiry and reason. For example, in their account of democracy at work in a rehabilitation unit, Benbow and Bowers (1998) report how service users set the guidelines about television watching and smoking times. Service user participation in decision making communicates an expectation of healthy behaviour. This practice is therapeutic insofar as it recognizes the strengths of service users, and facilitates interaction and understanding. In order to achieve this aim, the traditional institutional hierarchies of authority are flattened. According to Watson (1992), democratization is not to be confused with egalitarianism. In a bureaucratic organization, it is not possible for everyone to have a say about everything and it is not always appropriate for service users to attend business meetings (Benbow and Bowers, 1998). Furthermore, service users will vary in their ability to contribute to decision making according to the severity of their symptoms. Staff and management need to take care that they do not delegate decisions they feel they cannot live with.

Reality confrontation

Staff and service users contribute to reality confrontation by reflecting individuals' behaviour back to them. The confrontation spoken of here is not about creating conflict or being critical, although it may result from a conflict or crisis, but the giving of information and sharing of feelings in an acceptable way (Watson, 1992). Confrontation makes possible the expression of feelings and thereby contributes to social interaction and social learning.

Permissiveness

In a therapeutic community, staff and service users need to learn to tolerate deviant behaviour. People with mental health problems may often exhibit unconventional behaviour. It is important that staff withhold judgement and not exhibit fear or prejudice, although at times they will exert authority and control. Service users need to learn self-regulation and this lesson is best learned in contact with others, where peers and staff can influence and limit behaviour rather than through physical means such as locked doors and medications. Benbow and Bowers (1998) provide an example of how permissiveness can provoke change in service users' behaviour. Service users were provided with a range of activities that gave them a reason to get out of bed and get dressed in the morning, rather than being forced to get up by nursing staff.

Group cohesion

Group cohesion is important in order to create a climate of support and involvement in therapeutic communities. Sharing among staff and service users of daily duties and unit resources facilitates communalism. Developing group cohesiveness has become increasingly difficult since the advent of very short lengths of stay (Watson, 1992). Short lengths of stay also mean service users rarely know about the progress of their peers and are therefore not in a position to provide feedback.

INPATIENT MENTAL HEALTH SERVICES

The principles outlined above remain relevant to contemporary mental health settings, although there are few formal therapeutic communities in the UK. However, the principles have been influential in the development of modern mental health inpatient facilities and modifications and additions have been made to develop a therapeutic milieu given the modern challenges to the provision of mental healthcare.

CRITICAL THINKING CHALLENGE 21.2

In what ways do you feel that the principles of a therapeutic community have been incorporated in the day-to-day practice of adult mental health inpatient facilities?

Since Maxwell Jones there have been numerous and far-reaching changes in the mental healthcare system. The drivers of these changes are multiple, and they include attempts to increase efficiency and reduce costs, the rise of community mental health, increasing numbers of seriously unwell service users with complex needs, new psychotherapeutic interventions and greater professionalization of mental health workers. Furthermore, brief hospitalization may be an appropriate method of treatment for some service users. A consequence of these changes to the length of stay is rapid service user turnover and more inpatients with complex needs.

In the UK the main inpatient facilities are acute admission services, Psychiatric Intensive Care Units (PICUs) and forensic services (including medium and high secure services). Acute inpatient facilities utilize two-thirds of the budget allocated to mental healthcare and are often seen as the mainstay of care for people experiencing disabling mental distress (Baguley et al., 2007). There are 69 NHS trusts in the UK which provide mental health acute inpatient services comprising 554 acute mental health wards with a total of 9885 beds (Healthcare Commission, 2008).

PICUs are low secure environments which specialize in the care and treatment of people who are '…compulsorily detained usually in secure conditions, who are in an acutely disturbed phase of a serious mental disorder. There is an associated loss of capacity for self-control, with a corresponding increase in risk, which does not enable their safe, therapeutic management and treatment in a general open acute ward' (Department of Health, 2002, p. 3).

Medium and high secure services provide assessment, care and treatment of people who are subject to legal proceedings and have, or who are suspected of having, a mental health problem. The core tasks of a forensic service include:

- '...the assessment, management and treatment of high-risk mentally disordered offenders in the community, in hospitals (particularly hospitals using security) and in prisons,
- the assessment, support and treatment of victims, especially those who develop dangerous behaviour,
- the provision of advice to and collaborative working with other psychiatrists, GPs, lawyers, police officers, prison staff, social workers and especially probation officers,
- the provision of evidence and reports for legal purposes' (Department of Health, 2007, p. 7).

A key aspect of forensic settings is that of public safety which will often include an emphasis on risk assessment and risk management and containment. There are three interrelated aspects of security in secure mental healthcare settings (Department of Health, 2010a):

- procedural security (the policies and procedures in place to maintain safety and security),
- physical security (the physical design of buildings, secure perimeter fences, locked doors, airlocks, personal alarms, specialist security staff and so on),
- relational security (which involves engaging with service users and the development of professional boundaries and safe and therapeutic effective relationships).

Goals of the therapeutic milieu

The goals of the modern inpatient therapeutic milieu are containment, structure, support, involvement, validation (Gunderson 1978, cited in Delaney, 1992), symptom management (Delaney, 1992; Delaney et al., 2000), maintaining links with the service user's family or others and developing and maintaining links with the community (Greene, 1997) (see Box 21.4). More recently the tasks of the modern inpatient ward have been identified: keep service users safe, assess problems and needs, treat service users' mental health concerns, meet service users' basic care needs and provide physical healthcare (Bowers et al., 2005).

To varying degrees all inpatient services aim to create a therapeutic milieu within which the service user's recovery can be supported and promoted. However, nurses working in secure inpatient environments require specialist skills to engage service users and develop therapeutic relationships within the context of physical and procedural security.

According to Hummelvoll and Severinsson (2001, pp. 163–164) 'the greatest challenge is to revitalize the aims and content of the milieu therapy within the given frames

---

> **Box 21.4 Goals of the therapeutic milieu**
>
> Containment
> Structure
> Support
> Involvement
> Validation
> Symptom management
> Maintaining links with the service user's family or others
> Developing and maintaining links with the community

(time, high service user turnover, the complexity of service users' needs and suffering) enabling them to make the most of the interhuman and environmental experiences on the ward'.

Containment

One of the major goals of inpatient mental health facilities is to provide a place of safety. For many mental health service users, inpatient care is 'a refuge from self-destructiveness' (Thomas et al., 2002). Inpatient services seek to secure the physical wellbeing of service users and to compensate for their lack of internal controls. These goals are encoded in policies; for example, the precautions to be taken with service users deemed to be a risk to self or others, such as isolating them from other service users and the general public or ensuring constant supervision in the case of actively suicidal service users (Delaney et al., 2000). Measures taken include locked areas, the use of rapid tranquillization, seclusion, locked doors, screened windows and balconies, medical care and the provision of food and shelter. Paradoxically, some mental health service users experience the confinement of the mental health facility as 'freeing' (Thomas et al., 2002). The idea is to reassure the service user and others that mental distress will not overwhelm them or the care environment.

Shorter stays in the acute setting and service users with more complex needs mean that greater emphasis is placed on ensuring safety in the inpatient milieu. The two major nursing techniques to ensure safety are *limit-setting* and *observation*. A therapeutic milieu needs sufficiently experienced nursing staff to maintain a continuous watchful presence in a nonthreatening, non-intrusive manner and to set reasonable limits on behaviour. Such watchfulness is not necessarily perceived by service users as intrusive. Many appreciate it, perceiving close monitoring as indicative of staff competence (Thomas et al., 2002). On the other hand, Thomas et al. (2002) also report that service users value opportunities to converse with peers away from staff eyes. Nurses also monitor the level of environmental stimulation and provide service users with suitable activities and milieu treatments such as relaxation groups, drug and alcohol groups, medication groups, discussion groups, cooking classes and exercise classes. For a discussion of observation in mental health inpatient units see Box 21.5.

ETHICAL DILEMMA

Duffy (1995) argues that the ethic driving the procedure of closely observing suicidal and self-harming service users is that of paternalism, which in turn is based on an assumption of irrationality; that is, any person who decides to harm themselves is by definition irrational.

1. What is the ethical basis of paternalism? Do you agree that it applies in the case of close observation? Why or why not?
2. Do you agree that anyone who desires death is irrational? Are there any circumstances under which you could imagine that such a choice would be rational? Why or why not?

CRITICAL THINKING CHALLENGE 21.3

Close observation, and special observation in particular, raises ethical and professional issues for nurses. For example, how would you go about developing a therapeutic relationship with a service user under these circumstances?

ETHICAL DILEMMA

Duffy (1995) reports that although nurses dislike the intrusiveness of close observation, few question their role in performing it. He also suggests that there is a deep contradiction in this activity; that is, although nurses endorse an ethic of service user autonomy, their role in close observation necessarily infringes it.

1. What do you think of Duffy's argument that close observation infringes service user autonomy?
2. Do you think close observation is a nursing role? Why or why not?

Structure

The structure of the milieu refers to how time, people and places are organized. A predictable structure provides order and stability; it establishes routines and schedules for individual service users and the group as a whole. A sound structure is achieved by ensuring that service users

---

Box 21.5 Nursing observation in an inpatient milieu

A major nursing activity in mental health facilties is observation. Service users admitted to a facility are usually required to inform the nurse of their whereabouts, if they are intending to leave the unit, either in person or by writing in a purpose-designed book in an easily accessible part of the ward. The level of observation is based on an assessment of the service user. For example, where service users are assessed as posing no risk to themselves or others, then normal observation applies. If a service user's behaviour is assessed as a cause of concern, then that service user will be under what is termed *continuous observation* or *close observation*. Where a service user is assessed at definite risk for self-harm, suicide or violence, then that service user will require *special observation*. Special observation is also referred to as *maximum observation, constant observation* and *constant supervision* (Duffy, 1995, p. 944).

In the cases of close and special observation, the idea is that the service user's freedom of movement will be restricted to varying degrees. When a service user is under close observation, the nurse locates the service user's whereabouts in a specified time period, usually every 10 or 15 min, but it might also be half-hourly or hourly. The nurse also then usually signs an observation sheet to the effect that the service user has been sighted and might also comment on the service user's behaviour and location. Contrary to expectations, two studies have found that service users experience close observation as reassuring rather than intrusive (see Jones et al., 2000; Thomas et al., 2002).

When a service user is under constant observation, the nurse is usually required to keep the service user in sight at all times, even when the service user goes to the toilet and showers. The nurse is also required to be close enough to the service user to be able to prevent self-harm. This requirement is often practised by the nurse being within arm's reach of the service user.

---

are orientated to the ward's physical layout, as well as being informed about mealtimes, particular policies, such as no smoking in public areas, and any special requirements, such as informing staff of their whereabouts. The physical environment includes colours, lighting, furniture and unit design and layout. The architecture of a setting, through the provision of spaces for both private contemplation and social interaction, influences activities such as eating, talking, receiving visitors and using the telephone, as well as helping to ensure that service users maintain some control over their lives. Some inkling of the value service users place on structure can be gleaned from their approval of hospital cleanliness, and well-stocked refrigerators and snack cabinets (Thomas et al., 2002).

Support

The goals of support are to help service users feel safe, and to promote hope, a sense of wellbeing and self-esteem. Support is achieved by being emotionally available to service users, allowing and helping them to express their emotions, and interacting in a respectful way. Support can be conveyed by listening to service users, providing attention, praise and reassurance, providing assistance in using and developing coping skills and providing education and direction. However, in providing support it is important that service users have the opportunity to interact with a wide social network and not be confined to a primary therapeutic relationship. In a supportive milieu, the service user learns to resocialize and to relate to others in new ways. Support also involves assessing the service user's social network and education of and interaction with the family (Delaney et al., 2000).

Involvement

In the therapeutic milieu all relationships are regarded as potentially therapeutic. Therapeutic outcome is considered a function not just of the service user's relationship with the nursing team but of the total social organization. The goal of involvement requires service users to attend to and take responsibility for maladaptive behaviours. Everyone in the therapeutic milieu is required to provide and accept constructive feedback from others on behaviours. Involvement encourages service users to be actively involved in their treatment and counsels against service user passivity. The desires and interests of the service user in terms of their treatment are highly valued.

Validation

Validation means that treatment is individualized and that it is the nurse's responsibility to try to understand the meaning of individual behaviour. Each service user is treated as worthy and as able to openly discuss values, feelings and goals. Service users learn to view themselves, through validation of past negative experiences, not as 'sick' or 'bad' but as injured parties (Norton and Bloom, 2004). Validation requires flexibility in the application of rules. Too-rigid adherence to structural issues such as ward routine or policies can undermine the goal of validation.

Symptom management

Relationships with service users in the acute mental healthcare setting tend to be short and symptom-oriented. With shorter lengths of stay there is more focus on 'symptom stabilization in preparation for less restrictive levels of care and a more extensive utilization of ambulatory services' (Munich, 2000). LeCuyer (1992) also suggests that after an inpatient stay the service user's coping mechanisms will be increased or at least restored to pre-hospitalization levels. In order to achieve these goals, the emphasis is on communication that is practical and supportive. Accurate assessment of symptoms might require the use of symptom scales, and nurses document both their nature and changes to their character. Nurses also administer and provide information about medications, assess their efficacy in controlling symptoms and consider the service user's ability to follow the prescribed regimen (Delaney et al., 2000). Service user behaviours are described in terms of whether they are typical or suggest an escalation in symptomatology. Also recorded are the nursing actions that assist the service user to reorganize successfully and which cognitive deficits are experienced and contribute to their inability to function.

In the contemporary therapeutic milieu the principal mechanism for biopsychosocial assessment and intervention in collaboration with service users and their families is the multidisciplinary team (MDT). The MDT:

> *...consists of individuals from multiple disciplines and acts as an embodiment of the neo-biopsychosocial model, with each team member providing not only a unique perspective on viewing the service but also offering unique opportunities to aid in creating an environment that is conducive to change.*

> (Tobias and Haslam-Hopwood, 2003)

The professionals who comprise the MDT usually include a psychiatrist, a psychologist, mental health nurses, social workers and occupational therapists. While every discipline has a specific role to fill, their roles often overlap which can be observed most clearly in the conduct of various therapies including individual, group and family therapies, where any member of the team may take the lead role.

Maintaining links with the service user's family or significant others

In the contemporary short-stay environment, with the concomitant drive to return service users to the community as soon as possible, links with the service user's family and significant others need to be nurtured and maintained (Greene, 1997). However, maintaining links with service users' families and friends is an important aspect of all inpatient care, including care provided in secure services. Families might be confused, fearful, fed-up, anxious or relieved when one of their members is admitted to a mental healthcare facility. They often need to be provided with information about the nature of mental health disorders, treatment and prognosis. They often want to know how they can best help the person on the road to recovery. It is important to try and involve the family in the treatment process. They should be encouraged to visit the service user in hospital and the service user should be allowed to take leave with the family as soon as they are able. Such leave might begin with short outings with family members and extend to overnight and weekend passes home. The family should also be involved in the discharge process.

Developing and maintaining links with the community

Developing and maintaining links with the community ensures that the service user has access to and knows about appropriate, available resources. Inpatient mental health nurses can ensure this continuity of care by finding out about service users' support networks, and the service user's understanding about their diagnosis and their treatments. When informed consent from the service user is required before administering medication, service users are given a sense of hope and direction for their treatment after discharge (LeCuyer, 1992). Community links can be developed by inviting and including staff at community agencies in ward meetings. However, there is some evidence that nurses do not do enough to prepare service users for their return to the community (Thomas et al., 2002).

Criticisms of acute inpatient care

There have been many reports which have highlighted concerns about the quality of care and unmet needs of service users in acute mental health facilities which have threatened the development of the therapeutic milieu (Healthcare Commission, 2008; Sainsbury Centre for Mental Health, 2006). For Rethink (2006, p. 4) '...there is a crisis in psychiatric inpatient care with wards over-crowded, treatment taking place in "bleakness and squalor" and staff left feeling demoralised and unsupported.'

There is a reported wide variation of the quality of acute inpatient care across the UK (Healthcare Commission, 2008). While it is important to recognize that much good practice does exist, such as health promotion activities (such as smoking cessation, physical activity and advice on healthy eating and diet) and regular community meetings which offer feedback from service users on the day-to-day running of the ward (Healthcare Commission, 2008), service users receiving care on acute mental healthcare facilities have often reported feeling unsafe, threatened or even physically assaulted (Healthcare Commission, 2008). There is also an apparent wide variation in the delivery of therapeutic interventions on acute mental healthcare facilities, with poor engagement with nothing to do, inconsistent provision of talking therapies or interventions for substance misuse (Healthcare Commission, 2008; Rethink, 2006).

There have also been changes to acute mental healthcare over the last 30 years which have lead to a movement away from inpatient care to more care in the community. This has meant a reduction in the number of beds and a raising of the criteria threshold for admission, which has increased the pressure on staff working in such environments. Baguley et al. (2007) argues that there has been an increase in the acuity of service user problems in such settings, with the inpatient population largely comprising people with serious and ensuring mental health problems: '...great deal of evidence suggests inpatients have greater levels of disadvantage, social exclusion, homelessness, and a much wider and more complex set of needs than they did in the past' (SNMAC, 1999, p. 8). However, it seems that there are systemic problems, meaning that the nursing profession has not kept pace with change, and there have been concerns that mental health nursing has responded by becoming increasingly custodial in its function (SNMAC, 1999). Baguley et al. (2007, p. 49) highlight the impact of systemic problems on the provision of mental health nursing care:

The negative reports from service users about nursing attitudes and shortages in acute inpatient care may be viewed from a hierarchical perspective in which nurses feel disempowered by the inpatient system. The nursing duty of care embraces safety and therapy. However, within traditional services, nurses are preoccupied with risk assessment and containment. A large element of the nursing role involves servicing consultants' ward rounds and implementing the decisions that are made.

A frequent criticism of the modern inpatient facilities is that there is insufficient engagement by mental health nurses to deliver individual care (Thomas et al., 2002). However, there are some actions nurses can take to minimize barriers to staff–service user interaction. Service users can have a primary nurse who they know by name, and nurses can ensure their availability by being visible on the ward.

Morrison et al. (1997) found that the design and layout of hospital and ward environments can shape behaviour in profound, anti-therapeutic ways. For example, service user's privacy can be severely compromised if their possessions are taken away from them or inspected, and if they are expected to adhere to routines and schedules not of their making. These routines are anti-therapeutic to the extent that they conflict with the stated aim of many mental healthcare settings to restore patients to the community, where self-regulation is the rule. Some hospital layouts are also conducive to the creation of a crowd (Lee 1976, cited in Morrison et al., 1997): for example, large dining rooms might provoke anxiety in many service users.

Morrison et al. (1997) also found that the practices of confining service users to certain areas during the day, such as day rooms, and restricting their access to other areas, such as dormitories and bedrooms, were associated with both high staff control/low service user autonomy and higher incidents of aggression and disturbed behaviour, which in turn led to higher rates of seclusion. The problem appears to be that confining service users together for long periods in small spaces significantly increases the chances of negative interactions occurring.

Cleary et al. (1999) also found that ward layout profoundly affected the amount of time nurses spent interacting with service users. Because they spent so much time looking for service users, they spent little actual time with service users. They also noted the importance of specially designated spaces such as interview rooms, rather than day rooms, as facilitators of interaction. Cleary et al. (1999) also found that rapid service user turnover meant that much nursing time was now spent on a large number of administrative tasks and evaluating the service.

What is clear is that acute mental healthcare settings require effective leadership and research which clarifies the role and function of mental health nursing care (Bowers 2005, SNMAC, 1999).

COMMUNITY CARE

The previous section considered the goals of the therapeutic milieu, which have been modified over time to take account of shorter hospital stays as well as more acutely unwell service users. The focus up until this point has been on the therapeutic milieu in inpatient units. However, the changes and ideas that led to the development of modern therapeutic communities led not only to changes within psychiatric asylums themselves, but also to the development of therapeutic communities in community settings. Foremost among the needs of service users making the transition to community living is accommodation. Without adequate shelter, the shift from institutional to community care cannot succeed.

A wide range of support services are required by people with serious mental health needs in the community. One of the main criteria used to assess the level of support needed by a particular service user is that of the least-restrictive environment. Mental health settings can be ranked according to their degree of restrictiveness (Krauss and Slavinsky, 1982). The most restrictive environment is the secure inpatient facility, while living with the family of orientation is the least restrictive. In between are institutional environments such as nursing homes, private psychiatric hospitals and wards within general hospitals, whereas in the community there are hostels, boarding houses, hotels, group homes and the family of origin.

Homelessness and loneliness are common experiences for many people who suffer from a mental health problem (Chesters et al., 2005). There is a dearth of suitable housing for people with mental health problems (Singh and Castle, 2007), most of whom would prefer to live independently in ordinary housing (Chesters et al., 2005). However, the level of support many require and the lack of community acceptance mean that this goal will not always be achieved. Furthermore, people diagnosed with a mental disorder are over-represented in prisons (Singh and Castle, 2007). In helping service users acquire accommodation it is useful to keep in mind some of the goals of community living such as the freedom to have visitors, to come and go as one pleases, and a private space to call one's own.

In recent times the concept of *therapeutic community* has tended to be used mainly to refer only to those innovations existing outside of hospitals; for example, Richmond Fellowship, which was begun by Elly Jansen in 1959 (Jansen, 1980). Jansen (1980, pp. 32–33) defines the therapeutic community as an environment that 'should provide a communal living experience which encourages open communication, and promotes intrapsychic and social adjustment to the maximum capacity of the individual'. Therapeutic communities are often nonmedical, unlike milieus, which are often associated with hospitals. They are often located in a residential setting, rather than a hospital.

The therapeutic community defines mental disturbance as a problem in relationships rather than a health problem (Jansen, 1980). The goal of the therapeutic community is to foster therapeutic relationships so as to enable the transition, usually from an inpatient unit, to independence. Therapeutic communities like Richmond Fellowship were based on the premise of normality; that is, a person is considered a functioning human being rather than a mental disorder or disability. Richmond Fellowship provides accommodation, aftercare and counselling. Residents stay for 6 months or longer. They learn survival skills such as finding a job and accommodation. In this environment there are no service users, but residents. On this assumption of function, residents are expected to share accommodation, rent and housework on an egalitarian basis and to get up in the mornings and look for work. Therapeutic communities like Richmond Fellowship can only accommodate very few service users. However, not all service users require this level of support on discharge.

Therapeutic communities are often very demanding of staff. Apart from commitment and expertise, they need the skills to empower service users (O'Brien et al., 2001; Prebble and McDonald, 1997) and develop partnerships with them (Creedy and Crowe, 1996; Prebble and McDonald, 1997). Empowerment in this context involves assisting in decision making and developing incremental decision making (O'Brien et al., 2001). Residents are initially encouraged to make decisions on a range of matters, from small things such as taking responsibility for particular tasks like washing up, to large decisions such as how much to budget for special activities. Developing collaborative partnerships is achieved through sharing responsibility for such things as household tasks. However, it also involves finding out what attributions/beliefs service users have about their problems: Why did they have problems? What do they think will make them better? Which treatments do they think work or not? How effective do they believe certain treatments to be?

Although the origins of these residentially based therapeutic communities can still be traced to Thomas Main and Maxwell Jones, some practitioners believe the community is the best place for implementing therapeutic community principles. For example, Murray and Baier (1993, p. 11) argue that the 'therapeutic milieu is an integral, vital treatment modality for mental illness in transitional living facilities for homeless, chronically mentally ill persons'. They further argue that it is easier to implement a therapeutic community in the community setting 'because some of the institutional attitudes and constraints are absent' (Murray and Baier, 1993, p. 14). For O'Brien et al. (2001), implementing therapeutic community principles in a hospital is impossible because of the dominance of the medical model. They intend the term to apply to residences within the community, not wards within hospitals. For them, a therapeutic community provides more than a place to live: it 'should be a living and learning environment structured to enhance a person's opportunity to develop social skills necessary to live independently of the health system' (O'Brien et al., 2001, p. 5). Their perspective on the concept of therapeutic community is interesting in that it derives from the theory of antipsychiatry as expounded in David Cooper's *Psychiatry and Anti-Psychiatry* (1967). This orientation emphasizes the provision of shelter, and independence, personal growth and recovery from ill health. The aim is to value the person's experience rather than focusing on the symptoms of mental disorder, to avoid labels such as 'mental illness' and to reduce reliance on medication.

Although accommodation is critical, more than this is required for service users to successfully negotiate the transition from hospital to community. Mental health policy in the UK has promoted the shift from institutionally based care to care in the community. As part of this shift, the large psychiatric institutions have been gradually closed down or much reduced in size, and inpatient mental health services have been moved into mainstream health services. Although this process is ongoing and has gathered momentum, how best to deliver community services is still under review. At first, the shift to community care simply meant a change in location. Those services that were originally provided by a single institution were provided by many services. One of the flaws in this approach was that many servicer users were unable to negotiate multiple services without a great deal of help. Consequently, many people suffering from severe and longstanding mental health problems have often experienced gaps in care. Furthermore, because the services were intended only for people with mental health problems,

they became marginalized and excluded from normal community life. In order to facilitate access and continuity of care, the MDT and care coordination through the Care Programme Approach (CPA) (see below) are the preferred mechanisms for the coordination of the range of services necessary to meet the identified needs of service users.

The next sections will explore the types of community mental health services provided in the UK and the models underpinning these ways of working.

COMMUNITY MENTAL HEALTH SERVICES IN THE UK

Primary care

The majority of people who have mental health problems will initially seek help from their GP. They may also receive first-line support from help line services such as NHS Direct or the Samaritans. Over 90% of people with mental health problems continue to be treated in primary care, including approximately one in four people receiving treatment for psychosis (National Mental Health Development Unit, 2011). GPs and other health professionals working in primary care therefore need the skills to detect mental health problems and offer the best evidence-based treatment. The National Service Framework (NSF) for Mental Health (Department of Health, 1999b) aimed to improve the consistency and availability of services provided to people with mental health problems in primary care.

For common mental health problems such as mild to moderate depression, panic and anxiety disorders, GPs will often instigate pharmacological treatment in conjunction with a referral for counselling or cognitive behavioural therapy. The introduction of the Improving Access to Psychological Therapies (IAPT) programme has been enhancing treatment choice in primary care settings (National Mental Health Development Unit, 2011). GPs also signpost service users to NICE-guideline-recommended self-help websites based on the principles of cognitive behavioural therapy, for common mental health problems.

Community Mental Health Teams

The NSF for Mental Health (Department of Health, 1999b) stipulated that specialist mental health services must ensure that interventions are provided in a timely and effective manner to people who require more support than is available in primary care. This is essential with service users who have complex presentations, comorbid disorders or dual diagnoses.

Community Mental Health Teams (CMHTs) are the foundation for secondary mental healthcare. CMHTs provide care and support for adults with severe, and/or enduring, mental health problems. Such problems are those which have a major impact on someone's ability to cope with everyday life due to a mental disturbance that is not primarily due to drugs, alcohol or organic illness. These include schizophrenia, bipolar affective disorder, severe anxiety disorders and severe depression. CMHTs also provide support and guidance for carers of people with severe and enduring mental health problems.

CMHTs receive referrals primarily from GPs, but also from other agencies such as housing, police, probation services and drug and alcohol services. People can also refer themselves to the team or they may be referred by a concerned family member or friend. Mental health units also refer to CMHTs for community follow-up of service users when they are discharged from hospital.

A multidisciplinary assessment will be offered to determine whether the CMHT is the right service to provide help and support. The assessment may involve more than one professional depending on the needs of the service user. Following an assessment, service users can expect a clear decision about any support that can be given. This may be short-term care and support by a duty worker or, if needs are ongoing and more complex, allocation of a care coordinator would be indicated, for longer-term support and monitoring of mental health needs. Should the CMHT not be appropriate, then the person will be informed about more suitable services.

Assertive Outreach Teams

Assertive Outreach Teams (AOTs) work in a similar way to CMHTs, but the care coordinators have a smaller caseload of around 12 service users, with whom they work with very intensively. Some AOTs provide a more flexible and responsive service with extended working hours including evenings and weekends. AOTs work with service users who are often at the highest risk of unplanned hospital admissions. These service users will have complex mental health and social issues and are difficult to engage into CMHT services. AOT is based on the US case management model of Assertive Community Treatment (ACT). This evidence-based model was developed in the 1960s and has been implemented in many countries around the world (Shives, 2008) The ACT model most closely 'mirrors the medical model of care in which psychiatrists and nurses have critical roles' (Schaedle et al., 2002, p. 210). However, clinicians share a caseload rather than assuming individual responsibility for service users.

An important feature of this model, and from where it derives its description as assertive, is case finding or *outreach* to those individuals in greatest need. These are often the service users who have had multiple hospital admissions. The clinician will try to find ways to interrupt the

process that leads to hospitalization (Witheridge, 1989). This might involve the use of relapse-prevention techniques or supported accommodation for service users. Outreach involves developing and maintaining working relationships with hospitals and other community agencies that might come into contact with this clientele.

Assertive outreach working is useful for service users with whom it is very difficult to have sustained contact. Care coordinators often liaise with a variety of other agencies to help with issues such as housing, benefits and activities of daily living. Services are provided in a variety of community locations dependant on the service user's preferences. This may include the home, local cafes, parks or community centres. Outreach working can help service users establish a more stable and secure community base, and reduce the number of necessary hospital admissions (Department of Health, 1999b). This model has been found to be most effective in reducing hospitalization for service users diagnosed with schizophrenia whose disorder is unstable, or treatment resistant and have nowhere to live (Drake et al., 2001).

Ford and King (2005) highlighted that whereas the AOT model adopts the main principles of the ACT model, the concept has not been as readily transferable to the UK system as was previously thought, with less positive results than have been found in the USA. There appear to be difficulties in delivering the AOT model in different localities in the UK, including lack of resources and barriers in integrating service users into mainstream facilities. It has been suggested that while still integrating the essential principles of the original ACT model, asserting outreach working in the UK needs to be delivered in a flexible manner that is sensitive to local needs.

Older Persons Services

Currently Older Persons Services (or OPS) provide support and care for persons over the age of 65 who have severe and enduring mental health disorders, including organic conditions such as dementia and Alzheimer's disease. These teams work in a similar way to CMHTs but provide specialized care for older persons.

Home Treatment/Crisis Resolution Teams

Crisis situations require urgent and appropriate action to be taken to reduce risk of relapse and prevent harm to both the service user and the public. Home Treatment Teams (HTTs) or Crisis Resolution Teams (CRTs) are community-based services that provide crisis intervention. HTTs provide an alternative to hospital admission, giving service users care in the comfort and privacy of their own homes. This affords service users more choice and control over the management of their mental health condition, and allows them to stay with supportive family members. There is also a cost benefit in treating people at home. Studies demonstrate the cost efficiency and effectiveness of home treatment services, with a saving of up to £700 per service user per month in comparison with hospital admission (Centre for the Economics of Mental Health, 2007).

However, there has also been criticism of the HTT model of care. Allen (2010) emphasizes the lack of continuity of care service for users under the care of HTTs. The service user may be faced with different members of staff every day and continually have to repeat their story, making it difficult to establish a therapeutic relationship. Other issues include a lack of time for engaging in meaningful sessions, and a lack of support with practical and social issues. Service users often wish for more support with such issues rather than just basic emotional support and assistance with medication. Apart from the demonstrated cost benefits, it has been highlighted that research evidence for the efficacy of HTTs is sparse. The existence of HTTs has also been seen as a reason for the increasingly disturbed nature of inpatient mental health wards, with only the most acutely unwell service users being treated in hospital as opposed to at home (Allen, 2010).

Accident and emergency mental health liaison

Mental health liaison nurses work closely with HTTs, or indeed may share the role for assessing people presenting to accident and emergency departments with mental health concerns. Mental health liaison nurses carry out psychosocial assessments for people presenting in crisis, working closely with the service user to determine the most appropriate services for their needs. This may be a hospital admission, a referral to the HTT or signposting to other more appropriate community agencies.

Child and Adolescent Mental Health Services

Child and Adolescent Mental Health Services (CAMHS) are specialized in providing support and treatment for children and young people up to the age of 18, with developmental, behavioural, emotional, relationship and mental health problems. Specialized multidisciplinary assessments are offered and appropriate treatment is provided. This may include psychosocial interventions, individual, family and group therapy and, if required, pharmacological treatment.

Research has provided evidence that failing to address mental health concerns in young people leads to an increased future risk of suicide, deliberate self-harm, substance misuse and poorer achievements in education and employment; therefore, timely and effective interventions by CAMHS teams are crucial (Richards et al., 2009)

Early Intervention Service

Early Intervention teams usually work with people between the ages of 14 and 35 (although the qualifying age varies between different services) who are at risk of, or presenting with, the first signs of psychosis. Early Intervention Services aim to foster engagement and work together with educational, youth and social services to promote recovery. Services follow the same principle of care coordination as CMHTs but usually have smaller caseloads to assertively engage service users.

There is growing evidence that early assessment and prompt treatment with antipsychotic medication and psychosocial intervention can lead to improved longer term mental health and reduced suicide rates. Studies also show that specialist early interventions in psychosis lead to more reduced relapses and hospital stays than generic mental health teams, leading to a greater cost efficiency in the long term (Singh, 2010).

In addition to the above services, there are also specialist community-based services that work with service users with specific needs. These include outpatient counselling and psychotherapy for eating disorders and post-traumatic stress disorder.

COMMUNITY MENTAL HEALTH SERVICE MODELS

The Care Programme Approach

Mental illness places demands on services that no one discipline or agency can meet alone. It is logical that a system of effective co-ordination is required if all services are to work in harmony to the benefit of the service user.

(Department of Health, 1999a, p.2)

The Care Programme Approach (CPA) was introduced to the UK in 1990 for working-age adults in contact with secondary mental health services. The CPA aims to address the above-quoted issue with a 'whole-systems approach'. It sets requirements for Health Authorities in collaboration with social services to put in place arrangements for the care and treatment of people with severe mental health problems in the community (Department of Health, 1991).

Historical development of the CPA process

The CPA process is underpinned by four key elements:

- assessment: systematic arrangements for assessing the health and social needs of service users,
- care plan: written plan that addresses the identified health and social care needs, and outlines how they will be implemented and achieved,

- care coordinator: the appointment of a care coordinator to keep in close touch with the service user and monitor care,
- regular review: and, if need be, agreed changes to the care plan.

In 1999, the Government undertook a timely review of the CPA process. This review followed the introduction of the NSF for Mental Health (Department of Health, 1999b) which, along with public concern following several high-profile incidents in the community, further highlighted the importance of integrating health and social care. The review resulted in the publication of *Effective Care Coordination in Mental Health Services: Modernising the CPA* (Department of Health, 1999a). The key changes were focused on Integration of the CPA and care management models and creating a 'seamless service'. The CPA incorporated and replaced the social services model of care management. In effect, the CPA *is* care management for people of working age in contact with specialist mental health services. A joint assessment process prevents duplication and repetition, which can be confusing and distressing for the service user and carer, and ensures that services are allocated from whichever sources that match the persons need (Department of Health, 1999a).

Fully integrated services will have a single operational policy, shared processes of risk assessment, complaints procedures and serious incident reviews, joint staff training and shared information systems across both health and social care (Department of Health, 2005). The integrated approach requires that all new referrals are received at a single point of entry with one assessment to access a health or social service resource (Department of Health, 2005). A care coordinator is then appointed from either health or social care, to act as point of contact and to see that care plans are devised, implemented and reviewed at appropriate intervals. The requirement to review care plans six-monthly was changed, stipulating that this should now be an ongoing process.

Two levels of the CPA were introduced – standard and enhanced – to reflect the differing complexity of cases. However, this has since been reviewed back to a single level of CPA, to which service users are either subject or not. The NSF for Mental Health (Department of Health, 1999b) set a standard requiring that those under the CPA should be able to access services 24 h a day, 365 days a year. They should receive a written copy of their care plan, including a collaboratively formulated crisis and contingency plan which lays out the actions to be taken in the event of a crisis. Care plans should be holistic and promote partnership working with other services, such as housing, education, employment and, if indicated, drug and alcohol teams and criminal justice.

Despite the shift towards fully integrated health and social care services, there are arguments that current practice does not represent true integration. Barre and Evans (2005) draw attention to the tensions that remain between different disciplines, impacting on interprofessional working. Professional groups continue to have different policies, budgets, remuneration packages, working conditions, sickness management and entitlement to leave, which can lead to confusion, perceived differences in power or authority, and potentially resentment. Conversely, integration of health and social care services can also lead to fear of losing one's professional identity due to role overlap and generic ways of working.

The principles of caring for people in the community are based on the recovery model and include self-determination, normalization, a focus on service user strengths and recruiting environmental agencies. These principles are the topic of the next section.

Principles and models underlying mental healthcare in the community

The recovery approach is a broad, values-based approach that should underpin good professional practice and guide the process of any psychosocial interventions (Department of Health, 2006b; National Institute for Mental Health in England, 2005). Recovery is not about a cure, but an individual process which encourages the development of new meaning and purpose, and the integration of the experience into ones future life. The recovery approach is person-centred and focuses on the therapeutic relationships between service user and healthcare professionals. The relationships developed with individual service users in the community are often long-lasting, unlike the short relationships developed in the hospital setting. It is not sufficient to simply empathize with the service user. These relationships are more like partnerships: service users are empowered by being helped to find their own solutions to problems, and given hope through optimism and a recognition of their abilities. Some of the principles that can assist in achieving this are self-determination, normalization, a focus on service user strengths and recruiting environmental agencies and forces (Cnaan et al., 1990). Implementing these principles might involve a great variety of interventions, some of which may seem alien to those trained in professional disciplines. The mental health system itself can also be a barrier to the full implementation of these principles.

Self-determination

One of the major aims of the shift to community care was to foster service user self-determination. Service users have consistently demonstrated their desire to be informed about their treatment and to make decisions about it. This independence can be supported by helping service users to identify and pursue their own goals, and to take responsibility for their actions and behaviour, and respecting their decisions about medication. However, there is still progress to be made in improving service user participation in treatment and recovery plans (SCESNMHP, 2002).

Service user self-determination is the key to developing a partnership, as their goals and aspirations become the centre of the relationship. Self-determination can best be catered for by engaging in activities such as ensuring that the service user's consent to involve their family or others in the treatment plan is obtained, getting the service user to help plan the activities they want to engage in, encouraging the service user to set their own goals and ensuring that the service user can refuse, if they wish, to participate in activities. Success is gauged by the pursuit of the service user's goals, not by the extent to which the service user has conformed to the expectations of the mental health system or service providers. From this perspective the emphasis is on trying to achieve the goal, rather than on whether or not the service user succeeds.

The imposition of controversial Supervised Community Treatment (SCT) for some service users conflicts with the goal of service user self-determination and choice. SCT and the Community Treatment Order (CTO) were introduced in the 2007 reform of the Mental Health Act, as a way of safely treating and promoting recovery of service users in the community, as opposed to being detained in hospital. SCT is seen as particularly relevant for 'revolving-door' service users who experience frequent relapses and compulsory hospital admissions. Such service users often historically disengage from community services and/or become nonconcordant with their treatment plans following hospital discharge (Care Quality Commission, 2010). National statistics reveal that many more service users have been subject to SCT than was previously anticipated. The Care Quality Commission (2010) found that since their introduction there have been an average of 367 CTOs imposed every week. Indeed, 4107 CTOs were imposed in 2009/2010, which virtually doubled from the previous year (Care Quality Commission, 2010). Approximately 30% of the service users subjected to CTOs have no history of disengaging or refusing treatment (Care Quality Commission, 2010).

Excessive use of CTOs has an impact on the way service users view the mental health system, and their relationship with their care coordinators, who are required to closely monitor service users' adherence to their treatment order conditions. This can lead to difficulties in maintaining the therapeutic relationship, when service users may feel coerced, and lacking in choice and control. In such situations professionals also report perceiving themselves as more authoritarian and less able to work collaboratively towards true service user self-determination. The Mental Health Alliance (2010) highlights that many service users feel that SCT is stigmatizing, unsupportive and intrusive in nature. The most positive views from service users who have been made subject to a CTO are from those who have been actively involved in the planning of their treatment conditions, and given appropriate and consistent support in the community.

Supervised Community Treatment is a topic that will no doubt be of increasing interest and criticism in the near future, given its perceived coercive nature and the current limited evidence for good outcomes and improved quality of life for service users.

Normalization

Another principle of community care is normalization. Normalization can be achieved by encouraging service users to set the rules for behaviour, engaging in trips and excursions with service users, setting expectations for appropriate behaviour and expressing disapproval of deviant behaviour and encouraging a normal routine in matters such as hygiene, housework and dressing. Service users can be helped to integrate into the community by helping them develop social networks, for example by introducing them to community groups. Some services provide a minivan whereby service users can be transported to various community venues such as local social, cultural and sporting clubs and participate alongside other community members. However, care must be taken that this strategy does not increase social isolation by identifying the service users as a homogeneous group (Evans and Moltzen, 2000). Integration into the community can also be assisted by encouraging service users to use mainstream health services such as the local GP for their medication rather than specialist mental health services. Service users may also need help in developing work and leisure skills. For example, a service user may demonstrate artistic aptitude and skills, and wish to use their leisure time more meaningfully. The system response to this desire might be to provide a professional in a day hospital setting to teach the service user a craft such as leatherwork. An alternative would be to find a group of service users with similar wants and then advertise for volunteers to teach the service users particular skills for a limited period. Volunteers could be drawn from art schools and colleges, or they might be practising or retired artists, who could be asked to teach specific skills to the service users for half a day weekly, for 10 weeks. One of the great advantages of this method is that service users would be helped to better integrate into the community, rather than being marginalized and identified as a 'special' group.

Focus on service user strengths

A focus on service users' strengths rather than their problems and weaknesses can enhance motivation. When considering strengths, the nurse, in collaboration with service user, assesses what the service user wants, rather than their needs (Rapp, 1998). For example, if the service user wants to live independently of their family, then what they need to do to achieve this goal – such as adhering to their medication regimen or learning to budget – can be placed in a context relevant to the service user.

Recruiting environmental agencies

People with mental health concerns are one of the most socially excluded groups in society, having greater difficulty in accessing employment, education, recreational activities and quality healthcare (Social Exclusion Unit, 2004). This group is vulnerable to social isolation, poverty, physical ill health and stigmatization. Recruiting environmental agencies involves working effectively with community services, with the aim of promoting social inclusion of people who have a mental health disorder. Mental health professionals should engage in partnership working with services including GPs, housing departments, local employment agencies, voluntary work providers, education services and leisure facilities. Through this way of working, healthcare professionals can strive to break down barriers and help reduce stigma, which is one of the greatest barriers to social inclusion for people with a mental health disorder (Social Exclusion Unit, 2004). Service users may require assistance in procuring housing and work or education. They might need help in using public transport, shopping, budgeting, cooking and accessing mainstream leisure activities. Once these needs have been assessed, care coordinators can assist service users in achieving their goals by recruiting environmental agencies to provide the level of support that is required. This may range from simply liaising with local services and helping people access local activities of interest to them, to arranging a travel buddy or taxi card, or accompanying a service user to a medical or housing appointment if they find this particularly challenging or do not feel their views are being taken seriously.

More intensive, longer-term support could involve a floating support worker who can provide individualized support in the home or the community for a period of up to 2 years. Different levels of supported accommodation are also available for service users who require additional support to manage their activities of daily living. These include sheltered accommodation, group home facilities with drop in support staff, housing projects that are staffed 9 a.m.–5 p.m. and 24-hour-staffed high-support residences. These services are provided by organizations such as Richmond Fellowship, Supporting People, Hestia Housing and the Cyrenians.

Recruiting community forces also means taking account of the families of people with mental health problems. In the community, family and significant others are often expected to shoulder a large burden of care for their relatives. It is not uncommon for families to feel they are being blamed for their relative's problems, and

they have often been ignored when it comes to being informed about diagnoses and treatment. They have not been able to participate fully and meaningfully in treatment and recovery planning (SCESNMHP, 2002). However, carers are usually keen to be involved. They want up-to-date information and need to be confident that support will be prompt and available when needed. Mental health professionals should provide families and caregivers with advice and education about mental disorder and its treatment, and offer support to them in the management of any problems. Family education has been found to be one of the core interventions that help service users achieve quality of life (Drake et al., 2001). Although caring for a person with a mental health disorder can be rewarding, it can also be very stressful and tiring at times. The NSF for Mental Health (Department of Health, 1999b) called for greater attention to be given to the needs of carers. It stipulated that all carers who provide regular and substantial support are entitled to an assessment of their own needs. The carer's assessor can then discuss what could be provided to support the carer with any challenges in their role, to enhance the balance in their lives and maintain their own health and wellbeing. Services provided may include support groups, signposting to voluntary agencies, information about government services to which they are entitled and direct payments for carers and residential respite services. Carers should have their own care plan which is to be reviewed on an annual basis.

The strengths model

The strengths model (Rapp, 1998; Rapp and Goscha, 2006) was developed in response to a perceived emphasis in other models on the problems associated with mental disorder, rather than the service user's strengths and talents. In this model individual professionals work closely with individual service users. The relationship between care coordinator and service user, which is the first linking activity, is considered paramount and also provides a vehicle for the monitoring function. In this model the community is conceptualized as a resource, and as being full of resources capable of meeting the diverse needs of a wide variety of service users (for further discussion of the strengths model see Ch. 2).

The rehabilitation model

The rehabilitation model (Anthony et al., 1993), as with the strengths model, emphasizes the need to deliver services that service users want, rather than the goals of the mental health delivery system. However, the focus of this model is on assessing and developing the skills service users require to lead a normal, satisfying life. Through the development of skills the person is helped to create a meaningful identity that fosters hope (McQuistion et al.,

2000). This focus is in keeping with a philosophy that is centred on service user wellbeing and quality of life, not just keeping the person out of hospital. It is rehabilitative in that it focuses on wellness and competence rather than illness and disability. The type of training offered is usually training in daily living tasks. These tasks might include such things as how to work the washing machine or where to go to pay the rent. This training is best provided in the service user's place and with their own materials and tools, known as 'in vivo'. In vivo training overcomes problems with the transfer of skills from one setting to another and ensures that the service user can function in their particular environment.

The type of care offered should be determined by service user needs and goals. Too often the focus is on what the mental health delivery system is able to provide. When service users are asked about the goals they seek for themselves, they indicate that these are, in order of priority: money, availability of healthcare, a decent place to live, transportation, socialization and help if needed (Rapp, 1998). These goals contrast with those of the mental health service delivery system, which seeks reduced hospital inpatient stays, integration, mainstreaming and continuity of care. They also contrast with those of many service providers, who often simply want the service user to adhere to their medication regimen.

Service users in the community require a wide range of support services according to their varying needs at any one time. Care in the community seeks to encourage the development of the service user as a person in interaction with others, rather than as someone suffering from a health problem or disability. The focus of care is more on day-to-day functioning and less on 'illness' management. The major goals of community care are to assist people towards independent living, and to help them fit into the community and develop a sense of belonging. In the community, the service user needs functional skills such as being able to budget, plan meals and manage their medication. He or she also needs social competencies, such as being able to establish and use relationships with family and peers, and to express feelings without losing control (Yurkovich and Smyer, 1998).

The MDT in the community

A team approach is most often preferred in community settings. According to Yurkovich (1989, p. 19) a community setting is made therapeutic by 'an interdisciplinary team working together in collaboration with the service user, using a community–service user setting, to provide a microcosm of the "real" world'. A team approach is expensive and is often considered to be best confined to the care of people with the most complex problems (Onyett and Ford, 1996). Like its hospital counterpart, the MDT in the community is the vehicle for the delivery of care and consists of many professional disciplines. The principles guiding the operation of MDTs are shared tasks and the provision of complementary competencies by different professionals (Onyett, 1999). The MDT is more than a group of professionals who interact with one another as necessary. Unlike the conventional medical model of team working, the MDT 'is a mechanism for case allocation, clinical decision making, teaching, training and supervision, and the application of the necessary skill mix for the best outcomes for service users' (Renouf and Meadows, 2001).

NURSE'S STORY: A SERVICE USER IN THE COMMUNITY

One of the biggest difficulties I face is whether to admit someone to hospital or to care for them in the community when they relapse. John is a 36-year-old service user of mine who was dual-diagnosed with schizophrenia and substance abuse problems with whom I have been working for 2 years.

About 6 weeks ago he started to develop psychotic symptoms again. He believed the men who were renovating a block of flats next door to him were entering his flat at night and interfering with him sexually. His symptoms weren't helped by the fact that he was taking a variety of drugs including marijuana and possibly speed. I was having a hard time knowing what to do with him, because he has always been reluctant to accept mental health services. Although he agrees to letting me visit him about every 6–8 weeks, he's never very forthcoming about what he has been up to. This reluctance, along with the fact that he had always had to be detained in hospital under the Mental Health Act, made me think he would be unwilling to go to hospital voluntarily if it came to that. So I had to think of some way in which I could respect his preferences, while at the same time ensuring he was taking his prescribed medication and not so much of the unprescribed stuff. The other issues I had to keep in mind were that if his mental state continued to deteriorate he might pose a danger to himself or, more likely, other people. However, because he wasn't violent or abusive at this stage, I decided to continue to manage him in the community if I could get him to agree to more frequent visits, which he did. I also arranged to do a joint visit with one of my colleagues, a social worker, so as to get another person's perspective and to ensure that someone else was familiar with his current condition in case a crisis situation arose. During my visits, which I had gradually increased to twice a week, we talked about his prescribed medication and it emerged that he was having problems with side effects. Although he hadn't stopped taking it completely, he was taking it erratically. I suggested that the psychiatrist might be able to help and he eventually agreed to visit him at the clinic.

At this stage John is still psychotic but I'm pretty sure he's taking his medication as prescribed and seeing the psychiatrist weekly for the moment, and I visit him once a week to monitor how he's doing.

In this model of team work, each professional brings specialist skills, which, for nursing, are often skills in relation to medication management. This diversity of professional expertise is one of the great strengths of the MDT, because people with severe and long-term mental health problems have many needs that cannot be met satisfactorily by a single discipline. However, in order for the team to function effectively there is also much overlap in what are termed core skills, such as risk assessment, intervening in crises and forming trusting relationships with service users. Therefore, its potential weaknesses are that because of the blurring of responsibilities among community mental health professionals all need to be aware of the unique contribution of each to ensure effective care for service users, and information about service users needs to be shared in a timely way. The team method of working has been criticized on the grounds that it is basically 'an institutional model delivered in the community that limits service users' choices and options' (Pyke, 1999, p. 79). However, it does offer the advantage of continuity of care. When a staff member goes on leave there is always someone else who can fill in.

Despite the existence of the MDT, working in the community can be professionally isolating at times (Witheridge, 1989). Individual professionals often work alone. They may visit individual service users in their home, which might be a boarding house, hostel, the street or even a prison. Or they might meet the service user in some other community setting such as a park or a coffee shop. They often also lack easy access to other professionals and, if a crisis occurs, must decide how best to act, so sound clinical judgement and sound training in risk assessment are required. For example, the police might need to be involved in helping admit a service user to hospital, and distressed family and neighbours comforted. In the event of hospitalization, the professional would liaise with the inpatient team to devise a workable discharge plan. They might also have to arrange for the care of animals and plants while the service user is in hospital.

THE FUTURE OF MENTAL HEALTH SERVICES IN THE UK

There is an ongoing national move to reconfigure mental health service provision in the UK with a shift towards more personalized, efficient and cost-effective care as indicated by recent White Papers and policies such as *Liberating the NHS* (Department of Health, 2010b), *No Health Without Mental Health* (Department of Health, 2011) and *Our Health, Our Care, Our Say* (Department of Health, 2006a). Mental health currencies or tariffs will allow contracting and payment for services in a consistent way. All service users will be clustered into one of 21 groups (plus five forensic pathways) based on their presenting mental health problems and needs. Each cluster is linked to a package of care that a typical service user might expect to be offered, and commissioners of

mental health services will then pay a nationally set tariff for various inpatient or outpatient treatments (Department of Health, 2011).

A process of Payment by Result is being implemented to support the modernization of the NHS, whereby service providers are paid for the care they give and rewarded for efficiency. *Liberating the NHS* calls for these tariffs to be implemented by 2013 and for similar currencies to be developed for CAMHS in future (Department of Health, 2010b). Existing services are changing to meet this new agenda, with some areas of the UK already reconfigured and others in the planning stages for change.

Assessment services (or early access services) will see and assess all new referrals for acute, severe and enduring mental health problems for people aged 18 and older. The service will incorporate older persons over the age of 65, excluding those with an organic condition. The service will provide follow up and treatment for service users who are likely to respond to treatment for a period of up to 6 months.

CMHTs are being reconfigured into Community Recovery Teams. The aim of recovery teams is to support service users with severe and enduring mental health disorders who are aged 18 and over. The focus will be on recovery, enhanced mental wellbeing and social inclusion. Community Recovery Teams will also incorporate existing Assertive Outreach Services, with most AOT staff bringing their own caseloads and working within the recovery team. These services will also incorporate service users over the age of 65 providing they have a diagnosis of a functional, nonorganic mental health disorder. Separate dementia services for older persons with cognitive impairment are being introduced, replacing current Older Person Services.

These changes are also reflected in inpatient services, with generic acute wards being reconfigured as assessment and recovery wards. Assessment wards treat newly admitted service users who are in some form of crisis, usually for a maximum of up to 3–4 weeks. Assessment wards will link closely with the Community Assessment Teams. Recovery wards will treat service users who require longer term care, especially those well known to services. In some areas, two different types of recovery ward have been implemented – acute and complex – to meet the different needs of service users requiring extended periods of hospitalization. Recovery wards will have strong links with the Community Recovery Teams.

CONCLUSION

In this chapter it has been argued that the quality of the environment in which service user care takes place is important to their recovery and rehabilitation. Environmental strategies in the care of people with mental health problems have a long history, but their application over time has been patchy. These strategies reached their peak in the eighteenth century, when it was noticed that service users were more 'manageable' in a pleasant environment. In the twentieth century, Thomas Main and Maxwell Jones pioneered the concept of the hospital and environment as treatment tools. The principles on which the therapeutic milieu is based include open communication, democratization, reality confrontation, permissiveness, group cohesion and the MDT. The goals of the inpatient therapeutic milieu are containment, structure, support, involvement, validation, symptom management and maintaining links with family and the community.

The preferred contemporary setting for the provision of mental healthcare is the community, which accords best with the principle of caring for people in the least-restrictive environment. The predominant form of service delivery in the community is the CPA, and there are a variety of community-based services for service users with different needs. The principles of caring in the community are based on the recovery approach, and include self-determination, normalization, a focus on service user strengths and the community as a resource. There is an ongoing national move to reconfigure mental health service provision in the UK with a shift towards more personalized, efficient and cost-effective care. Major changes in the structure of community and inpatient services have already been implemented, and further changes are on the horizon.

EXERCISES FOR CLASS ENGAGEMENT

Discuss the following questions with your tutorial group.

◆ How can an emphasis on safety in the inpatient setting promote or detract from the development of therapeutic relationships?

◆ How can nurses in an inpatient setting provide support to families?

◆ Is it possible and/or desirable to maintain a nursing identity when working in a community setting?

◆ What services are available in your community to assist mental health service users?

REFERENCES

Allen, D., 2010. Community services vs crisis resolution teams. Ment. Health Pract. 14 (1), 26–28.

Anthony, W.A., Forbess, R., Cohen, M.R., 1993. Rehabilitation oriented case management. In: Harris, M., Bergman, H. (Eds.), Case Management for Mentally Ill Patients: Theory and Practice. Harwood Academic, Chur.

Baguley, I., Alexander, J., Middleton, H., Hope, R., 2007. New ways of working in acute inpatient care: a case for change. J. Ment. Health Train., Educ. Pract. 2, 43–52.

Barre, T., Evans, R., 2005. Integration: holy writ or shibboleth? Ment. Health Pract. 9 (3), 40–43.

Benbow, R., Bowers, L., 1998. Rehabilitation using therapeutic community principles. Nurs. Times 94 (1), 56–57.

Bowers, L., Simpson, A., Alexander, J., et al., 2005. The nature and purpose of acute psychiatric wards: the Tompkins acute ward study. J. Ment. Health 14 (6), 625–635.

Care Quality Commission, 2010. Monitoring the Use of the Mental Health Act in 2009/10. Care Quality Commision, London.

Centre for the Economics of Mental Health, 2007. Model to Assess the Economic Impact of Integrating CRHT and Inpatient Services. Health Service and Population Research Department King's College, London.

Chesters, J., Fletcher, M., Jones, R., 2005. Mental illness recovery and place. Aust. e-J. Adv. Ment. Health 4 (2), 1–9.

Cleary, M., Edwards, C., Meehan, T., 1999. Factors influencing nurse–patient interaction in the acute psychiatric setting: an exploratory investigation. Aust. N. Z. J. Ment. Health Nurs. 8 (3), 109–116.

Cnaan, R.A., Blankertz, L., Messinger, K.W., et al., 1990. Experts' assessment of psychosocial rehabilitation principles. Psychosoc. Rehabil. J. 13 (3), 59–73.

Cooper, D., 1967. Psychiatry and Anti-Psychiatry. Tavistock, London.

Creedy, D., Crowe, M., 1996. Establishing a therapeutic milieu with adolescents. Aust. N. Z. J. Ment. Health Nurs. 5 (2), 84–89.

Delaney, K.R., 1992. Nursing in child psychiatric milieus. Part 1: what nurses do. J. Child Psychiatr. Nurs. 5 (1), 15–19.

Delaney, K.R., Pitula, C.R., Perraud, S., 2000. Psychiatric hospitalization and process description: what will nursing add? J. Psychosoc. Nurs. Ment. Health Serv. 38 (3), 7–13.

Department of Health, 1991. The Care Programme Approach for People with a Mental Illness, Referred to Specialist Psychiatric Services. Department of Health, London.

Department of Health, 1999a. Effective Care Coordination in Mental Health Services: Modernising the CPA. Department of Health, London.

Department of Health, 1999b. National Service Framework for Mental Health – Modern Standards and Service Models for Mental Health. Department of Health, London.

Department of Health, 2002. Mental Health Policy Implementation Guide: National Minimum Standards for General Adult Services in Psychiatric Intensive Care Units (PICU) and Low Secure

Environments. <http://www.dh.gov.uk/prod_consum_dh/groups/dh_digitalassets/@dh/@en/documents/digitalasset/dh_4060440.pdf>.

Department of Health, 2005. Building Bridges: A Guide to Arrangements for Inter-agency Working for the Care and Protection of Severely Mentally Ill People. Department of Health, London.

Department of Health, 2006a. Our Health Our Care Our Say. Department of Health, London.

Department of Health, 2006b. From Values to Action: The Chief Nursing Officers Report of Mental Health. Department of Health, London.

Department of Health, 2007. Best Practice Guidance Specification for Adult Medium-Secure Services Health Offender Partnerships 2007. <http://www.rcpsych.ac.uk/pdf/Guidance%202.pdf>.

Department of Health, 2010a. See Think Act: Your Guide to Relational Security. <http://www.dh.gov.uk/prod_consum_dh/groups/dh_digitalassets/documents/digitalasset/dh_113671.pdf>.

Department of Health, 2010b. Liberating the NHS. Department of Health, London.

Department of Health, 2011. No Health Without Mental Health. Department of Health, London.

Drake, R.E., Goldman, H.H., Leff, H.S., et al., 2001. Implementing evidence-based practices in routine mental health service settings. Psychiatr. Serv. 52 (2), 179–182.

Duffy, D., 1995. Out of the shadows: a study of the special observation of suicidal psychiatric in-patients. J. Adv. Nurs. 21 (5), 944–950.

Evans, I.M., Moltzen, N.L., 2000. Defining effective community support for long-term psychiatric patients according to behavioural principles. Aust. N. Z. J. Psychiatry 34, 637–644.

Ford, K., King, M., 2005. A model for developing assertive outreach: meeting local needs. Ment. Health Pract. 8 (10), 34–39.

Goldstein, J.L., Godemont, M.M.L., 2007. The legend and lessons of Geel, Belgium: a 1500-year-old legend, a 21st-century model. Commun. Ment. Health J. 29 (5), 441–458.

Greene, J.A., 1997. Milieu therapy. In: Johnson, B.S. (Ed.), Psychiatric-Mental Health Nursing: Adaptation and Growth. Lippincott-Raven, Philadelphia, pp. 221–231.

Healthcare Commission, 2008. The Pathway to Recovery: A Review of NHS Acute Inpatient Mental Health Services. <http://www.cqc.org.uk/_db/_documents/The_pathway_to_recovery_200807251020.pdf>.

Hummelvoll, J.K., Severinsson, E., 2001. Coping with everyday reality: mental health professionals' reflections on the care provided in an acute psychiatric ward. Aust. N. Z. J. Ment. Health Nurs. 10 (3), 156–166.

Jansen, E., 1980. Editor's discussion. In: Jansen, E. (Ed.), The Therapeutic Community: Outside the Hospital. Croom Helm, London, pp. 19–51.

Jones, J., Ward, M., Wellman, N., et al., 2000. Psychiatric inpatients' experience of nursing observation: a United Kingdom perspective. J. Psychosoc. Nurs. 28 (12), 10–20.

Jones, M., 1953. The Therapeutic Community. Basic Books, New York.

Kahn, E.M., 1994. The patient–staff community meeting: old tools, new rules. J. Psychosoc. Nurs. 32 (8), 23–26.

Krauss, J.B., Slavinsky, A.T., 1982. The Chronically Ill Psychiatric Patient and the Community. Blackwell Scientific Publications, Boston.

LeCuyer, E.A., 1992. Milieu therapy for short stay units: a transformed practice theory. Arch. Psychiatr. Nurs. 6 (2), 108–116.

McQuistion, H.L., Goisman, R.M., Tennison Jr, C.R., 2000. Psychosocial rehabilitation: issues and answers for psychiatry. Commun. Ment. Health J. 36 (6), 605–616.

Main, T., 1946. The hospital as a therapeutic community. Bull. Menninger Clin. 10, 66–70.

Main, T., 1980. Some basic concepts in therapeutic community work. In: Jansen, E. (Ed.), The Therapeutic Community: Outside the Hospital. Croom Helm, London, pp. 52–63.

Mental Health Alliance, 2010. Mental Health Alliance Briefing Paper 2: Supervised Community Treatment. The Mental Health Foundation, London.

Mills, J.A., Harrison, T., 2007. John Rickman, Wilfred Ruprecht Bion, and the origins of the therapeutic community. Hist. Psychol. 10 (1), 22–43.

Morrison, P., Lehane, M., Palmer, C., et al., 1997. The use of behavioural mapping in a study of seclusion. Aust. N. Z. J. Ment. Health Nurs. 6 (1), 11–18.

Munich, R.L., 2000. Leadership and restructured roles: the evolving inpatient treatment team. Bull. Menninger Clin. 64 (4), 482–494.

Murray, R.B., Baier, M., 1993. Use of therapeutic milieu in a community setting. J. Psychosoc. Nurs. 31 (10), 11–16.

National Institute for Mental Health in England, 2005. NIMHE Guiding Statement on Recovery. National Institute for Mental Health in England, London.

National Mental Health Development Unit, 2011. Improving Access to Pscychological Therapies. National Mental Health Development Unit, England.

Norton, K., Bloom, S.L., 2004. The art and challenges of long-term and short-term democratic therapeutic communities. Psychiatr. Q. 75 (3), 249–261.

O'Brien, A.P., Woods, M., Palmer, C., 2001. The emancipation of nursing practice: applying anti-psychiatry to the therapeutic community. Aust. N. Z. J. Ment. Health Nurs. 10 (1), 3–9.

Onyett, S., 1999. Community mental health team working as a socially valued enterprise. J. Ment. Health 8 (3), 245–251.

Onyett, S., Ford, R., 1996. Multidisciplinary community teams: where is the wreckage? J. Ment. Health 5 (1), 47–55.

Porter, R., 2002. Madness: A Brief History. Oxford University Press, Oxford.

Prebble, K., McDonald, B., 1997. Adaptation to the mental health setting: the lived experience of comprehensive nurse graduates. Aust. N. Z. J. Ment. Health Nurs. 6 (1), 30–36.

Pyke, J., 1999. Community services and supports. In: Clinton, M., Nelson, S. (Eds.), Advanced Practice in Mental Health Nursing. Blackwell Science, Oxford.

Rapp, C., 1998. The Strengths Model: Case Management with People

Suffering from Severe and Persistent Mental Illness. Oxford University Press, New York.

Rapp, C., Goscha, R.J., 2006. A beginning theory of strengths. In: Rapp, C.A., Goscha, R.J. (Eds.), The Strengths Model: Case Management with People with a Psychiatric Disability, second ed. Oxford University Press, New York.

Renouf, N., Meadows, G., 2001. Teamwork. In: Meadows, G., Singh, B. (Eds.), Mental Health in Australia: Collaborative Community Practice. Oxford University Press, London.

Rethink, 2006. Behind Closed Doors: Acute Mental Health Care in the UK. <http://www.rethink.org/mental_health_shop/products/rethink_publications/behind_closed_doors.html#>.

Richards, M., Abbott, R., Collis, G., et al., 2009. Childhood Mental Health and Life Chances in Post-War Britain: Insights from Three National Birth Cohort Studies. SCMH/The Smith Institute/Unison & MRC, London.

Sainsbury Centre for Mental Health, 2006. The Search for Acute Solutions: Improving the Quality of Care in Acute Psychiatric Wards. <http://www.centreformentalhealth.org.uk/publications/search_acute_solutions.aspx?ID=476>.

SCESNMHP (Steering Committee for the Evaluation of the Second National Mental Health Plan), 2002.

Evaluation of the Second National Mental Health Plan. SCESNMHP, Canberra.

Schaedle, R., McGrew, J.H., Bond, G.R., 2002. A comparison of experts' perspectives on assertive community treatment and intensive case management. Psychiatr. Serv. 53 (2), 207–210.

Sedgwick, P., 1982. Psychopolitics. Pluto Press, London.

Shives, L., 2008. Basic Concepts of Psychiatric-Mental Health Nursing. Lippincott, Williams and Watkins, Philadephia.

Shorter, E., 1997. A History of Psychiatry: From the Era of the Asylum to the Age of Prozac. John Wiley & Sons, New York.

Singh, B.S., Castle, D.J., 2007. Why are community psychiatry services in Australia doing it so hard? Med. J. Aust. 187 (7), 410–412.

Singh, S., 2010. Early intervention in psychosis. Br. J. Psychiatry 196, 343–345.

SNMAC (Standing Nursing and Midwifery Advisory Committee), 1999. Mental Health Nursing: "Addressing Acute Concerns". <http://www.dh.gov.uk/en/Publicationsandstatistics/Publications/PublicationsPolicyAndGuidance/DH_4008476?ssSourceSiteId=ab>.

Social Exclusion Unit, 2004. Mental Health and Social Exclusion. Office of the Deputy Prime Minister, London.

Thomas, S.P., Shattell, M., Martin, T., 2002. What's therapeutic about the therapeutic milieu? Arch. Psychiatr. Nurs. 16 (3), 99–107.

Tobias, G., Haslam-Hopwood, G., 2003. The role of the primary clinician in the multidisciplinary team. Bull. Menninger Clin. 67 (1), 5–17.

Tuck, I., Keels, M.C., 1992. Milieu therapy: a review of development of this concept and its implications for psychiatric nursing. Issues Ment. Health Nurs. 13, 51–58.

Watson, J., 1992. Maintenance of therapeutic community principles in an age of biopharmacology and economic restraints. Arch. Psychiatr. Nurs. 6 (3), 183–188.

Witheridge, T.F., 1989. The assertive community treatment worker: an emerging role and its implications for professional training. Hosp. Commun. Psychiatry 40, 620–624.

Yalom, I.D., 1983. Inpatient Group Therapy. Basic Books, New York.

Yurkovich, E., 1989. Patient and nurse roles in the therapeutic community. Perspect. Psychiatr. Care 25 (3/4), 18–22.

Yurkovich, E., Smyer, T., 1998. Strategies for maintaining optimal wellness in the chronic mentally ill. Perspect. Psychiatr. Care 34 (3), 17–24.

Chapter | 22 |

Person-centred approaches to managing risk

Kim Usher, Kim Foster, and Lauretta Luck

CHAPTER POINTS

- Communication is a skill that underpins all mental health nursing interventions and is central to assessing and managing risk.
- Self-harm and suicidal behaviour need to be differentiated.
- Assessment of risk behaviours is an essential part of assessment.
- Effective interventions can be implemented when working with people who exhibit aggressive, violent, self-harming and suicidal behaviour.
- Service user choice and informed consent underlie care considerations in regard to people who exhibit challenging behaviour.
- The individual strengths and limitations of the nurse and service user must be recognized and considered in care planning and delivery.

KEY TERMS

- aggression
- anger
- capacity
- communication skills
- counter-transference

DOI: http://dx.doi.org/10.1016/B978-0-7020-4493-9.00022-6

- empathy
- ethicolegal issues
- informed choice
- informed consent
- limit-setting
- professional boundaries
- risk
- seclusion
- self-harm
- suicide
- therapeutic relationship
- transference
- violence

LEARNING OUTCOMES

The material in this chapter will assist you to:

- define the key terms related to communicating with individuals,
- describe the key communication skills necessary to establish and maintain a therapeutic nurse–service user relationship and to engage effectively with families and carers,
- outline a strengths approach to working with families and carers when a person has a mental health problem,
- understand nursing assessment and management of distressed service users who may be aggressive,
- understand the principles of teaching anger management/impulse control,
- understand nursing strategies for service users who are suicidal and service users who self-harm,
- outline the skills nurses use to work with service users who demonstrate risk behaviours such as aggression, violence, self-harm and suicide,
- distinguish between the terms used in regard to suicide and self-harm,
- outline the relevant ethicolegal issues related to informed consent and seclusion.

INTRODUCTION

This chapter outlines person-centred and interpersonal skills related to mental health nursing. It is based on a perspective that values the strengths and skills of both the mental health nurse and the person who is the service user, while recognizing that both can have vulnerabilities (Hem and Heggen, 2003). The chapter is divided into three sections. It begins with an overview of the communication

and person-centred skills that underpin the therapeutic nurse–service user relationship and nurses' interactions with families and carers. These are the essential underlying skills that the mental health nurse needs when working with service users in special situations. Issues related to nurse vulnerabilities are discussed in this section, particularly in relation to use of self. A strengths approach to working with families and carers is also outlined. The second section of the chapter discusses risk. In this section the management of service users at risk of self-harm, suicide, aggression and violence is addressed. Special attention is given to risk assessment. Tools to aid assessment, and subsequent nursing interventions, are included. Section three introduces the ethicolegal issues of service user choice and consent, which are important when planning and implementing nursing skills.

COMMUNICATING WITH SERVICE USERS AND FAMILIES

Arguably, mental health nurses use 'self' as their most essential therapeutic tool, and the nurse–service user relationship is one of the most vital clinical components of nursing practice (Fourie et al., 2005; Lauder et al., 2002; Stein-Parbury, 2005). 'Self' in this context relates to self-awareness and the need for the mental health nurse to understand and be aware of their own subjective and experiential world while using specialist skills. This use of self includes professional detachment, self-awareness and understanding of personal emotions, beliefs and values (see Ch. 1). This personal understanding is used to facilitate the therapeutic relationship, where the outcome is a focus on the needs of service users and their families (Fontaine, 2003; Horsfall et al., 2000). The therapeutic relationship is a balance between the personal self, offering human closeness and professional distance (Hem and Heggen, 2003; Welch, 2005). What does this mean for nurses practising in this specialty? It challenges nurses to review who they are in ways that may not be as rigorously required in other nursing specialties. In addition, there is an increased emphasis on interpersonal communication skills. It is understandable that some novice nurses have difficulty with the notion that communication is a 'skill' and that these skills require theory, understanding, practice and personal reflection. One of the activities we all engage in throughout our lives is communication: we communicate with others individually, in groups, via the telephone, via electronic means, in writing and in a variety of social, informal and formal situations. It could therefore be claimed that this amount of understanding, practice and personal involvement would mean that we already have expertise in communication. Although this argument seems reasonable, there are many indicators to suggest that we are not always good at communicating.

Communication as it applies to mental health nursing has other attributes in addition to those with which we are most familiar. Mental health nurses use communication skills to develop a therapeutic relationship with service users and their families. Additional focused communication skills are required with respect to communication theory, skills and practice, and these are discussed below.

Therapeutic relationships

A cornerstone skill for initiation, development and maintenance of a therapeutic relationship between nurse and service user is interpersonal communication (Cameron et al., 2005; Lauder et al., 2002; Stickley and Freshwater, 2006). Further, there is increasing evidence that supports a positive link between the efficacy of a therapeutic relationship and improved outcomes for service users diagnosed with mental health problems (Howgego et al., 2003). A therapeutic relationship is an enabling relationship that supports the needs of the service user. The nurse is entrusted to understand the service user, to enable them to understand their own needs and therefore become empowered in their life (Lauder et al., 2002; McAllister et al., 2004). Mutually agreed goals for nursing practice are enhanced by the therapeutic relationship. A therapeutic relationship is based on *rapport* – establishing a connection with the person and developing trust – and is distinct from interviewing, counselling and education (McAllister et al., 2004). Therapeutic relationship differs from other interactions in its structure, purpose and intent. The value of the relationship is exhibited by improvement in the service user's wellbeing and capacity to take control of their life (Borg and Kristiansen, 2004; Lauder et al., 2002). Therapeutic relationships also differ from social relationships and intimate relationships (Horsfall et al., 2000). While establishing and engaging in a therapeutic relationship, the mental health nurse focuses his or her skills on the service user and judiciously uses self-disclosure. In addition, contemporary mental health services are now focusing more on the context in which the service user exists, and there is a developing emphasis on providing family-focused care, as opposed to the traditional focus on the individual service user. Therefore the principles of therapeutic rapport also need to be extended to include families and carers of people with mental health problems.

Empathy

Empathy is not sympathy. *Sympathy* is about pity, compassion, commiseration and condolence, and while there are social situations where the offering of sympathy may be culturally and socially relevant, still it is not empathy. Nor is sympathy appropriate for the therapeutic relationship. Five conceptualizations of empathy have been proposed: empathy as a human trait, a professional state, a communication process, caring and a special relationship (Kunyk and Olson, 2001). Empathy as a communication process and a professional state can offer us a clear understanding of what we mean by 'empathy' and a theoretical basis for our understanding (see Ch. 1).

Empathy is about observing, listening, understanding and attending. It is 'being' with the person physically, cognitively and emotionally, and understanding their story, thoughts, feelings, beliefs and emotions. It is an ability to understand the person as fully as we can, and from their subjectively expressed view. It means not making judgements and not giving advice, but genuinely striving to understand the service user's subjective experience and communicating this understanding to the person. Here empathy is conceptualized as both a communication process and a professional process (Kunyk and Olson, 2001).

Empathy involves perceptiveness, listening to meaning, listening to feelings and listening in context, attending, responding appropriately and maintaining presence with the service user (Boggs, 2007). In this sense, empathy is linked to the therapeutic use of self. The mental health nurse is able to actively listen to both the cognitive content of the service user's story and the subjective meaning this has for the service user. Nurses need to be honest about their own experiences and subjective responses, so they are able to clearly hear, respect and understand the experience of the service user. This means that the service user's experience is acknowledged (Collins and Cutcliffe, 2003). Empathy is one of the important building blocks of a constructive therapeutic alliance between nurse and service user.

Earlier research suggested that rather than the five conceptualizations of empathy listed above, there are two types of empathy (Alligood, 1992, cited in Evans et al., 1998). The first is *basic empathy*. This is our trait capacity to understand and feel for others. This personal characteristic is shaped by our family, social environment and culture, and is contextually and culturally expressed. The second type of empathy is *trained empathy*

(Evans et al., 1998). Trained empathy is a professional skill that is taught, learnt and developed. Trained empathy enables the nurse to create a trusting relationship in which the service user feels able to discuss their feelings and thoughts, thus facilitating the nurse's understanding of the service user, their responses and health needs (Reynolds and Scott, 2000). These two types of empathy are reflected in the five conceptualizations and can be aligned with 'empathy as a human trait' and 'empathy as a professional state' (Kunyk and Olson, 2001, p. 319).

Two personal characteristics of the nurse that contribute to the skill of empathy are the capacity for immediacy and the ability to be open-minded. The skill of *immediacy* refers to the capacity of the mental health nurse to respond to the service user and their feelings in the 'here and now' with warmth and genuineness (Kneisl et al., 2004; Reynolds and Scott, 2000). It is a combination of both an appropriate physical presence and the clinical use of communication skills, such as those discussed in this book. *Open-minded* people tend to have a dynamic or fluid (rather than static) world view. Open-mindedness conveys the nurse's attitude of acceptance and capacity to 'take the person as they are'.

Active listening

Active listening requires attention, genuineness and an ability to 'hear' what the service user has to say and validate the meaning of the service user's perceptions. This does not mean that the nurse overtly or inadvertently agrees, or disagrees, with delusions or hallucinations; rather, the service user's perception and experience are heard and acknowledged. The skilful use of active listening requires practice and reflection on the part of the mental health nurse and contributes to the capacity of the nurse to maintain presence with the service user. As discussed in Chapter 1, the examined 'self' affects the 'micro' skills that are valuable in the therapeutic relationship.

Listening to service users is improved by being available, in the here and now, in the best environment for communication: in a therapeutic space with reduced distractions and noise (Stickley and Freshwater, 2006). The ideal may not always be possible, but consideration of the safety and privacy of the environment demonstrates good communication skills on behalf of the nurse. Often when we first start working with people in the mental health context we are overly worried about what we will say next rather than what the service user is saying. A good way to increase your skills and be more effective is to concentrate on what the service user is saying and become an effective and active listener.

Mental health nurses' communication skills are a combination and purposeful extension of a number of personal and professional communication strategies (Rydon, 2005). While the skills discussed here are not exhaustive, they offer some explanation and description of communication strategies, including closed and open-ended questions, reflective listening, paraphrasing, summarizing, body language and touch, influence and transference and counter-transference.

Closed and open-ended questions

Closed and open-ended questions elicit different types of responses from the service user, and both are useful in mental health nursing. A *closed question* is one that elicits a brief answer, often a single word. Asking many closed questions in a row can seem like an interrogation, but there is value in asking closed questions in order to gather specific information. An *open-ended question* allows the respondent to answer more fully. Open-ended questions have the advantage of not narrowing down or directing the response, and so the answer can give you information that you may not have expected. This style of questioning also allows the service user to tell their subjective experiences, an important communication strategy that enhances the nurse–service user therapeutic relationship. Individuals will nevertheless share information at the level they feel comfortable or safe with, so a closed question might elicit a detailed response or an open-ended question might be answered with a single word. Ordinarily, however, these questioning styles are a good guide for communication (see Table 22.1).

Reflective listening

Reflective listening means literally echoing the service user's communication. The purpose of this skill is to redirect the content or feelings back to the service user. Reflective listening can include reflecting the content of the communication or reflecting the service user's feelings (Stickley and Freshwater, 2006). Reflection of feelings, however, requires prudent, skilful use and a good

Table 22.1 Examples of closed and open-ended questions

Closed	Open-ended
Are you feeling good today?	How are you feeling today?
Are you still getting side effects from your medication?	How are your medications affecting you now?
Do you want to come to group?	What would you like to do today?
Does feeling stressed still make you feel like harming yourself?	How does your stress affect you now?

therapeutic relationship. Over-use of reflective listening can seem contrived and stilted:

Service user:	*I feel really sad about my family.*
Nurse:	*You feel really sad about your family?*
Service user:	*I want to go home.*
Nurse:	*You want to go home?*

Paraphrasing

Essentially, paraphrasing is confirming the main points made by the service user – either the content of the communication or the feelings – by restating them (Arnold, 2007). Restating these main points can be a combination of your own words or the same phrases that the service user has used. Paraphrasing is a useful communication skill that is different to, but can overlap with, other skills. Paraphrasing can be used to confirm that you have heard and understood the service user's subjective experience or perception. Any misunderstandings can also be clarified with the use of paraphrasing (Stein-Parbury, 2005). It indicates that you have been actively listening to both content and feelings.

Service user:	*I'm sorry for the mess I'm in. It's just that some days I can't find the energy to tidy up or do anything.*
Nurse:	*I see. You're feeling distressed about your lack of energy.*
Service user:	*If they do that to me one more time I'm just going to have to tell them, that's all.*
Nurse:	*It sounds like you're feeling angry about this issue and think it's time to let people know.*

Summarizing

Summarizing means putting together the main issues and ensuring that you have understood them from the service user's perspective. The main issues could be focused on the content, perceptions or feelings of the service user. This communication strategy can be useful for clarifying what you have shared, or for gaining some new perspectives or insights, or it can be used to conclude your current communication with the service user (Arnold, 2007).

Nurse:	*So, the important issues for you are finding suitable accommodation, repaying your car loan and getting organised so you can return to your university studies.*

The use of 'rote' learnt responses ('Tell me about that') or reflective paraphrasing ('So you say you feel down')

might impede the development of the nurse–service user relationship, as the nurse may not convey genuine concern and empathy (Rydon, 2005). Clearly there are times when active listening is the best response, and silence or minimal verbal responses enable the service user to better express their perceptions and feelings. The point here is that when the emphasis of communication is restricted to 'rote' and learned responses, the nurse is unable to express genuine concern and empathy, and this in turn impedes the development of the therapeutic relationship. Skilful therapeutic communication with service users and their families requires practice and self-awareness so that the nurse can use a variety of responses that are congruent with who she or he is as a person.

Body language and touch

Communication, of course, is not only verbal exchanges. Body language is an integral part of how we send and receive messages. Both verbal messages and messages sent via our body language can be misunderstood or misinterpreted. Body language, or nonverbal signals, include all the cues we send with our body: how we stand, our facial expressions, how close to other people we position ourselves, what we wear, how much we move our hands, whether we cross our arms and any other physical movement that can be interpreted (or misinterpreted) by the recipient of our communication (Stein-Parbury, 2005). There may be times when we communicate one message verbally but give a conflicting message with our body language. Nurses need to consider both the impact of their body language alone (a raised eyebrow or hands on hips) and the congruence between their body language and their verbal communication. Congruence between verbal messages and body language is important.

Body language and the issue of touch have particular significance in the mental health setting. Regard for the service user's perceptions includes understanding the possible impact of 'touch' (Rydon, 2005). The nurse touching the service user may have significance for the service user beyond that intended by the nurse. In some circumstances touch may be perceived fearfully, as a threat, or as seduction. It may also be culturally inappropriate. Remaining sensitive to service user feedback about the level of eye contact is also important in therapeutic nurse–service user communications. Inappropriate eye contact, in particular a fixed gaze or stare, may also be misinterpreted or culturally inappropriate. Touch and eye contact are two important considerations when communicating with service users with mental health problems and reinforce the necessity of competently and skilfully understanding the particular health problem and needs of the service user.

Influence

We influence other people by what we say, what we do not say, what we focus on (feelings, content, context), our body language and our attitude to the other person's communication. That is, we have interpersonal and mutual influence. This is particularly so when we are in a professional role caring for service users who have perceptual, emotional, linguistic or cognitive impairment concomitant with their mental health problems. Service users will feel more able to trust a nurse who demonstrates that he or she understands the service user's needs and feelings (Borg and Kristiansen, 2004; Reynolds and Scott, 2000). In addition to the many micro skills that we can learn and practise to improve our communication skills, attitudes and values are important elements of therapeutic communication. Treating service users with respect, dignity, genuineness and honesty are among the characteristics that interweave with trained empathy to enhance the therapeutic relationship and build trust (Rydon, 2005; Stickley and Freshwater, 2006; Welch, 2005). Talking and approaching situations in a calm manner is also an important feature of effective and therapeutic communication in the mental health setting (Cowin et al., 2003). These skills require nurses to recognize their own strengths and limitations and seek appropriate resources and/or mentors.

Transference and counter-transference

So far we have looked at the impact of our communications on the service user, their perceptions and feelings. What of the impact of the service user on our perceptions and feelings? In order to understand the issues of transference and counter-transference, it is important to gain some insights into where these concepts originated. Sigmund Freud (1856–1939) was the founder of the psychoanalytic model and it is from Freud's work that these concepts emerged (see Ch. 7) (Howgego et al., 2003). Without detailing his work, it is important to grasp Freud's notion of the 'unconscious'. Unlike the way we use this idea in everyday language, the 'unconscious' in psychoanalytic terms means that the person is not aware, or not conscious, of the motivation for their thoughts, feelings or actions. This is pivotal to the idea of transference and counter-transference.

The process of *transference* occurs when a person transfers beliefs, feelings, thoughts or behaviours that occurred in one situation, usually in their past, to a situation that is happening in the present. Traditionally it was meant to refer to the service user with unconscious feelings or beliefs about someone in their past, transferring these feelings or beliefs onto the psychoanalyst. Past issues and conflicts experienced by the service user are carried into the therapeutic relationship (Cameron et al., 2005; Pearson, 2001). These can include issues with authority, sibling rivalry, anxiety and dependence. The service user brings these unresolved issues from the past into the present one-to-one relationship with the nurse. These

feelings in the therapeutic relationship may be triggered by the nurse's manner, look, position or speech. The transference may be displayed by covert or overt hostility, contempt for the nurse, lack of cooperation, or deference and submissiveness.

The service user's self-awareness is reduced as a result of transference. Helping the service user to identify the past issues, deal with the feelings and emotions, and to examine their meaning in the present, is an effective way to support the service user to work through the transference. This supportive strategy develops the service user's capacity to make choices. Dealing with transference in an empathic and honest manner, through judicious and skilful reality-based self-disclosure, can effectively disengage the transference (Pearson, 2001).

Counter-transference is regarded as the response of the analyst to the service user. It also includes the response of the analyst to the service user's transference (Cameron et al., 2005). Generally the nursing perspective is that counter-transference is the response of the nurse to the service user (whether this is due to unconscious or conscious reasons). One cue that you might be experiencing counter-transference is having strong feelings towards a service user, either negative or positive. For instance, the service user may have similarities to you in their age, gender, family relationships, life situation or personal issues that generate strong positive feelings for you. Alternatively, you may experience a strong feeling of dislike or avoidance of a particular service user related to their behaviours, such as aggressive or self-harming behaviours, or you may feel a lack of understanding of their behaviours and communications due to their mental health problems, particularly service users with personality disorders (Deans and Meocevic, 2006).

Boundaries

Finally, one salient feature of a working therapeutic relationship involves respecting the needs of the service user while remaining professional, and that includes the setting of boundaries (Horsfall et al., 1999). The core aim of the therapeutic relationship is to engage in a collaborative relationship with the service user with the aim of providing nursing care that is goal-directed, planned and purposeful (see Chs 1 & 2). The nurse's aim should be to facilitate and engage in activities that help achieve the service user's healthcare goals, not social goals or the nurse's own needs. Here the issues of professionalism, therapeutic relationship, counter-transference and boundaries intersect. Confusing the highly personal nature of the nurse–service user relationship with that of a social relationship may result in difficulties ranging from a negative treatment outcome for the service user through to charges of unprofessional, unethical or illegal behaviour. Boundary transgressions can range from inappropriately disclosing personal information (including personal telephone numbers or home address), agreeing to meet with the service user on a social level (in any context or manner), exchanging gifts and breaching service user confidentiality, through to inappropriate touching, verbal abuse, physical abuse or sexual abuse (Cleary et al., 2002). Keeping service user information to yourself, or not documenting some of the information that the service user discloses, may indicate that boundary issues need to be reflected upon or monitored. It is important for nurses to remain self-reflective around issues of nurse–service user boundaries and ethical practice. Some avenues of support for these issues include seeking peer support, engaging in clinical supervision sessions, remaining current with professional groups, being informed about current education developments and fostering an ethical culture in the work environment or organization.

Issues in working with families and carers

Over the past few decades, deinstitutionalization has seen the care of people with mental health problems shift increasingly from large psychiatric institutions out into the community. This marked change to service provision has led to growing numbers of people with chronic mental health problems living with families and carers in the community. As Kinsella et al. (1996) recognize, by their very nature mental health problems can be understood as a familial experience. Although an individual may have symptoms of mental disorders and receive treatment for them, due to the interconnected nature of families this can affect every member of the family.

In recognition of the changing needs of families, more recently there has also been a paradigm shift in service provision so that the focus of care provided to families has moved to a strengths approach rather than the previous deficit approach. From this perspective, there is an openness to recognizing the positive attributes of families (Darbyshire and Jackson, 2005). This is also in keeping with the idea that rather than seeing families as damaged, they are viewed as challenged (Walsh, 1996). This approach acknowledges that it is more constructive to consider the strengths that a family has, and foster further positive growth and development for family members, than to continue focusing only on the difficulties they face (Usher et al., 2005). This offers us a framework for communicating and working together with families. It also means that when we assess a service user we continue to recognize the need to assess the context in which they live.

Such an approach includes the principle that while we do not ignore the problems and challenges the family may have, we also attend to the diversity of the individual and family responses to adverse circumstances. The approach also acknowledges that while problems exist, families are the best judge of their circumstances, and can be supported by us to find their own solutions and ways of coping. This approach assists us as nurses to work with families with a focus on their strengths, competencies and the resources they need to deal with the particular issues they face. So, using a strengths-based framework moves us away from the idea of trying to fix individual or family deficits and towards recognizing their existing protective attributes and abilities, and encourages the development of further skills in managing their own situation. This in turn encourages nurses to view families as active agents and decision-makers in their own care rather than as passive recipients of the services we provide.

SKILLS IN SPECIFIC RISK SITUATIONS

Risk assessment and management

The term *risk* is commonly used in mental health practice and refers to the possibility of a (usually) adverse outcome occurring when a person engages in destructive behaviour. Risks can be seen in mental health settings for both service users and staff. In the broadest sense of the term, behaviours related to risk include the risk of violence or harm to self and/or others, various forms of physical, emotional and sexual abuse, gambling, promiscuity, reckless behaviours such as dangerous driving of a car, nonadherence (to medications and/or treatment recommendations), substance abuse and the failure to achieve one's potential. Other risks that can affect staff and/or family/carers include the risk of emotional trauma or stress and/or physical injury (Kelly et al., 2002).

Risk assessment and management refers to the need to identify and estimate risk so that structured decisions can be made as to how to manage the risk behaviour(s). As the most common forms of risk in mental health settings include the risk of violence and harm to self, the following section explores the assessment and management of the person who is aggressive, the prevention of violence and the assessment and management of the person who is self-harming and/or suicidal.

Managing aggressive behaviour

Managing violent and aggressive behaviour is becoming an increasing responsibility for mental health nurses (Owen et al., 1998; Shepherd and Lavender, 1999), who are often the target of aggression because of their frequent and direct contact with service users in the inpatient and community settings (Fry et al., 2002). While the level of aggression and violence towards mental health nurses is said to be increasing, the extent of the problem is largely underestimated (Fry et al., 2002). It is therefore important for the nurse to have sound background knowledge about aggression and its determinants as well as an understanding of the best ways to manage such behaviour should it occur.

Aggression is an action or behaviour that can range from violent physical acts such as kicks and punches, through to verbal abuse, insults and nonverbal gestures (Garnham, 2001). People who are *aggressive* behave in a way that demonstrates their anger. For example, aggressive people may invade the personal space of others, shout or talk loudly, bang their fists, stomp their feet, shake their hands, stare until others feel uneasy or stand over people (Distasio, 2002). The overall feeling projected is an attempt to dominate. *Violence*, on the other hand, can be defined as a serious physical attack where the intent is to cause harm to an individual or object (Garnham, 2001; Littrell and Littrell, 1998).

Aggressive behaviour is multifactorial. It may be caused by internal, external or situational factors. *Internal* causes, or causes related to the individual, can be the presence of a serious mental disorders such as acute phases of schizophrenia, intoxication, age and gender, with young males being more likely to be involved in aggression and violence (Lanza, 1988; Linaker and Busch-Iversen, 1995; Pearson et al., 1986). A previous history of violence is a strong, perhaps the strongest, predictor of future violence (Blair, 1991; Tardiff, 1998). *External* predictors are the environment, such as crowding or limited space, certain hospital shifts, staff gender (with males more likely to be attacked than females) and timing, where 'hotspots' such as handover or other busy periods have been identified as likely times for violent episodes to occur (Aquilina, 1991; Nijman et al., 1999; Turnbull and Patterson, 1999; Vanderslott, 1998; Whittington and Wykes, 1994). There has also been a higher incidence of violence where the treatment setting was perceived by the service user as coercive, controlling, threatening or frightening (Quintal, 2002). Both internal and external risk factors can be identified as those that are *static* (that is, not changeable and based on past history, e.g. age and gender) or *dynamic* (that is, changeable and can be treated, e.g. intoxication) (Ignelzi et al., 2007). Clearly, the dynamic factors are those that nurses and other health professionals can intervene with.

Managing aggressive behaviour can be challenging for any nurse. The main goal in managing aggressive behaviour is the prevention of an escalation, or de-escalation, into violence towards self, others and the environment. One way to prevent the escalation of aggression into violence is to know the predictors of violence and have the capacity to recognize these in your service users. Observable behaviour and cues that may indicate a person's potential for violence (see also Box 22.1) can be identified using a framework based on the acronym STAMP. This stands for:

*S*taring and eye contact: includes prolonged glaring or absence of eye contact,

Tone and volume of voice: includes sharp or caustic tone, demeaning inflection, increased volume,
Anxiety: includes flushed appearance, hyperventilation, rapid speech, dilated pupils and physical indicators of pain such as grimacing, writhing and clutching the body, confusion and disorientation,
Mumbling: includes talking under the breath, criticizing staff, repeating the same or similar questions/requests, slurred speech,
Pacing: includes walking around confined spaces, walking back and forth (Luck et al., 2007).

A further way to prevent violence is to know the service user well. This requires the nurse to assess each service user thoroughly and to be aware of any history of violence. The nurse needs to look for signs of escalating aggression and be aware of potential triggers of aggression and violence in the environment. This is where the nurse makes an assessment of the risk the service user poses for an aggressive or violent act.

A number of risk assessment tools have been developed and tested. These tools can be useful in clinical practice as they help identify potential risks and offer a link between assessment and management of aggressive incidents (Doyle and Dolan, 2002). A useful tool for assessing aggression is the overt aggression scale for the objective rating of verbal and physical aggression (Yudofsky et al., 1986). This scale measures aggression in four areas: verbal aggression, and physical aggression against self, objects and other people. The modified overt aggression scale measures verbal aggression, physical aggression against property and/or aggression against self on a five-point ordinal scale.

The ultimate goal of assessment and management of the risk of violence is the effective management and prevention of violence. In addition to thorough assessment, the nurse's use of respectful and effective communication aimed at managing the risk, protecting self and others and enhancing recovery is vital (Ignelzi et al., 2007). The management of aggressive behaviour is a process that may develop according to the level of risk the person poses. If the service user is verbally aggressive, the nurse must use verbal techniques for de-escalation in the first instance (Department of Health, 2008). However, if the person does not respond to these techniques, or is already threatening or acting out aggressive behaviour, intervention may need to increase to include physical intervention and/or the use of medication (see Box 22.2).

When faced with an angry or verbally aggressive service user, remain calm and talk softly but clearly. It is important to intervene early in an attempt to de-escalate the situation (Delaney et al., 2001). The following strategies are usually helpful in this instance.

- Use non-judgemental communication and be aware of the service user's feelings. Remain in control of your own emotions.
- Attempt to uncover the source of the distress and engage the service user in questions that might help identify the problem area.
- Do not try to talk when they are shouting or talking loudly, and do not argue or become defensive.
- Use open-ended questions to elicit additional information from the service user but do not attempt to interrogate.
- Attempt to help the service user identify ways to deal effectively with the situation.
- Most importantly, know when you need help, and when you do need it, call for it.

If the service user's anger continues to escalate then you may need to set limits: these help the service user establish appropriate boundaries, which can increase their sense of security. Limit-setting is a means by which the service user is told what behaviour is acceptable, what is unacceptable and the consequences of behaving in an unacceptable way. It is one way to avoid aggressive incidents. Limits are often placed on behaviours prior to their occurrence. That is, the nurse and service user discuss the outcomes if certain behaviour occurs in the future. If this is the case, it is important that such outcomes do occur in the event of the unwanted behaviour. It is therefore imperative that all staff are aware of the plan and that everyone agrees to follow through with the action in the event of the unwanted behaviour. However, remember that some inpatient environments are perceived as coercive and controlling and, because of limited space, may make the service user more likely to become violent (Quintal, 2002).

If the service user's behaviour continues to escalate, other interventions such as medication, restraint or seclusion may be required (Department of Health, 2008; NICE, 2005). *Medications* such as antipsychotic drugs and/or anti-anxiety drugs can be useful in assisting the service user to become calm. The National Institute for Health and Clinical Excellence (NICE) has issued guidance on the use of medication in emergency situations in *Violence: The Short-Term Management of Disturbed/Violent Behaviour in In-Patient Psychiatric Settings and Emergency Departments* (NICE, 2005). The guidance indicates that oral medication should be offered before parenteral medication wherever possible and the drug of choice here is oral lorazepam. If the aggressive person is experiencing a psychotic episode, then oral haloperidol may also be offered (NICE, 2005). Where oral therapy is refused or not effective, and rapid tranquillization is indicated, then a combination of an intramuscular antipsychotic (intramuscular haloperidol) and an intramuscular benzodiazepine (intramuscular lorazepam) is recommended (NICE, 2005). In the event of the use of haloperidol then an antimuscarinic drug must be available to respond to any extrapyramidal side effects or dystonic reactions. In the event of rapid tranquillization, attending staff must monitor vital signs and pulse oximeters should be available. Blood pressure, pulse rate, temperature, respiratory rate and hydration should be taken and regularly and accurately recorded, at appropriate intervals, until the service user regains consciousness (NICE, 2005).

Restraint involves the safe immobilization of a person who may be at risk from harming themselves or others (NICE, 2005). The *Code of Practice: Mental Health Act 1983* (Department of Health, 2008) stresses that if physical restraint is used it should:

- be reasonable, justifiable and proportionate to the risk posed by the patient,
- be used for only as long as is absolutely necessary,

- involve a recognized technique that does not depend on the deliberate application of pain (the application of pain should be used only for the immediate relief or rescue of staff where nothing else will suffice),
- be carried out by those who have received appropriate training in the use of restraint techniques (Department of Health, 2008, p. 118).

Throughout restraint, nursing staff should continue attempts to verbally de-escalate the situation and be alert to any signs of respiratory or cardiac distress (Department of Health, 2008; NICE, 2005)

Seclusion (see next section) is usually only used when other measures such as those above have not been successful in reducing the service user's aggression and/or there is a strong risk of harm to self or others.

In the event of the use of rapid tranquillization, restraint or seclusion a 'crash bag' or 'crash trolley' should be available within 3 min (which must include a bag valve mask, oxygen, automatic external defibrillator (AED), cannulas, suction, fluid and first-line medications for use in resuscitation) (NICE, 2005). A doctor should be quickly available when requested by nursing staff (Department of Health, 2008). Any aggressive or violent situation requires a post-incident review, which should take place as soon as possible after the event, and no later than 72h afterwards (NICE, 2005). The review should attempt to learn any lessons from the incident, and to ensure that staff and service users are appropriately supported so that the therapeutic milieu may be maintained. If physical restraint has been used, nurses should evaluate the service user's care plan(s) and take steps to assit the person reintegrate back into the ward environment (Department of Health, 2008).

Seclusion

An Australian study (Wynaden et al., 2002) found that when managing difficult behaviours, nurses used a management hierarchy that had seclusion at the bottom. The hierarchy included things like distraction, the use of outdoor areas to separate service users, encouraging the service user to regain control of their behaviour, and communication techniques. They also found that the nurses used intuitive judgements when deciding whether to seclude a service user, and would use seclusion if it had been successful in a similar situation in the past.

Why use seclusion?

People admitted to acute mental health units may at times become distressed, irritable, aggressive, violent or pose a danger to themselves. Nurses use various interventions in an attempt to reduce harm to the service user or others including the use of de-escalating techniques, sedating medications, special observations, acute care units and seclusion. Seclusion is usually instigated in such instances when the other methods have failed

(Bowers et al., 2006; Muir-Cochrane et al., 2002). Its use is based on the therapeutic principles of containment, isolation and decrease in sensory input (Gutheil, 1978). One study found that the most common reason nurses gave for using seclusion was the immediate control of violent behaviour. Other reasons given were to protect the safety of staff and other service users (Terpstra et al., 2001). Even though aggression and violence are the most common reasons for seclusion in the inpatient setting (Meehan, 1997; Muir-Cochrane, 1995), service users have in the past reported being secluded for inappropriate reasons, such as refusing to attend an activity or refusing to take medications (Heyman, 1987).

Seclusion is '…the supervised confinement of a patient in a room, which may be locked. Its sole aim is to contain severely disturbed behaviour which is likely to cause harm to others' (Department of Health, 2008, p. 122). Muir-Cochrane et al. (2002) explain that this practice, although long considered an important practice in the treatment and control of people with mental health problems, is controversial. The controversy is said to focus on legal, ethical, professional, attitudinal and safety issues (Wynaden et al., 2002). Seclusion raises issues of nursing 'control' and there are questions regarding how these issues are ethically balanced with service users' rights. Differences in staff levels of experience, nurses' perceptions of seclusion and individual nurses' perceptions of the seriousness of service users' behaviours also affect the practice of seclusion (Lowe et al., 2003; Muir-Cochrane, 1996). The implementation of and preference for seclusion in a consistent and appropriate manner is also of concern to mental health nurses. Issues of staff–service user ratio are also reported to have a statistical relationship with the use of seclusion (Donat, 2002). A decreased use of service user seclusion follows a focused effort to increase staffing numbers. This strategy was concurrent with supportive service user behavioural treatment plans and staff training. Because of the controversy, the use of seclusion continues to be varied, with some facilities using it routinely, some sparingly and others not at all. The practice continues to be recognized as an acceptable tool for the management of certain behaviours (Muir-Cochrane et al., 2002), even though current practice in mental healthcare is based on use of the least-restrictive environment wherever possible.

Holmes (1998), however, explains how the term 'seclusion' refers to different things, such as time out, open seclusion, isolation, quiet room and so on. Whichever way it is conceived, seclusion still tends to be perceived in a negative way by service users (Farrell and Dares, 1996; Griffith, 2001).

Service user perspectives on seclusion

It would be assumed that all service users would regard seclusion as punitive; however, some service users have reported that they felt seclusion aided their recovery (Heyman, 1987; Soliday, 1985). Others, of course, have reported the opposite. These service users reported that seclusion made them feel helpless, punished, depressed, disgusted, afraid, vulnerable and worthless (Heyman, 1987; Martinez et al., 1999; Norris and Kennedy, 1992; Soliday, 1985). In a study by Meehan (1997), service users supported the use of seclusion in the inpatient unit but claimed it was over-used. They also reported that rather than helping a service user feel safe, seclusion can actually make a person feel vulnerable, neglected and punished. An Australian qualitative study of service users' perspectives on the experience of seclusion found that most service users perceived the experience in a negative way. The service users reported similar feelings to those reported in earlier studies, such as abandonment, fear and isolation; however, they also reported feeling under-informed about the seclusion process (Meehan et al., 2000). Service users continue to perceive nursing staff as reactive rather than preventative where aggressive behaviour is concerned. This suggests that many nurses continue to resort to traditional ways of managing difficult behaviours, such as seclusion and medication, rather than adopt early intervention techniques (Meehan et al., 2006).

Nurse perspectives on seclusion

Staff attitudes to seclusion have been the focus of a number of studies (Bowers et al., 2006; Terpstra et al., 2001, for example). Some mental health staff defended the use of seclusion as an acceptable way to manage the destructive or violent behaviour of severely disturbed service users. Not all healthcare professionals, however, believe seclusion to be desirable or efficacious; females have been found to be less approving of seclusion in general (Bowers et al., 2006). Some say its use is a violation of freedom and dignity and that it may in fact be counter-therapeutic and lead to dependency on staff, cause hallucinations due to sensory deprivation, and cause feelings of abandonment (Tooke and Brown, 1992). One study of staff attitudes to containment found that the factor with the greatest influence over a nurse's preparedness to use seclusion was whether it was considered safe for the service user and whether it was considered effective. An earlier study found that 85% of nurses prefer to use medication rather than seclusion as they consider it to be less restrictive (Terpstra et al., 2001).

Policy perspectives on seclusion

The *Code of Practice: Mental Health Act 1983* (Department of Health, 2008) provides the legal framework for the use of seclusion and health services will also have local policies to govern the use of seclusion. Seclusion must only be used as a last resort and for the shortest possible time and should not be used if there is a danger of suicide or self-harm (NICE, 2005). If seclusion is used a suitably qualified and trained person must be in attendance outside of the seclusion room at all times, and a documented report must be made every 15 min (Department of Health, 2008). Nurses must be aware of the relevant local policy related to their place of work. The relevant policy should be referred to, to determine such aspects as when seclusion can be used, who can instigate seclusion and under what conditions, the timing of observations of the service user in seclusion, how long seclusion can be used and when seclusion should be terminated.

CASE STUDY: MARIA (PART A)

Maria, a 23-year-old female, was brought to the accident and emergency department by the police after threatening to stab her boyfriend with a knife, and acting 'quite bizarrely' when the police attended. At the time of the Crisis Resolution Team's arrival she was pacing up and down and yelling in a threatening manner at all staff who passed. The police were still in attendance.

The staff initially approached Maria by introducing themselves and explaining their role in being present. (Only one person spoke to Maria.) The staff ensured that in interacting with Maria they maintained an open posture. Direct eye contact was maintained as was appropriate to the situation. Staff explained the situation to Maria. During this time a constant assessment was made of Maria's response to the assessors, and her level of arousal.

As Maria stopped pacing and appeared to be engaging with the staff, she was asked if she would like to sit down and talk about what had occurred. Maria agreed to this.

CRITICAL THINKING CHALLENGE 22.2

In part A of the case study, what are the immediate management priorities for Maria? Consider the context of her presentation, the current setting and the available staff.

From the information provided in the case study, identify the strategies the staff used to defuse Maria's aggression. In your opinion, do they seem to have been effective? How do you know this?

CASE STUDY: MARIA (PART B)

By being open and honest with Maria, and acting in an assertive but nonaggressive manner, staff were able to reduce Maria's hostility enough to engage in an assessment process. After the interview, Maria expressed her appreciation that someone wanted to listen and hear her side of the story. Maria does have a mental health problem, which is currently well controlled with the medication she takes. Unfortunately her relationship is volatile, due partly to her boyfriend's over-protectiveness. He is always checking on what she has been up to, and whether she has taken her medication. Today they had been arguing about housework, when he started to blame her anger with him on her not taking her medication. At this point Maria became extremely frustrated and picked up a knife from the kitchen bench. Maria denies any intention to use the knife, stating that she was just frustrated and wanted to get her point across. Maria agreed that this was not the best response to the situation.

Following discussion with Maria's case manager it was agreed that her case manager would help her to develop more effective communication strategies, and would provide support and psychoeducation for Maria's boyfriend. Maria was discharged home.

The authors would like to acknowledge Kym Park for this case study.

CRITICAL THINKING CHALLENGE 22.3

In part B of the case study, does the situation seem to have ended successfully? Provide rationales for your responses.

Applying the principles of developing a therapeutic rapport with service users, identify the strategies staff used in this situation that enhanced rapport and trust.

In this situation, there was a precipitating factor and psychosocial issues surrounding the event. What were they? Does the management plan developed by the staff adequately address them?

This situation may have been handled differently if the staff had responded differently to Maria's aggression. What other strategies may have been used to manage Maria's behaviour? Consider the viability of the use of psychotropic medication and restraint.

Self-harming behaviours and suicide risk

A number of terms are used to describe behaviour that may be damaging to the self. Note that suicidal behaviour can be seen to exist on a continuum. For instance, there is a clear risk that the person who deliberately self-harms may eventually go on to commit suicide (Holdsworth et al., 2001; Slaven and Kisely, 2002). Some of the terms are used interchangeably, although there are distinctions to be made between them. The terms listed in Box 22.3 are in order of increasing level of harm or risk.

Box 22.3 Terms used to describe self-harm and suicide

- Self-harm or injury/deliberate self-harm: any intentional damage to the person's body, without a conscious intention to die. Includes the use of cutting, burning, carving, branding, head-banging, scratching, biting, bruising, abrasions and pulling skin and hair. This is distinct from suicidality and self-harm that results from psychosis.
- Parasuicidal behaviour: actions that are intended to cause self-injury but not intended to be lethal (e.g. cutting wrists or taking an overdose of a drug in low doses and/or drugs that will not cause death). Note: this term is no longer routinely used.
- Self-poisoning: intentionally ingesting a substance in more than the recommended dose, either through accident or to deliberately self-harm.
- Suicidal ideation: thoughts or ideas about suicide.
- Lethality of suicide threat: the seriousness of the threat or attempt to suicide and the degree to which the action is likely to result in death.
- Suicide: the deliberate and conscious attempt to kill oneself. May be either completed (results in death) or attempted.

The issues of suicide and deliberate self-harm or injury will almost certainly be encountered by nurses in their practice, whether in a community mental health setting, inpatient mental health unit, emergency department or other health setting. In one study, for example, 96.3% of nurse respondents had experience with people who deliberately self-harm (McAllister et al., 2002a). Suicide and/or self-harm may engender concern and anxiety in the nurse due to personal attitudes, and the moral, ethical, legal and practical requirements of care. The care of service users who are suicidal or self-harming may necessitate the provision of support and clinical supervision to the mental health nurse by experienced staff, to enable them to continue working with these service users and to develop the necessary attitudes, knowledge and skills needed to care for them (Cutcliffe and Barker, 2002).

Working with the person who self-harms

Self-harm may be distinguished from suicidal behaviour in that self-harm is a nonlethal, sometimes impulsive, method of alleviating emotional distress where the person deliberately inflicts injury on himself or herself. The person may self-harm without having suicidal intent (Holdsworth et al., 2001). Rates of self-harm vary but it has been estimated by NICE that between 4.6 and 6.6% of people have self-harmed (NICE, 2004) while the Adult

Psychiatric Morbidity Survey (APMS) (NHS Information Centre, 2009) found that 4.9% of people surveyed said they had engaged in self-harm.

A recent study of nurses' attitudes towards service users who self-harmed found that nurses who saw themselves as skilled in working with these service users were more likely to feel positive towards them and less likely to demonstrate negative attitudes. This highlights the importance of nurses having relevant intervention and therapeutic skills in this area (McAllister et al., 2002b).

Reasons for self-harming behaviour

There are complex reasons why service users self-harm. Self-harm is generally considered a negative or self-destructive act, yet it can be viewed from another perspective. It may be empowering or affirming of the person's individuality and strength in expressing themselves and/or dealing with strong emotions. The use of self-harm can therefore be interpreted as an act of power rather than the more common perception of it as an act of emotional pain and/or the inability to cope with feelings or experiences.

It may be that self-harm actually reveals the person's will to live or survive, as the service user's use of self-harm can be seen as a way of maintaining psychological integrity through releasing unbearable feelings and thereby easing an urge towards suicide. It may be a rite of passage for some young people; for instance, where body scars from cutting reveal a sense of 'tribal belonging' (Martin, 2002). Some people use physical self-injury to deal with overwhelming emotions or situations, and to relieve tension.

It is common for people who self-harm to have a history of abuse, and to be anxious and/or depressed, and/or diagnosed with borderline personality disorder or dissociative identity disorder. Episodes of self-harm have also been associated with recreational substance use (Holdsworth et al., 2001). The self-harm behaviour of the person can be a way to express and 'release' psychic pain through the flow of blood. It can represent a destructive way of dealing with perceived uncontrollable negative feelings such as intense anger or desperation. The perception that self-harm is used as a way of attention-seeking has not been found to be accurate. People who self-harm often do so in private as a secret and shameful practice (McAllister et al., 2002b) as they may feel that there is no other option available to them. It can be seen as a method of expressing deep needs that require skilful help (Hopkins, 2002).

Providing care and communicating with the person who self-harms

Research has found that nurses generally hold more negative than positive attitudes towards service users who self-harm. The reasons for this include their own feelings of anxiety about the act of self-injury, and frustration that other care priorities prevent them from giving these service users the time and space needed to explore their use of self-harm. Nurses can find it stressful and can feel helpless to prevent repetitive self-harm attempts (Holdsworth et al., 2001; Hopkins, 2002; McAllister et al., 2002b; McKinlay et al., 2001; Smith, 2002). The nurse may end up being ambivalent towards the person, and resent the demands placed upon them (Hopkins, 2002). This can interfere with the development of therapeutic rapport, so the ability to empathize is compromised and engagement becomes more difficult. The healthcare context that can lead to a more transient connection between nurse and service user may also make it difficult for nurses to find the time or energy to subjectively engage with service users, so their hearing of service user stories remains incomplete. There is a need for nurses to work with this ambiguity through reflective practice and to navigate between the positions of neutrality, distance and empathy (Holdsworth et al., 2001; Hopkins, 2002; McAllister, 2001).

Comprehensive assessment of the person who self-harms

The lack of structure to guide assessment, management and discharge planning for the service user who is self-harming is a significant issue raised by nurses working with these service users (Slaven and Kisely, 2002). The five-dimensional nursing assessments model (Rawlins et al., 1993) covers physical, intellectual, emotional, social and spiritual aspects of the service user and is a comprehensive tool for use in assessment of service users who self-harm. This model goes beyond the more traditional biopsychosocial model as it considers all dimensions of the person, including the spiritual.

It is important that assessment also focuses on the person's strengths as well as problems or needs. As the previous discussion has highlighted, this approach provides a more accurate and comprehensive overview of the service user than simply viewing them and their behaviour from a pathogenic or illness perspective (McAllister and Estefan, 2002).

Interventions for self-harming behaviour

Service users report that it is helpful for a nurse to sit down and talk with them. One complaint service users have is that nurses do not necessarily understand the reasons for the self-harm, and that they offer medication rather than making themselves available to talk (Smith, 2002). These are important messages to consider when working with service users who self-harm. Box 22.4 outlines some useful skills for dealing with a service user who has self-harmed.

NURSE'S STORY: SELF-HARM

I was working in the accident and emergency department one day when Sally arrived for assessment. Sally is pretty. When she is wearing long sleeves you wouldn't think she had a care in the world. In short sleeves, however, the picture isn't so pretty. There are about 50 self-inflicted scars running laterally across both inner arms from each radial pulse up to the biceps. We can't use her left arm for taking a blood pressure: the drum of the stethoscope won't sit flat on all the lumpy scar tissue.

Sally is wearing a tank-top; the scars are reminders that our work as mental health nurses is important. Using the language of a mental health professional, I said that talking through things is a safe alternative to cutting herself, but now that she's talking I feel afraid … I have no idea what she, or I, will say. How can I relate to her experiences? How can I understand her life? What if I mess things up?

Sally is doubtful too. She speaks of the release that cutting offers: 'When I slash-up I'm not trying to kill myself. I just want to feel something: anything's better than nothing.' It doesn't hurt to slash-up; the blood-letting takes some of the pain and the anger away, she says. Sally feels embarrassed and sore afterwards. That's why she's running an 'experiment' with me to see if talking helps.

Months later I realize something that I probably should have known. Not knowing and not experiencing self-harm, I start to realize that Sally's life isn't a disadvantage to her. She needs to tell her story, without somebody interrupting with their story or with clichés. She needs somebody who knows what counter-transference is, and tries not to let it get in the way. She needs somebody to challenge her unrealistic beliefs, but still believe in her. She needs support and being listened to without judging, not rescuing.

Paul McNamara

CRITICAL THINKING CHALLENGE 22.4

How do you think you would feel if you were working with a service user who had deliberately self-harmed?

What factors in your life may have led to your opinions and feelings on this issue? Consider your own background in terms of religion, family beliefs about the value of life, etc.

What measures could you take to protect the therapeutic relationship if you found you were experiencing either very negative or overly positive counter-transference feelings towards a service user who self-harmed?

Box 22.4 Nursing skills used with the person who is self-harming

- Approach the person with an open mind and a supportive attitude.
- Encourage the person to share their thoughts and feelings regarding the self-harm.
- Remove potentially harmful objects such as razors, glass, pins, scissors, knives and lighters.
- Assess for any precipitating factors prior to self-harm and remove/reduce them if possible.
- Assess for risk of suicide.
- Convey a sense of calm, control and safety to the person.
- If the person is distressed, reassure them of their safety.
- Remain available to the person for emotional support.
- Explore alternative coping methods for expressing negative feelings.
- Follow the setting's protocol with regard to level of observation.
- Use restraint and/or medication only if absolutely necessary and according to the setting's policy.
- Review the episode with the person afterwards and develop with them a mutually agreed plan for managing possible future episodes, e.g. note what factors precipitate self-harm and try to reduce or eliminate them.
- Gain the service user's agreement that they will contact a staff member if they feel overwhelming negative feelings that may lead to self-harm behaviours.
- Agree to spend time with the person and support them when they require emotional support.

Sources: Horsfall et al. (2000); Whitehead and Royles (2002).

Working with the person who is suicidal

Many people experience temporary or fleeting thoughts of suicide at some point in their lives, but most of us do not go on to try it (Pirkis et al., 2002). The Adult Psychiatric Morbidity Survey (APMS) (NHS Information Centre, 2009) found that 16.7% of people surveyed said that they had thought about ending their lives, and 5.6% said that they had made a suicide attempt. In the UK there were 5675 suicides in 2009, 31 fewer than those recorded in 2008 (5706) (Office of National Statistics, 2011). More males than females in all age groups commit suicide, although this is greatest in the 20–44-year age group. However, the overall suicide rate has declined over the past 10 years. In 2000, the male suicide rate was 19.9 per 100 000 reducing to 17.5 per 100 000 in 2009. For women, the rates also show a downward trend from 6.2 per 100 000 in 2000 reducing to 5.2 per 100 000 in 2009 (Office of National Statistics, 2011).

The likelihood of committing suicide is dependent, at least to some extent, on the ease of access to, and knowledge of, effective means (Office of National Statistics, 2003). In young adult men aged 15–44 in 2001, 'hanging, strangulation and suffocation' was responsible for almost 50% of all suicides while drug-related poisoning was the second most common cause of death by suicide. For men, 'other poisoning' (mostly comprised of motor vehicle exhaust fumes) accounted for 10%. In men over 75 years 'hanging, strangulation and suffocation' was the most common method of suicide, accounting for over 40% in 2001. Drug poisoning accounted for almost 50% of suicide deaths in all age groups in women, while the second most common method was 'hanging, strangulation and suffocation' (Office of National Statistics, 2003).

Reasons for suicidal behaviours

Although the reasons for attempting suicide vary, it is commonly related to an effort to deal with relationship difficulties and to the presence of mental health disorders such as schizophrenia, depression and dual diagnosis of both severe mental disorder and substance abuse (Gournay and Bowers, 2000; Pirkis et al., 2002). An attempt to suicide is often reported by service users as reflecting their feelings of powerlessness or the experience of loss and disappointment, where they want freedom from the psychic pain they feel rather than actually wanting to die (Talseth et al., 2001). It is this ambivalence, where the person wants to escape from their feelings but retains an underlying desire to live, that nurses can try to understand and access when they work with the person who is suicidal.

Assessing for risk of suicide

If the nurse is concerned about a person they think may be suicidal, it is important that they talk directly with them about suicide. Prevention of suicide is far better than having to treat the consequences of a suicidal act. However, the nurse may be concerned about directly asking the person about suicide for fear of unintentionally causing the person to become suicidal. Discussing suicide will not make the person more likely to attempt suicide. Talking openly about the possibility of it and giving the service user a chance to talk about it may lead to the person realizing that it is not the best solution for their problem (see Box 22.5).

As well as conducting a comprehensive mental state and psychosocial assessment, using the six broad areas shown in Box 22.6, which each reveal an escalating level of risk, the nurse can specifically structure their questioning of suicide risk (see Box 22.7).

Therefore, if a person has thoughts about committing suicide, has a plan to take pills and has the pills in their home with the immediate intention of acting out their plan, they are at an acute and high level of suicide risk. A person who has thoughts about committing suicide and a vague plan of taking some pills, but is not sure what pills

---

Box 22.5 **Risk factors for suicidal behaviour**

Risk factors associated with suicide include:

- being male and aged between 15 and 30 years,
- previous deliberate self-harm,
- previous history of suicide attempts,
- mental disorder: primarily depression and schizophrenia,
- substance/alcohol abuse,
- dual diagnosis of mental disorder and substance abuse,
- recent stressful events such as divorce, loss of job, breakdown of relationship or death of a loved one,
- anniversaries of previous losses.

Box 22.6 **Assessment of suicidality: questions**

Examples of questions for assessing risk for suicide:

- Has the person been having thoughts about ending their life?
- Does the person intend to end their life?
- Is there a plan about how they would go about ending their life? (e.g. taking pills, hanging, etc.)
- Is there a means to carry out the plan? (e.g. does the person have access to these pills, do they have a rope or other device?)
- What is the timeframe for their plan? (e.g. is it immediate, or is it something they have thought about for the future?)
- Has the person ever tried to end their life before?

---

they might take and does not have any pills available, is not at as high a risk of suicide. There is obviously a need for regular reassessment of risk for suicide as the person's risk level may change at any time.

Caring for and communicating with the person who is suicidal

As highlighted throughout this chapter, the nurse–service user relationship is pivotal in the provision of care in a mental health setting, and particularly in providing care for the person who is suicidal. The key aspects of providing interpersonal care for the person who is suicidal may be seen as inspiring hope, communication and engagement (Cutcliffe and Barker, 2002; Samuelsson et al., 2000). However, nurses can struggle to understand why a person would want to try and kill themselves or injure themselves through self-harm. It may be seen as irrational and/or be mystifying to them (Hopkins, 2002). Some

Box 22.7 **Assessment of suicidality: direct questions**

Examples of direct questions that may be used for assessing suicidal ideation:

- Have you been feeling 'down' or depressed for a few days at a time?
- Do you ever feel that life is not worth living?
- When you feel like this, have you ever had thoughts of ending your life?
- What do you think you might do to end your life?
- Have you taken steps towards doing this (e.g. buying pills)?
- Have you thought about when you might end your life?
- What has stopped you from doing this so far?
- What could help make it easier for you to deal with your problems?
- What are your hopes for the future?

nurses may feel distressed and find that they either avoid working with these people or become overly involved in their care and extremely upset if the person eventually commits suicide (McLaughlin, 1999). It is understandable that when the nurse has cared for a service user and worked closely with them over time, their personal sense of loss can be significant if the service user commits suicide. It is important that nurses are able to respect the individual's particular situation, beliefs and right to self-determination. Although the provision of hope is crucial and the vast majority of service users will eventually overcome their suicidal feelings, the realistic understanding that not all service users will survive is a difficult but ultimately essential realization for the nurse.

The nurse can use a number of support strategies when working with suicidal service users. These include receiving ongoing professional clinical supervision in order to increase their professional skills and coping skills. Clinical supervision may also provide a safe avenue for nurses to express their feelings. Nurses can ensure that they attend in-service and/or regularly update their knowledge of suicidality and management through professional journals and/or texts. Use of collaborative care planning with the service user, which results in individualized care (Samuelsson et al., 2000), can also improve the nurse's sense of self-efficacy and the service user's experience of receiving comprehensive and relevant care.

Service user perspectives on being cared for while suicidal

Service users who are suicidal report that the most distressing aspects of their experience are the loneliness, suffering and despair they feel, and the need to feel respected as people and given responsibility for their own lives. They ask to be cared for as human beings. Nurses need to have an understanding of the meaning of this experience for the person as well as a deeper understanding of their own experiences in taking care of the person, rather than simply understanding suicide in terms of theories or models (Samuelsson et al., 2000; Talseth et al., 2001). Service users can feel ashamed of being a mental health service user and embarrassed that they require treatment. They may sense a lack of respect from staff and feel that staff do not trust them. However, they have also reported positive experiences of care received. Feeling cared for and secure with staff who were friendly, welcoming, accepting of them and allowed them to talk about their problems contributed to positive experiences (McLaughlin, 1999; Samuelsson et al., 2000). The skills and attitudes of the nurse clearly play an important role when working with service users who are suicidal.

Nursing interventions for the person who is suicidal

Nurses themselves consider that effective communication is the most important skill a mental health nurse must have when working with service users who are suicidal (McLaughlin, 1999). Throughout this chapter the need for effective communication has been highlighted as the basis from which the nurse can be therapeutic when working with the service user. Nevertheless, the major focus of care for suicidal service users in the inpatient setting seems to be that of observation, albeit often linked with therapeutic communication and engagement (Cutcliffe and Barker, 2002; Horsfall and Cleary, 2000). Observation includes terms such as *one-to-one care*, *'specialling'* or *close observation*. Observation usually ranges from intensive 24-hour care where the nurse is never more than an arm's length away from the service user, through to lower-level 'category' observations where there are periodic and regular 'checks' of the service user's whereabouts and wellbeing. Observation has the aim of preventing the service user attempting suicide by reducing risk (Bowers et al., 2000; Cutcliffe and Barker, 2002; Horsfall and Cleary, 2000). Although observation may be commonly used as a strategy it also needs to be implemented consistently and appropriately (Bowers et al., 2000). The issue of service user rights and the use of power by staff need to be considered (Horsfall and Cleary, 2000). It is imperative for nurses to be aware that nursing engagement could be more effective than observation as a way of inspiring hope in the person through use of the interpersonal relationship. The engagement approach advocates the use of the nurse–service user therapeutic relationship where the nurse attempts to explore with the service user the issues that led to their suicidal behaviour. An understanding of these issues by another

Box 22.8 Nursing strategies for use with the service user who is suicidal

- Approach the person calmly and maintain a non-judgemental attitude.
- Provide reassurance of safety.
- Develop rapport and genuine regard for the person.
- Enable regular time and space to allow the person to talk freely about their thoughts and feelings.
- Maintain a safe environment by removing potentially injurious objects including knives, glass and razor blades.
- Follow local protocol concerning regular observation of person's safety and location.
- Judiciously use self-control options that the person can use when they are feeling on the verge of attempting suicide, e.g. contact the nurse or other staff member.
- Involuntary admission may need to be considered for the person who is in the community.
- Ensure the person has 24-hour access to help.

person may help to address the service user's need for physical and emotional security (Cutcliffe and Barker, 2002). Box 22.8 lists nursing strategies for use with service users who are suicidal.

NURSE'S STORY: MANAGING THE PERSON WHO IS AT RISK

I have been a mental health nurse since 1988 and have worked mainly in acute settings. One of the most difficult clinical situations I have encountered is known as constant observation. This means being no further than an arm's length away from the service user at all times, including bathroom activities. The fact that it is done to prevent the person from coming to harm, either by their own hand or due to their altered judgement, makes it no less difficult. The service user gets cross at times because they feel that their space is being invaded and that the nurse is stopping them from doing what they want to do. If the service user is responding to hallucinations or delusional beliefs, you can become a part of these thoughts, and the service user can become paranoid about you.

I remember looking after a young man (18 years old) who was transferred to our inpatient unit for reasons of safety. It was late in the evening (10 p.m.) and at this time he was under constant observation. He had presented with suicidal ideation, delusions and auditory hallucinations, and this was his first admission to a mental health unit. On arrival on our unit, he was hypervigilant and restless. He was given some PRN medication (valium) to help reduce his agitation, and then settled into his room. I found it difficult to relax about this young man, chose to observe him closely, and discussed my feelings and observations with my colleague. I couldn't voice

my exact concerns, but he just didn't 'feel right' to me. He wasn't expressing any suicidal ideation to us, but he remained restless. I observed him looking perplexed and walking up to the exits. My colleague agreed with my observations and we decided between us to observe him closely overnight. We decided to continue to observe him at 10-minute intervals while he was asleep, and constantly when he was awake. Throughout the next day he became increasingly distressed and at greater risk of self-harm. He was placed on constant observations.

Once his pharmacotherapy levels were established, his symptoms decreased. The degree of observation lessened and supportive therapy was commenced. He was later discharged home into the care of his family, with community case management.

As a mental health nurse, I think the important thing about close observation is that it requires the use of personal qualities such as empathy, patience, warmth and being able to understand and tolerate anxiety and anger.

Observation is a situation where the nurse really needs, and uses, interpersonal skills such as listening, reflecting, observing and building rapport. This can be a tense and uncomfortable situation, but it can also provide a unique opportunity to work closely with a service user, supporting them through this time so they can stay safe and eventually get well. I think it is one of the most important things we can do for our service users.

Donna-Maree Bates

The use of the *no-suicide contract* is another strategy used by nurses working in crisis assessment teams, inpatient mental health settings and community mental health settings. It is used for both assessment of risk and as a management strategy (Farrow, 2002). The contract addresses the prevention of a suicide attempt by the service user and may be a written contract, although it is more often a verbal agreement between the nurse and service user. It usually includes an agreement that when the service user feels they may attempt suicide, they agree instead to contact the nurse (or other agreed person) and discuss their feelings rather than acting on them. If the service user does not comply with the agreed contract, the consequence may be that they face a more restrictive level of care, such as involuntary admission under the Mental Health Act. Therefore, there are significant ethical and legal implications for their use. Although they are commonly used internationally, research has indicated that no-suicide contracts may be more a protective strategy for nurses or a result of a lack of available alternatives or resources such as inpatient facilities or nursing skills, rather than necessarily being the best decision regarding care (Farrow, 2002). In summary, the commonly accepted use of observation and no-suicide contracts by nurses working with the person who is suicidal needs to be thoughtfully considered before implementation.

CASE STUDY: BEN (PART A)

Ben is a 47-year-old man who is transported by ambulance to the accident and emergency department of the local hospital accompanied by the police. He has been unwillingly brought in to hospital and presents as combative and uncooperative, and seems confused. The ambulance officer reports that they were called out by Ben's ex-wife Amelia, after she received a call from him, where he sounded intoxicated, was crying and expressing remorse about their relationship breakdown. Ben told her he had taken an overdose of paracetamol, sertraline and diazepam and wanted to die. This is the second time in the past month that Ben has presented at the emergency department with a suicide attempt.

CRITICAL THINKING CHALLENGE 22.5

In part A of the case study, what rights do the police and ambulance officers have to take Ben to hospital against his will?

What are the immediate nursing priorities for Ben? Consider issues such as the drugs taken, his repeat suicide attempt and his aggression and confusion.

Ben is combative, confused, uncooperative and noncompliant, but the doctor will not prescribe sedation. What likely reason(s) are there for this decision?

How would you feel about nursing a person who had made repeated suicide attempts? Consider factors such as your own beliefs and background.

CASE STUDY: BEN (PART B)

Ben is nursed overnight in the hospital and is administered activated charcoal via nasogastric tube and intravenous acetylcysteine, with regular observations including Glasgow Coma Scores and vital signs. A nurse constantly observes Ben during this time. Ben is angry and uncooperative with the nurse. Towards the end of the shift, Ben says to the nurse, 'What the f... is wrong with you? You haven't saved my life. You've just delayed the inevitable. I'll top myself the moment I get out of here.'

The nurse from the Crisis Resolution Team later interviews Ben and conducts a full assessment. The findings include the fact that Ben is employed full time but has some current financial stressors, has a large network of friends and no significant medical history. He shows signs of depression and is overweight, with poor self-care and diet. He has been drinking large amounts of alcohol lately, and appears to have low self-esteem. However, he has good communication skills and a good rapport is developed during the interview. Ben agrees to be transferred as a voluntary service user to the mental health inpatient unit 'for a night or two'.

The authors would like to acknowledge Paul McNamara.

CRITICAL THINKING CHALLENGE 22.6

In part B of the case study, if you were the nurse constantly observing Ben, how would you feel about him swearing at you and saying he would kill himself? How could you best respond to his statements?

What are the aims of constant observation of the person who is suicidal? Explore the benefits and disadvantages of such obervation for both the service user and the nurse.

Explore the skills and strategies the nurse could use to develop rapport with Ben.

Based on the information provided, identify Ben's likely strengths and vulnerabilities. How could these be addressed in terms of risk management?

If Ben had not agreed to transfer to the unit as a voluntary service user, should he be made an involuntary service user under mental health legislation? Consider issues such as service user rights, dignity, empowerment, duty of care and risk assessment.

When planning is made for Ben to be discharged from hospital, what issues need to be considered? How might these be best addressed?

ETHICOLEGAL ISSUES

Service user choice in the therapeutic setting

Nurses and other health professionals are often called upon to make decisions that affect the care of the service user. Even though there may not be a right or wrong answer to ethical questions, there are ways of arriving at a decision that are more inclusive than others. Being involved in choices about their treatment is also part of the service user's right to self-determination. So, both health professionals and service users in any type of hospital or healthcare setting can be called upon to make or be involved in decisions about the service user's care. There is ever-increasing pressure from service user groups, the profession and the government for nurses to encourage service user participation in decision making related to their care. The nurse is often the person the service user will turn to for advice when such choices need to be made. Participation by the service user promotes autonomy and indicates health professionals' respect for the rights of the service user. Involving the service user in choices about their care and assisting them to make choices in the role of advocate has additional therapeutic advantages. The respect shown to the service user when involving them in decisions about their care may result in enhanced self-esteem and a reduction in helplessness (Brabbins et al., 1996). It may also lead to mutual respect and regard between the nurse and the service user (Munhall, 1991).

Informed consent

Everyone has the right to be informed about and to give consent to any form of treatment. Unfortunately, it is often assumed that consent is only required when major clinical interventions are to be undertaken or where the proposed intervention presents a significant risk to the person. However, consent should be obtained for all procedures, including nursing procedures, wherever service user autonomy is at stake (Aveyard, 2002). Procedures where a recognized risk of side effects or adverse effects exists, as is the case with many medications used in psychiatric treatment, is also an area where consent is required (Wallace, 2001). Further, information sharing in situations involving consent has in the past been viewed as a one-way process where the information was 'aimed at' rather than 'shared with' the service user. Shared information giving and decision making, which maintains the autonomy and interests of the service user as its central focus, is now the preferred approach to consent (Kerridge et al., 2005).

In mental health facilities there are times when consent may not be necessary: for example, when a service user is involuntarily detained and prescribed a course of treatment against his or her will according to the relevant Mental Health Act. However, a person having a mental health problem or being detained in a mental health facility does not mean they cannot retain some role in consenting to treatment. In fact, service users who are involuntarily detained may be considered capable of consenting to some things, and should be informed about treatment decisions and given the opportunity to participate in treatment planning. Even though a service user's wishes may be overruled at times, this does not excuse the failure to involve them in making the decisions (Kerridge et al., 2005).

Nurses need to be aware that the administration of interventions or procedures without the appropriate application of the Mental Health Act and/or consent of the service user can result in legal action being taken against the healthcare provider and/or the healthcare facility. Therefore, obtaining informed consent prior to nursing interventions is an important practice. Nurses also need to be aware of the service user's consent status, of any orders that have been made, and of the need to inform the service user about the treatment they are to receive and to encourage the service user's cooperation in decision making (Wallace, 2001).

Informed consent assumes that the following requirements have been satisfied:

- a fair description of the procedure to be followed has been supplied,
- the possible risks and discomforts have been explained,
- the benefits to be expected have been described,
- any alternative procedures that might be advantageous have been disclosed,
- an offer to answer any queries has been made,

- it has been clearly explained that the person is free to refuse or withdraw consent at any time (Usher and Arthur, 1998; Wallace, 2001).

For consent to be informed it must be voluntary, specific and come from a competent person. The last of these is often the problematic area for mental health nurses. We will examine each aspect in detail.

Consent must be voluntary

For consent to be voluntary it must be given freely without any form of duress. Care must be taken when working with service users who have a mental health problem, as persistent persuasion is often considered to be a reasonable part of mental healthcare, yet may be perceived by the service user as duress. For example, if the nurse uses persuasion to ensure a service user takes their medication and if the service user understands or believes that he or she has no other choice but to follow the advice of the prescriber, this does not constitute informed consent (Brabbins et al., 1996). In other words, if the service user is of the opinion that she or he has no other choice but to take the medication, then informed consent is not achieved.

Consent must be specific

For consent to be specific the service user must be aware of what it is he or she is consenting to. In other words, service users must be given sufficient information to make decisions about the proposed treatments.

Capacity to give consent

Mental capacity is a key issue in any healthcare context where judgements of competency are critical to deciding: whether a service user can or should decide and/or be permitted to decide for themselves; and the point at which another or others will need to, or should, decide for the service user. This issue becomes even more complicated when it is realized that a service user deemed to be 'rationally incompetent' can still be capable of making self-interested choices and, further, that even if these choices are deemed irrational, they may not necessarily be harmful (Wallace, 2001).

In England and Wales, the legal framework that guides decisions about capacity among adults over the age of 16 is the Mental Capacity Act 2005. This Act specifies that there must exist a presumption of capacity (that is that a person has the right and is able to make decisions) unless this is proved otherwise. The Act also requires that:

- individuals must be supported to make their own decisions, for example with the help of counselling or medication, and be given all appropriate information before it is decided they do not have capacity,
- people have a right to make decisions others may see as eccentric or unwise. Anything done for someone without capacity must be in their best interests,
- anything done for someone without capacity must be the least restrictive of their basic rights and freedoms.

Neither the existence of a diagnosed mental disorder nor hospitalization is sufficient grounds to deny an individual's right to make informed choices about their care. The hospitalized mental health service user may have been considered (at least temporarily) incompetent to care for themselves outside the inpatient setting. However, it does not automatically follow that the service user is generally incompetent to make any treatment or other decisions related to their care (Schafer, 1985). Competence to make decisions may vary for one person across time and across tasks; that is, a person may be held competent to make one decision but not another. That is, under the Mental Capacity Act 2005 assessments about capacity are 'decision-specific'; for example, a person may be deemed to have capacity to decide their dietary preferences but not able to manage a large sum of their own money. The Mental Capacity Act 2005 identifies a two-part test of assessment of capacity, where:

1. it has to be determined whether the person's ability to make decisions is impaired or disturbed, and
2. if so, whether the disturbance is so great that they lack judgement to make the particular decision.

The recognition of decision-specfic capacity potentially creates a problem for those who work with people who experience mental health problems, as failure to assess capability accurately has potentially serious ramifications as it may violate a person's autonomy and lead to situations where they are subjected to interventions that are against their wishes (Kerridge et al., 2005).

Ongoing consent

A further process has been considered necessary to ensure that informed consent is current and that it involves the service user in a mutual decision-making process (Usher and Arthur, 1998). The authors argue that consent should not be seen as static, but rather as an ongoing dynamic process in which the service user has a vital role. An ongoing consensual process keeps the service user involved at each step of the therapeutic process. It also keeps them up to date and informed about treatment decisions and, further, it requires that the service user's competency to make decisions and choices is not considered static.

ETHICAL DILEMMA

If a voluntary service user is prescribed medication but refuses to take it, what should the nurse do? If the nurse uses persuasion or coercion to get the service user to take the medication, this could be said to rest on the principle of paternalism; that is, the nurse believes they know the best for the service user. Does this persuasion make the consent invalid? What do you think is the right thing to do in this situation?

What if the service user had an involuntary treatment order according to the Act? Do they have the right to refuse to take medications? This situation may present an ethical dilemma for the nurse who, while believing the service user will benefit from the medication, realizes that any form of coercion could make the consent invalid (Gallagher and Usher, 1993).

CONCLUSION

This chapter has focused on the nursing skills that underpin the provision of therapeutic care for service users in the specialty of mental health nursing. In particular, the chapter has discussed selected communication and nursing skills surrounding service users at risk, issues of violence, aggression and seclusion, and ethicolegal considerations including consent. These are important skills for the nurse to develop when working with people who have a mental health problem, as each nurse–service user encounter is a unique interaction with the potential to heal and support. As stated, these nursing issues have acknowledged the service user and the family as having strengths, vulnerabilities and opportunities. In other words, the interaction between nurse, service user and/or family is an opportunity for all to learn and grow.

EXERCISES FOR CLASS ENGAGEMENT

The personal qualities of the nurse are a significant factor in determining the nature of the therapeutic relationship they form with their service users. Describe your own qualities and explain how they might assist or impede the development of therapeutic rapport. In a small group, outline ways in which you could develop therapeutic qualities.

Identify the specific communication skills you will need in order to develop and maintain an effective therapeutic nurse–service user relationship. As a group, choose the three skills you believe are critical.

Describe the elements of risk assessment. How can a comprehensive risk assessment assist in the management of people identified as being at risk?

Management of aggressive behaviour can be challenging for the nurse. Describe some effective verbal strategies that may be used to defuse the person's aggression before it escalates.

Differentiate between the terms 'self-harm' and 'suicide'. Outline the major nursing issues and strategies for the person who is self-harming, and the person who is suicidal. What beliefs do you hold concerning people who self-harm and people who are suicidal? How can you manage these in order to provide effective nursing care?

Describe your understanding of the term 'informed consent'. What aspect(s) of informed consent may be affected when the person has a mental health problem and how can this/these be addressed ethically and legally? How might the issue of choice be relevant to informed consent?

REFERENCES

Aquilina, C., 1991. Violence by psychiatric inpatients. Med. Sci. Law 31, 441–447.

Arnold, E.C., 2007. Developing therapeutic communication skill in the nurse-client relationship. In: Arnold, E.C., Boggs, K.U. (Eds.), Interpersonal Relationships: Professional Communication Skills for Nurses, fifth ed. Elsevier, St Louis.

Aveyard, H., 2002. Implied consent prior to nursing care procedures. J. Adv. Nurs. 39 (2), 201–207.

Blair, T., 1991. Assaultive behaviour: does provocation begin in the front office? J. Psychosoc. Nurs. Ment. Health Serv. 29 (5), 21–26.

Boggs, K.U., 2007. Bridges and barriers in the therapeutic relationship. In: Arnold, E.C., Boggs, K.U. (Eds.), Interpersonal Relationships: Professional Communication Skills for Nurses, fifth ed. Elsevier, St Louis.

Borg, M., Kristiansen, K., 2004. Recovery-orientated professionals: helping relationships in mental health services. J. Ment. Health 13 (5), 493–505.

Bowers, L., Gournay, K., Duffy, D., 2000. Suicide and self-harm in inpatient psychiatric units: a national survey of observation policies. J. Adv. Nurs. 32 (2), 437–444.

Bowers, L., van der Werf, B., Vokkolainen, A., et al., 2006. International variation in containment measures for disturbed psychiatric inpatients: a comparative questionnaire survey. Int. J. Nurs. Stud. 44, 357–364.

Brabbins, C., Butler, J., Bentall, R., 1996. Consent to neuroleptic medication for schizophrenia: clinical, ethical and legal issues. Br. J. Psychiatry 168, 540–544.

Cameron, D., Kapur, R., Campbell, P., 2005. Releasing the therapeutic potential of the psychiatric nurse: a human relations perspective of the nurse-patient relationship. J. Psychiatr. Ment. Health Nurs. 12 (1), 64–74.

Cleary, M., Jordan, R., Horsfall, J., 2002. Ethical mental health nursing practice. In: Horsfall, J. (Ed.), Mental Health Nursing: Shaping Practice. Central Sydney Area Health Service, Nursing Division, Sydney.

Collins, S., Cutcliffe, J.R., 2003. Addressing hopelessness in people with suicidal ideation: building upon the therapeutic relationship utilizing a cognitive behavioural approach. J. Psychiatr. Ment. Health Nurs. 10 (2), 175–185.

Cowin, L., Davies, R., Estall, G., et al., 2003. De-escalating aggression and violence in the mental health setting. Int. J. Ment. Health Nurs. 12 (1), 64–73.

Cutcliffe, J.R., Barker, P., 2002. Considering the care of the suicidal client and the case for 'engagement and inspiring hope' or 'observations'. J. Psychiatr. Ment. Health Nurs. 9, 611–621.

Darbyshire, P., Jackson, D., 2005. Using a strengths approach to understand resilience and build health capacity in families. Contemp. Nurse 18, 211–212.

Deans, C., Meocevic, E., 2006. Attitudes of registered psychiatric nurses towards patients diagnosed with borderline personality disorder. Contemp. Nurse 21 (1), 43–49.

Delaney, J., Cleary, M., Jordan, R., et al., 2001. An exploratory investigation into the nursing management of aggression in acute psychiatric settings. J. Psychiatr. Ment. Health Nurs. 8, 77–84.

Department of Health, 2008 Code of practice: the Mental Health Act 1983. <http://www.dh.gov.uk/en/Publicationsandstatistics/Publications/PublicationsPolicyAndGuidance/DH_084597>.

Distasio, C.A., 2002. Protecting yourself from violence in the workplace. Nursing 32 (6), 58–64.

Donat, D.C., 2002. Impact of improved staffing on seclusion/restraint reliance in a public psychiatric hospital. Psychiatr. Rehabil. J. 25 (4), 413–416.

Doyle, M., Dolan, M., 2002. Violence risk assessment: combining actuarial and clinical information to structure clinical judgements for the formulation and management of risk. J. Psychiatr. Ment. Health Nurs. 9, 649–657.

Evans, G.W., Wil, D.L., Alligood, M.R., et al., 1998. Empathy: a study of two types. Issues Ment. Health Nurs. 19 (5), 453–461.

Farrell, G., Dares, G., 1996. Seclusion or solitary confinement: therapeutic or punitive treatment? Aust. N. Z. J. Ment. Health Nurs. 5 (4), 171–179.

Farrow, T., 2002. Owning their expertise: why nurses use 'no suicide contracts' rather than their own assessments. Int. J. Ment. Health Nurs. 11 (4), 214–219.

Fontaine, K.L., 2003. Mental Health Nursing, second ed. Pearson Education, NJ.

Fourie, W.J., McDonald, S., Connor, J., et al., 2005. The role of the registered nurse in an acute mental health inpatient setting in New Zealand: perceptions versus reality. Int. J. Ment. Health Nurs. 14 (2), 134–141.

Fry, A.J., O'Riordan, D., Turner, M., et al., 2002. Survey of aggressive incidents experienced by community mental health staff. Int. J. Ment. Health Nurs. 11 (2), 112–120.

Gallagher, F., Usher, K., 1993. Informed consent in mental health nursing. Proceedings of the 20th Annual Convention of the Australian College of Mental Health Nurses, Sydney.

Garnham, P., 2001. Understanding and dealing with anger, aggression and violence. Nurs. Stand. 16 (6), 37–42.

Gournay, K., Bowers, L., 2000. Suicide and self-harm in inpatient psychiatric units: a study of nursing issues in 31 cases. J. Adv. Nurs. 32 (1), 124–131.

Griffith, L., 2001. Does seclusion have a role to play in modern mental health nursing? Br. J. Nurs. 10 (10), 656–661.

Gutheil, T., 1978. Observations on the theoretical bases for seclusion of the psychiatric inpatient. Am. J. Psychiatry 135 (3), 325–328.

Hem, M.H., Heggen, K., 2003. Being professional and being human: one nurse's relationship with a psychiatric client. J. Adv. Nurs. 43 (1), 101–108.

Heyman, E., 1987. Seclusion. J. Psychosoc. Nurs. 25 (11), 9–12.

Holdsworth, N., Belshaw, D., Murray, S., 2001. Developing A&E nursing responses to people who deliberately self-harm: the provision and evaluation of a series of reflective workshops. J. Psychiatr. Ment. Health Nurs. 8 (5), 449–458.

Holmes, C.A., 1998. The Policies and Practices of Seclusion: an Advisory Report for the Western Sydney Area Mental Health Service. Western Sydney Area Health Service, Parramatta, New South Wales.

Hopkins, C., 2002. 'But what about the really ill, poorly people?' An ethnographic study into what it means to nurses on medical admissions units to have people who have harmed themselves as their clients. J. Psychiatr. Ment. Health Nurs. 9 (2), 147–154.

Horsfall, J., Cleary, M., 2000. Discourse analysis of an 'observation levels' nursing policy. J. Adv. Nurs. 32 (5), 1291–1297.

Horsfall, J., Cleary, M., Jordan, R., 1999. Towards Ethical Mental Health Nursing Practice. Australian and New Zealand College of Mental Health Nurses, South Australia.

Horsfall, J., Stuhlmiller, C., Champ, S., 2000. Interpersonal Nursing for Mental Health. McLennan & Petty, Sydney.

Howgego, I.M., Yellowlees, P., Owen, C., et al., 2003. The therapeutic alliance: the key to effective patient outcome? A descriptive review of the evidence in community mental health case management. Aust. N. Z. J. Psychiatry 37 (2), 169–183.

Ignelzi, J., Stinson, B., Raia, J., et al., 2007. Utilizing risk-of-violence findings for continuity of care. Psychiatr. Serv. 58 (4), 452–454.

Kelly, T., Simmons, W., Gregory, E., 2002. Risk assessment and management: a community forensic mental health practice. Int. J. Ment. Health Nurs. 11 (4), 206–213.

Kerridge, I., Lowe, M., McPhee, J., 2005. Ethics and Law for the Health Professions, second ed. Federation Press, Sydney.

Kinsella, K., Anderson, R., Anderson, W., 1996. Coping skills, strengths, and needs as perceived by adult offspring and siblings of people with mental illness: a retrospective study. Psychiatr. Rehabil. J. 20 (2), 24–32.

Kneisl, C.R., Wilson, H.S., Trigoboff, E., 2004. Contemporary Psychiatric–Mental Health Nursing. Pearson Education, NJ.

Kunyk, D., Olson, J.K., 2001. Clarification of conceptualizations of empathy. J. Adv. Nurs. 35 (3), 317–325.

Lanza, M.L., 1988. Factors relevant to client assault. Issues Ment. Health Nurs. 9 (3), 239–257.

Lauder, W., Reynolds, W., Smith, A., et al., 2002. A comparison of therapeutic commitment, role support, role competency and empathy in three cohorts of nursing students. J. Psychiatr. Ment. Health Nurs. 9 (4), 483–491.

Linaker, O.M., Busch-Iversen, H., 1995. Predictors of imminent violence in psychiatric inpatients. Acta Psychiatr. Scand. 92 (4), 250–254.

Littrell, P., Littrell, S., 1998. Current understanding of violence and aggression: assessment and treatment. J. Adv. Nurs. 41 (2), 154–161.

Lowe, T., Wellman, N., Taylor, R., 2003. Limit-setting and decision-making in the management of aggression. J. Adv. Nurs. 41 (2), 154–161.

Luck, L., Jackson, D., Usher, K., 2007. Stamp: components of observable behaviour that indicate potential for patient violence in emergency departments. J. Adv. Nurs. 59 (1), 11–19.

McAllister, M.M., 2001. In harm's way: a postmodern narrative inquiry. J. Psychiatr. Ment. Health Nurs. 8 (5), 391–397.

McAllister, M.M., Estefan, A., 2002. Principles and strategies for teaching therapeutic responses to self-harm. J. Psychiatr. Ment. Health Nurs. 9 (5), 573–583.

McAllister, M.M., Creedy, D., Moyle, W., et al., 2002a. Nurses' attitudes towards clients who self-harm. J. Adv. Nurs. 40 (5), 578–586.

McAllister, M.M., Creedy, D., Moyle, W., et al., 2002b. Study of Queensland emergency department nurses' actions and formal and informal procedures for clients who self-harm. Int. J. Ment. Health Nurs. 8 (4), 184–190.

McAllister, M., Matarasso, B., Dixon, B., et al., 2004. Conversation starters: re-examining and reconstructing first encounters within the therapeutic relationship. J. Psychiatr. Ment. Health Nurs. 11 (4), 575–582.

McKinlay, A., Couston, M., Cowan, S., 2001. Nurses' behavioural intentions towards self-poisoning clients: a theory of reasoned action, comparison of attitudes and subjective norms as predictive variables. J. Adv. Nurs. 34 (1), 107–116.

McLaughlin, C., 1999. An exploration of psychiatric nurses' and clients' opinions regarding inpatient care for suicidal clients. J. Adv. Nurs. 29 (5), 1042–1051.

Martin, G., 2002. Self-injury in context. Ausinetter 16 (3), 9.

Martinez, R.J., Grimm, M., Adamson, M., 1999. From the other side of the door: client views on seclusion. J. Psychosoc. Ment. Health Nurs. 37 (3), 13–22.

Meehan, T., 1997. Nurse Researchers Investigate Effect of Seclusion on

Mentally Ill. Nursing Review, February. Royal College of Nursing, London.

Meehan, T., Vermeer, C., Windsor, C., 2000. Clients' perceptions of seclusion: a qualitative investigation. J. Adv. Nurs. 31 (2), 370–377.

Meehan, T., McIntosh, W., Bergen, H., 2006. Aggressive behaviour in the high-secure forensic setting: the perceptions of patients. J. Psychiatr. Ment. Health Nurs. 13, 19–25.

Muir-Cochrane, E., 1995. An exploration of ethical issues associated with the seclusion of psychiatric clients. Collegian 2 (3), 14–20.

Muir-Cochrane, E., 1996. An investigation into nurses' perceptions of secluding clients on closed psychiatric wards. J. Adv. Nurs. 23 (3), 555–563.

Muir-Cochrane, E., Holmes, C., Walton, J., 2002. Law and policy in relation to the use of seclusion in psychiatric hospitals in Australia and New Zealand. Contemp. Nurse 13 (2/3), 136–145.

Munhall, P.L., 1991. Institutional review of qualitative research proposals: a task of no small consequence. In: Morse, J.M. (Ed.), Qualitative Nursing Research: a Contemporary Dialogue. Sage, CA, pp. 258–271.

NHS Information Centre, 2009. Adult psychiatric morbidity in England, 2007: results of a household survey. <http://www.ic.nhs.uk/webfiles/publications/mental%20health/other%20mental%20health%20publications/Adult%20psychiatric%20morbidity%202007/APMS%202007%20(FINAL)%20Standard.pdf>.

NICE (National Institute for Health and Clinical Excellence), 2004. Self harm: the short-term physical and psychological management and secondary prevention of self-harm in primary and secondary care. <http://guidance.nice.org.uk/CG16/Guidance/pdf/English>.

NICE (National Institute for Health and Clinical Excellence), 2005. Violence: the short-term management of disturbed/violent behaviour in in-patient psychiatric settings and emergency departments. <http://www.nice.org.uk/CG25>.

Nijman, H.L., Camp, J.M., Ravelli, D.P., et al., 1999. A tentative model of aggression on inpatient psychiatric wards. Psychiatr. Serv. 50 (6), 832–834.

Norris, M., Kennedy, C., 1992. The view from within: how clients perceive the seclusion process. J. Psychosoc. Ment. Health Nurs. 30 (3), 7–13.

Office of National Statistics, 2003. Health statistics quarterly. <http://www.statistics.gov.uk/downloads/theme_health/HSQ20.pdf>.

Office of National Statistics, 2011. Suicide rates in the United Kingdom, 2000–2009. <http://www.statistics.gov.uk/statbase/Product.asp?vlnk=13618>.

Owen, C., Tarantello, C., Jones, M., et al., 1998. Violence and aggression in psychiatric units. Psychiatr. Serv. 49 (11), 1452–1457.

Pearson, L., 2001. The clinician–client experience: understanding transference and countertransference. Nurse Pract. 26 (6), 8–11.

Pearson, M., Wilmot, E., Padi, M., 1986. A study of violent behaviour amongst inpatients in a psychiatric hospital. Br. J. Psychiatry 149 (2), 232–235.

Pirkis, J., Francis, C., Warwick Blood, R., et al., 2002. Reporting of suicide in the Australian media. Aust. N. Z. J. Psychiatry 36 (2), 190–197.

Quintal, S.A., 2002. Violence against psychiatric nurses: an untreated epidemic? J. Psychosoc. Ment. Health Serv. 40 (1), 46–55.

Rawlins, R.P., Williams, S.R., Beck, C.K. (Eds.), 1993. Mental Health–Psychiatric Nursing: a Holistic Life-Cycle Approach, third ed. Mosby-Year Book, St Louis.

Reynolds, W.J., Scott, B., 2000. Do nurses and other professional helpers normally display much empathy? J. Adv. Nurs. 31 (1), 226–234.

Rydon, S.E., 2005. The attitudes, knowledge and skills needed in mental health nurses: the perspective of users of mental health services. Int. J. Ment. Health Nurs. 14 (2), 78–87.

Samuelsson, M., Wiklander, M., Asberg, M., et al., 2000. Psychiatric care as seen by the attempted suicide client. J. Adv. Nurs. 32 (3), 635–643.

Schafer, A., 1985. The right of institutionalized psychiatric clients to refuse treatment. Canada's Ment. Health 33 (3), 12–16.

Shepherd, M., Lavender, T., 1999. Putting aggression into context: an investigation into contextual factors influencing the rate of aggressive incidents in a psychiatric hospital. J. Ment. Health 8 (2), 159–170.

Slaven, J., Kisely, S., 2002. Staff perceptions of care for deliberate self-harm clients in rural Western Australia: a qualitative study. Aust. J. Rural Health 10 (5), 233–238.

Smith, S.E., 2002. Perceptions of service provision for clients who self-injure in the absence of expressed suicidal intent. J. Psychiatr. Ment. Health Nurs. 9 (5), 595–601.

Soliday, S.M., 1985. A comparison of client and staff attitudes toward seclusion. J. Nerv. Ment. Dis. 173 (5), 282–286.

Stein-Parbury, J., 2005. Patient and Person: Interpersonal Skills in Nursing, third ed. Elsevier, Sydney.

Stickley, T., Freshwater, D., 2006. The art of listening in the therapeutic relationship. Ment. Health Pract. 9 (5), 12–18.

Talseth, A.-G., Jacobsson, L., Norberg, A., 2001. The meaning of suicidal psychiatric inpatients' experiences of being treated by physicians. J. Adv. Nurs. 34 (1), 96–106.

Tardiff, K., 1998. Prediction of violence in clients. J. Pract. Psychiatry Behav. Health 4 (1), 12.

Terpstra, T.L., Terpstra, T.L., Pettee, E.J., et al., 2001. Nursing staff's attitudes toward seclusions and restraint. J. Psychosoc. Nurs. Ment. Health Serv. 39 (5), 20–28.

Tooke, S.K., Brown, J.S., 1992. Perceptions of seclusion: comparing client and staff reactions. J. Psychosoc. Nurs. Ment. Health Serv. 30 (8), 23–26.

Turnbull, J., Patterson, B., 1999. Aggression and Violence. Macmillan, London.

Usher, K., Arthur, D., 1998. Process consent: a model for enhancing informed consent in mental health nursing. J. Adv. Nurs. 27 (4), 692–697.

Usher, K., Jackson, D., O'Brien, L., 2005. Adolescent drug abuse: helping families survive. Int. J. Ment. Health Nurs. 14, 209–214.

Vanderslott, J., 1998. A study of violence towards staff by clients in an NHS Trust hospital. J. Psychiatr. Ment. Health Nurs. 5 (4), 291–298.

Wallace, M., 2001. Health Care and the Law: A Guide for Nurses, third ed. Law Book, Sydney.

Walsh, F., 1996. The concept of family resilience: crisis and challenge. Fam. Process 35, 261–281.

Welch, M., 2005. Pivotal moments in the therapeutic relationship. Int. J. Ment. Health Nurs. 14, 161–165.

Whitehead, L., Royles, M., 2002. Deliberate self-harm: assessment and treatment interventions. In: Regel, S., Roberts, D. (Eds.), Mental Health Liaison: A Handbook for Nurses and Health Professionals. Baillière Tindall, London.

Whittington, R., Wykes, T., 1994. An observation of associations between nurse behaviour and violence in psychiatric hospitals. J. Psychiatr. Ment. Health Nurs. 1, 85–92.

Wynaden, D., Chapman, R., McGowan, S., et al., 2002. Through the eye of the beholder: to seclude or not to seclude. Int. J. Ment. Health Nurs. 11, 260–268.

Yudofsky, S., Silver, J., Jackson, W., et al., 1986. The overt aggression scale for the objective rating of verbal and physical aggression. Am. J. Psychiatry 143 (1), 35–39.

Chapter | 23 |

Therapeutic interventions

Christine Palmer

CHAPTER POINTS

- Mental health nurses use a range of therapeutic interventions when they work with people who have mental health problems.
- You will be more therapeutic in a mental health context if you understand yourself.
- Being able to identify the stressors in your life will enable you to help others with their stress.
- Relaxation skills and assertiveness skills can be learned and are useful for all nurses.
- Risk assessment and crisis-intervention strategies are used in a range of environments or settings.
- Psychotherapies include individual psychotherapy, brief therapies, motivational interviewing, cognitive behavioural therapy and dialectical behaviour therapy.
- Behaviour is learned, and so it can be unlearned through behaviour therapy.
- Group therapy is a cost-effective and therapeutic way to treat larger numbers of people at the same time.
- Family therapy is an intervention that works to effect change in the family system.
- Psychoeducation is a family-orientated intervention designed to empower and engage families in the care of people with mental health problems.
- Service user-centred ideas of recovery indicate that people will not engage with rehabilitation programmes unless they have hope for a better life.
- Social skills training helps people to learn or relearn social skills.

- The Care Programme Approach helps to ensure that service users receiving care in secondary services have their needs identified and met with an identified professional taking responsibility for coordinating their care.
- Electroconvulsive therapy is an intervention with attendant nursing responsibilities.

KEY TERMS

- activity groups
- assertiveness skills
- behaviour therapy
- brief therapies
- Care Programme Approach (CPA)
- cognitive behavioural therapy (CBT)
- crisis intervention
- dialectical behaviour therapy
- electroconvulsive therapy
- family therapy
- group therapy
- individual psychotherapy
- instilling of hope
- interviewing
- motivational interviewing
- psychoeducation
- psychosocial rehabilitation
- psychotherapy
- relaxation skills
- risk assessment
- social skills training
- stress management
- telephone counselling

LEARNING OUTCOMES

The material in this chapter will assist you to:

- identify stressors and learn strategies for managing stress,
- understand the implications of accurate risk assessment and crisis intervention,
- differentiate between aggressive, passive and assertive response styles,
- recognize fundamental concepts related to a range of psychotherapeutic intervention strategies such as individual psychotherapy, brief therapies, motivational interviewing, cognitive behavioural therapy and dialectical behaviour therapy,
- describe how behaviour is learned, maintained and extinguished,

- recognize the therapeutic factors as they occur within therapy and activity groups,
- understand family-centred approaches to treatment,
- realize how psychosocial rehabilitation contributes to recovery from mental health problems,
- consider how nurses can influence the recovery of people with enduring mental health problems,
- understand how working alongside or with the service user contributes to better outcomes for the service user,
- consider the ethical issues related to electroconvulsive therapy.

INTRODUCTION

This chapter provides an overview of a range of therapeutic interventions used by mental health nurses working with people with mental health problems. Some of the content here will require you to review material in other chapters to help your understanding. Working through this chapter will not give you the skills to be expert in any of these techniques, but it will enable you to understand some fundamental concepts. You may even begin to understand yourself better. When you are working with people with mental health problems, a deeper understanding of yourself will help you to be more therapeutic. One aspect of self-understanding and the understanding of others involves culture; throughout this chapter, it is important to consider the specific cultural perspective and needs of the person.

We all experience stress and the outcomes of living stressful lives. Being able to identify the stressors in your life will enable you to better manage your own stress before you can begin to help others with their stress. There are many stress-management strategies from which to choose. This chapter considers relaxation skills and assertiveness skills. Relaxation is a simple physical skill that can be learned with practice, and assertiveness skills are particularly useful for nurses in any area of clinical specialty.

Mental health nursing requires accurate assessment of risk to ensure good outcomes, because a person may represent a risk not only to themselves, but also to others in the community. Crisis intervention also requires specific skills that aim to ensure risk minimization. Crisis intervention can occur in a range of environments or settings, and telephone counselling is just one of these.

Many therapies or therapeutic endeavours have been developed to help people with their psychological problems. Among those discussed briefly here are the psychotherapies, such as individual psychotherapy, brief therapies, motivational interviewing (MI), cognitive behavioural therapy (CBT) and dialectical behaviour therapy (DBT). In addition, behaviour therapy, group therapy (including activity groups) and family therapy (including psychoeducation) are briefly reviewed.

Psychosocial rehabilitation is a term used to describe the kind of rehabilitation that is provided particularly for those with chronic and enduring mental health problems. According to service user-centred ideas of recovery from mental health problems, people will not engage with rehabilitation programmes unless they have hope for a better life. While people can arrive at a sense of hope without the input of nurses, we are also able to contribute to a person's sense of hope so that a more desired life can be achieved. Social skills training is also an aspect of psychosocial rehabilitation that will help people relearn the skills they need in order to engage more actively in the communities in which they live.

Finally, this chapter considers the roles of interviewing, care coordination and electroconvulsive therapy (ECT) in contemporary mental health nursing. Taking a more collaborative approach to interviewing supports the orientation towards service user-centred care. The Care Programme Approach (CPA) is also a service user-centred approach ensuring personalized care emphasizing the role of a coordinator of care, and on promoting and supporting self-care to assist the person to live their life as independently as possible (Department of Health, 2008). Although ECT remains a contentious intervention, it is a valid treatment strategy with attendant nursing responsibilities. While providing information on all these topics, this chapter also asks you to reflect on who you are, and what you believe and value.

STRESS MANAGEMENT

Before considering how to manage stress, it is important to understand how stress manifests and affects the body. Among the effects of stress are increased blood flow to skeletal muscles, decreased blood flow to other organs, increased heart rate, raised blood pressure, rapid breathing and increased arousal so that vision and hearing are more acute. This is the body's way of preparing for fight or flight. That is, the body prepares to fight and defend against, or flee, the stress-causing situation. For example, say when walking back to your car after finishing work late at night, you hear footsteps behind you. In order to prepare you for fight or flight, all of the responses described above occur. They are all essential and automatic physical responses designed to keep you alive.

These responses occur in part because adrenaline is released into the bloodstream. Stress is a normal part of life today but if we have too much stress, or if it is prolonged or too intense, we experience a range of unpleasant symptoms. These include a dry mouth, tremor, palpitations, sleep disturbance, shoulder and neck pain, irritability, indigestion, uncertainty and confusion. Having high levels of adrenaline and other hormones circulating through the body much of the time is bound to affect our functioning, as we should only be in a state of hypervigilance or hyperalertness for a brief period of time.

It is also important to consider what causes stress. It is not usually a particular event or situation that causes stress, but your perception of and reaction to the event. For example, two people coming across a dog in the street might experience the situation quite differently. One person might view the dog as 'man's best friend' and experience pleasure in seeing the animal. The other person might view the dog as a potential threat, perhaps because of a dog attack during childhood, and subsequently experience fear and anxiety, resulting in stress. Also, although we all experience stress, not all stressful situations have a detrimental effect on us. This is because of a range of internal and external factors that help to mediate the impact of stress. Internal factors might include effective coping skills and a relaxed personal style. External factors might include strong social support and a comfortable living environment. Nevertheless, the inability to manage stress ultimately leads to difficulties in living and, for some, mental health problems.

Escot et al. (2001, p. 273) examined the stress levels of nursing staff working in an oncology setting and found that 'stress is primarily related to inadequate training, lack of time to deal with the psychological component of caregiving, especially terminal care, and relationships with other medical staff'. Edwards et al. (2002, p. 213) found that 'mental health workers are likely to experience stress as a result of working closely with service users over an extended period of time'. Other workplace difficulties causing stress that these authors identified included increased workload, increased administration, lack of resources and problems with management.

It is important to remember that the stresses we experience in one part of our lives, such as at work, will overlap into others, such as relationships, and vice versa. There are many opportunities for us to experience stress at work. Simply working a variety of shifts during the week can be stressful. The responsibilities that nurses are expected to take on, often without the necessary experience, also contribute to stress. Personal relationships provide their own challenges and we all experience these at some time. Before you can focus on managing stress, you need to identify what causes stress for you (see the first exercise at the end of this chapter).

Once you are aware of the major stressors in your life, you can begin to think about how to manage them or, more correctly, manage the *effects* of the stress you are experiencing. Remember, it's not the stress itself that is the problem; it's how you react to the stress that is crucial.

According to Battison (1997, p. 24) there are four main techniques people use to manage stress. You can:

- change the situation,
- increase your ability to deal with the situation,
- change your perception of the situation,
- change your behaviour.

Notice that there is a definite call for change in your life. However, many of us find change stressful. If you have a perception or belief that change will be difficult, you are much more likely to find it stressful. If you believe that change presents opportunity, you are less likely to find it stressful. Nevertheless, if we do not change the behaviour that results in stress, stress will remain a part of our lives and we will ultimately suffer ill health: mental, physical or both.

Skills such as time management, being assertive, relaxation, yoga, visualization, managing change, meditation and correct breathing can all be learned relatively easily, and some of these skills are addressed in this chapter. Changes to your lifestyle such as healthy eating, reducing alcohol, drug and tobacco consumption, and exercising require considerable commitment. It is important to find out what works well for you in addition to lifestyle changes so that you can use these strategies whenever you feel the effects of stress.

Relaxation training

Relaxing is an excellent way to manage your body's responses to stress. It works because you can't be both tense and relaxed at the same time. When you experience tension, relaxation is a certain way to alleviate it. It is also important to use relaxation to prevent the adverse effects of stress, not just manage these symptoms. Relaxation can involve simply setting aside some time to sit back and listen to soothing music, read a good book or take a stroll around the park (Battison, 1997). Listening to music and reading might also be done from the comfort of a hot bath combined with aromatherapy. Learning to breathe more effectively will also lead to relaxation.

Progressive muscle relaxation (PMR; also known as deep muscle relaxation) can be carried out reasonably quickly and with great effect. It can be done independently or by following the instructions on a CD (available in a range of outlets including music stores). Because PMR is a skill, it will take practice. You won't develop the skill overnight. PMR involves the progressive relaxation of the major muscles of the body while making a conscious effort to distinguish muscle tension from muscle relaxation. It has been found that PMR also relaxes the mind and internal organs (Romas and Sharma, 1995). Ultimately, you will be able to relax groups of muscles at will, which can be done anywhere. PMR has been shown to be effective in treating a range of physical and psychological conditions such as headaches and anxiety disorders and in preventing the effects of stress (Ayers et al., 2007; Romas and Sharma, 1995; Rausch et al., 2006).

To begin to learn how to use PMR, you will need to set aside some time every day to practise. You can do this sitting in a comfortable chair, or preferably lying down. Find a quiet place where you won't be interrupted. Avoid PMR immediately after food as relaxation of the stomach may occur, resulting in delayed digestion (Patel, 1991). If lying flat on the floor or bed, be sure that you let your feet flop loosely and, if in a chair, let your arms hang loosely. Above all, be sure that you are comfortable or you will find it difficult to relax. You can either follow written instructions until you have memorized them or you could record the instructions with a digital voice recorder and play it through each day. This way you can devote your attention to relaxation.

Before beginning muscle relaxation, it is important to take a few slow, deep breaths to prepare yourself. PMR involves working the major muscle groups, starting with the lower limbs and working through to the head (although some authors don't follow this directional flow). Begin by flexing the feet, holding the flexion for a few seconds, then releasing the tension. Focus on the difference between the tension resulting from flexion and the relaxation resulting from releasing the muscles. Repeat this action for each muscle group and take a short break between each action. Alternatively, tense and relax the calves, thighs, buttocks, back, chest, shoulders, hands, arms, neck, jaw, eyes (face) and forehead (Battison, 1997). Finishing the session should involve acknowledging freedom from tension, resting quietly for a few minutes and counting backwards from 10. Then take a deep breath and get up quietly. To effectively help others develop relaxation skills you need to be able to do this well for yourself. This will also lead to a belief in the benefits of relaxation.

Assertiveness training

Assertion is about being able to communicate clearly to others and avoiding misunderstandings that might contribute to stress. Assertiveness, therefore, is a communication skill that will enhance your interpersonal effectiveness and make social situations more comfortable (Gambril, 1995). As our personalities develop, we tend to learn a pattern of responding that is aggressive, passive or assertive (see Table 23.1). The passive person's rights are often violated by others. Being taken advantage of inevitably leads to frustration, anxiety and unhappiness. At the other end of the continuum, the aggressive person violates the rights of others and takes advantage of them. The aggressive person is generally defensive and humiliating, perhaps resulting in social isolation. The assertive person, however, protects the rights of each party and achieves goals without hurting others. This results in self-confidence and the ability to express oneself appropriately in emotional and social situations.

Table 23.1 Comparing passive, assertive and aggressive styles

Passive	Assertive	Aggressive
Communicates indirectly; can have human rights violated	Communicates directly and clearly; protects own rights and the rights of others	Communicates critically and explosively; violates the rights of others
Does not achieve goals	Achieves goals without hurting others	Achieves goals at the expense of others
Allows others to make choices or decisions	Chooses for self	Intrudes on others' choices
Doesn't manage problems	Addresses problems and negotiates	Unwilling to listen to others and acts on problems too quickly

Source: Adapted from Davis (1989).

Central to these ways of responding is the consideration of basic human rights. We all have the basic right to be treated with respect, for example, and the right to say no without feeling guilty. Making your situation understood by others in a non-aggressive way enables you to feel comfortable without violating the rights of the other person. It is important that your verbal and nonverbal behaviours match. Appropriate nonverbal behaviour to support your verbal message includes good eye contact, a firm voice (don't apologize or shout) and open body posture to show sincerity (Patel, 1991). So, what is your communication style?

CRITICAL THINKING CHALLENGE 23.1

You've had a number of stressful situations within your family recently, and so you have been unable to complete your essay on time. You approach your lecturer to ask for an extension on your essay return date.

Decide which of the following responses would best describe your pattern of responding.

You would say:

- If it's okay with you... If it's not too much trouble ... um, would it be okay ... this essay that's due ... I'm sorry ...
- I've had a number of stressful situations lately and I'm going to need an extension on the essay. Would it be all right if I have another week to return it to you?
- Look, I can't get that essay done on time. You haven't given us enough time. You should schedule these things better.

The first response is non-assertive or passive and the last response is aggressive. As you can see from the assertive response, the message is honest, direct and clear. The problem is clearly addressed and the desired outcome openly negotiated.

Being assertive is a skill that anyone can develop with practice. Learning to be assertive means that you will have a choice about how you respond to others. It is important to be aware that you are under no obligation to be assertive all the time. When you have assertion skills, you have the choice to be assertive or to say nothing at all. Many of us have never learned to be assertive and may find it difficult to change patterns of responding that are passive or aggressive. For example, women in some cultural and religious groups learn to defer their thoughts and feelings to those of others, particularly men. These early and strong patterns of responding might be difficult to alter in the short term. However, it is important to determine what your pattern of responding is so that you can acknowledge it and work on changing specific aspects of your behaviour.

There are many types of assertion skills that can help you to handle situations you will encounter either personally or professionally. Some difficult situations can include making or refusing requests, accepting and giving compliments, expressing opinions, giving negative feedback or being confrontational, initiating conversations, sharing intimate feelings and experiences with others, and expressing affection. Examples include conveying a nursing assessment to other members of the multidisciplinary team, and refusing a request to care for a service user with complex needs when you are a novice nurse. Indeed, nurses' concerns about advocating on behalf of service users have been found to be a factor that supports the use of assertiveness skills in the workplace (Timmins and McCabe, 2005). Many of us find it hard to refuse unwanted requests and this can make life difficult. Just as often, a person might be unable to accept a compliment without countering it by minimizing it. For example, when someone says, 'You look nice today,' it is important to say 'Thank you'. It's quite a different response to say, 'Thanks, but this old dress/suit belongs in a clothing bin'.

Teaching assertiveness skills to others is usually done in groups involving people who need to develop assertion skills. There are a number of workbooks available that can be used to work through and learn how to develop assertiveness skills. A simple and easy text by Davis et al. (2000) can help you to assess your interpersonal style and your difficulties before guiding you though some strategies for changing your behaviour if you see the need to do so. Once you learn some of these skills you'll be able to support others to recognize their non-assertiveness or aggressiveness and help them to learn new ways of behaving.

RISK ASSESSMENT

Risk assessment involves determining whether a person has the potential for self-harm, either actively or passively, or is considered to pose a risk for hurting someone else. Whenever a person with a mental health problem seriously hurts or kills another person, this usually elicits a strong reaction from the media and the public. When the result is an official enquiry into organizations and individual mental health practitioners, the outcome is usually a tightening of risk assessment and risk management strategies as well as considerable anxiety among staff. Where the service user involved in violent behaviour has been treated in a secure environment such as a forensic mental health service, the need for accurate risk assessment skills is heightened (Kelly et al., 2002). Risk assessment is designed to *prevent* rather than predict self- or other-directed violence. It is a continuous and dynamic process that is affected by the person's changing mental state and the environment at the time. Therefore, risk assessment is a critical clinical skill in practising as a competent beginning mental health nurse.

CRITICAL THINKING CHALLENGE 23.2

When a service user is at risk due to self-neglect, we refer to this as passive self-harm. How might you assess the risk for passive harm?

Risk assessment is not straightforward and it is inevitable that mistakes will be made. According to Doyle and Dolan (2002, p. 651), 'clinical risk predictions are only slightly above chance and the competence varies greatly between clinicians'. This means that risk assessment depends on the skills of individuals rather than on the outcome of focused education. Because nurses spend more time with service users than do other health professionals, we are able to gather important information that will inform the multidisciplinary team regarding a person's risk. So, if during your interactions with a service

user you feel concerned about the person's potential risk, acknowledge your role and responsibility to report this to the team and write about it in the service user's file.

Risk for violence

Some risk factors for violence identified by Doyle and Dolan (2002) include a history of violence, recent verbal threats, a lifestyle that is violent (such as belonging to a gang or trafficking illicit drugs), and being a victim of childhood physical and sexual abuse. The presence of alcohol or other substance use problems and/or personality traits that are antisocial, explosive or impulsive also increases the risk for violence. Although many believe that marijuana is a safe drug, a belief assisted by its description as a 'recreational drug', it has been found to contribute significantly to violence (Mullen, 2002). Fear, hallucinations, agitation, anger and suspiciousness revealed through a mental status examination will also alert you to an increased potential for violence. There has been considerable research into specific diagnostic groupings (Axis I disorders) considered to have a greater or lesser potential for violence, with significant variation among the results (Monahan et al., 2001). However, an Axis II diagnosis of antisocial personality disorder is predictive of future violence (see Ch. 16 for more information about personality disorders). A tool might be useful in helping to predict the risk for violence, depending on your level of expertise. Abderhalden et al. (2004) offer a tool for use in the acute inpatient setting, whereas Murphy (2004) points out that community mental health nurses tend to rely more on their experience than on the use of an assessment tool.

Self-harm and suicide

Some people carry out acts of deliberate self-harm without aiming to commit suicide. Some attempt suicide unsuccessfully and may therefore fall into the category of self-harm. Risk factors for self-harm or suicide include the presence of suicidal ideas, feelings of hopelessness, having a plan for committing suicide and having the means to carry out that plan. Demographic factors such as age, being male, being single and having no social support increase the risk for suicide. Young people have their own set of risk factors, largely related to what is going on in their home, school and social environments (Murray and Wright, 2006). Diagnoses of depression or borderline personality disorder carry with them an increased risk for self-harm and suicide. In addition, 10% of people with schizophrenia will commit suicide and 15% of people with alcohol- or substance-dependence problems will also kill themselves, although alcohol is implicated in up to 65% of successful suicides (Varcarolis, 1998). Ultimately, having a mental health problem increases the risk for suicide (see Chs 9, 10 and 22). Using a tool to guide your suicide risk assessment is suggested, particularly for novice nurses (Cutcliffe and Barker, 2004).

Factors that protect against violence or self-injury include a safe environment, strong social support, a good relationship with staff and an acceptance of the current treatment approach (Doyle and Dolan, 2002). Clearly, nurses have a role in preventing violence or self-harm. Given that nurses are in the best position to assess and manage risk, we need to be sharpening our risk assessment skills. But these are skills that tend to be taken for granted and learned 'on the job' rather than formally. Understanding risk factors and protective factors will help you to better assess risk. However, more accurate risk assessment comes from deeper knowledge and extensive experience.

Crisis intervention

What represents a crisis for one person might not have the same impact on another person, but no one is immune to crisis (see Ch. 9). Situational life crises such as unwanted pregnancy, death of a loved one, serious physical illness and assault are frequently the cause of emotional disequilibrium or imbalance requiring crisis intervention. Being able to intervene effectively during a crisis is a critical clinical skill required by the mental health nurse.

Crisis intervention has developed as a specialty area in mental health nursing that largely involves responding to people in the community who are overwhelmed by problems or difficulties with life. Often people are referred by a primary healthcare provider (such as a general practitioner or nurse practitioner), accident and emergency staff or sometimes by a family member. Some individuals will make direct contact with crisis resolution services, often because they have no one else to turn to for help.

We invariably respond to crisis with our usual ways of coping. However, because of the magnitude of the problem or a distorted perception of the problem, our usual coping behaviours might fail to resolve it. As a result, we might try other means of coping (such as alcohol or other drug abuse, eating excessively or not eating at all) and these are usually even less effective. Crisis intervention involves interrupting a maladaptive or ineffective pattern of responding and supporting the person to return to the pre-crisis level of functioning (Greenstone and Leviton, 2002). Therefore, the focus is on current difficulties and the timeframe is brief.

Crisis intervention is quick, short term and based in the here and now. 'Management of the crisis, not resolution, is the goal of crisis intervention' (Greenstone and Leviton, 2002). Crisis intervention helps the person in crisis to locate or develop the resources from within or externally in order to return to the pre-crisis level of functioning (Myer, 2001). At times, following resolution of

a crisis, an individual may actually develop new coping skills that will help him or her deal more effectively with future crises. Conversely, lack of resolution of a crisis may result in more disabling psychological problems and subsequent crises will not be well managed.

In order to work effectively in crisis intervention, it is important to have a model to direct your actions. The model will ensure that no relevant information is missed, so the best possible outcome is achieved for the service user. There are many available models [for example, see the work of Slaikeu (1990) and the model offered by Greenstone and Leviton (2002)] but they all reflect the need to act quickly and to base interventions on an accurate assessment of the situation and of risk. Aguilera (1994) offers a simple model for assessing and managing crises. She asserts that there are three factors that, when present, defend against the development of crisis. These are the presence of social support, intrinsic coping skills (such as the ability to solve problems) and a realistic perception of the event, resulting in the belief that you can manage. Consequently, if your assessment reveals a lack in any of these areas, you would direct your interventions to meet the area of need.

CASE STUDY: SUE

Sue is a 29-year-old woman who is distressed about her relationship breakdown. She had been married for 2 years before her husband began seeing another woman. He informed her 2 days ago that he is leaving her for the other woman. While talking with you about her feelings of betrayal and helplessness, she mentions that her father sexually abused her as a child. She realizes that the same feelings have been generated through this experience. One of the aims of crisis intervention in Sue's case would be to stay focused on the current issue that has precipitated the crisis, in this case the relationship breakdown. The sexual abuse issue can be dealt with at a later time and potentially over a longer timeframe.

Well-practised communication skills, particularly listening and helping the person to tell their story, are fundamental to crisis intervention. Without being clear about what the problem is, it is unlikely that you will be able to intervene effectively in a crisis. Crisis intervention is one time when you, as the helper, take some control and provide direction because the person in crisis is usually unable to do so for him or herself. Myer (2001) suggests that we take control and determine the direction of the therapy without causing dependence. 'The more severe the reaction to the crisis situation, the more active the crisis worker must be' (Myer, 2001, p. 6). The focus is on ensuring both physical and psychological safety.

Telephone counselling

Counselling by telephone is designed to support people in crisis, so it usually involves a single session. It often occurs after hours and at no cost to the recipient. In addition, telephone counselling affords anonymity to the caller at a time when the person is experiencing vulnerability. As with any counselling session, the telephone counsellor helps the person cope with the crisis by working through feelings and by problem-solving. Outcomes include resolution of the problem, referral for further treatment or, if the counselling is unsuccessful, lack of engagement. Interestingly, it has been found that most calls to crisis centre call lines are from people seeking social support rather than crisis intervention (Watson et al., 2006), which may require an adjustment to the way that telephone services are offered. However, telephone counselling might also be set up for the convenience of the service user; for example, for people with physical disabilities who might otherwise have difficulty accessing an office. In addition, some counsellors might augment face-to-face counselling sessions with telephone sessions (Sanders, 1996).

Nurses working with crisis resolution services are frequently required to interview and counsel people by telephone. Their goal is to make an accurate assessment and to ensure safety for the caller and others. Others at risk might include spouses or children in cases where the caller is expressing anger against them. Nurses working in mental health inpatient units and emergency departments may also do telephone counselling, often by accident rather than design. Often people in crisis will contact these services for help when they are at a loss to know what else to do. Nevertheless, whenever you are called upon to counsel someone by telephone, you will require a process to help you work through the situation.

There are many models for crisis intervention by telephone (Egan, 1998; Lester, 2002; Slaikeu, 1990) but they all follow a similar problem-solving plan. There needs to be initial engagement or the development of rapport through a caring, honest and open approach before the problem can be explored and analysed. The same counselling skills used for face-to-face counselling are used, but with greater emphasis on listening. Following engagement, it is important to determine the person's safety before moving on to explore their needs. Once the person's needs have been thoroughly explored, a plan of action would be developed that includes a follow-up appointment.

CRITICAL THINKING CHALLENGE 23.3

How do you make psychological contact when you don't have eye contact? Role play a counselling session by telephone. In pairs, sit back-to-back or side-by-side and begin to work through a mock crisis situation. Begin by introducing yourself. Continue for 5–10 min.

Report back to the larger group:

♦ What specifically helped with engagement?
♦ How did you overcome the barrier of no eye contact?
♦ How did you know how comfortable the service user felt?
♦ How did the service user know that the counsellor was interested?

When working on the telephone, more frequent verbal responses are necessary. It is important to let the service user know that they are being heard and that you are there, listening to the story. Typical verbal encouragers include: uh-huh, yes, sure, go on, mmmm, right, okay, I see, Do you want to say more about that? and Please tell me more about that. These verbal encouragers let the service user know that they are being listened to, and this enables further elaboration of the story about the current crisis.

Listening carefully is also very important. When telephone counselling, there are no visual cues to attend to so you must focus your listening skills more acutely. This enables a more accurate assessment of what the service user is thinking and feeling, which enables you to reflect that understanding to the service user in a truly empathic way. The telephone counsellor needs to listen for voice tone, pitch and volume, and breathing noises that might indicate anxiety, grief or anger. It is important to listen for crying and other noises like snorting, groaning, grunting, sighing, laughter, sarcasm and silences (Sanders, 1996). These will need to be interpreted in the context of what is being said.

PSYCHOTHERAPY

Psychotherapy is concerned with 'the complex messy nature of the human experience. This includes the problematic domains of the aesthetic, the ethical, and the spiritual' (Petchkovsky et al., 2002, p. 330). The term *psychotherapy* is used to describe a number of interpersonal models, each with its own individual philosophy and set of techniques. Examples of psychotherapeutic models include individual psychotherapy, brief therapies, MI, CBT and DBT. To be able to practise any of these psychotherapies, you would need to undertake a specialized programme of study that might include supervised practice, but nurses can and do conduct psychotherapy.

Individual psychotherapy

The early work of Sigmund Freud (1938/1965) revealed that much of what motivates us and influences our behaviour occurs at an unconscious level. Despite some of his work being challenged over the years, it is this understanding that underpins psychotherapy. Although psychotherapy can occur in groups, it most commonly occurs individually. The goal of psychotherapy is to effect change in the person's character, as difficulties of living are viewed as linked to childhood development of the psyche. 'Psychodynamic theory is rooted in the belief that we develop a sense of self during childhood' (Gallop and O'Brien, 2003, p. 216).

Psychotherapy occurs between service user and therapist, usually over a lengthy period of time (time-unlimited). It provides the service user with opportunities to examine the historical experiences that have shaped who they are and influenced their life decisions. This happens when the service user brings those past experiences into the present relationship with the therapist and re-enacts them (transference). Transference is an unconscious process; that is, the person is unaware that he/she is doing it. According to Evans (2007, p. 191), 'transference is about one's fundamental ways of relating to those one loves, fundamental ways that repeat throughout one's life, although new experiences do provide the possibility for change in this pattern'. The person may begin to relate to you as the nurse in one of these patterned ways: for example, as someone who can be trusted, loved and respected. From this place, the service user might be able to talk more deeply about the things that concern them. Alternatively, the service user might respond to you as someone who is unlikeable and untrustworthy, reflecting that person's earlier experiences. This negative transference is quite common and needs to be immediately recognized as such rather than taken personally.

The therapist is also responsible for recognizing what he or she brings to the therapeutic relationship and the counter-transferences that support the service user's re-enactment of earlier relationships. For example, it is important to recognize that reciprocal love or dislike for the service user is counter-transference and that expressing this would be counter-therapeutic and potentially destructive. Counter-transference can be viewed as a natural and expected response in some instances (for example, responding as the caring and nurturing mother), but it is important to recognize this response as counter-transference, as it has the potential to be damaging to the service user. For example, an adult who struggled as a child to get confirmation of love from a parent might re-enact that struggle in the service user–therapist relationship (transference). The therapist who doesn't recognize the transference and allows the service user to continue to seek affirmation (without challenging it) is demonstrating counter-transference. So, the therapist is responding to a situation that is rooted in the service user's past and causing the situation to be repeated in the present. The appropriate response on the part of the therapist would be to explore the service user's need for love and to help the service user gain insight into

how this is related to experiences from an earlier time in his or her life. Counter-transference can be viewed as a natural and expected response in some instances (for example, responding as the caring and nurturing mother), but it is important to recognize our response as counter-transference, as it has the potential to be damaging to the service user (see Ch. 22 for more information on these terms).

Gallop and O'Brien (2003) argue that nurses need to deepen their understanding of psychodynamic theory, not just at the cognitive level, but at the affective level: the level of emotions. We need to be aware that our own developmental experiences determine who we are and that we re-enact our personal histories in everyday relationships, professional or personal. Much of this occurs unconsciously and puts us at risk of behaving inappropriately. 'Our history that creates the self is replayed in every interaction and decision throughout our lives. So that when we respond to our clients and they respond to us, we in the present bring with us our past' (Gallop and O'Brien, 2003, p. 219). This is particularly important to acknowledge when we are working with people who are already distressed by mental health problems and are vulnerable.

Brief therapies

Brief therapies began in the 1960s when efforts were made to make the psychotherapeutic model of counselling available to greater numbers of people. Access to psychotherapy was limited due to the time-unlimited nature of early psychotherapy. However, the brief therapies expanded as it became clear that they could be very effective (Bloom, 1997). Brief therapies include interpersonal psychotherapy, solution-focused therapies, CBT and MI. Effectiveness, efficiency and economy have therefore led to an explosion in brief therapies.

The goal of brief therapies is to manage problems in the here and now (the present). The duration of the short-term therapies ranges from a single session through to around 20 interviews, as compared with individual psychotherapy, which occurs regularly over at least a 2-year period. Given the fiscal environment in healthcare services, improved access to forms of treatment that provide value for money is welcomed. Furthermore, brief therapies can be, in general, as effective and long-lasting as time-unlimited psychotherapy (Bloom, 1997, p. 7).

Motivational interviewing

Motivational interviewing (MI) is a relatively modern psychotherapeutic model, having been conceptualized in 1982 by Bill Miller and Steve Rollnick. It is an intervention that was initially developed for work with people with substance abuse and dependence problems. Indeed, Miller (1998) defines addiction as fundamentally a problem of motivation. You may be aware that many people with these problems tend to use the defence mechanism of denial; that is, they initially refuse to acknowledge that a problem exists. Once the person begins to acknowledge that there may be a problem, they may still be reluctant to engage in treatment. This indecision is known as *ambivalence* and MI essentially aims to change the substance use problem by helping people to explore and resolve this ambivalence (Rollnick and Miller, 1995).

MI is described as a directive form of counselling. It is not directive in terms of the therapist telling the service user what to do and how to behave, because it is also defined as a service user-centred counselling strategy. It is directive in that it is goal-directed and the therapist provides guidance in an attempt to resolve ambivalence. When the service user begins to see that there is a problem with substance use, resistance is expressed or experienced. This is normal and expected, and is accepted as part of the MI approach. The therapeutic relationship is more like a partnership where two people work together, rather than a professional relationship where the therapist is acknowledged as the expert. It is thought that the nature of this type of relationship is also empowering. This gives the service user a sense of self-control and personal power, which contributes to the recovery process.

Rollnick and Miller (1995) differentiate what they call the spirit of MI from the techniques they recommend to support it. Central to MI is the need for the therapist to resist persuading the service user to make changes in behaviour. Motivation to change is determined to come from the service user. Readiness to change, however, is a result of interpersonal interaction rather than being a personality attribute of the service user (trait). Any attempts to persuade or coerce the service user will only lead to increased resistance. The counselling style is described as quiet and involves guiding the service user towards considering the options and their consequences. It is not confrontational. The therapist would never tell the service user what he or she should be doing. According to Rollnick and Miller (1995):

> It is inappropriate to think of motivational interviewing as a technique or set of techniques that are ... 'used on' people ... rather it is an interpersonal style. It is a subtle balance of directive and service user-centred components, shaped by a guiding philosophy and understanding of what triggers change. If it becomes a trick or a manipulative technique, its essence has been lost.

(Rollnick and Miller, 1995, p. 326)

The wheel of change or transtheoretical model developed by Prochaska and DiClemente (1983) is used to support the philosophy of MI. The model outlines five stages related to the readiness to change behaviour; in this case, abstaining from addictive substances like alcohol.

1. Precontemplation: the individual does not intend to change. The person is often not aware that there is a problem, and is not actively looking for an alternative life.
2. Contemplation: there is acknowledgement that a problem exists, and so the person begins to think about change. There is a developing awareness of the advantages of change, but the disadvantages are also recognized (Prochaska, 2001).
3. Preparation: the person begins to learn new skills and gather information as the readiness to change develops. At this stage the plans are for change to take place within the next month (Finnell, 2003).
4. Action: significant behaviour change occurs as the person begins to engage in new behaviours.
5. Maintenance: permanent changes in behaviour are now sought. The person works towards establishing the change, by adjusting their lifestyle and actively avoiding returning to old patterns of behaviour.

According to the philosophy of MI, the therapist guides the service user through these stages at a pace determined by the service user. Changing destructive patterns of substance abuse and dependence does not happen all at once. Motivated by relevant and meaningful goals, the change occurs progressively (Finnell, 2003). As relapse is viewed as part of the process of change, a return to earlier stages in the process is considered normal.

In addition to the spirit of MI, five principles underpin the model, as outlined by Miller et al. (1992).

1. Avoid argumentation: there should not be any confrontation or arguing with the service user. This will only result in the service user returning with argumentation and withdrawing from the therapy. If the service user were to deny having a problem with alcohol, despite the overwhelming evidence, the therapist would not argue about the evidence with the service user.
2. Express empathy: this is considered critical to the approach. Expression of empathy gives service users the message that they are heard and understood. This is important because it is unlikely to have occurred within the family or the community. This leads to service users being more open to therapy and to sharing their stories. Service users are also more likely to be open to the gentle challenges from the therapist about their beliefs about substance use. Change occurs because service users are more comfortable in working with their ambivalence.
3. Support self-efficacy: supporting a person's sense of self-efficacy contributes to the service user's belief that change is possible. Self-efficacy is supported through

acknowledging the person's past ability to change and by supporting the person to choose his or her own plan for change. Observing others who have made changes in their lives is also a powerful motivator for change.

4. Roll with resistance: resistance from the service user is considered normal and not to be contested. The counsellor rolls with the resistance by encouraging the service user to find his or her own solutions to problems. Because there is no differentiation between the therapist and service user, there is nothing for the service user to fight against. The counsellor might offer new perspectives, but these are not imposed on the service user.

5. Develop discrepancy: this involves helping service users to see the discrepancies between what they hope to achieve (their goals) and how they are currently behaving. Recognizing that their actions are leading them away from rather than towards the achievement of their important goals provides the motivation for change.

MI has been found to be very effective, particularly where a person's suffering from the effects of the addiction has increased, as it does over time. People have changed their patterns of substance dependence after as little as 1–2 h of MI. And a single session of MI prior to embarking on a rehabilitation programme has been found to double the chances of a person's abstinence continuing 3 months later (Miller, 1998). And this is possible because someone has actively listened to the service user's problems, helped the service user to acknowledge and resolve ambivalence and supported them in achieving their goal of a changed life. But problems with motivation and behaviour change are not limited to the addictions field and not to mental health problems alone. MI has been found to be effective in working with people with eating disorders (Carels et al., 2007; Treasure et al., 2007), with sexual health concerns (Byrne et al., 2006), with criminal offenders (Clark et al., 2006) and in improving general health (Butterworth et al., 2006; Knight et al., 2006).

Cognitive behavioural therapy

Cognitive behavioural therapy (CBT) grew out of behavioural therapy. Originally designed as a treatment approach for people with depression, CBT is now used for a range of disorders, and has been found to be a cost-effective approach (Myhr and Payne, 2006; Vos et al., 2005). It is usually conducted over around 16–20 sessions. Its premise is that there is an interrelationship between thoughts, feelings, behaviour, biology and the environment. That is, each factor influences the others. This has been understood for centuries. The Roman emperor Marcus Aurelius wrote:

If some external object distresses you, it is not the object itself but your judgement of it which causes pain. It is up to you to change your judgement. If it is your behaviour which troubles you, who stops you from changing it?

(Blackburn and Davidson, 1990, p. 16)

In the cognitive model, our thoughts are classified into three layers: the outer layer holds our automatic thoughts, the middle layer contains our intermediate beliefs or underlying assumptions and the inner layer stores our core beliefs. The core beliefs develop during childhood as a result of experience and the influence of significant others. CBT aims to cause change at each of these levels. The goal of treatment is to bring into conscious awareness the service user's negative automatic thoughts, which are specific to certain situations, and the person's underlying assumptions, and to challenge them.

We all have negative automatic thoughts that are present when we are awake. They are responsible for many of our behaviours. An example of a negative automatic thought is: 'I can't cope'. This leads to the person behaving in a helpless way. The underlying assumption might be: 'If I can't work this out, then I'm no good'. The core belief for this person might be: 'I'm a failure'. The negative automatic thoughts are the most superficial and are more likely to be acknowledged. Once challenged, the service user learns to develop new or revised beliefs. These are considered during therapy and practised in real life (or 'in vivo').

Assessment for suitability to engage with the CBT model is carried out initially. This assessment will determine whether the service user has the motivation to change and whether he or she has the ability to engage and to problem-solve. The model is prescriptive; that is, there is a distinct process for engaging in therapy with the service user. Regardless of the person's difficulties, the same specific techniques and strategies central to the model are used. These include Socratic questioning (Calvert and Palmer, 2003) and homework, such as charting behaviours and mood using a visual analogue scale, and keeping automatic thought records. Keeping an automatic thought record alerts the service user to the negative automatic thoughts that continue to affect their feelings and behaviour, ultimately maintaining mental health problems. Homework is set after each session to ensure that the service user remains motivated and learns the skills to take over their own therapy.

Initially, service users are given an overview of CBT and shown how a five-part model – based on the interrelationships between thoughts, feelings, behaviour, biology and environment – is used to identify the more serious problems. Service users are asked to identify a situation that caused a strong negative emotional response. Then service users identify their specific emotional responses to that situation as well as their cognitions, physical responses and behaviours. The fifth aspect of the model, the environment, provides the context within which these responses occurred, including culture and personal history. Organizing the person's experiences into the categories of thoughts, feelings, behaviour and physical responses is fundamental to CBT (Dattilio and Padesky, 1990).

An example of this might be if an employee, 'Jane', received negative feedback about her work performance from her employer and had a strong emotional response. The emotions, thoughts, actions and physical responses that occurred within the work environment for Jane during this scenario would be described and sketched out.

The therapeutic relationship in CBT is collaborative. The service user is an active participant in the process and is responsible for learning new ways of responding. There is also an emphasis on empiricism, which is the gathering of data to provide evidence to challenge current beliefs. Service users are taught to identify their dysfunctional thoughts and the therapist then tests the validity of those beliefs. For example, in the situation described above, Jane believes that everyone thinks she is stupid. The therapist would ask Jane for evidence of this. It is most unlikely that Jane would have any evidence. Ultimately, service users learn to evaluate their own thoughts and manage their own responses (Dattilio and Padesky, 1990).

CBT has been found to be very effective in the treatment of depression over many years and is now used for a range of health conditions. Its efficacy has been strongly reported for the anxiety disorders (e.g. Barlow et al., 2005; Rosser et al., 2004) and for the management of medication non-adherence (Rodrigues, 2007). CBT has also been found to be useful in working with people with learning disabilities (Brown and Marshall, 2006) and for people requiring cancer and palliative care (Mannix et al., 2006; Semple et al., 2006).

Dialectical behaviour therapy

Dialectical behaviour therapy (DBT) was developed by Marsha Linehan and first published in 1993. It is a therapeutic technique designed specifically to help people manage deliberate self-harming behaviours where the intention is not to kill oneself. These people are frequently women with a diagnosis of borderline personality disorder. DBT is highly structured, goal-orientated and time-limited, and is based on a cognitive behavioural approach.

The service user's involvement in DBT is voluntary. Indeed, the service user needs to be committed to working towards the behaviour change that is necessary to alter her or his lifestyle and subsequent difficulties. This is known as the pretreatment phase of DBT. Without commitment from the service user, DBT will not proceed. In particular, 'the service user must agree to work

on decreasing self-harming behaviours and interpersonal styles that interfere with therapy and on increasing behavioural skills' (Swales et al., 2000, p. 10). The core intervention strategies involved are 'validation' and 'problem-solving'. The main work is carried out in weekly individual therapy sessions that focus on targeted behaviours. The therapist accepts the service user as a valid human being while at the same time expecting change. The most important behaviour to be addressed is the self-harming behaviour. Once this has been brought under control, other issues are addressed.

The group therapy aspect of DBT occurs concurrently with individual therapy and involves skills training. The person with borderline personality disorder has not developed effective coping skills, and so learning how to solve problems effectively is very important. There are four groups of skills, or modules (Linehan, 1993):

- core mindfulness skills (derived from Buddhist meditation),
- interpersonal effectiveness skills,
- emotion modulation skills,
- distress tolerance skills.

As skills are learned in the group sessions they are applied in the real world and also addressed in individual counselling sessions. The therapist acts as coach to support the use of these new skills as they are learned, both within sessions and over the telephone as problems arise (Wolpow, 2000). It is the combination of acceptance or validation and active change or problem-solving that brings about the alteration in personality style that enables these service users to lead more fulfilling lives.

Before considering DBT, it is important to consider what borderline personality disorder means (see also Ch. 16), especially in the context of DBT. People with borderline personality disorder are very challenging to work with because of their personality style, which often develops as the result of a very difficult childhood. According to Linehan (1993), the experiences and responses of the child who develops borderline personality disorder were 'invalidated' or disqualified by the significant others around the child. This means that the child's experiences were not acknowledged or accepted as real. Sexual abuse is considered the ultimate form of invalidation and is frequently an aspect of the history of the person with borderline personality disorder. At the same time, Linehan argues that, for these people, there exists a biological predisposition within the autonomic nervous system to react poorly to stress. It is important to note that the majority of people who are given the diagnosis of borderline personality disorder are women.

The person with borderline personality disorder classically has a dysfunctional lifestyle and staggers from one crisis to the next. Linehan points out that these service users are unable to regulate their emotions (have extreme emotional reactions to situations), have chaotic interpersonal relationships, have a disturbed sense of self and are unable to regulate their thoughts and behaviours. They lack problem-solving skills and so respond to life haphazardly. They frequently engage in self-damaging behaviours such as substance abuse, promiscuity and over-eating, but the most common behaviour is self-mutilation. According to the DBT approach, the diagnosis relates to a certain pattern of behaviours and so, once these behaviours cease, the diagnosis also no longer exists (Swales et al., 2000).

DBT was originally designed as an individual therapy approach combined with group skills training, telephone contact between sessions and a strong emphasis on therapists also receiving DBT from each other. Therapist consultation is fundamental due to the risk of therapist burnout when working so intensively with service users with such challenging patterns of behaviour. Aspects of DBT can now be applied in a range of settings using the principles of treatment rather than these specific modes (Wolpow, 2000), and for a range of conditions (Linehan et al., 1999). However, success is determined by the quality of the service user–therapist relationship. In particular, the service user learns that their own needs and the therapist's needs are both important.

CASE STUDY: GEORGIA

Georgia was a 21-year-old woman admitted to hospital due to self-harming behaviour. She had repeatedly cut her arms and body with razor blades. She said she did this because it helped with her emotional pain. It eventually transpired that when Georgia was a young girl, she had been sexually abused by a neighbour. She was deeply ashamed and embarrassed about what had happened to her and was also worried about how her parents would react once they knew. Georgia's experience was validated by her parents and friends and by the nurses working with her. Rather than staff feeling anger towards her continued self-harming, it was important for Georgia to be acknowledged as a young person struggling to manage her emotional responses to past traumatic experiences. She needed time and patience before she could begin to learn new ways of responding. Several years on, Georgia is a different person, undertaking postgraduate studies, working and having a life worth living.

BEHAVIOUR THERAPY

The behavioural model developed from the early work of Pavlov at the turn of the nineteenth century and Skinner during the early twentieth century. Pavlov's early experiments involving dogs showed that involuntary behaviours can be conditioned to occur (classical conditioning) and that, ultimately, this learned response can be unlearned (extinguished). It is normal for salivation to occur in response to the presentation of food, but it is not normal for salivation to occur at the sound of a tuning fork. Pavlov paired the presentation of food with the sound of a tuning fork until eventually salivation occurred at the sound of the tuning fork without the presence of food. The dogs had been conditioned to salivate at the sound of the tuning fork. Persistent sounding of the tuning fork without the presentation of food eventually led to extinction of this learned response; that is, the dogs no longer salivated at the sound of the tuning fork.

CRITICAL THINKING CHALLENGE 23.4

What are some of your conditioned responses? For example, consider how the sound of the school bell at the end of the day results in a lightening of mood for both students and teachers! What happens when you smell toast cooking in the kitchen?

Skinner later developed the early work of Thorndike (1911, cited in Barker and Fraser, 1985). He called this *operant conditioning* and showed that behaviours can be learned and unlearned through processes of positive and negative reinforcement. That is, behaviours can be strengthened through positive reinforcement or the presentation of rewards, and weakened through negative reinforcement involving the removal of rewards. Removing a reinforcer to a behaviour, such as walking away from the child having a temper tantrum, results in extinction of the temper-tantrum behaviour. Be aware, though, that initially ignoring a behaviour will result in an increase in that behaviour before it begins to subside.

Punishment can also be used to change behaviour. When defined in behavioural terms, punishment refers to procedures designed to suppress behaviours, not the infliction of physical or psychological pain or harm. Punishment decreases the strength of certain behaviours rather than eliminating them (Sundel and Sundel, 1993). Punishment can involve applying a punishing stimulus immediately after the unwanted behaviour is performed. An example of this is when the teacher humiliates a student verbally for arriving late at class. Alternatively, punishment might involve the removal of a positive reinforcer. Examples of this include a child being placed in time out following a temper tantrum, or a service user with anorexia who loses weight or doesn't gain weight according to a prescribed schedule, losing the privilege of calling their friends for 48 h. To be effective, the punishment needs to be applied consistently; that is, each time the behaviour presents, the punishment is applied. Punishment is most effective when applied immediately after the undesirable behaviour. It is also important to specify alternative behaviours that are more appropriate (Sundel and Sundel, 1993). There are, of course, professional and ethical issues which must be considered in the application of such techniques in nursing practice.

Behaviour therapy has been found to be particularly useful in explaining the development of phobias, anxieties and fears and the ways in which these are generalized to a range of stimuli. For example, a person who has a fear of spiders may well find that the fear generalizes to a range of crawling insects as well as toys and pictures of spiders. The events that occur prior to or after behaviours determine whether those behaviours will be learned, maintained or changed. For example, the presence of a spider will result in heightened anxiety. Moving away from the spider causes the anxiety to subside. Therefore, the person learns that spiders are to be feared and to avoid spiders. Unfortunately, this will result in avoidance of environments that have the potential to contain spiders, causing constriction of the person's social world.

It is important to point out that in the case study about George, he is not aware that his avoidance of anxiety-provoking situations actually increases his anxiety. He will not accept the idea that staying within an anxiety-provoking situation will be helpful in managing his anxiety and in preventing future panic attacks. George believes that he would 'freak out' and that this would be the most awful outcome for him. He would feel vulnerable and he might never get back home. Combined with education, staying with George and verbally supporting him to stay within the anxiety-provoking situation will show him that his most feared outcome will not be realized. Once he recognizes that avoidance only worsens the situation, that he can cope with his anxiety and that terrible things won't happen to him, he can begin to change his behaviour.

CASE STUDY: GEORGE

George suffers from symptoms of schizophrenia but is more disadvantaged by his social and panic anxiety (see Ch. 17). Using Truax's (2002) model for behavioural case conceptualization, the reinforcers and punishments that cause his anxieties to occur and persist, resulting in increasing social isolation, are as follows.

- Positive reinforcement: an increase in a consequence leads to an increased probability that panic attacks will happen in the future. For example, George's family members carry out his weekly grocery shopping and manage his finances and bill-paying for him. This reinforcement increases the likelihood of George not engaging in these behaviours and increases the probability of panic attacks occurring should he engage in these behaviours.

- Negative reinforcement: a decrease in an uncomfortable or aversive consequence or outcome leads to increased avoidance of anxiety-provoking situations in the future. When George stays at home rather than engaging in social situations or using public transport, it reduces his anxiety, thereby increasing his avoidance of these anxiety-provoking situations.

- Positive punishment: an increase in a negative consequence leads to decreased engagement in anxiety-provoking situations in the future. For example, when George goes for long walks far from his home but within his suburb, his anxiety increases because he fears 'freaking out'. He has now limited his walks to a small radius from his home, and so his social world is shrinking even further.

- Negative punishment: a decrease in a consequence leads to a decreased probability that he will stay in anxiety-provoking situations in the future. For example, George is unable to use positive self-talk to manage his anxiety and is therefore unable to stay in anxiety-provoking situations. He is so certain that he will 'freak out' that he no longer puts himself at risk.

In George's case, the target behaviour, the behaviour we wish to change, is the social isolation that George suffers as a result of his avoidance of anxiety-provoking situations. It is important to point out that 'the target behaviour is the behaviour to be observed and measured; it is the focus of modification' (Sundel and Sundel, 1993, p. 4). The target behaviour can be the behaviour we want to increase (e.g. acceptable or appropriate social behaviour), or the behaviour we want to minimize (e.g. lying on the bed all day). George has hopes and goals that include working and living in a small beachside community. In order to achieve these goals, George needs to be able to cope with driving a vehicle or using public transport, meeting new people and widening his social world without fear of losing control.

Prior to working with George and his problems, the nurse would need to carry out a behavioural assessment. This requires George to record the triggers, both internal and external to his anxiety, and to identify his physical, cognitive, emotional and behavioural responses. The frequency and duration of anxiety responses would also need to be recorded. This helps to identify specific cues to certain behaviours and also to determine improvement or deterioration. Treatment should address both his behavioural (e.g. social avoidance) and cognitive responses (e.g. believing that he will lose control and perhaps his life). This is because his beliefs continue to limit his ability to act.

After determining what causes and maintains certain behaviours, it is possible to develop a treatment plan together that specifies goals, what will need to be done to achieve those goals, how goal achievement will be measured, and a timeline for goal achievement. For example, George may set being able to travel into the city in a car as his goal. A plan involving systematically working from sitting in a stationary car to driving short distances in the car, to travelling into the city, will need to be laid out. The plan will also need to indicate how many weeks or months this process will take.

GROUP THERAPY

Group therapy involves the engagement of two or more people in therapy at the same time. This mode of therapy is more cost-effective than individual therapies because more people can be treated at once. Group counselling is also more efficient if the group is composed of people with similar problems (the homogeneous group); for example, a psychoeducational group for families of people with schizophrenia. However, efficiency and cost-effectiveness are not the most important reasons for engaging people in group therapy. There are immense benefits for service users who come together with others who are experiencing the same or similar difficulties. Often the benefits are derived from interactions with others in the group rather than through the therapeutic efforts of the counsellor (Byrne and Byrne, 1996).

There are as many approaches that can be taken in group therapy as there are for individual therapy. Group therapy provides an opportunity for people to explore their thoughts, feelings and behaviours and the impact they have on others. This is achieved through facilitation by the therapist/nurse therapist and through feedback from the other group members. Ultimately, learning occurs about relating to others. One thing that is certain is that almost everyone benefits from healthy interpersonal relationships. We are all social beings and we thrive on relating to others. An important outcome of any type of group is the relationships developed with others and the opportunity to learn better or more effective ways of relating.

Therapeutic groups can be divided into two main categories: general-purpose groups and problem-focused groups (Earley, 2000). Addressing specific issues such as grief, sexual abuse or alcohol abuse is the goal of problem-focused groups. They aim to impart information and provide support to people in crisis and consequently are time limited. General-purpose groups attempt to facilitate deeper character change by addressing problems that arise from the interpersonal processes that occur in groups (Earley, 2000). This involves the expression of transference and counter-transference as early relationships and customary interpersonal difficulties are re-enacted in the group with other group members. These processes occur unconsciously and interactions within the group provide opportunities for other group members or the therapist to gently make the person aware of what has been happening.

Yalom (1995) determined that there are 11 curative or therapeutic factors that occur in psychotherapy groups. When a psychotherapeutic group is working effectively, these curative factors are operating and group members are benefiting from them. The factors work interdependently; that is, they don't occur or function separately but interrelate with each other. The same factors operate in every type of group but their interplay and importance can vary widely from group to group. In addition, people from within the same group can benefit from differing clusters of therapeutic factors. These factors are:

- instilling of hope: people are inspired by the improvements that others have made and the group provides opportunity for the therapist to point out the improvements people have made;
- universality: entering a group enables people to see that they are not alone in their struggles. Hearing that others have the same difficulties is reassuring because people realize that their problems are not beyond solving;
- imparting information: this might include learning about their health problems or how to cope. Education might be an explicit or implicit part of the group;
- altruism: in giving to and supporting others, group members also receive. Finding that they are valuable to others boosts self-esteem;
- corrective recapitulation of the family group: the therapy group represents the family in many ways. This provides the opportunity to act out old family relationships and to recognize how earlier relationships continue to be acted out in current relationships;
- development of socializing techniques: learning social skills might be an explicit part of the group or it may be more indirect, as people observe the socially acceptable behaviour of others;
- imitative behaviour: group therapists influence the communication patterns in members by modelling certain behaviours such as self-disclosure or support;
- interpersonal learning: the group becomes a social microcosm so that members are able to re-enact interpersonal behaviours typical of their lives outside the group. Feedback from others enables a person to see that their behaviours are responsible for their interpersonal difficulties;
- group cohesiveness: cohesiveness is essential for the other curative factors to operate. It involves members feeling warmth and comfort in the group and feeling that they belong and are accepted and supported by others;
- catharsis: this is the expression and mutual working through of strong emotions that have not been previously expressed. The group provides a safe environment for this to happen. Therefore, catharsis will only occur once group cohesiveness develops;

- existential factors: these are the elements in the group process that help members to develop an understanding of their individual existences. This is more likely to occur in groups where there is a focus on thinking, talking and feeling.

Some of these factors are self-evident, while others are more subtle and take an understanding of psychotherapy to enable their facilitation and expression. Nevertheless, when setting up a group therapy programme, it is important to plan it well (Sharry, 2001) and to consider the expectations or goals you have for the group. If you are the therapist you will need to decide whether it will be a closed group – that is, one that has a set number of members for a set period of time – or an open group. An open group allows different membership each time the group meets and the group membership at each session will determine to some extent the direction the group takes. Whichever type of group you facilitate, there will be a specific process of coming together or initial engagement, reaction and resistance to working, developing trust, working through issues, and termination or closure (Fehr, 1999). In an open group, trust may take longer to develop as membership fluctuates.

Activity groups

Activity groups grew out of the perceived need to occupy people during the long hospital stays of the past. Ultimately, activity groups became a part of psychosocial rehabilitation programmes and are also often part of an organized therapy programme in mental health facilities today. While the task of organizing an activity programme has been taken on largely by occupational therapists, this role was historically a nursing responsibility. Given the amount of time that nurses spend with service users, nurses need to once again embrace this responsibility. Activity groups involve gathering together a group of people interested in a particular activity or those who need to develop skills in a particular area.

Examples of activity groups include those based on cooking skills, gardening, art, walking, newspaper discussion, reminiscence and games and sporting groups. Many inpatient mental health units hold daily 'community meetings' designed to engage service users in daily planning and organization. Originally developed to help construct a therapeutic milieu – that is, a physical and emotional ward environment that is therapeutic and empowering for service users – these community groups might also be viewed as activity groups in some respects. Despite the perception that activity groups are not particularly challenging and that they only serve the purpose of keeping people occupied, many of Yalom's curative factors (outlined above) can operate. Not least of these are the development of socializing techniques and imitative behaviour.

NURSE'S STORY: FACILITATING A GROUP

I used to facilitate a discharge planning group in an acute inpatient setting. This was an open group due to the nature of the rapid turnover of clients in this setting. While I might plan for a reasonably structured group with specific goals, the members inevitably determined the direction of the group. I always began with introductions and gave each person an opportunity to identify short- and long-term goals. I also attempted to discuss any concerns about medications, accommodation, family relationships, employment and money management. However, the acuity of the mental health problems of the group members dictated the issues addressed. For example, a group member with a bipolar mood disorder and somewhat elevated in mood will inevitably find it difficult to stay 'on track'. As the group facilitator, it's important to allow everyone to participate in the group. It may be necessary to gently point out the domination by a group member or to encourage others to have some say. Despite this challenge to the group process, it enables several of the curative factors to operate. These include and are probably not limited to universality, instillation of hope, altruism, interpersonal learning and the development of socializing techniques. So, despite the concerns of nurses that group therapy might not be effective or appropriate in an acute inpatient setting, coupled with the challenges that these groups will pose, group therapy is valuable at a range of levels, not least of which is clients having the opportunity to relate more effectively with others.

FAMILY THERAPY

Family therapy developed in the 1950s from the belief that the family was responsible for causing schizophrenia. In particular it was believed that certain communication styles within families were responsible for causing the problem (the skewed and schismatic families). A further belief centred on the communication style of the mother, the so-called *schizophrenogenic mother*. Although these ideas have long since been rejected, a group of interventions known as family therapy had been born (Goldenberg and Goldenberg, 2000). Family therapy shifted the focus on therapy directed at unconscious material (psychotherapy) 'to a focus on the interpersonal process – that is, how family members interact with each other' (Kadis and McClendon, 1998, p. 6).

Family therapy is an approach to treatment that is based on the fundamental premise that when a person has a problem, it usually involves the whole family (Eisler et al., 2007; Mellor et al., 2000). Family interactions might be causing the problem or prolonging the problem for the identified service user, or the problem or behaviours of the service user might be affecting other members of the family. Family therapists aim to effect change in the entire family system. Family therapy usually involves multiple family members, not necessarily the same family members each time, or therapy might involve a single family member (Meech and Wood, 2000).

Even when therapy involves a single individual, its impact will be experienced by the wider family. This might be demonstrated through an improvement in family functioning and/or through the alleviation of symptoms (Mellor et al., 2000). Unlike individual therapists who believe that problems reside within the person, family therapists believe that 'the dominant forces within our lives are located externally, within the family' (Nichols and Schwartz, 2001, p. 6). Therapy concentrates on the family and the way it is organized. Ultimately this affects the lives of each family member in some way. That is, the whole system is affected.

Nichols and Schwartz (2001) maintain that family therapy is particularly useful in working with children who are having problems. This is because they are strongly influenced by the family and must remain within its influence. Marital problems, family feuds and difficulties that develop in people when there has been a major family transition are also particularly amenable to family therapy. The role of the family therapist is to understand the dynamics that occur within families and then to help the family members to reconsider the ways in which they interact with each other. The family therapist then motivates the family members to change.

When working with families, the problem is viewed as dysfunction in the relationship between family members. The relationship therefore becomes the focus of attention. Sometimes the person identified as 'the problem' behaves in that way in order to hold the family together. For example, consider the child who misbehaves when his or her parents begin fighting. The misbehaviour distracts the parents from their conflict and so further fighting is averted. The parents then work together to manage the child's problem behaviour. Ultimately the problem is not with the child but with the marital relationship.

The two-way mirror is a useful tool in family therapy. While there is a therapist in the room with the family, behind the mirror sit a number of other members of the team observing the therapy in progress. This allows immediate feedback, as the observers call into the therapy room by telephone to give feedback or direction to the therapist and/or family. Observers may see things (communication styles, body language) that the therapist does not, so these can be communicated *during* the session rather than following it.

Another tool used in family therapy is the genogram, which is a graphic representation of the family and its patterns across generations. The genogram is drawn up with the involvement of the family, helping to engage all family members, as the mapping process seeks input

from everyone. Enduring and broken relationships, illegitimate and legitimate children, blended and nuclear family relationships are all depicted on the same page, revealing the emotional processes of the family to both the therapist and the family members (McGoldrick et al., 1999).

CASE STUDY: BILL AND JOAN

Bill and Joan have been married for 30 years. Joan has a diagnosis of bipolar affective disorder and had been moderately depressed for around 2 years. At around the time that Joan became well, Bill was made redundant from his job after a very lengthy period of employment with the company. Bill had always been the breadwinner and the caregiver in the family. Now his wife was supporting him emotionally and was independent of him. This role transition resulted in a great deal of conflict in the family. Bill had difficulty adjusting to his new role and in accepting that his wife no longer relied on him. Their teenage daughter blamed her mother for causing the conflict. Although Joan was being held responsible for the problems, no doubt due to her history of mental health problems, essentially the expected roles of family members had been reversed and there was now confusion about how to function. The therapy concentrated on the patterns of communication within the family and on accepting that Joan was now well and functioning in different and unexpected ways.

Psychoeducation

Initially designed to help families develop skills to understand and cope with a family member diagnosed with schizophrenia, psychoeducation is now used with families with any type of problem, including families with relationship problems (Goldenberg and Goldenberg, 2000). In the mental health field, psychoeducation refers to the provision of information about a person's mental health problems to that person and/or his or her family. Psychoeducation grew out of the belief that people with mental health problems, particularly those diagnosed with schizophrenia, are vulnerable to stress and that excessive stress in the person's life is likely to exacerbate the disorder; that is, too much stress will cause the person to become unwell or relapse. Therefore psychoeducation is considered an intervention designed to reduce the impact of the disorder on the service user. For example, it has been found to be effective in reducing the number and duration of relapses for service users with bipolar affective disorders (Colom et al., 2003).

The early work of Brown (1958, cited in Bland, 1986) claimed that some families contribute to stress through the ways they communicate and behave. These families were deemed to have high levels of expressed emotion (EE) and high EE was considered detrimental to the wellbeing of the service user. Expressed emotion was originally defined as consisting of five constructs, namely critical comments, hostility, emotional over-involvement, warmth and positive remarks (Jenkins and Karno, 1992). Today, however, EE in families tends to be assessed only in terms of the first three, negative, constructs. The level of EE in families is determined through a face-to-face interview with family members, known as the Camberwell Family Interview. Once a family is deemed to indicate high EE, psychoeducation is considered the appropriate intervention.

Psychoeducation programmes can be run in multifamily groups over several weeks but may also be organized around the needs of individual families. The benefit of several families coming together in a group is the sharing of information, the support they provide each other and the experience of universality; that is, the recognition that they are not alone in having these problems. Supportive family education programmes need to attempt to reinforce strengths and promote resilience. Psychoeducation will also enable families in particular to understand medical jargon and to appreciate the experience from the perspective of others, including the service user. A comprehensive psychoeducation programme will provide information not only about the specific mental health problems, but also about the available resources in the community, as well as information on and practice in applying problem-solving skills (Palmer, 1996).

Families and service users need to be provided with information about mental health problems, just as they would if the diagnosis was a physical health problem. Indeed, Mullen et al. (2002) argue that family interventions need to be considered 'core business' for mental health services. When there is an emphasis on providing information to support service users and their families, they are more likely to benefit from the intervention. A collaborative approach that recognizes the experiences of families and service users and their unique knowledge of the disorder will convey to them that they are not to blame and that they have something to contribute to the overall care plan. Family problems need to be viewed as normal responses to very difficult situations that tax the family's usual coping resources (Kavanagh, 1992).

Providing psychoeducation to families is designed to alert them to the need to reduce stress at home and to change the ways in which they relate to the person with mental health problems. This is thought to reduce relapse rates, which is argued to be a cost-effective way of managing mental health problems. Ultimately, though, the psychoeducation approach designed to reduce EE in families maintains a philosophy that families are responsible for the mental health problems or, at least, are responsible for contributing to hospitalization and subsequent healthcare costs. While historically families were blamed for directly causing mental health problems, the shift to assessing EE and providing psychoeducation can be seen as a more subtle form of blaming families. Families experience considerable burden in taking care of family members with mental health problems in the community. This perception of responsibility for the service user's health problems has the potential to add to that burden.

PSYCHOSOCIAL REHABILITATION AND RECOVERY

Psychosocial rehabilitation is a treatment approach designed for people who are severely disabled by long-term mental health problems. Most people with enduring mental health problems have a diagnosis of schizophrenia. However, many people with bipolar affective disorder and depression also have long-term needs (Ekdawi and Conning, 1994). The cognitive and emotional problems experienced by people with enduring mental health problems result in social disability, which in turn results in their needing help and support to negotiate the social world (Perkins and Repper, 1996). In line with the shift from inpatient to community mental healthcare, most psychosocial rehabilitation is now carried out in the community (see also Ch. 2 for issues related to service users, recovery and rehabilitation).

Psychosocial rehabilitation is the process of assisting people to tap into and learn the internal and external skills, supports and resources necessary to be successful (Vandevooren et al., 2007). Success is measured by the individual's satisfaction in living, learning and working in the environment(s) of their choice. At its most basic level, psychosocial rehabilitation seeks to help people determine and prioritise their goals, identify the pathways for achieving these goals, and develop the necessary skills and supports to achieve these goals (Anthony et al., 1991; Legere, 2007). The concept of recovery from physical illness and disability does not mean that the suffering has disappeared, all the symptoms have been removed and/or functioning has been completely restored. For example, as Deegan (1988) points out, a person with paraplegia can recover even though the spinal cord cannot. Recover is what *people* with disabilities do. Similarly, a person with mental health problems can recover even though this may not equate to a 'cure' in a medical sense.

It is argued that before a person actively engages the rehabilitation services offered, they will need to have embarked on their personal journey of recovery (Anthony, 1993). Psychosocial rehabilitation efforts designed to have a positive impact on severe mental health problems can do more than leave the person less impaired, less dysfunctional, less disabled and less disadvantaged. These interventions can result in the person gaining more meaning, purpose, success and satisfaction with their life. Recovery outcomes include more subjective outcomes such as self-esteem, empowerment and self-determination.

Curtis (1997, p. 16) has identified a number of recovery principles that, she argues, need to be reflected in the rehabilitation programmes offered, as follows.

- Recovery is an active, ongoing and individual process.
- Recovery is not linear; it entails growth, plateaus, setbacks, side tracks and fast tracks.
- Recovery relates not only to the experience of symptoms, but also to the secondary assaults of stigma, discrimination and abuse.
- Hope is the most fundamental factor in recovery.
- Recovery requires the presence of people who believe in and stand by the person.
- Recovery can occur without professional intervention.
- The establishment of a sense of control or free will is critical to recovery.
- 'Remembering your track record', or learning from observing your own mental and emotional behaviour, is critical to coping.
- Self-directed coping strategies are effective and can be learned.
- Maintaining or developing connections to valued activities and people is critical to the recovery process.
- Connecting with other people on a human level is important.
- Recovery is a process of 'finding meaning in your experience'.

There are a number of possible stimulants to recovery. These may include other service users who are in recovery or recovering effectively. Books, films and therapy groups may lead to unexpected insights into possible life options. Visiting new places and talking to various people are other ways in which the recovery process might be triggered. Critical to recovery is regaining the belief that there are options from which to choose, a belief perhaps even more important to recovery than the particular option one initially chooses (Curtis, 1997). Therefore, we need to structure our settings so that recovery 'triggers' are present. Boring day treatment programmes and inactive inpatient programmes do not stimulate recovery (Anthony, 1993). We need more creative programming. The strongest recovery-orientated programmes identified to date are those that arise from and are operated by skilled service user providers (Curtis, 1997).

We cannot presume to know what a person hopes to achieve in life. We are all individuals and have different desires and needs. As nurses, we may think we know what is best for a person, but this is at best naive and at worst paternalistic. Before engaging someone in rehabilitation services it is important to find out what they hope to achieve. A rehabilitation programme designed to be completed by everyone is unlikely to suit the needs of all service users.

Instilling hope

There has been a great deal of research into what helps people with long-term mental health problems to recover in such a way that they can live relatively normal and productive lives despite the re-emergence of symptoms of health problems from time to time. It has been found that hope is considered fundamental before a person can embark on recovery. Curtis (1997) identified a number of factors considered critical to recovery reported by service users. The factor that was ranked as the most important was having 'just one person who believed in me'. This is one of the ingredients thought to be important in promoting a sense of hope. Morse and Penrod (1999) offer a process model for the development of hope following a critical life experience, such as being told that you have breast cancer or that you have a mental disorder. This model was developed out of qualitative enquiry exploring emotional responses to the experience of ill health.

NURSE'S STORY: GOALS

Goals are integral to living. Without goals we merely react to what happens in our lives. I used to routinely invite into the classroom two people with bipolar affective disorder who lived independently in the community. They talked about their experiences with mental health services to groups of postgraduate nursing students. While one of these people valued himself according to his ability to remain employed, the other accepted that work was too stressful for him. He gained his sense of self-worth from his ability to be a good husband and a good father to his two young daughters. Although the two held different goals, their goals allowed each of them to survive and thrive in the community.

To help identify clients' goals I routinely started my inpatient predischarge group therapy sessions with introductions and a request for people to identify their short-term and 5-year goals. The goals were almost always quite different from each other. For some, at this stage of their illness, a 5-year projection into the future was impossible. However, everyone has a dream and this should be tapped into, as dreams provide the impetus for goals. Further, it is not our place to decide whether the goals are realistic or not. If a goal seems unachievable, it might be wise to break it down into smaller and more achievable sub-goals. I would usually say, 'That sounds like a great goal. What do you think you'll need to do to achieve that?' From there, people are able to contemplate a way forward with something to live for and work towards.

The Morse and Penrod (1999) model has a number of overlapping phases that begin with a critical life event. People inevitably experience uncertainty, suffering, hope and the challenge of despair and, ultimately, the achievement of a 'reformulated self'. At each of these phases, a different level of knowing or perceiving is experienced.

- Enduring: after a critical life experience we initially focus on cultivating our powers of endurance, which involves suspending or suppressing emotions and remaining in control. We do this because we worry that we will 'lose it' or disintegrate. The level of knowing here is awareness.
- Uncertainty: this is evident when we recognize what has happened and know what our goals are for the future, but we are unable to choose a course of action from a range of options. This state of uncertainty paralyses hope. At this time we simply exist in an emotional state and suffer as a result of not being able to act. When we are in a state of uncertainty, we have no other choice but to tolerate the present.
- Suffering: the level of knowing here is acknowledgement. We begin to grasp the situation and consequently suffer emotionally. Morse and Penrod (1999, p. 148) comment that 'the depth of the state of suffering is despair, utter hopelessness'. Out of this overwhelming emotional experience, we begin to piece together reality and develop a perception of the future. 'This process of piecing together a new future begins in small incremental pieces, eventually building to … acceptance of the event and identification of both a goal and the means to attain it, which eventually leads to hope' (Morse and Penrod, 1999, p. 148). So suffering is viewed as integral to moving on and ultimately to repair.
- Hope: the level of knowing is now acceptance and we become future-orientated. We are able to develop an action plan designed to achieve desired goals. When we have hope, we understand the reality of the event while also understanding the real possibility of negative outcomes. Indeed, 'bracing for negative outcomes is a powerful motivating force for developing hope' (Morse and Penrod, 1999, p. 148). Supportive relationships are now sought and hope is bolstered.
- Reformulated self: there is now a sense of becoming a 'better person' for having suffered. This state has been labelled the 'reformulated self', where the past is accepted and we also accept that the future has been irrevocably changed and a choice is made to 'make the most of life'.

Understanding the process involved in developing a sense of hope for one's future is fundamental to helping nurses know how to respond to people during the phases of enduring, uncertainty and suffering. If these phases are acknowledged as normal or expected, we won't make the mistake of attempting to force people to have hope when they are not ready to accept it. The trauma involved in dealing with a critical life experience, such as the diagnosis of a mental disorder, results in a range of responses. These responses are part of a process that is not linear: we move back and forth between these phases. Understanding this may also explain the delays for some in developing hope. These are normal responses, and so should not be assessed as being part of a disorder.

Deegan, (1996, 1997) was diagnosed with schizophrenia at 17 years of age and is very clear about the need for health professionals to treat people with mental health problems as human beings. Although this may seem like a simple thing to do, the medically dominant model of 'disease' reinforces the notion of the person as 'illness'. Deegan (1993, p. 9) says: 'it is as if the whole world has put on a pair of warped glasses that blind them to the person you are and leaves them seeing you as an illness'. Stocks (1995, cited in Hayne and Yonge, 1997, p. 319) agrees, saying, 'once our personal identities are transformed into a psychiatric label, we are objects that are never allowed to be people again'.

It is clearly important to see the person as separate from the mental health problem. However, there are many ways in which we maintain the view of the person as an 'illness'. These include a tendency to focus predominantly upon problems, interpreting all behaviour as part of the illness, over-emphasizing assessment, diagnosis and prognosis, and neglecting to consult the service user (Palmer, 1999). These are all things that are likely to stifle hope. If nurses cannot accept people with mental health problems as human and social beings, who else in society will? After all, we are all human beings with unique abilities, shortcomings and, often, disabilities. We are all a psychological 'work in progress' and having a mental health problem does not make one 'weak' or imperfect.

Social skills training

There are many types of skills training designed to improve problem-solving skills, relaxation skills, assertion skills and coping skills. Similarly, social skills can be learned. We are not born with them. How do you know how to greet someone in a culturally appropriate way? How do you know how to behave when you walk into a university classroom? These are behaviours that we take for granted and therefore tend not to think about before doing them. They are also examples of social skills that we have learned as we were socialized into our culture. Much of this learning took place during childhood and adolescence, and so by adulthood we pretty much have these skills well developed.

However, the development of a mental health problem during childhood or adolescence is likely to have implications for the development of sound social skills. Mental health problems can distort communication with family members and peers, and the separations that ensue if a child or adolescent is hospitalized can disrupt family life, social life and schooling, where we learn many early social skills. If you develop a long-term mental disorder later in life, it is likely that you will have fewer opportunities to practise learned social skills, and if you don't use them, you will lose them. Social isolation often occurs for people with serious mental health problems because of the stigma and discrimination that result and because it is harder to communicate with others when you have bizarre thoughts and experiences. These interfere with the ability to sustain relationships and develop new ones. Social skills deficits have also been shown to be related to poor vocational (work) outcomes for people with severe mental health problems (Cheung et al., 2006).

Much of the social skills training in mental health services focuses on working with people diagnosed with schizophrenia (Bellack, 2004). People diagnosed with social phobia and depression are also often in need of social skills training (O'Donohue and Krasner, 1995). Essentially, though, most people with mental health problems will have social and interpersonal problems as part of their overall picture. A lack of attention to social skills development may have a negative impact on social functioning (Saravanamuttu and Pyke, 2003).

Social skills training is centred on teaching people the skills necessary to communicate effectively with others. There are some general approaches to teaching people social skills. As with most skills training packages, social skills training is usually carried out in groups. However, there are opportunities at almost every encounter to teach skills and to reinforce those skills already taught and being practised. When we role model appropriate social skills we provide opportunities for learning. However, O'Donohue and Krasner (1995) recommend using a model similar in presentation to the group members so that the behaviour has more relevance to them. That is, the role model for a group of adolescents learning how to present for a job interview should be an adolescent who has suffered similar life problems.

Most social skills training groups combine instruction, modelling, rehearsal or role playing as well as coaching, feedback and reinforcement. Rehearsal and role playing involve practising the skill once instruction has been provided. Coaching involves having an instructor or teacher help the group members to practise the skill accurately by giving feedback on performance and praise (positive reinforcement) when the skill is performed well. Homework is an essential component of training packages because without practice in the real world, the goal of improved social skills will never be achieved. That is, social skills are not simply taught, they are developed through practice and the more practice, the more socially able the person will be.

INTERVIEWING

While the skill of interviewing might not strictly be considered an intervention, the nurse's interviewing style may have considerable impact on therapeutic outcomes. When you meet with a service user to carry out a clinical interview, you need to engage or connect with that person in the same way that you might when being therapeutic. That is, it is important to develop rapport by being open, thoughtful, caring and honest, both verbally and nonverbally. Interviewing a person to attempt to find out what is happening is likely to be viewed as threatening if the approach taken is to fire off a list of questions that seek to arrive at a medical diagnosis. As part of the process of empowering people with mental health problems, the assessment process (usually undertaken via clinical interview) needs to be collaborative and shared (see Ch. 10).

It is the service user who has the knowledge or information required for them to move towards identifying problems and planning care. As nurses, we currently ask questions from a power base rather than a discovery base. However, the service user is the expert in his or her experience of mental health problems, so we can share in the discovery of an understanding of the person's experience through the way in which we ask questions. At the outset, set the scene by letting the service user know that your goal is to work together with them to arrive at some conclusion regarding what is going on at the moment. You might say something like, 'Let's talk about what is happening for you. You'd probably like to get a clearer idea of what is going on and I need to hear your story so that we can better know what to do next.' Ask questions that help people to understand themselves and, through this, also arrive at some understanding of what is happening. Asking questions that recognize the expertise of the service user and summarizing that information is a collaborative approach to guided discovery (Palmer, 1999).

NURSE'S STORY: THE THERAPEUTIC ENCOUNTER

As a worker in the community, most of my time with people was spent talking through any current concerns, from weight gain to marital difficulties. These are the personal issues that contribute to difficulties in living and they are the mental health issues that we all experience and need an active listener for. However, most of us don't have the additional burden of serious mental health problems. The therapeutic encounter is designed to provide support and to enable people to solve their problems through exploring their difficulties in greater depth. When a person has a recurrence of symptoms, we attempt to manage the symptoms together in the community with more frequent visits and telephone contact. Whenever someone required hospitalization, I would liaise with staff working in the ward and visit the person there throughout the hospitalization. I was also involved in discharge planning and family meetings. This clearly communicated to people that I was there with them throughout the ordeals that they experienced. This is particularly important if you, as the nurse, were responsible for affecting their admission in the first place.

CARE COORDINATION

The Care Programme Approach (CPA) describes a pattern of service delivery for engaging and supporting service users to live their lives as fully and independently as possible. The overall aim of CPA is that of promoting social inclusion and recovery. The *care coordinator* assumes primary responsibility within a multiprofessional team for engagement with the service user and the '…quality of the relationship between service user and the care coordinator is one of the most important determinants of success' (Department of Health, 2008, p. 7).

The care coordinator is often a nurse but can also be a social worker, an occupational therapist, psychologist or psychiatrist; that is, anyone from the multidisciplinary team. They are considered to have generic skills or a core group of skills that allow them to provide a particular service to service users.

CPA takes an holistic approach, seeing the individual themselves and their families and carers as being central to the assessment and care planning process. The person is therefore seen in their various life roles and needs assessments must aim to nurture mental and physical health and wellbeing while encompassing such diverse elements as:

- family,
- parenting,
- relationships,
- housing,
- employment,
- leisure,
- education,
- creativity,
- spirituality,
- self-management and self-nurture (Department of Health, 2008).

Staff who act as care coordinators may also deliver a range of services to service users including counselling, assistance with social and financial needs and supervision of medication (Johnston et al., 1998). In addition, care coordinators are responsible for ongoing mental state assessment as well as risk assessment to ensure the person's safety and the safety of others. Because care coordination may often be carried out in the person's own home, there is often greater contact with family members and, therefore, greater opportunity to work with families. Further information on the CPA can be found in Chapter 21.

ELECTROCONVULSIVE THERAPY

Invented in 1938 in Italy by two eminent psychiatrists (Ugo Cerletti and Lucio Bini), electroconvulsive therapy (ECT) was investigated at a time when a number of physical treatments were developed, including insulin coma therapy, metrazole convulsive therapy and psychosurgery. ECT is the only one of these treatments used routinely today. Much of the controversy surrounding ECT grew out of its initial indiscriminate use and abuse. At first ECT was used without anaesthetic or muscle relaxation, with many adverse effects such as fractures, pain and cardiovascular problems.

Today, however, once a person is considered a candidate for ECT – that is, the person has a mental health problem that may respond well to ECT – a full psychological and physical assessment is carried out. Wherever possible, consent for treatment is sought from the service user. If this is not forthcoming, and the person is assessed as not being capable of giving consent, the Mental Health Act allows for treatment to proceed, but only with a second opinion (see Ch. 4 for further information). Section 58 A of the Mental Health Act 1983, amended 2007 (http://www.opsi.gov.uk/acts/acts2007/ukpga_20070012_en_1), allows the administration of ECT without consent only if it is considered necessary to save the person's life or to prevent serious damage to the person's health.

ECT involves the application of two metal electrodes to the head, through which an electric current is delivered. The electrodes can be applied either bilaterally (one on each side of the head, usually in the frontotemporal region) or unilaterally (both on the same side of the head). Whether applied bilaterally or unilaterally, the treatment is almost equally effective. However, different adverse effects can be experienced. According to Endler and Persad (1988, p. 26), 'unilateral ECT to the non-dominant hemisphere is less stressful for the service user than bilateral; it minimizes confusion and memory loss; and it is almost as efficacious as bilateral in terms of alleviating the symptoms of depression'.

Indeed, in a more recent study, high-dosage right unilateral ECT showed an equivalent response rate (Sackeim et al., 2000). This study also supported other findings that bilateral ECT results in greater impairment in memory (both anterograde and retrograde amnesia). These authors concluded that: 'right unilateral ECT at high dosage is as effective as a robust form of bilateral ECT, but produces less severe and persistent cognitive effects' (Sackeim et al., 2000, p. 425). And, in response to concerns about the effects of ECT on cerebral function, a study by Ende et al. (2000, p. 941) found evidence that ECT does not cause tissue damage and that 'there is no hippocampal atrophy, neuronal damage, or cell death induced by ECT'. Nevertheless, ECT has been found to cause memory impairment that cannot be attributed to the original illness state (MacQueen et al., 2007; Watkinson, 2007).

ECT is widely accepted as an effective intervention in the treatment of severe depression, catonia or a prolonged and severe episode of mania (NICE, 2003), although its use remains controversial (Persad, 2001). There is contention not only among the public regarding ECT (Teh et al., 2007), but also within the mental health professions, as many professionals question its efficacy (Barker, 2003; Challiner and Griffiths, 2000). However, recent publications support earlier conclusions that anti-depressants and ECT are effective and safe treatments for older people diagnosed with depression (Salzman et al., 2002) and for people who are suicidal (Persad, 2001).

In the past, ECT has been used to treat a wide range of mental disorders, including schizophrenia. An examination of both older and more recent research has revealed that ECT is as effective as antipsychotic medications in the treatment of schizophrenia, particularly with people experiencing an acute episode. When used in combination with antipsychotic medications, it has been found to be more effective than ECT or medication used alone (Keuneman et al., 2002). However, the National Institute for Health and Clinical Excellence (NICE) does not recommend the use of ECT in the management of schizophrenia (NICE, 2003).

Whether conducted in a general theatre or a specialized ECT suite attached to an inpatient mental health unit, ECT remains a physically intrusive treatment that requires specialised nursing skills. Generally, though, the role of the nurse in working with a person preparing for ECT is to support the person and to prepare them for the procedure, both physically and psychologically, just as you would for any procedure requiring a general anaesthetic. Other responsibilities for the nurse are also the same as for any operative procedure conducted under general anaesthesia. For example, you may be required to provide close observation to ensure that the service user does not eat or drink prior to the procedure. You would also need to ensure that make-up and jewellery have been removed. These are basic safety measures to prevent complications and to ensure an accurate assessment of skin colour during the anaesthetic.

ECT remains a controversial intervention in psychiatry today. Much of this controversy stems from the historical use of ECT and from its representation in films such as *One Flew Over the Cuckoo's Nest* (Vermeulen, 1999). This is despite substantial research and descriptive evidence testifying to its effectiveness. Those who have not observed ECT and who base their understandings on historical and media representations of it are likely to be surprised at how innocuous it is. A positive attitude to ECT has been found to be directly related to greater exposure to and knowledge about ECT (Endler and Persad, 1988; Gass, 1998). Nevertheless, concern persists because we are not entirely certain how ECT works and because of the cognitive side effects experienced. Ultimately, service users and families still express fears about the long-term effects on brain function.

CONCLUSION

This chapter has given some fundamental information about a number of therapeutic intervention strategies that will assist you in being with and working with people with mental health problems. Some of these intervention strategies apply to specific situations or service user difficulties, but there is always a way of working effectively with people experiencing challenging mental health problems. Some are more technical than others and require further education and practice to master. But many of the skills outlined here can be learned and applied to the interactions you will experience now as a novice nurse and later, as your experience develops.

NURSE'S STORY: ECT

A woman in her mid-thirties with whom I had worked many years ago left a lasting impression on me regarding the efficacy of ECT. She was a very attractive woman with a supportive husband and two young children. However, she suffered from symptoms of major depression. When depressed she experienced feelings of hopelessness and delusions of worthlessness. She believed that she was so worthless that her family would be better off without her and that we really shouldn't bother helping her. As with any delusion, her thoughts could not be countered.

She began treatment with ECT at the usually prescribed rate of three times each week. She had a very quick recovery and I recall her saying to us not long before she was discharged home, 'Thank you for keeping me alive until I got well'. She was also overheard recommending ECT to other depressed clients in the hospital.

This was a very important lesson for me as a mental health nurse. I was able to see someone move from a very distressed and debilitated state. She had been profoundly suicidal, but came to find pleasure in her life again following ECT. While ECT has the usual risks associated with a general anaesthetic, the risk of suicide from major depression seemed to be far greater for this woman. Every person needs individual assessment when making clinical decisions about treatment and certainly current ECT research has been more explicit in relation to its adverse effects, but this experience and many others testify to its continued utility.

Novice nurses have frequently expressed their concern to me that they might 'say the wrong thing' and make the situation more challenging for the service user. If you take a caring and thoughtful approach that avoids the generous delivery of advice, it is unlikely that you will cause harm. However, if you take with you some specific skills and models for your practice, you are likely to feel more confident and to understand the goals of your interaction. It is also hoped that, through reading this chapter, you have developed a sense of the importance of treating people with mental health problems as valid human beings who require your support and help through a particularly troubling time.

EXERCISES FOR CLASS ENGAGEMENT

A number of exercises are presented here to help you to engage with and consolidate what you have learned from this chapter. You should discuss the issues raised with your group or class members. Some of these activities also ask you to reflect on your personal values, beliefs and actions so that this greater insight into yourself will help you to be more effective in your interactions with others.

♦ What are the main stressors in your life? Consider relationship problems, difficulties with children, problems with parents, financial worries, physical conditions, environmental factors, study pressures, work factors, nutrition and exercise, in addition to chemical factors such as nicotine, alcohol, caffeine and other substances. Identify those that you can learn to manage and list the stressors in terms of their importance or greatest impact.

♦ Using the written text from a book or CD, follow the instructions for carrying out PMR. Were you able to relax? What effect did the exercise have on your respiratory and heart rates?

♦ Which of the assertion skills (making requests, refusing requests, accepting and giving compliments, expressing opinions, giving negative feedback or being confrontational, initiating conversations, sharing intimate feelings and experiences with others and expressing affection) do you find difficult to manage? Why do you think this is? Of the situations that you find difficult to manage, which one in particular presents the greatest challenge to you? How do you feel whenever you fail to manage these situations assertively?

♦ Consider the kinds of life events that might cause an individual to experience crisis, such as rape, loss of a job, unplanned pregnancy or death of a loved one. How would you respond to being admitted to hospital for colorectal surgery? How would you respond to being admitted involuntarily to an acute mental health unit?

♦ Mark is a 25-year-old single male. He has just been diagnosed with genital herpes and is extremely distressed. Although he is intelligent and has coped well with previous life crises and has good relationships with family and friends, he feels so ashamed that he can't discuss this with anyone he knows well. He believes that life is no longer worth living as he believes he will never have a normal sex life or a meaningful relationship again. What do you make of Mark's perception of his problem? Which interventions do you think are necessary according to Aguilera's model for crisis intervention?

♦ What are your short-term goals (that is, what do you hope to achieve over the next few weeks or months)? What is your main 5-year goal? What will you need to do over the next 5 years to achieve that goal? What is likely to interfere with your achievement of that goal? What is likely to support your achievement of that goal?

♦ As a group, rent and watch a DVD of *One Flew Over the Cuckoo's Nest*. What stereotypes are portrayed in this movie? Which of these persist today? How does the portrayal of ECT in this movie make you feel about ECT? In addition, what are your thoughts about the nurse–service user and doctor–service user relationships as portrayed for that era? How do you think a movie made today would portray these things?

♦ Consider your values concerning health and wellness as well as self-determination. What issues might arise for you if you were responsible for preparing a service user for ECT against that person's wishes? How would you deal with this situation?

REFERENCES

Abderhalden, C., Needham, I., Miserez, B., 2004. Predicting inpatient violence in acute psychiatric wards using the Broset Violence Checklist: a multicentre prospective cohort study. J. Psychiatr. Ment. Health Nurs. 11 (4), 422–427.

Aguilera, D., 1994. Crisis Intervention: Theory and Methodology, seventh ed. Mosby, St Louis.

Anthony, W.A., 1993. Recovery from mental illness: the guiding vision of the mental health service system in the 1990s. Psychosoc. Rehabil. J. 16 (4), 11–23.

Anthony, W.A., Cohen, M., Farkas, M., 1991. Psychiatric Rehabilitation. Centre for Psychiatric Rehabilitation, Boston.

Ayers, C.R., Sorrell, J.T., Thorp, S.R., et al., 2007. Evidence-based psychological treatments for late-life anxiety. Psychol. Aging 22 (1), 8–17.

Barker, P., 2003. Barker's beat. Ment. Health Pract. 6 (10), 38–39.

Barker, P.J., Fraser, D. (Eds.), 1985. The Nurse as Therapist: A Behavioural Model. Croom Helm, London.

Barlow, J.H., Ellard, D.R., Hainsworth, J.M., et al., 2005. A review of self-management interventions for panic disorders, phobias and obsessive-compulsive disorders. Acta Psychiatr. Scand. 111 (4), 272–285.

Battison, T., 1997. Beating Stress. Allen & Unwin, London.

Bellack, A.S., 2004. Skills training for people with severe mental illness. Psychiatr. Rehabil. J. 27 (4), 375–391.

Blackburn, I., Davidson, K., 1990. Cognitive Therapy for Depression and Anxiety. Blackwell Scientific, New York.

Bland, R., 1986. Family Support Program. Occasional paper 86(1). University of Queensland, Brisbane.

Bloom, B.L., 1997. Planned Short-Term Psychotherapy: A Clinical Handbook, second ed. Allyn & Bacon, Boston.

Brown, M., Marshall, K., 2006. Cognitive behavioural therapy and people with learning disabilities: implications for developing nursing practice. J. Psychiatr. Ment. Health Nurs. 13 (2), 234–241.

Butterworth, S., Linden, A., McClay, W., et al., 2006. Effect of motivational interviewing-based health coaching on employees' physical and mental health status. J. Occup. Health Psychol. 11 (4), 358–365.

Byrne, J., Byrne, D.G., 1996. Counselling Skills for Health Professionals. MacMillan Education, Melbourne.

Byrne, A., Watson, R., Butler, C., et al., 2006. Increasing the confidence of nursing staff to address the sexual health needs of people living with HIV: the use of motivational interviewing. AIDS Care 18 (5), 501–504.

Calvert, P., Palmer, C., 2003. Application of the cognitive therapy model to initial crisis assessment. Int. J. Ment. Health Nurs. 12 (1), 30–38.

Carels, R.A., Darby, L., Cacciapaglia, H.M., et al., 2007. Using motivational interviewing as a supplement to obesity treatment. Health Psychol. 26 (3), 369–374.

Challiner, V., Griffiths, L., 2000. Electroconvulsive therapy: a review of the literature. J. Psychiatr. Ment. Health Nurs. 7 (3), 191–198.

Cheung, L.C.C., Tsang, H.W.H., Tsui, C.U., 2006. A job-specific social skills training program for people with severe mental illness: a case study for those who plan to be a security guard. J. Rehabil. 72 (4), 14–23.

Clark, M.D., Walters, S., Gingerich, R., et al., 2006. Motivational interviewing for probation officers: tipping the balance toward change. Fed. Probat. 70 (1), 38–44.

Colom, F., Vieta, E., Martinez-Aran, A., et al., 2003. A randomised trial on the efficacy of group psychoeducation in the prophylaxis of recurrences in bipolar patients whose disease is in remission. Arch. Gen. Psychiatry 60 (4), 402–407.

Curtis, L., 1997. New Directions: International Overview of Best Practices in Recovery and Rehabilitation Services for People with Serious Mental Illness. New Zealand Mental Health Commission, Wellington.

Cutcliffe, J.R., Barker, P., 2004. The nurses' global assessment of suicide risk (NGASR): developing a tool for clinical practice. J. Psychiatr. Ment. Health Nurs. 11 (4), 393–400.

Dattilio, F.M., Padesky, C.A., 1990. Cognitive Therapy with Couples. Professional Resource Exchange, Sarasota, FL.

Davis, C.M., 1989. Patient–Practitioner Interaction. Slack, Thorofare, NJ.

Davis, M., Robbins Eshelman, E., McKay, M., 2000. The Relaxation and Stress Reduction Workbook, fifth ed. New Harbinger, Oakland, CA.

Deegan, P., 1988. Recovery: the lived experience of rehabilitation. Psychosoc. Rehabil. J. 11 (4), 11–19.

Deegan, P., 1993. Recovering our sense of value after being labelled mentally ill. J. Psychosoc. Nurs. 31 (4), 7–11.

Deegan, P., 1996. Recovery as a journey of the heart. Psychiatr. Rehabil. J. 19 (3), 91–97.

Deegan, P.E., 1997. Recovery and empowerment for people with psychiatric disabilities. Soc. Work Health Care 25 (3), 11–24.

Department of Health, 2008. Refocusing the care programme approach: policy and positive practice guidance. <http://www.dh.gov.uk/en/Publicationsandstatistics/Publications/PublicationsPolicyAndGuidance/DH_083647>.

Doyle, M., Dolan, M., 2002. Violence risk assessment: combining actuarial and clinical information to structure clinical judgements for the formulation and management of risk. J. Psychiatr. Ment. Health Nurs. 9 (6), 649–657.

Earley, J., 2000. Interactive Group Therapy: Integrating Interpersonal, Action-Oriented, and Psychodynamic Approaches. Brunner/Mazel, Philadelphia.

Edwards, D., Hannigan, B., Fothergill, A., et al., 2002. Stress management for mental health professionals: a review of effective techniques. Stress Health 18 (5), 203–215.

Egan, G., 1998. The Skilled Helper: a Problem-Management Approach to Helping, sixth ed. Brooks/Cole, Pacific Grove, CA.

Eisler, I., Simic, M., Russell, G.F.M., et al., 2007. A randomised controlled treatment trial of two forms of family therapy in adolescent anorexia nervosa: a five-year follow-up. J. Child Psychol. Psychiatry 48 (6), 552–560.

Ekdawi, M.Y., Conning, A.M., 1994. Psychiatric Rehabilitation: A Practical Guide. Chapman & Hall, London.

Ende, G., Braus, D.F., Walter, S., et al., 2000. The hippocampus in patients treated with electroconvulsive therapy: a proton magnetic resonance spectroscopic imaging study. Arch. Gen. Psychiatry 57 (10), 937–943.

Endler, N.S., Persad, E., 1988. Electroconvulsive Therapy: The Myths and the Realities. Hans Huber, Toronto.

Escot, C., Artero, S., Gandubert, C., et al., 2001. Stress levels in nursing staff working in oncology. Stress Health 17 (5), 273–279.

Evans, A.M., 2007. Transference in the nurse–patient relationship. J. Psychiatr. Ment. Health Nurs. 14 (2), 189–195.

Fehr, S.S., 1999. Introduction to Group Therapy: A Practical Guide. Haworth Press, New York.

Finnell, D.S., 2003. Use of the transtheoretical model for individuals with co-occurring disorders. Community Ment. Health J. 39 (1), 3–15.

Freud, S., 1938/1965. The Basic Writing of Sigmund Freud. Modern Library, New York.

Gallop, R., O'Brien, L., 2003. Re-establishing psychodynamic theory as foundational knowledge for psychiatric/mental health nursing. Issues Ment. Health Nurs. 24 (2), 213–227.

Gambril, E., 1995. Assertion skills training. In: O'Donohue, W., Krasner, L. (Eds.), Handbook of Psychological Skills Training: Clinical Techniques and Applications. Allyn & Bacon, Boston.

Gass, J.P., 1998. The knowledge and attitudes of mental health nurses to electroconvulsive therapy. J. Adv. Nurs. 27 (1), 83–90.

Goldenberg, I., Goldenberg, H., 2000. Family Therapy: An Overview, fifth ed. Brooks/Cole, Belmont, CA.

Greenstone, J.L., Leviton, S.C., 2002. Elements of Crisis Intervention: Crises and How to Respond to Them, second ed. Brooks/Cole, Pacific Grove, CA.

Hayne, Y., Yonge, O., 1997. The lifeworld analysis of the chronically mentally ill: an analysis of 40 written personal accounts. Arch. Psychiatr. Nurs. 11 (6), 314–324.

Jenkins, J.H., Karno, M., 1992. The meaning of expressed emotion: theoretical issues raised by cross-cultural research. Am. J. Psychiatry 149 (1), 9–21.

Johnston, S., Salkeld, G., Sanderson, K., et al., 1998. Intensive case management: a cost-effectiveness analysis. Aust. N. Z. J. Psychiatry 32, 551–559.

Kadis, L.B., McClendon, R., 1998. Concise Guide to Marital and Family Therapy. American Psychiatric Press, Washington.

Kavanagh, D.J., 1992. Recent developments in expressed emotion and schizophrenia. Br. J. Psychiatry 160, 601–620.

Kelly, T., Simmons, W., Gregory, E., 2002. Risk assessment and management: a community forensic mental health practice model. Int. J. Ment. Health Nurs. 11 (4), 206–213.

Keuneman, R., Weerasundera, R., Castle, D., 2002. The role of ECT in schizophrenia. Australas. Psychiatry 10 (4), 385–388.

Knight, K.M., McGowan, L., Dickens, C., et al., 2006. A systematic review of motivational interviewing in physical health care settings. Br. J. Health Care Psychol. 11 (2), 319–332.

Legere, L., 2007. The importance of rehabilitation. Psychiatr. Rehabil. J. 30 (3), 227–229.

Lester, D., 2002. Crisis Intervention and Counselling by Telephone, second ed. Charles C Thomas, Springfield, IL.

Linehan, M.M., 1993. Cognitive Behaviour Therapy of Borderline Personality Disorder. Guilford Press, New York.

Linehan, M.M., Schmidt, H., Dimeff, L.A., et al., 1999. Dialectical behaviour therapy for patients with borderline personality disorder and drug-dependence. Am. J. Addict. 8, 279–292.

McGoldrick, M., Gerson, R., Shellenberger, S., 1999. Genograms: Assessment and Intervention, second ed. W W Norton, New York.

MacQueen, G., Parkin, C., Marriott, M., et al., 2007. The long-term impact of treatment with electroconvulsive therapy on discrete memory systems in patients with bipolar disorder. J. Psychiatry Neurosci. 32 (4), 241–249.

Mannix, K., Blackburn, I.M., Garland, A., et al., 2006. Effectiveness of brief training in cognitive behaviour therapy techniques for palliative care practitioners. Palliat. Med. 20 (6), 579–584.

Meech, C., Wood, A., 2000. Reconnecting past, present and future lives: therapy with a young person who experienced severe childhood privation. Aust. N. Z. J. Fam. Ther. 21 (2), 102–107.

Mellor, D., Storer, S., Firth, L., 2000. Family therapy into the 21st century: can we work our way out of the epistemological maze? Aust. N. Z. J. Fam. Ther. 21 (3), 151–154.

Miller, W., 1998. Toward a motivational definition and understanding of addiction. Motivational Interviewing Newsletter 5 (3), 2–6.

Miller, W.R., Zweben, A., DiClemente, C.C., et al., 1992. Motivational Enhancement Therapy Manual: A Clinical Research Guide for Therapists Treating Individuals with Alcohol Abuse and Dependence. National Institute on Alcohol Abuse and Alcoholism, Rockville.

Monahan, J., Steadman, H.J., Silver, E., et al., 2001. Rethinking Risk Assessment: The MacArthur Study of Mental Disorder and Violence. Oxford University Press, Oxford.

Morse, J., Penrod, J., 1999. Linking concepts of enduring, uncertainty, suffering, and hope. Image J. Nurs. Sch. 31 (1), 145–150.

Mullen, P., 2002. Marijuana and mental illness. Paper presented at the Mental Health Services Conference Inc. of Australia and New Zealand (The MHS), Sydney, 21 August.

Mullen, A., Murray, L., Happell, B., 2002. Multiple family group interventions in first episode psychosis: enhancing knowledge and understanding. Int. J. Ment. Health Nurs. 11, 225–232.

Murphy, N., 2004. An investigation into how community mental health nurses assess the risk of violence from their clients. J. Psychiatr. Ment. Health Nurs. 11 (4), 407–413.

Murray, B.L., Wright, K., 2006. Integration of a suicide risk assessment and intervention approach: the perspective of youth. J. Psychiatr. Ment. Health Nurs. 13 (2), 157–164.

Myer, R.A., 2001. Assessment for Crisis Intervention: A Triage Assessment Model. Wadsworth, Toronto.

Myhr, G., Payne, K., 2006. Cost-effectiveness of cognitive-behaviour therapy for mental disorders: implications for public health care funding policy in Canada. Can. J. Psychiatry 51 (10), 662–670.

NICE (National Institute for Health and Clinical Excellence), 2003. Guidance on the use of electroconvulsive therapy. <http://guidance.nice.org.uk/TA59/Guidance/pdf/English>.

Nichols, M.P., Schwartz, R.C., 2001. Family Therapy: Concepts and Methods, fifth ed. Allyn & Bacon, Boston.

O'Donohue, W., Krasner, L., 1995. Handbook of Psychological Skills Training: Clinical Techniques and Applications. Allyn & Bacon, Boston.

Palmer, C.J., 1996. Education and Support for Families and Friends of People with Schizophrenia. Masters dissertation, Queensland University of Technology, Brisbane.

Palmer, C.J., 1999. Recovery-focused mental health nursing: a model for the future? Paper presented at the Scientific Meeting of the Australian and New Zealand College of Mental Health Nurses (ANZCMHN), Tasmania, 9–12 September.

Patel, C., 1991. The Complete Guide to Stress Management. Plenum Press, New York.

Perkins, R.E., Repper, J.M., 1996. Working Alongside People with

Long Term Mental Health Problems. Chapman & Hall, London.

Persad, E., 2001. Electroconvulsive therapy: the controversy and the evidence. Can. J. Psychiatry 46 (8), 702–703.

Petchkovsky, L., Morris, P., Rushton, P., 2002. Choosing a psychodynamic psychotherapy model for an Australian public sector mental health service. Australas. Psychiatry 10 (4), 330–334.

Prochaska, J.O., 2001. Treating entire populations for behaviour risks for cancer. Cancer J. 7 (5), 360–368.

Prochaska, J.O., DiClemente, C.C., 1983. Stages and processes of self-change of smoking: toward an integrative model of change. J. Consult. Clin. Psychol. 51 (3), 390–395.

Rausch, S.M., Gramling, S.E., Auerbach, S.M., 2006. Effects of a single session of large-group meditation and progressive muscle relaxation training on stress reduction, reactivity, and recovery. Int. J. Stress Manag. 13 (3), 273–290.

Rodrigues, L.J., 2007. A closer look: the benefits and effectiveness of CBT on a female-specific unit for treatment of bipolar disorder. Issues Ment. Health Nurs. 28 (5), 533–542.

Rollnick, S., Miller, W.R., 1995. What is motivational interviewing? Behav. Cogn. Psychother. 23, 325–334.

Romas, J.A., Sharma, M., 1995. Practical Stress Management. Allyn & Bacon, Boston.

Rosser, S., Erskine, A., Crino, R., 2004. Pre-existing antidepressants and the outcome of group cognitive behaviour therapy for social phobia. Aust. N. Z. J. Psychiatry 38 (4), 233–239.

Sackeim, H.A., Prudic, J., Devanand, D.P., et al., 2000. A prospective, randomised, double-blind comparison of bilateral and right unilateral electroconvulsive therapy at different stimulus intensities. Arch. Gen. Psychiatry 57 (5), 425–434.

Salzman, C., Wong, E., Wright, B.C., 2002. Drug and ECT treatment of depression in the elderly, 1996–2001: a literature review. Biol. Psychiatry 52 (3), 265–284.

Sanders, P., 1996. An Incomplete Guide to Using Counselling Skills on the Telephone, second ed. PCCS Books, Manchester.

Saravanamuttu, R., Pyke, J., 2003. Interaction: case managers and social skills teaching. Psychiatr. Rehabil. J. 27 (1), 79–82.

Semple, C.J., Dunwoody, L., Sullivan, K., et al., 2006. Patients with head and neck cancer prefer individualised cognitive behaviour therapy. Eur. J. Cancer Care (Engl) 15 (3), 220–227.

Sharry, J., 2001. Solution-Focused Groupwork. Sage, London.

Slaikeu, K.A., 1990. Crisis Intervention: a Handbook for Practice and Research, second ed. Allyn & Bacon, Boston.

Sundel, S.S., Sundel, M., 1993. Behaviour Modification in the Human Services: A Systematic Introduction to Concepts and Applications, third ed. Sage, Newbury Park, CA.

Swales, M., Heard, H.L., Williams, J.M.G., 2000. Linehan's dialectical behaviour therapy (DBT) for borderline personality disorder: overview and adaptation. J. Ment. Health 9 (1), 7–23.

Teh, S.P.C., Helmes, E., Drake, D.G., 2007. A Western Australian survey on public attitudes toward and knowledge of electroconvulsive therapy. Int. J. Soc. Psychiatry 53 (3), 247–273.

Timmins, F., McCabe, C., 2005. Nurses' and midwives' assertive behaviour in the workplace. J. Adv. Nurs. 51 (1), 38–45.

Treasure, J., Sepulveda, A.R., Whitaker, W., et al., 2007. Collaborative care between professionals and nonprofessionals in the management of eating disorders: a description of workshops focused on interpersonal maintaining factors. Eur. Eat. Disord. Rev. 15 (1), 24–34.

Truax, P., 2002. Behavioural case conceptualisation for adults. In: Hersen, M. (Ed.), Clinical Behavioural Therapy: Adults and Children. John Wiley & Sons, New York.

Vandevooren, J., Miller, L., O'Reilly, R., 2007. Outcomes in community-based residential treatment and rehabilitation for individuals with psychiatric disabilities: a retrospective study. Psychiatr. Rehabil. J. 30 (3), 215–217.

Varcarolis, E.M., 1998. Foundations of Psychiatric-Mental Health Nursing, third ed. WB Saunders, Philadelphia.

Vermeulen, J., 1999. A personal reflection by a psychiatric nurse: electroconvulsive therapy: history, perception, knowledge and attitudes. Paper presented at the Scientific Meeting of the Australian and New Zealand College of Mental Health Nurses (ANZCMHN), Launceston Tasmania, 9–12 September.

Vos, T., Gorry, J., Haby, M.M., et al., 2005. Cost-effectiveness of cognitive behavioural therapy and drug interventions for major depression. Aust. N. Z. J. Psychiatry 39 (8), 683–692.

Watkinson, A., 2007. ECT: a personal experience. Ment. Health Pract. 10 (7), 32–35.

Watson, R.J., McDonald, J., Pearce, D.C., 2006. An exploration of national calls to Lifeline Australia: social support or urgent suicide intervention? Br. J. Guid. Counc. 34 (4), 471–482.

Wolpow, S., 2000. Adapting a dialectical behaviour therapy (DBT) group for use in a residential program. Psychiatr. Rehabil. J. 24 (2), 135–141.

Yalom, I.D., 1995. The Theory and Practice of Group Psychotherapy, fourth ed. Basic Books, New York.

Chapter | 24 |

Psychopharmacology and medicines management

Kim Usher, Kim Foster, Lauretta Luck, and Reuben Pearce

CHAPTER POINTS

- Psychotropic medications play an important role in the treatment of mental health problems. The nurse plays a pivotal role in medication administration and service user education. It is also important for the nurse to be aware of the potential side effects and interactions of these drugs.
- Assisting the service user to understand the importance of taking psychotropic medication as prescribed and the issues surrounding medication concordance as an important skill for the mental health nurse.
- Polypharmacy is to be avoided where possible, especially the tendency to use drugs from different classes at the same time. Its use with older people is not advised.
- Issues related to 'as-needed' (PRN) medication administration is of contemporary relevance.
- Nursing assessment and interventions related to psychopharmacological side effects is important knowledge for the mental health nurse.

LEARNING OUTCOMES

The material in this chapter will assist you to:

- describe the role of the nurse in the administration of psychotropic medication and related interventions, including medication indications, interactions, side effects and precautions,
- identify the important classes of psychotropic medications and the disorders for which they are used,
- understand the issues for service users requiring psychotropic medications,
- understand the action, use and side effects related to anti-anxiety/sedative-hypnotic, antidepressant, mood-stabilizing and antipsychotic drugs,
- understand the issues related to the as-needed (PRN) administration of psychotropic medication and related interventions,
- outline the relevant legal and ethical issues related to the administration of psychotropic medication.

INTRODUCTION

This chapter provides an overview of the principles of psychopharmacology, which is the study of drugs used to treat mental health problems. The chapter provides important information related to drug indications, interactions, side effects and precautions, and discusses service user education and the issues of adherence, concordance and as-needed (PRN) medication administration.

The use of drugs that have a demonstrated ability to relieve the symptoms of mental health problems has become widespread since the mid-1950s (Baldessarini and Tarazi, 2001). The pharmacological agents used in current psychiatric practice are the anti-anxiety sedatives, antidepressants and mood-stabilizing, neuroleptic and antipsychotic drugs. Collectively, these drugs are referred to as **psychotropic** medications and are the focus of discussion in this chapter.

It is important to remember that psychotropic medications are just one part of the service user's treatment and on their own should not be considered a 'quick fix' or cure-all. In fact, psychotropic medications are not helpful to all people who experience symptoms of mental disorder and have many untoward effects that can cause discomfort and distress.

Skillful mental health nursing encompasses an understanding of the particular pharmacological actions of the psychotropic agents as well as an empathic understanding of the potential issues for the person taking these medications. Regardless of the treatment setting, which can range from inpatient to community, mental health nurses play a pivotal role in working with service users and their families as they grapple with the issues surrounding these medications. It is important that the nurse develops a comprehensive understanding of both the medications and their impact on an individual as well as developing an understanding of the supportive and therapeutic nursing interventions that promote medication concordance.

IMPORTANT PHARMACOLOGICAL PRINCIPLES

Supportive and therapeutic nursing interventions enable the service user to develop and maintain medication concordance and foster the service user's understanding of their medications. As the mental health nurse plays an important role in the administration of psychotropic medications, especially within mental health inpatient units, it is essential to have a sound working knowledge of psychotropic medications, including their pharmacology and relevant neurochemistry. This knowledge is important for the nurse when offering medication education to the service user and their family.

All drugs are prescribed for particular effects or target symptoms that the prescriber hopes to change. Therefore it is important for the nurse to be aware of the symptoms that particular drugs target as well as the symptoms experienced by individual service users. The correct identification of symptoms is a key component of a thorough nursing assessment. Side effects, on the other hand, are the expression of effects for which the drug was not intended. Not all side effects are harmful, but some can be, so the nurse needs a sound working knowledge of this area of practice. Nurses also need to be aware of **polypharmacy**. Polypharmacy implies the use of multiple psychotropic drugs at the same time. Essentially it is defined as the use of two or more psychotropic drugs, or two or more drugs from the same chemical class or two or more drugs with the same or similar pharmacological action to treat different conditions (Kingsbury et al., 2001). Although it might be useful at some stage for the medical treatment of people diagnosed with serious mental health problems, polypharmacy is generally not advisable as it can increase the chance of adverse drug side effects and interactions. It can also be extremely problematic with certain groups of vulnerable people, including older people (Shupikai Rinomhota and Marshall, 2000).

An understanding of how psychotropic drugs work is important for mental health nurses so that they can better understand the issues surrounding the prescription and administration of these drugs. The neuron is the basic functional unit of the brain and central nervous system (CNS) and all communication in the brain involves neurons communicating across synapses at receptors. Receptors are the targets for the **neurotransmitters** or chemical messengers necessary for communication between neurons. The neurotransmitters acetylcholine, noradrenaline (norepinephrine), dopamine, serotonin (5HT) and gamma-aminobutyric acid (GABA) are implicated in the development of mental disorder. Table 24.1 offers a brief overview of the role of these transmitters in relation to their function and mental disorders as referred to by Galbraith et al., 2007):

The psychotropic drugs produce their therapeutic action by altering communication among the neurons in the CNS. In particular, they alter the way neurotransmitters work at the synapse by modifying the reuptake of a neurotransmitter into the presynaptic neuron, activating or inhibiting postsynaptic receptors or inhibiting enzyme activity (Shupikai Rinomhota and Marshall, 2000). One of the difficulties that is widely associated with the use of psychotropic drugs is how specific they are at targeting a particular brain function. For example, a psychotropic drug may target an area of the brain that dopamine plays a part in mediating. As dopamine has multiple functions in different pathways of the brain, the drug may affect more than one function and there is currently no way of restricting which part of the brain the psychotropic drug takes action upon. This is why there can be unwanted side effects associated with certain psychotropic drugs (Galbraith et al., 2007).

Table 24.1 The role of neurotransmitters in relation to their function and mental disorders

Transmitter	Functions	Related mental/ neurological disorders
Acetylcholine	Cognition, skeletal muscle movement, memory, consciousness	Dementia, Parkinson's disease
Dopamine	Skeletal muscle movement, behaviour, emesis (vomiting), hormone release	Psychosis, Parkinson's disease, inhibition of hormone release, aberrant behaviour, i.e. disinhibition, mania
Noradrenaline (norepinephrine)	Arousal, sleep, mood, appetite, hormone release, body temperture	Eating disorders, depression, insomnia
Serotonin	Arousal, sleep, mood, appetite, hormone release, body temperture, behaviour and transmission of pain	Eating disorders, depression, insomnia, mania
Glutamate	Learning and memory	Epilepsy, excititoxicity, i.e. after traumatic brain injury, neurodegenerative disease
Gamma-aminobutyric acid (GABA)	Motor control, memory, consciousness	Anxiety, aberrant behaviour, i.e. disinhibition, insomnia

From: Fundamentals of Pharmacology: An Allied Approach for Nursing and Health, 2e, Galbraith A, Bullock S, Manias E, Hunt B, Richards A © 2007. Reproduced by permission of Taylor & Francis Books UK.

IMPORTANT PSYCHOTROPIC DRUGS

This section explores the most important groups of psychotropic drugs in current use: the anxiolytics (anti-anxiety) drugs, antidepressants, mood stabilizers and antipsychotics (neuroleptics). These groups of drugs are listed in Table 24.2 with common examples from a local perspective.

Table 24.2 Classification of psychotropic drugs

Type	Drug group	Example
Antipsychotic: traditional	Phenothiazines	*Group 1*
		Chlorpromazine
		Levomepromazine
		Promazine
		Group 2
		Pericyazine
		Pipotiazine
		Group 3
		Fluphenazine
		Perphenazine
		Prochlorperazine
		Trifluoperazine
	Thioxanthines	Flupenthixol
	Butyrophenones	Haloperidol
		Benperidol
	Diphenylbutylpiperidines	Pimozide
	Substituted benzamides	Sulpride
Antipsychotic: atypical		Clozapine
		Risperidone
		Olanzapine
		Quetiapine
		Aripiprazole
		Amisulpride
		Paliperidone
Antidepressant	Tricyclic and related drugs	Amitriptyline
		Lofepramine
		Trazodone
		Mianserin
		Nortriptyline
		Trimipramine
		Imipramine
		Dosulepin
		Clomipramine
		Doxepin
	Selective serotonin-reuptake inhibitors (SSRIs)	Citalopram
		Escitalopram
		Fluoxetine
		Fluoxamine
		Paroxetine
		Sertraline
	Serotonin- and noradrenaline-reuptake inhibitors	Venlafaxine
		Duloxetine
	Selective inhibitors of noradrenaline	Reboxetine

(continued)

Table 24.2 Continued

Type	Drug group	Example
	Monoamine oxidase inhibitors	Isocarboxazid
		Phenelzine
		Tranylcypromine
	Presynaptic alpha$_2$-adrenoreceptor antagonists	Mirtazipine
Mood stabilizing	Lithium	Lithium carbonate
	Anticonvulsants	Carbamazipine
		Valproate
		Lamotrigine
Anti-anxiety	Benzodiazepines	Chlordiazepoxide
		Diazepam
		Clonazepam
		Alprazolam
		Lorazepam
	Azapirones	Buspirone
	Beta-adrenergic blockers	Propanolol
Sedative-hypnotic	Benzodiazepines	Flurazepam
		Temazepam
	Cyclopyrrolones	Zoplclone
	Imidazopyrimidines	Zolpidem

Anti-anxiety or anxiolytic medications

Anxiety is a common human experience that is a normal reaction to a threat of some kind. It leads to a flight-or-fight response in the individual. Anxiety is also the feature of many mental health problems. When anxiety becomes disabling, anti-anxiety medications may be useful (Shupikai Rinomhota and Marshall, 2000). Anti-anxiety drugs can be divided into benzodiazepines and nonbenzodiazepines. The benzodiazepines are probably the most commonly prescribed drugs in the world today and are the drug of choice for the short-term treatment of anxiety states.

Indications for use

The benzodiazepines are thought to reduce anxiety because of their **potentiation** of the inhibitory neurotransmitter GABA, which results in a clinical decrease in the individual's anxiety by an inhibition of neurotransmission (Shupikai Rinomhota and Marshall, 2000). Clinically they are used to treat anxiety, insomnia, alcohol withdrawal, skeletal muscle relaxation, seizure disorders, anxiety associated with medical disease and psychotic agitation (Ballanger, 2000; Battaglia et al., 1997;

Table 24.3 Managing benzodiazepine side effects

Side effect	Intervention
Drowsiness	Encourage appropriate activity but warn against engaging in activities such as driving or operating machinery
Dizziness	Observe and take steps to prevent falls
Feelings of detachment	Encourage socialization
Dependency, rebound insomnia/anxiety	Encourage short-term use; educate to avoid other drugs such as alcohol; plan for withdrawal

Garza-Trevino et al., 1989). Therefore, although the discussion here is primarily related to the use of these drugs as anti-anxiety agents, they also have a sedative effect and are often used for that purpose.

Side effects

Side effects from the benzodiazepine drugs (Table 24.3) are common, dose-related, usually short-term and almost always harmless. They include drowsiness, reduced mental acuity and impaired motor performance. However, other effects such as headache, dizziness, feelings of detachment, nausea, hypotension and restlessness may also be experienced. Therefore the service user should be warned of the risk of accidents and cautioned about driving a car or operating dangerous machinery. These drugs generally do not live up to their reputation of being strongly addictive, especially if they have been used for appropriate purposes, if their use has not been complicated by other factors such as the addition of other medications and if their withdrawal is planned and gradual. However, if addiction does occur with these medications the resulting physical dependence can lead to development of tolerance and onset of a withdrawal syndrome (Box 24.1) if they are ceased abruptly.

It is also important to remember that older service users are more vulnerable to side effects because the ageing brain is more sensitive to the action of sedatives (Shupikai Rinomhota and Marshall, 2000).

Contraindications/precautions

Benzodiazepines should not be taken in conjunction with any other CNS depressants including alcohol. Their use in pregnancy is not recommended due to a possible risk of teratogenicity (birth defects). Should a woman be planning a baby or find that she is pregnant then the medication should be gradually withdrawn. A risk/benefit analysis may need to be undertaken should there be concern for withdrawal of a benzodiazepine in relation to her mental health (Taylor et al., 2009).

Interactions

Interactions may occur with alcohol, monoamine oxidase inhibitors, phenytoin, antacids and agents with anticholinergic activity.

Box 24.1 Symptoms of benzodiazepine withdrawal syndrome

Agitation
Anorexia
Anxiety
Autonomic arousal
Dizziness
Hallucinations
Insomnia
Irritability
Nausea and vomiting
Seizures
Sensitivity to light and sounds
Tinnitus
Tremulousness

Service user education

The service user should be educated about the following:

- driving or operating machinery should be avoided until tolerance develops,
- alcohol and other CNS depressants potentiate the effects of benzodiazepines, and therefore should be avoided,
- benzodiazepine use should not be stopped suddenly,
- the use of benzodiazepines during pregnancy is not recommended.

Nonbenzodiazepine anti-anxiety drugs

Buspirone is a potent nonbenzodiazepine anxiolytic drug with no known addictive or sedative properties. It is effective in the treatment of anxiety and it has no muscle-relaxant or anticonvulsant properties. It is of no use in the management of alcohol or other drug abuse or panic disorder. Generally it takes about 3–6 weeks before maximum anxiolytic effects are achieved.

Propanolol is a beta-blocker that is useful in the treatment of anxiety. It blocks **beta-noradrenergic receptors** centrally as well as in the peripheral cardiac and pulmonary systems. Beta-noradrenergic receptors play an important role in regulating the rate of the heart beat. When a person is stressed and anxious the body produces noradrenaline, resulting in an increased heart rate, hypervigilance and other physiological responses often associated with the flight-or-fight response. When anxious for psychological reasons that might not be associated with, for example, being chased by a lion or faced by an intruder with nowhere to run (i.e. out of context with their actual situation), then it can be helpful to reduce the physiological effects of extra noradrenaline production to reduce those flight-or-fight reactions in the body. These flight-or-fight physiological reactions can be very unpleasant and lead to increasing anxiety further through a vicious circle of anxious thoughts influencing physiological reaction and back again. It is an everyday occurrence to get similar feelings when people enter uncomfortable situations such as sitting an examination, or going to a job interview; however, these normally pass after the event. Beta-blockers reduce certain physiological symptoms of anxiety, especially tachycardia, rather than working directly on the anxiety. For this reason it is important to remember that while the drug can help with those physiological symptoms of anxiety the psychological support needs to be put in place to address the causes of the difficulties with a view to developing coping strategies that aim to prevent future episodes.

Antidepressant drugs

Depression is a disorder characterized by symptoms such as depressed mood, lack of pleasure or interest, appetite disturbance, sleep disturbance and fatigue. Depression is thought, at least in part, to be a result of dysregulation of neurochemicals, particularly serotonin and noradrenaline. The physiological understanding of antidepressant drug action offers some support for this theory. Antidepressant drugs enhance the transmission of these neurochemicals in a number of ways: they block the reuptake of the neurotransmitters at the synapse, inhibit their metabolism and destruction and/or enhance the activity of the receptors. The action of these drugs at the synapse is immediate but it takes several weeks for antidepressants to have an effect on mood.

Indications for use

Antidepressant medications are indicated in the treatment of dysthymic disorders (chronic and persistent low mood), major depression, maintenance treatment of depression and prevention of relapse and anxiety disorders such as panic disorder and obsessive–compulsive disorder. The drugs elevate mood and alleviate the other symptoms experienced as part of depression. Choice of a particular antidepressant medication will depend on its symptom profile, side effects, comorbid medical conditions, concurrent medications and risk of drug interactions, and the individual's drug history. If the service user responds to the course of treatment with a particular drug they should continue taking the drug at the same dosage for up to 9 months. If they remain symptom-free during this time then the drug will be gradually withdrawn. Service users whose depressive symptoms return after withdrawal of medication may need long-term maintenance (Treatment Protocol Project, 2000).

Side effects

Tricyclic antidepressants

The tricyclic drugs, available on the market for many years now, are chemically similar, so their effects and side effects tend to vary little between individual drugs. They work primarily by serotonin- and noradrenaline-reuptake inhibition. The blockade of reuptake leads to extra transmitters available for receptor binding. Underlying this pharmacological approach is the hypothesis that depression is linked to a depletion in the synaptic levels of noradrenaline and serotonin. Antidepressant drugs then act by raising the levels of one or both of these neurotransmitters. They achieve this by blockade of the presynaptic reuptake of one or both of these neurotransmitters thus increasing synaptic levels and treating the depression. Side effects include sedation, dry mouth, constipation, blurred vision, seizures and urinary retention. They may also cause postural hypotension and serious cardiac problems such as heart block and arrhythmias. Because of their serious side effects these drugs can lead to life-threatening consequences if taken in large quantities, such as in suicide attempts, and if this is suspected then immediate action to support life must be instigated. (Box 24.2 lists

signs of overdose.) In the case of service users experiencing symptoms of severe depression and where a potential for suicide is predicted, supervision is required and when the person is not an inpatient the dispensing of small, sublethal quantities is recommended (Baldessarini, 2001).

Monoamine oxidase inhibitors

Monoamine oxidase inhibitors (MAOIs) were the first group of antidepressant drugs discovered. They remain very effective antidepressants; however, due to their potentially serious side effects their use has mostly been replaced by the newer antidepressant drugs. The MAOIs work by inhibiting both types of the enzyme (monoamine oxidase A and B) that metabolize serotonin and noradrenaline. Service users taking these drugs must avoid noradrenaline **agonists**, which include its dietary precursor, **tyramine**. Adverse effects include drowsiness or insomnia, agitation, fatigue, gastrointestinal disturbances, weight gain, hypotension and dizziness, dry mouth and skin, sexual dysfunction, constipation and blurred vision. The major concern with the use of these drugs is their potential to interact with specific foods that contain tyramine, and other amine drugs such as those found in any cough preparation (Box 24.3). Such an interaction can result in excessive and dangerous elevation in blood pressure, known as a hypertensive crisis.

Box 24.2 Signs of tricyclic overdose

Agitation
Confusion, drowsiness, delirium
Convulsion
Bowel and bladder paralysis
Disturbances with the regulation of blood pressure and temperature
Dilated pupils

Source: Treatment Protocol Project (2000).

Box 24.3 Food and drugs to be avoided by service users taking MAOIs

Cheeses, especially matured cheeses
Pickled herrings, cured meats and beef extracts such as marmite
Liver and chicken livers
Whole broad beans, avocados (especially if overripe), soybean paste
Figs, especially if overripe
Large numbers of bananas
Alcoholic drinks, especially Chianti and other red wines
Other antidepressant drugs, nasal and sinus decongestants, narcotics, adrenaline (epinephrine)
Stimulants, hayfever and asthma drugs

Selective serotonin-reuptake inhibitors

The selective serotonin-reuptake inhibitor (SSRI) group of antidepressant drugs inhibit the reuptake of serotonin at the presynaptic membrane. This leads to an increased availability of serotonin in the synapse and therefore at the receptors, thereby promoting serotonin transmission. These drugs are as effective as the tricyclic antidepressants but safer, as they cause less-serious side effects and have decreased risk of death by overdose. While the actions and effectiveness of these drugs are similar, they are all structurally different from each other, resulting in differences in their side effects. Side effects are similar to those of the tricyclic group except that they do not have the cardiovascular, sedative and **anticholinergic** side effects. Nausea, diarrhoea, anxiety and restlessness, insomnia, sexual disturbances, loss of appetite, weight loss and headache are the most common. They should not be stopped abruptly; the withdrawal syndrome includes symptoms such as dizziness, paraesthesia, anxiety, sleep disturbance, agitation and tremor. They should not be combined with MAOIs (Shupikai Rinomhota and Marshall, 2000).

Contraindications/precautions

Caution is warranted in the use of all antidepressant drugs. Once the drugs start to take effect and the service user's mood lifts, the service user may become a risk for suicide. This has been of particular note with the treatment of children and adolescents under the age of 18. In particular citalopram, escitalopram, paroxetine, sertraline, mirtazapine and venlafaxine are not recommended for use with children. Clinical trials have suggested that these drugs have failed to show efficacy in this age group while demonstrating an increase in harmful outcomes such as increased risk of self-harm and suicide (Medicines and Healthcare Products Regulatory Agency, 2004). Fluoxetine is the antidepressant recommended for treating children and adolescents through clinical trials that have demonstrated its efficacy; however, it needs to be used with caution due to some similar risks to the drugs mentioned above (Taylor et al., 2009).

SSRIs should not be combined with MAOI therapy. MAOIs should not be started within 1 week of tricyclic therapy and, conversely, tricyclic drugs should not be commenced within 2 weeks of stopping a MAOI. The tricyclics are a special risk with people diagnosed with depression because of their severe cardiac toxicity if taken in large doses. Caution is warranted in service users with cardiac disease and with older service users. Tricyclics may also impair reaction times, especially at the beginning of treatment. Alcohol may increase the sedative effects of tricyclics.

Interactions

Tricyclics

Hyperpyretic crisis, seizures or serious cardiac events may occur if administered in conjunction with MAOIs. They may prevent therapeutic effect of some antihypertensives.

MAOIs

Hypertensive crisis may occur if administered with many other drugs including adrenaline (epinephrine), noradrenaline, reserpine, narcotic analgesics and vasoconstrictors. Service users may also experience hypertensive crisis if tyramine-rich foods are ingested.

SSRIs

Alcohol may potentiate effect. The use of an SSRI with **cimetidine** may result in increased concentrations of SSRIs in the bloodstream. A hypertensive crisis may occur if SSRIs are taken within 14 days of MAOIs.

Service user education

Inform the service user of the time it will take for a marked effect to be experienced from the medication and that it is important for them to keep taking the medication even though they have not noticed an initial improvement in their condition.

Other information which service users may need to be advised of include:

- warn of problems when driving or operating machinery if sedation is experienced,
- advise the service user to discuss with their prescriber if they become pregnant or intend to breastfeed,
- warn about the effect that alcohol may have if combined with antidepressant medication,
- inform about possible interactions with foods and other drugs if taking MAOIs.

Mood stabilizers

Lithium carbonate, a naturally occurring salt, is the drug of choice for the treatment of acute mania and for the ongoing maintenance of service users with a diagnostic history of mania. An Australian, John Cade, discovered its effectiveness as a treatment for mania in 1949. Just how lithium works is not clear, but it is known to mimic the effects of sodium, thereby compromising the ability of neurons to release, activate or respond to neurotransmitters. It does appear to reduce the sodium content of the brain, and increase central serotonin synthesis and noradrenaline reuptake (Shupikai Rinomhota and Marshall, 2000). A number of other drugs have also been used successfully, either alone or in combination with lithium, to control the symptoms of mania. The antidepressants and a number of anticonvulsant drugs have also been used very successfully to reduce symptoms of mania.

Indications for use

Lithium

Lithium is the drug of choice for the treatment of acute mania and the ongoing maintenance of people diagnosed with bipolar disorders (Baldessarini and Tarazi, 2001). It is also useful in the treatment of **unipolar** depression, aggressive behaviour, conduct disorder and schizoaffective disorder.

Antipsychotics

A few of the atypical antipsychotics such as olanzapine, quetiapine, aripiprazole and risperidone have demonstrated effectiveness in acute episodes of mania and hypomania. Olanzapine is also being used increasingly as **monotherapy** or in combination with a mood stabilizer such as lithium or valproate for long-term maintenance therapy for bipolar disorder (Taylor et al., 2009).

Anticonvulsants

A number of anticonvulsant drugs have also been used to treat mania, especially when lithium is ineffective. These drugs are now rapidly becoming the drug of choice for many service users. Carbamazepine and valproate are examples of commonly used anticonvulsants. These drugs have been found to have acute antimanic and mood-stabilizing effects. Carbamazepine and valproate are recommended treatments for mixed or bipolar states, secondary mania, rapid cycling and lithium refractoriness (Nassir Ghaemi et al., 2001; Shupikai Rinomhota and Marshall, 2000). Lamotrigine is an anticonvulsant drug which is widely used for bipolar depression both for treatment and for prophylaxis to aid prevention of further episodes. It can reduce the risk of inducing a rapid switch or cycle in mood that can be caused when treating bipolar depression with antidepressants. Antidepressants are often used but with caution for bipolar depression.

Side effects

Lithium

Side effects can include drowsiness, metallic taste in the mouth, difficulty concentrating, increased thirst, dizziness, headache, dry mouth, gastrointestinal upset, nausea/vomiting, fine hand tremor, hypotension, **arrhythmias**, **polyuria**, dehydration and weight gain.

Anticonvulsants

- Carbamazepine: blood **dyscrasias**, drowsiness, nausea, vomiting, constipation or diarrhoea, hives or skin rashes, hepatitis.
- Valproate: prolonged bleeding time, gastrointestinal upset, tremor, **ataxia**, weight gain, somnolence, dizziness, hepatic failure.

Contraindications/precautions

Lithium

Lithium is contraindicated with cardiac or renal disease, dehydration, sodium depletion, brain damage, pregnancy and lactation.

Care should be taken with thyroid disorders, diabetes, urinary retention and history of seizures. The therapeutic range for lithium is 0.6–1.2 mmol/L for acute mania and 0.6–0.8 mmol/L for maintenance, but more conservative levels are increasingly being used. Symptoms of lithium toxicity rarely appear at levels below 1.2 mmol/L but are common above 2.0 mmol/L (Treatment Protocol Project, 2000). Therefore, as the therapeutic and toxic levels are so close, extreme care must be taken in monitoring the service user's blood level regularly, especially during early phases of the treatment. If the level exceeds 1.5 mmol/L the next dose should be withheld and the doctor/prescriber notified. Levels are usually monitored weekly until stable and then monthly. The blood samples for testing should be taken 12 h after the last dose when lithium has been taken for at least 5–7 days.

Anticonvulsants

Anticonvulsants are contraindicated with MAOIs and during lactation. Caution is required in older service users, cardiac/renal disease and pregnancy.

Before commencing carbamazepine a range of tests should be performed, including blood film examination, electrolytes, liver and kidney function. An electrocardiogram (ECG) should be requested should a patient have a heart condition. This is so that patients with an atrioventricular block can be excluded from treatment with the drug as it can exacerbate congestion. Carbamazepine may also interfere with the metabolism and blood concentrations of other drugs, so care is needed with oral contraceptives and other drugs. There is risk of foetal malformation, so it should not be taken during pregnancy.

Valproate should not be taken with aspirin and some antipsychotics as it may reduce the convulsive threshold increasing the risk of seizures. There is an increased risk of neutropenia (low white blood cell count) when given with olanzapine. It can also enhance the effects of alcohol and other CNS depressants. There is also the risk of foetal malformation, so it should be avoided during pregnancy.

Interactions

Lithium

Diuretics, angiotensin-converting-enzyme inhibitors (**ACE inhibitors**), neuroleptics, nonsteroidal anti-inflammatory drugs, alcohol and caffeine may interfere with lithium absorption.

Anticonvulsants

- *Carbamazepine*: erythromycin, isoniazid, oral contraceptives, **theophylline**, fluoxetine.
- *Valproate*: may potentiate alcohol, carbamazepine and barbiturates; should not be taken with aspirin or antipsychotics.
- *Lamotrigine*: renal/liver disease, rash. Lamotrigine can induce reactions such as **Steven–Johnsons syndrome** and toxic epidermal **necrolysis**. Valproate can increase plasma levels of lamotrigine that can lead to serious dermatological conditions such as the two mentioned above; it may also potentiate alcohol.

Service user education

Lithium

- The service user must be informed about the side effects and signs of toxicity (see Box 24.4 and nurse's story), and informed of the need for regular blood levels.
- Encourage a regular intake of about 10 glasses of water every day (approx 2.5 L).
- Take medication regularly even when feeling well.
- Do not operate machinery until initial drowsiness subsides.
- Discuss risks of taking lithium during pregnancy or when considering pregnancy.

Box 24.4 **Signs of lithium toxicity**

Early stages: anorexia, nausea, vomiting, diarrhoea, coarse hand tremor, twitching, lethargy, **dysarthria**, hyperactive deep tendon reflexes, ataxia, tinnitus, vertigo, weakness, drowsiness.

Later stages: fever, decreased urinary output, decreased blood pressure, irregular pulse, ECG changes, impaired consciousness, seizures, coma, death.

Note: lithium toxicity is a medical emergency.

NURSE'S STORY: LITHIUM INTOXICATION

An older service user was admitted to an inpatient unit for an episode of manic behaviour. She had experienced mania before and was on continuous treatment with lithium. The lithium dose was increased during the admission. The nurse returned to the ward after 2 days' leave and noticed that the service user appeared unwell, had a coarse tremor, was confused, ataxic and had myoclonic jerks. She called the doctor on call, expressed her concern and told him she would withhold the evening dose of lithium. She asked him to see the service user as soon as possible and to organize to have blood taken for a lithium level. The doctor refused to come to the ward and disagreed with the nurse's concern about the service user. He insisted she give the evening dose of the medication and said he would see the service user the next morning. The nurse refused to accept his decision and called her immediate supervisor and explained her concern for the service user's wellbeing. The medication was withheld, and an urgent blood request determined that the service user's lithium level was 2.2 mEq/L. The nurse had correctly diagnosed lithium toxicity and taken the correct action to advocate best care for the service user.

Anticonvulsants

- Inform the service user about avoiding sudden cessation of the tablets.
- Encourage service user to report unusual symptoms to the doctor/prescriber, such as spontaneous bruising, unusual bleeding, sore throat, fever, malaise, and yellow skin or eyes.
- Take medications with meals if gastrointestinal upset occurs.
- Avoid taking alcohol or nonprescription drugs without consulting the doctor/prescriber.
- Pregnancy must be avoided while taking the medication.
- Alternative methods of contraception may be required if taking valproate, as oral contraception may not be effective.

Antipsychotic or neuroleptic drugs

The traditional neuroleptic or antipsychotic drugs (also known as the typical antipsychotics) have been an important treatment for psychotic disorders since their discovery in the 1950s. These drugs revolutionized the treatment of mental disorder and soon became the mainstay of treatment for most psychotic disorders. Each group of the traditional antipsychotics appears to be equally effective for the reduction or elimination of 'positive symptoms' of psychosis (for example delusions, hallucinations, motor disturbances) (Treatment Protocol Project, 2000). However, the side-effects profile of the traditional antipsychotics became cause for concern because of their effect on quality of life and their link with non-adherence. The newer second-generation antipsychotics, commonly referred to as the atypicals or novel antipsychotics, were introduced in the 1990s. These drugs are better tolerated and less likely to lead to problems with medication adherence (Davies et al., 1998). Apart from clozapine, which has superior efficacy to the traditional antipsychotics, their efficacy appears to be equal to that of the traditional antipsychotics (Therapeutic Guidelines, 2000), and they are more effective in reducing the negative symptoms of psychosis, such as blunting of affect, **anhedonia**, apathy and lack of volition.

The traditional antipsychotics are dopamine antagonists. They block the **postsynaptic** dopamine subtype 2 (D$_2$) receptors primarily but also exert other synaptic effects. They reduce the 'positive' symptoms of schizophrenia. Atypicals, on the other hand, have D$_2$- and serotonin receptor subtype 2 (5HT$_2$)-blocking action The affinity with the 5HT$_2$ receptors may be why there is a reduction in **extrapyramidal side effects** alongside differences in the affinity with various D$_2$ central receptors. This means that the atypicals might be seen as a little more specific in the effect that they have; that is, not only reducing the positive symptoms of schizophrenia but also having an effect on the negative symptoms without the serious extrapyramidal side effects.

Indications

Antipsychotics are indicated for the treatment of acute and chronic psychoses, delusional disorder and severe depression where psychotic symptoms are present. They are also increasingly indicated for treatment of acute mania. Schizophrenia and schizoaffective disorders are the most common indications for antipsychotic drugs. Some of the phenothiazine group have other uses, such as an anti-emetic in the case of prochlorperazine and the treatment of intractable hiccoughs in the case of chlorpromazine, for example. Many of the antipsychotic drugs, especially the lower-potency ones such as chlorpromazine and haloperidol, have a prominent sedative effect. This effect is particularly conspicuous early in treatment, although **tolerance** usually develops quickly.

Side effects: traditional antipsychotics

The side effects of the traditional antipsychotic drugs are varied. They can affect every system of the body and range from effects on the CNS, including movement disorders, sedation and seizures, through to potentially life-threatening side effects such as neuroleptic malignant syndrome (see Table 24.4 for an overview of the side effects of typical antipsychotics). The most troubling of the side effects are the extrapyramidal reactions. These result from the effects of the antipsychotic drugs on the extrapyramidal motor system. This is the same system responsible for the movement disorders of Parkinson's disease. Acute dystonia, parkinsonism and akathisia occur early and can be managed by a variety of medications including

Table 24.4 Side effects of the traditional antipsychotics

Side effects	Key features	Time of maximal risk	Interventions
CNS extrapyramidal side effects			
Acute dystonic reaction	Painful muscle spasms in head, back and torso; can last minutes to hours, occur suddenly; causes fear	1–5 days	Administer antiparkinsonian drug quickly, respiratory support if needed, reassure and remain with service user
Akathisia	Restlessness, leg aches, person cannot stay still	5–60 days	Administer antiparkinsonian drug, change drug
Parkinsonism	Rigid, mask-like facial expression; shuffling gait; drooling	5–30 days; can recur even after a single dose	Administer dopamine agonist, support service user
Tardive dyskinesia	Results from prolonged use of traditional antipsychotics; stereotyped involuntary movements (tongue, lips, feet)	After months or years of treatment (worse on withdrawal)	Assess service users often, change to atypical drugs, no other treatment available
Neuroleptic malignant syndrome	Potentially fatal with hyperthermia, severe extrapyramidal side effects, sweating, muscle rigidity, clouding of consciousness, elevated **creatine phosphokinase**	Weeks usually	Supportive therapy, cease all medications, treat with **bromocriptine** and **dantrolene**

(continued)

Table 24.4 Continued

Side effects	Key features	Time of maximal risk	Interventions
Seizures	Traditional antipsychotics reduce seizure threshold, risk about 1% but greater with rapid titration or history of seizures	Early in treatment	May need to stop drug, observe service user, or manipulate drug dose
Other side effects			
Sedation	May be beneficial in agitated service users, can be mistaken for cognitive slowing		Educate service user to avoid driving or operating machinery, rest periods, adjust dose
Photosensitivity	Skin hyperpigmentation		Avoid sun, wear protective clothing, sunscreen, sunglasses
Anticholinergic	Dry mouth, blurred vision, orthostatic hypotension, tachycardia, urinary retention, nasal congestion		Observe, educate service user, provide support where needed, may need to change drug
Endocrine	Weight gain, diminished libido, impotence, amenorrhoea, galactorrhoea		Educate service user, reduce caloric intake, may need to change drug

Box 24.5 Useful tools for assessing drug side effects

LUNSERS

The LUNSERS (Liverpool University Neuroleptic Side Effect Rating Scale) is a useful tool for assessing side effects. It is designed for self-administration but can also be a useful tool for nurses to help detect service user reactions to changes in treatment (Morrison et al., 2000). See Day et al. (1995).

AIMS

The AIMS (Abnormal Involuntary Movements Scale) is a widely used tool for use with people on long-term antipsychotic medications. It is designed to assess for signs of tardive dyskinesia. See Munetz and Benjamin (1988).

GASS

The GASS (Glasgow Antipsychotic Rating Scale) is increasingly used as a scale to measure the number and severity of side effects individuals experience related to antipsychotic medication. See Waddell and Taylor (2008).

Box 24.6 Neuroleptic malignant syndrome

Neuroleptic malignant syndrome is a rare disorder that resembles a severe form of parkinsonism with coarse tremor and **catatonia**, fluctuating in intensity, accompanied by signs of autonomic instability (labile pulse and blood pressure, hyperthermia), stupor, elevation of creatine phosphokinase in serum and sometimes **myoglobinaemia**. In severe forms it may persist for more than a week after ceasing the medication. The risk of death from this syndrome is high (more than 10%); therefore immediate medical intervention is required if suspected.

Source: Baldessarini and Tarazi (2001).

potentially life-threatening (see Box 24.6). More information on traditional antipsychotic side effects can be found in the following articles: Usher (2001) (for particular emphasis on the service user's perspective), Usher and Happell (1996, 1997) and Arana (2000).

NURSE'S STORY: ANTIPSYCHOTIC DRUG SIDE EFFECTS

I remember talking to a young man, diagnosed with schizophrenia, about the side effects he was experiencing as a result of taking a number of the traditional antipsychotics. The experiences he described made me

the antiparkinsonian and benzodiazepine drugs. Tardive dyskinesia generally occurs later and has no effective treatment. The Abnormal Involuntary Movements Scale (AIMS) (see Box 24.5) is a useful tool for nurses to detect movement disorders in their service users. Neuroleptic malignant syndrome, an idiosyncratic hypersensitivity to antipsychotic drugs, is a rare but serious reaction that is aware of the serious impact these drugs can have on a person's life. For example, he described how the akathisia he experienced was so extreme that he felt it was no longer worth living. The choice between taking the drug, which he experienced extreme pressure to do, and experiencing the side effects (especially akathisia, which was not resolved by any other treatment), or not taking the drugs and living with the symptoms of the disorder, caused him a great deal of confusion and distress. He said there were many times when he considered suicide the only option, as he could see no way out of the predicament. He believed that living with the side effects caused such a poor quality of life that it was possibly not worth being alive. Similarly, he also experienced suicidal thoughts when the symptoms of the disorder were at its worst. He also told me how he believed the drug side effects made him recognizable by others as 'mentally ill'. This also caused him a great deal of personal distress as he remembered times when he felt conspicuous due to the visible drug side effects. He also recalled a time when he visited his sister's house, where he believed his drug side effects caused the whole family embarrassment, as the side effects drew people's attention to him and to his behaviour. This man's experience of the side effects of psychotropic drugs made me realize the importance of listening to the service user's side of the treatment story and helped me to become more cognisant of the issues surrounding medication adherence.

Antiparkinsonian medications

Antiparkinsonian medications, also referred to as anticholinergics, are used to reduce the extrapyramidal side effects that are caused primarily by traditional antipsychotic medications. Antiparkinsonian drugs with a central anticholinergic action inhibit the action of acetylcholine and are presumed to decrease the cholinergic influence in basal ganglia, which helps symptoms associated with parkinsonism, acute **dystonia** and akathisia. This therefore helps counter the effects of blocking dopamine in the brain pathway that effects movement and is associated with extrapyramidal side effects (Therapeutic Guidelines, 2000). (See Table 24.5 for their action and side effects.)

However, antiparkinsonian drugs are not routinely administered, as many service users taking antipsychotic medication do not experience extrapyramidal effects. The antiparkinsonian medications also have their own set of unwanted effects and there is considerable intentional misuse of these drugs for euphoric and sometimes hallucinogenic effects.

Side effects: atypical antipsychotics

The atypical antipsychotics may have some annoying side effects such as weight gain, constipation, dizziness and paradoxical hypersalivation, which occurs primarily during

Table 24.5 Antiparkinsonian medication: action and side effects

Name	Action	General side effects (dose-related)
Benztropine mesylate	Antihistamine and sedating qualities, long-acting	(Anticholinergic) Dry mouth, dilated pupils, urinary hesitancy, constipation, blurred vision, nausea
Benzhexol	Specific anticholinergic action, stimulant properties	Dizziness, hallucinations
Biperiden	Anticholinergic action	Euphoria, hyperpyrexia
Orphenadrine	Anticholinergic action	Delirium in older people

sleep. They may also cause extrapyramidal side effects at higher doses. Seizures may also occur with too rapid a titration associated with increase in dosage. In addition, cardiac problems such as atrial fibrillation, atrial flutter or myocarditis early in treatment, although uncommon, may occur.

- Clozapine: a serious adverse effect is the potential for **agranulocytosis**, which occurs in approximately 1–2% of service users. Precautions must be taken to ensure swift detection of this side effect should it occur.
- Risperidone: insomnia, agitation, anxiety, headache, postural hypotension particularly at the commencement of treatment, drowsiness, weight gain, gastrointestinal upset, sexual disturbance and extrapyramidal side effects.
- Olanzapine: drowsiness, weight gain, postural hypotension, peripheral oedema, extrapyramidal side effects and anticholinergic side effects (dry mouth, hypotension, tachycardia).
- Quetiapine: mild somnolence, mild **asthenia**, dry mouth, limited weight gain, postural hypotension, tachycardia and occasional syncope.
- Aripiprazole: gastrointestinal disturbance, tachycardia, asthenia, insomnia, **akathisia** (inner restlessness), drowsiness, tremor, headache, blurred vision.

Contraindications/precautions

Traditional antipsychotics

Caution should be taken in administering these drugs to older people and to medically ill or diabetic people.

Safety in pregnancy and lactation is not clear. They are contraindicated in people with a known sensitivity to one of the phenothiazines as a cross-sensitivity is possible. People taking typical antipsychotics should avoid extremes of temperature.

Atypical antipsychotics: clozapine

People taking clozapine must be made aware of the potential risk of agranulocytosis and be monitored regularly. Due to the drug's link to agranulocytosis it is restricted to those who have not responded to at least two other antipsychotics (National Institute for Health and Clinical Excellence, 2009). Clozapine can only be prescribed through a strict service user-monitoring programme. The service user's blood should be monitored weekly for 18 weeks and monthly thereafter. An immediate differential blood count measures the percentage of each type of white blood cell (WBC) in the blood, which can reveal problems such as abnormal cells. The test must be ordered if the service user reports flu-like symptoms. If during treatment an infection occurs and/or the WBC count has dropped below 3500/mm^3, or has dropped by a substantial amount from baseline, a repeat WBC and differential count should be done. If the results confirm a WBC below 3500/mm^3 and/or reveal an **absolute neutrophil granulocyte count** of between 1500 and 2000/mm^3, the leucocytes and granulocytes must be checked at least twice weekly. If the WBC falls below 3000/mm^3 and/or the absolute neutrophil granulocyte drops below 1500/mm^3, clozapine must be withdrawn at once and the service user closely monitored. Care should be taken when using these drugs with older people.

Interactions

Traditional antipsychotics

Concurrent use with antidepressants, antihistamines and antiparkinsonian agents may result in additional anticholinergic effects. Antacids and antidiarrhoeals may disrupt absorption of the antipsychotic. Alcohol may cause additional CNS depression.

Atypical antipsychotics

Drugs known to have substantial potential to depress bone marrow function should be avoided concurrently with clozapine. Atypical antipsychotics may enhance the effect of alcohol and other CNS depressants.

Smoking

Smoking can speed up the metabolism of clozapine; should a service user decide to give up smoking then their dose may need to be adjusted to counter increased plasma levels of the drug following cessation.

Service user education

Traditional antipsychotics

The service user will need information about the drug side effects and help with maintaining adherence. People taking typical antipsychotics should be careful in the sun (due to the drugs' known effect of increasing photosensitivity) and in extremes of temperature.

Atypical antipsychotics

Advice about having regular blood levels should be provided. Service users should be told the importance of seeing a doctor/prescriber immediately for any flu-like symptoms while taking clozapine. Information on possible side effects and drug interactions should be provided.

PRN (AS-NEEDED) ANTIPSYCHOTIC DRUG ADMINISTRATION

The need to reduce agitation, distress or aggression rapidly often results in the prescription and administration of an as-needed (*pro re nata*, or PRN) antipsychotic medication (Whicher et al., 2002) in inpatient mental health services. Antipsychotics and benzodiazepines are the main classes of medications used in this way. Approximately three-quarters of inpatients receive PRN medications during the course of their admission and at least half of these receive more than one dose (Curtis and Capp, 2003; Dean et al., 2006; Thapa et al., 2003). These medications are usually administered orally or by intramuscular injection. Once a PRN regimen is instigated, it should be reviewed at regular interviews by an independent prescriber for its frequency of use and clinical effectiveness. Generally, most PRN medications are given in the first few days after admission and are most frequently administered during the evening shift, from 6 p.m. onwards, and at weekends (Fishel et al., 1994; Gray and Smedley, 1996; McKenzie et al., 1999; Usher et al., 2001). It appears that peaks in PRN administration coincide with regular medication and meal times (Gray et al., 1997; Stratton-Powell, 2001). Reasons given for administering the PRN medications in mental health settings often include agitation, irritability, insomnia and request by the service user (O'Brien and Cole, 2004; Usher et al., 2001). Environmental influences have also been suggested. The study by Usher et al. (2007) proposed that the physical and psychological environment in which the service users were cared for had an effect on the individual's sense of security and adversely affected their mental health, causing anxiety, agitation and frustration, and ultimately aggression, which in turn affected their need to resort to PRN medications.

When nurses give PRN they are often required to decide what to give from a range of medications, as well as the amount to give, and when to administer (Usher et al.,

2003). This allows for nurses to administer psychotropic medications rapidly in acute situations or at the request of the service user (Whicher et al., 2002). The drugs most often prescribed for PRN administration have been the traditional antipsychotics, particularly drugs like haloperidol. There is now evidence to suggest that the benzodiazepines are just as effective as the traditional antipsychotics in managing acute agitation and disturbed behaviour and should therefore be the drug of choice (Geffen et al., 2002; Usher and Luck, 2004). However, examination of current practice indicates that this is not happening and that the traditional antipsychotics are being used predominantly for PRN treatment of psychotic disturbance (Geffen et al., 2002; Usher et al., 2001).

NURSE'S STORY: USING PRN MEDICATION

I have worked in an inpatient mental health service for some time. I clearly remember working with Adam, a 30-year-old man diagnosed with chronic schizophrenia who had been a client of the mental health service for the past 10 years, and had had numerous admissions to hospital. Adam's admissions were usually precipitated by ceasing his medication, increased substance use, hostile behaviour towards others, damage to property including setting fire to clothes and furniture, and a deterioration in mental state with increased paranoid thinking and delusional beliefs about the government.

During one particular admission, Adam was verbally aggressive towards staff. Adam would respond to his delusional beliefs and paranoid ideas, and this resulted in damage to property as he believed that certain items were harmful to him or had cameras hidden in them.

Adam didn't like taking medication, as he believed he didn't need it. He said he had experienced side effects from haloperidol, chlorpromazine and zuclopenthixol decanoate. He had clear signs of increasing arousal prior to his violent outbursts: he would look agitated, and pace the unit and mutter to himself, and on occasions he would approach staff and be verbally abusive. The staff observed that Adam would settle with PRN clonazepam and haloperidol. However, Adam began refusing the haloperidol.

Some of the staff did not give PRN medication when he was pacing and agitated. There were a number of incidents where a PRN drug was not given and Adam physically assaulted staff and property, resulting in the use of seclusion and the administration of intramuscular medication.

I was concerned about this situation because I felt it just reinforced Adam's reluctance to take medication. I decided to talk with the staff about some strategies we could all use so that there was a consistent approach to Adam's need for PRN medication. I sat down with Adam and talked to him about his concerns and found that he was agreeable and willing to take PRN clonazepam, which was administered in liquid form. However, he was very clear that he wouldn't take haloperidol as he experienced quite a few side effects from it. After discussion with his psychiatrist regarding the antipsychotic component of the PRN medication, the staff eventually managed to get Adam to agree to taking PRN medication by developing a trusting relationship with him and educating him about his medication regimen.

The authors acknowledge this contribution from Corianne Richardson, Clinical Nurse Specialist

MEDICATION CONCORDANCE

Acceptance of, and agreement with, prescribed psychotropic medication is an ongoing problem for service users diagnosed with disorders such as schizophrenia. In the past, this issue has been referred to in the literature as noncompliance or nonadherence. However, the term compliance implies a power differential between the service user and the healthcare provider, and also implies passive rather than active participation by the service user in the management of their mental health. Adherence can be seen as the extent to which the patient's behaviour matches agreed recommendations from the prescriber. The accepted term is now *concordance*, it seeks to promote a collaborative, shared decision making framework in relation to medication. It can be seen as a process rather than a behaviour, acknowledging a service user's view and respecting it even if they make a decision that is different from the healthcare professional's recommendation.

Nonconcordance can often lead to relapse and readmission to hospital. In fact, concordance with an antipsychotic medication regimen has been claimed as the single most important factor in deferring admission (Fernando et al., 1990). The issue of medication concordance is complex and multifaceted (Happell et al., 2002) but rarely includes the voice of the service user (Happell et al., 2004).

Causes of nonconcordance are related to issues such as drug side effects, where the antipsychotic medication may have an adverse impact on the person's quality of life (Keks, 1996) and may even cause more distress than the symptoms of the disorder (Usher, 2001), insight into their mental health problems (Schwarz et al., 1998) and lack of education about the medications (Coudreaut-Quinn et al., 1992). Despite informed choice, people sometimes stop taking their medications and, because they do not relapse immediately, fail to see the connection between the medications and their health (Treatment Protocol Project, 2000). Box 24.7 demonstrates some factors that can influence concordance.

Box 24.7 **Factors affecting concordance**

Disorder-related	Treatment-related	Prescriber-related	Person-related	Environmental	Cultural
Denial of disorder	Unwanted side effects	Authoritative	Disorganized lifestyle	Support from family	Religious beliefs
Severity of disorder	Route of administration	Not explaining	Forgetting to take medication	Peer pressure	Family influences
Level of disability	Lack of satisfaction	Not having faith/confidence in prescriber	Beliefs about illness	Contact with other users	Peer pressure
Rate of disorder progression	Fear of side effects	Lack of access to prescriber	Beliefs about treatment	Media	Access to alternative treatments
Impact of disorder on lifestyle	Poor symptom control	Lack of follow-up	Embarrassment	Access to alternative treatments	The National Health Service
	Previous negative experiences	Prescriber overworked	Fear of being stigmatized		
	Not seeing immediate benefits	Service over-burdened	Cognitive deficits		
	Misunderstanding treatment	Lack of training in appropriate interventions to improve adherence	Low self esteem		
	Frequent changes in treatment		Poor motivation		
	Duration of treatment	Irregular medication review	Lack of perceived risk illness poses		
			Low treatment expectations		

To help overcome lack of concordance with antipsychotic medication, a number of strategies have been explored (see Box 24.8). Evidence suggests that an active relationship between the nurse and the service user is essential for improving concordance (Bebbington et al., 1996; Vivian and Wilcox, 2000). Other helpful strategies to aid concordance include education about the medications and their side effects (Coudreaut-Quinn et al., 1992), frequent follow-up and support (Phan, 1992) and motivational interviewing (Kemp et al., 1996). In 2007 The National Prescribing Centre set out a competency framework for shared decision making with patients (Figure 24.1). The aim of this framework was to support clinicians in improving concordance with medication. It outlined three core competency areas: building a partnership, managing a shared consultation and sharing a decision.

It appears that no strategy is sufficient on its own, and a mixed approach to concordance may in fact be the best approach. However, it is clear that concordance to the newer atypical antipsychotics is not such a problem (Davies et al., 1998), probably because many of their side effects are less likely to cause extrapyramidal side effects.

Box 24.8 **Interventions to help with concordance to medication**

- Get to know your service user well.
- Help your service user develop an understanding of why the medications have been prescribed.
- Spend time talking about medications and the decisions related to concordance.
- Ask about the side effects being experienced and offer strategies to manage side effects where possible.
- Help the service user discuss issues related to their medications with their prescriber, doctor or nurse.
- Provide information and teaching sessions for family or significant others.

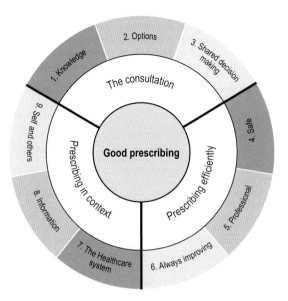

Figure 24.1 Competency framework for shared decision-making with patients.

National Prescribing Centre 2012. Adapted from page 9 'A single competency framework for all prescribers'. May 2012 London: NICE. Available from http://www.npc.co.uk/improving_safety/improving_quality/ resources/single_comp_framework.pdf. Reproduced with permission.

CASE STUDY: NONCONCORDANCE WITH PSYCHOTROPIC MEDICATIONS (PART A)

Tony was first diagnosed with paranoid schizophrenia 5 years ago. His symptoms were exacerbated by poor concordance to prescribed medications and 'self-medication' with cannabis. Despite it being objectively clear that cannabis use made him more paranoid, Tony felt that it helped him relax and was dismissive of education about harm-minimization or abstaining.

The main hurdle to concordance with prescribed medication for Tony was denial. Tony did not accept his diagnosis; consequently, he did not accept his treatment. If we accept that a diagnosis of schizophrenia would provoke a sense of loss (e.g. normalcy, altered levels of independence, re-evaluated life goals, decreased acceptance), we may be able to understand the denial as a component of grief. Tony certainly displayed other classic stages of grief, most notably anger (at his psychiatrist) and bargaining (with his community case manager regarding postponing or cancelling administration of depot medications).

Other contributing factors to Tony's nonconcordance included the disorder itself: paranoia is a barrier to building trust and rapport with clinicians; lack of education/ understanding about the disorder and its treatment; and side effects of prescribed medications.

CRITICAL THINKING CHALLENGE 24.1

Denial is a commonly used defence mechanism when a person is faced with issues they are not yet able to cope with on a conscious level. Discuss the concept of denial as a component of grief and loss in relation to the diagnosis of a chronic mental health problem. How does the concept of denial differ from that of insight? In part A of the case study, how could the nurse manage Tony's nonconcordance while recognizing the importance of denial as a coping mechanism?

Explore relevant strategies to address the other factors contributing to Tony's nonconcordance, such as his paranoia, lack of education and understanding, and unwanted side effects.

CASE STUDY: NONCONCORDANCE TO PSYCHOTROPIC MEDICATIONS (PART B)

A management plan was developed to address the factors contributing to Tony's nonconcordance. Tony's outpatient care was assigned to a community mental health nurse. This nurse administered and monitored prescribed medications and worked to build a therapeutic alliance with him. When Tony was an inpatient, as occurred frequently during the first 3 years of diagnosis, he was assigned a primary nurse on the mental health unit, who collaborated with the community nurse to provide continuity of care and another avenue for Tony to develop rapport.

Over time, Tony began to engage with his two primary carers, which provided an opportunity for education about his diagnosis and treatment options. In time, Tony became more accepting of the treating team as a whole, and would discuss medication issues freely with his psychiatrist.

As Tony's acceptance improved, medication options were no longer restricted to depot injections, and oral medications were trialled. Tony was very sensitive to traditional antipsychotics and developed extrapyramidal side effects at subtherapeutic doses. Trials of other atypical antipsychotic medications also had problems: poor symptom control and marked weight gain.

Twelve months ago a trial of clozapine commenced. It took 4 months to stabilize the dose at 450 mg *nocte* (at night). In doing so, Tony's mental state also stabilized. He developed considerable insight into his condition and treatment, and has developed a good degree of acceptance.

Nine months later, with encouragement from the community team, Tony undertook a trial of abstinence from cannabis. Tony says he has used cannabis only twice since. This hasn't been objectively checked through urine samples, but his community nurse has noted further improvement in symptom control and motivation to undertake activities of daily living and social interaction.

Tony has not required admission to the mental health unit for over 8 months now. If he remains stable until the new year, his community nurse intends to assist Tony in seeking work.

The authors acknowledge this contribution from Paul McNamara.

Table 24.6 Depot antipsychotic drugs

Name	Route	Typical maintenance dosage
Zuclopenthixol decanoate	Intramuscular	200–500 mg every 2–4 weeks
Fluphenazine decanoate	Intramuscular	12.5–100 mg every 2–4 weeks
Flupentixol decanoate	Intramuscular	50–300 mg every 2–4 weeks

CRITICAL THINKING CHALLENGE 24.2

In part B of the case study, Tony was trialled on atypical antipsychotics. How does this group of medications differ from typical antipsychotics? Identify the benefits and disadvantages of each of these drug groups.

The incidence of extrapyramidal side effects varies according to the particular antipsychotic medication used. Identify the various extrapyramidal side effects and explore the most effective management for these.

Tony was trialled on clozapine. What are the benefits and disadvantages of using this particular antipsychotic drug? Why is it not necessarily the first drug of choice for service users experiencing symptoms of psychosis?

Cannabis is commonly used by service users diagnosed with a mental health problem. What are the possible reason(s) for this? What does the term 'self-medicating' mean? Explore the effect(s) of cannabis when a person has a psychosis.

Critically analyse the strategies in the management plan used for Tony's nonconcordance. In your opinion, was the plan successful? If so (or not), explain the reason(s) for this.

DEPOT PREPARATION OF ANTIPSYCHOTIC DRUGS

Depot antipsychotic preparations, introduced in the 1960s, are useful where there might be problems with concordance with oral medications, where the service user is unable to take oral medications or if intestinal absorption is questioned. They are long-acting, injectable forms of the traditional antipsychotic drugs, produced mostly in the form of **decanoate esters** dissolved in an oily base. When administered by deep intramuscular injection, the drug is de-esterified to release the active drug, which slowly diffuses into the circulation. The injections are usually given every 2–4 weeks (Therapeutic Guidelines, 2000) (see Table 24.6) and generally the release of the drug must last at least 1 week to be considered a depot preparation (Dencker and Axelsson, 1996). However, it is important

to remember that a well-targeted nurse–service user relationship can help to promote medication concordance (Marland et al., 1999) and that the service user has a right to be involved in choosing the route of administration of prescribed medications wherever possible.

PSYCHOTROPIC DRUG USE IN SPECIAL POPULATIONS

Pregnant and lactating women

The care of women who are pregnant or lactating poses a significant challenge for the mental health nurse. The prescription and administration of psychotropic drugs, if required during pregnancy and lactation, presents many risks to the unborn foetus or the newborn child. Antipsychotic drugs, especially the atypical antipsychotics, commonly prescribed for women who experience psychoses during pregnancy or in the immediate postpartum period (Webb et al., 2004), have not been proved safe in pregnancy, and their use in pregnancy is not based on evidence from randomized clinical trials (Usher et al., 2005). However, the consequences of untreated mental health problems during pregnancy must be weighed against the risk of prenatal exposure to drugs, as antenatal psychological distress is known to be linked to premature labour, low birth weight, smaller head circumference and inferior functional assessments in the newborn (Viguera and Cohen, 1998). The evidence of the **teratogenic effects** of psychotropic drugs is mixed, and their use during pregnancy can expose the foetus to an increased risk of congenital malformation. Drugs such as lithium, valproate, lamotrigine and carbamazepine are known to have teratogenic effects in early pregnancy, as well as probable adverse effects.

- Antipsychotics, including depot injections, should be avoided in the first trimester.
- Women prescribed atypicals should change to traditional antipsychotics as soon as pregnancy is diagnosed.

- Pregnant and breastfeeding women should be prescribed the lowest possible dose.
- Depot injections should be avoided in breastfeeding women.
- Only infants born at full term should be exposed to the potential to ingest medication via breast milk.

Children

Although psychotropic drugs have been used with children for several decades, the use of these drugs with children should be carefully monitored. Children are particularly vulnerable to the cardiotoxic and seizure-inducing effects of high doses of tricyclic compounds. Deaths have been reported in children after accidental or deliberate overdosage with as little as a few hundred milligrams of a tricyclic drug (Baldessarini, 2001). Therefore, the nurse must be particularly vigilant if working with children who are prescribed psychotropic drugs.

Older people

Particular care must be taken when psychotropic drugs are considered for use with older service users (see Ch. 13). It is generally considered that older people will experience more adverse effects from psychotropic drug use, especially people over the age of 70, due to slower drug metabolism and excretion. For example, benzodiazepines are more likely to cause dizziness, which can lead to falls and serious injury (Shupikai Rinomhota and Marshall, 2000). Antidepressants in older people can be problematic and are more likely to cause dizziness, postural hypotension, constipation, delayed micturition, oedema and tremor (Baldessarini, 2001). It is important for mental health nurses to be aware of the special problems these drugs may pose when used with older service users and to be vigilant in supervising and monitoring side effects. Polypharmacy may have dire consequences for this group and should be avoided wherever possible.

NONMEDICAL PRESCRIBING

The beginnings of nurse prescribing go as far back as 1986 following the Cumberledge Report which made recommendations for community nurses to be able to prescribe a few items that would reduce the time for which it took service users to get access to those common treatments. Following these recommendations two reviews of prescribing by Dr July Crown gave way to the development of nonmedical prescribing in the UK (Nuttall, 2011). The first report was published in 1989 and made the recommendations that after special training district nurses and health visitors could prescribe from a very limited list. This report also led to nurses being able to administer certain drugs under 'group protocols'.

The second of the Crown reports was published in 1997 and group protocols were replaced with *patient group directions* (PGDs). PGDs were introduced in 2000. A PGD is a prewritten set of instructions for the supply and administration of certain service user groups; for example, a single dose of diazepam for agitation in someone who is acutely psychotic. PGDs are not the same as prescribing, but they do extend the powers of drug administration for nurses who have undergone the required training (National Prescribing Centre, 2009).

This second Crown report also introduced two types of nurse prescribing: independent prescribing and supplementary prescribing. Independent prescribing means that the nurse takes full responsibility for their prescribing practice and is accountable for the assessment of service users with both diagnosed and undiagnosed conditions: they can initialize, monitor and review treatment without support from a medical doctor. Supplementary prescribing is when a nurse enters partnership with a medical doctor/dentist and service user. They may prescribe under a clinical management plan (CMP) that has been agreed by all parties.

Since 1992 there have been various changes in the law which have seen a gradual development in the role of the nurse as a prescriber. In 1994 (following a 4-year pilot) nurses were able to gain a Nursing and Midwifery Council (NMC) recordable qualification that would allow them to prescribe from the *Nurse Prescribers' Formulary* once they had registered the qualification with the NMC. This formulary still exists for those original NMC-registered nurse prescribers and is now known as the *Nurse Prescribers' Formulary for Community Practitioners*. Another form of independent nurse prescribing was introduced in 2002 that allowed nurses who had received further training to prescribe from the *Nurse Prescribers' Extended Formulary*. This formulary extended the range of drugs that nurses could prescribe for specified conditions (Beckwith and Franklin, 2006).

The most significant change occurred in May 2006 when the full *British National Formulary* was permitted for use by nurses (excluding some controlled drugs). Nurses are only allowed to prescribe within their area of competence and must have completed a specific training programme in line with NMC standards. To enter a nurse prescribing programme nurses must have a minimum of 3 years post-qualifying experience and be signed off as competent in their assessment and diagnostic knowledge and skills. They also require sponsorship from a medical doctor who will act as a mentor throughout the 6-month training programme (NMC, 2006).

There are an increasing number of nonmedical prescribers working in mental health settings: the role increases the speed that service users get access to treatment, particularly out of hours, and can reduce hospital admission. Nursing skills can also bring benefit to the role in relation to concordance and therapeutic drug monitoring; this ultimately means better outcomes in terms of service user satisfaction and care (Latter, 2010).

NMC STANDARDS OF MEDICINES MANAGEMENT

In 2007 the NMC published their latest standards for medicines management. These standards aim to set a benchmark for which practice is measured in terms of the role of the nurse in medicines management. The NMC states that:

> *The administration of medicines is an important aspect of the professional practice of persons whose names are on the Council's register. It is not solely a mechanistic task to be performed in strict compliance with the written prescription of a medical practitioner [can now also be an independent and supplementary prescriber]. It requires thought and the exercise of professional judgement.*

(NMC, 2007, p. 1)

The standards cover the safe administration (including health and safety, checking and dispensing of drugs and the legal administration of controlled drugs) and the storage and transportation of medicines. The standards require that nurses who administer medication:

- are certain of the identity of the service user to whom the medicine is to be administered,
- are sure that the service user is not allergic to the medicine before administering it,
- know about the therapeutic uses of the medicine to be administered, its normal dosage, side effects, precautions and contraindications,
- are aware of the service user's plan of care,
- have checked both that the prescription or the label on the dispensed medicine is clearly written and unambiguous, and includes the expiry date (where it exists) of the medicine to be administered,
- have considered the dosage, the service user's weight where appropriate, method of administration, route and timing,

- administer or withhold in the context of the service user's condition (for example, if the service user is experiencing side effects),
- contacts the prescriber immediately where there are contraindications to the prescribed medicine, where the service user develops a reaction to the medicine or where the medicine is no longer suitable,
- makes a clear, accurate and immediate record of all medicine administered, intentionally withheld or refused by the service user, ensuring the signature is clear and legible (NMC, 2007).

Nurses are accountable for the administration of medication, even when this task has been delegated.

To see the full, in-depth guidelines, visit http://www.nmc-uk.org/Documents/Standards/nmcStandardsForMedicinesManagementBooklet.pdf.

CONCLUSION

This chapter has presented an overview of the issues related to psychopharmacology and medicines management, including the use of PRN psychotropic drugs, concordance with the drugs as prescribed and their use with special populations. To be effective practitioners, mental health nurses also need to be equipped with knowledge and understanding of the distinct drug indications, interactions, side effects and precautions related to the four major psychotropic medication groups (anti-anxiety, antidepressant, mood-stabilizing and antipsychotic). The skilled mental health nurse needs to have a working knowledge of psychopharmacology, as well as the related issues, as the administration of these drugs is a common but important nursing intervention. The information presented here will help to prepare the mental health nurse to make well-informed treatment decisions and engage in successful service user education. It will also help the nurse to detect and manage side effects from the psychotropic drugs, many of which can be harmful or even life-threatening.

EXERCISES FOR CLASS ENGAGEMENT

In a small group discuss the legal and ethical issues that a mental health nurse needs to consider when administering psychotropic medications. In particular, consider the issues related to concordance within inpatient settings.

As a group, outline what you believe are the important issues related to medication concordance. How might your beliefs differ from those of others? Larger group discussion to follow.

In small groups, debate and respond to the following questions.

- How would you manage a situation where you were of the opinion that a service user was being prescribed and administered a toxic level of a drug?
- Describe how polypharmacy can be a problem for people taking antipsychotic medications and for members of vulnerable groups, such as older people.

◆ Describe the signs of a tricyclic overdose and list those who might be at high risk of such an outcome.

◆ Anticonvulsant drugs are used in the management of people with bipolar disorders. Describe the action of these drugs and list their potential side effects.

◆ Lithium is commonly used as a mood-stabilizing drug. Outline why it is important to obtain regular blood tests for people taking this drug, and outline the therapeutic range and signs of lithium toxicity.

◆ The MAOIs, although used to treat depression, are no longer a popular choice. Outline the reasons why this is the case.

REFERENCES

Arana, G.W., 2000. An overview of side effects caused by typical antipsychotics. J. Clin. Psychiatry 61 (Suppl. 8), 5–13.

Baldessarini, R.J., 2001. Drugs and the treatment of psychiatric disorders: depression and anxiety disorders. In: Hardman, J.G., Limbard, L.E., Gilman, A.G. (Eds.), Goodman and Gilman's the Pharmacological Basis of Therapeutics, tenth ed. McGraw-Hill, New York, pp. 447–483.

Baldessarini, R.J., Tarazi, F., 2001. Drugs and the treatment of psychiatric disorders: psychosis and mania. In: Hardman, J.G., Limbard, L.E., Gilman, A.G. (Eds.), Goodman and Gilman's the Pharmacological Basis of Therapeutics, tenth ed. McGraw-Hill, New York, pp. 485–543.

Ballanger, J., 2000. Benzodiazepine receptor agonists and antagonists. In: Sadock, B., Sadock, V. (Eds.), Comprehensive Textbook of Psychiatry, seventh ed. Lippincott Williams & Wilkins, Philadelphia.

Battaglia, J., Moss, S., Rush, J., et al., 1997. Haloperidol, lorazepam, or both for psychotic agitation? A multicenter, prospective, double blind emergency department study. Am. J. Emerg. Med. 15 (4), 335–340.

Bebbington, P., Brewin, C.R., Marsden, L., et al., 1996. Measuring the need for psychiatric treatment in the general population: the community version of the MRC needs for care assessment. Psychol. Med. 26 (2), 229–236.

Beckwith, S., Franklin, P., 2006. The Oxford Handbook of Nurse Prescribing. Oxford University Press, Oxford.

Coudreaut-Quinn, E.A., Emmons, M.A., McMorrow, M.J., 1992. Self-medication during inpatient psychiatric treatment. J. Psychosoc. Nurs. 30 (12), 32–36.

Curtis, J., Capp, K., 2003. Administration of 'as needed' psychotropic medication: a retrospective study. Int. J. Ment. Health Nurs. 12, 229–234.

Davies, A., Adena, M.A., Keks, N.A., et al., 1998. Risperidone versus haloperidol: a meta-analysis of efficacy and safety. Clin. Ther. 20 (1), 58–71.

Day, J.C., Wood, G., Dewey, M., et al., 1995. A self-rating scale for measuring neuroleptic side effects: validation in a group of schizophrenic patients. Br. J. Psychiatry 166 (5), 650–653.

Dean, A.J., McDermott, B.M., Marshall, R.T., 2006. PRN sedation-patterns of prescribing and administration in a child and adolescent mental health inpatient service. Eur. Child Adolesc. Psychiatry 15 (5), 277–281.

Dencker, J.S., Axelsson, R., 1996. Optimising the use of depot antipsychotics. Cent. Nerv. Syst. Drugs 6 (5), 367–381.

Fernando, M.L., Velamoor, V.R., Cooper, A.J., 1990. Some factors relating to satisfactory post-discharge community maintenance of chronic psychotic patients. Can. J. Psychiatry 35 (1), 71–73.

Fishel, A.H., Ferreiro, B.W., Rynerson, B.C., et al., 1994. As needed psychotropic medications: prevalence, indications and results. J. Psychosoc. Nurs. 32 (8), 27–32.

Galbraith, A., Bullock, S., Manias, E., et al., 2007. Fundamentals of Pharmacology: An Applied Approach for Nursing and Health, second ed. Pearson Education, Harlow.

Garza-Trevino, E., Hollister, L., Overall, J., 1989. Efficacy of combinations of intramuscular antipsychotics and sedative hypnotics for control of psychotic agitation. Am. J. Psychiatry 146 (12), 1599–1601.

Geffen, J., Sorensen, L., Stokes, J., et al., 2002. Pro re nata medication for psychoses: an audit of practice in two metropolitan hospitals. Aust. N. Z. J. Psychiatry 36 (5), 649–656.

Gray, R., Smedley, N., 1996. Administration of PRN medication by mental health nurses. Br. J. Nurs. 5 (21), 1317–1322.

Gray, R., Smedley, N., Thomas, B., 1997. The administration of PRN medication by mental health nurses. J. Psychiatr. Ment. Health Nurs. 4 (1), 55–56.

Happell, B., Manias, E., Pinikahana, J., 2002. The role of the inpatient mental health nurse in facilitating patient concordance to medication regimes. Aust. N. Z. J. Ment. Health Nurs. 11 (4), 251–259.

Happell, B., Manias, E., Roper, C., 2004. Wanting to be heard: mental health consumers' experiences of information about medication. Int. J. Ment. Health Nurs. 13, 242–248.

Keks, N.A., 1996. Minimizing the non-extrapyramidal side effects of antipsychotics. Acta Psychiatr. Scand. 389 (Suppl.), 18–24.

Kemp, R., David, A., Hayward, P., 1996. Compliance therapy: an intervention targeting insight and treatment concordance in psychotic patients. Behav. Cogn. Psychother. 24 (4), 331–350.

Kingsbury, S.J., Yi, D., Simpson, M., 2001. Psychopharmacology: rational and irrational polypharmacy. Psychiatr. Serv. 52 (8), 1033–1036.

Latter, S., 2010. Promoting concordance in prescribing interactions. In: Courtney, M., Griffiths, M. (Eds.), Independent and Supplementary Prescribing: An Essential Guide, second ed. Cambridge University Press, Cambridge, pp. 107–118.

McKenzie, A., Kudinoff, T., Benson, A., et al., 1999. Administration of PRN medication: a descriptive study of nursing practice. Aust. N. Z. J. Ment. Health Nurs. 8 (4), 187–191.

Marland, G.R., Sharkey, V., Ward, E., 1999. Depot neuroleptics, schizophrenia and the role of the nurse: is practice evidence based? J. Adv. Nurs. 30 (6), 1255–1262.

Medicines and Healthcare Products Regulatory Agency, 2004. Report of the CSM Expert Working group on the safety of selective serotonin reuptake inhibitor antidepressants. <http://www.mhra.gov.uk/ home/groups/pl-p/documents/ drugsafetymessage/con019472.pdf>.

Morrison, P., Gaskill, D., Meehan, T., et al., 2000. The use of the Liverpool University neuroleptic side-effect rating scale (LUNSERS) in clinical practice. Aust. N. Z. J. Ment. Health Nurs. 9 (4), 166–176.

Munetz, M.R., Benjamin, S., 1988. How to examine patients using the abnormal involuntary movements scale. Hosp. Community Psychiatry 39 (11), 1172–1177.

Nassir Ghaemi, S., Manwani, S.G., Katzow, J.J., et al., 2001. Topiramate treatment of bipolar spectrum disorders: a retrospective chart review. Ann. Clin. Psychiatry 13 (4), 185–189.

National Institute for Health and Clinical Excellence, 2009. Schizophrenia: The NICE Guideline on Core Interventions in the Treatment and Management of Schizophrenia in Adults in Primary and Secondary Care (updated edition). Royal College of Psychiatry/The British Psychological Society, London.

National Prescribing Centre, 2007. A Competency Framework for Shared Decision-Making with Patients: Achieving Concordance for Taking Medications. NPC Plus, Liverpool.

National Prescribing Centre, 2009. Patient group directions: a practical guide and framework of competencies for all professionals using patient group directives. <http://www.npc.nhs.uk/non_ medical/resources/patient_group_ directions.pdf>.

NMC (Nursing and Midwifery Council), 2006. Standards of proficiency for nurse and midwife prescribers. <http://www.nmc-uk. org/Documents/Standards/ nmcStandardsofProficiencyFor NurseAndMidwifePrescribers.pdf>.

NMC (Nursing and Midwifery Council), 2007. Standards for Medicines Management. Nursing and Midwifery Council, London.

Nuttall, D., 2011. Prescribing in context. In: Nutall, D., Rutt-Howard, J. (Eds.), The Textbook of Non-Medical Prescribing. Wiley-Blackwell, Oxford, pp. 1–33.

O'Brien, L., Cole, R., 2004. Mental health nursing practice in acute psychiatric close-observation areas. Int. J. Ment. Health Nurs. 13, 89–99.

Phan, T.T., 1992. Enhancing client concordance to psychotropic medication regimens: a psychiatric community trial. Aust. J. Ment. Health Nurs. 2 (3), 94–104.

Schwarz, H.I., Vingrano, W., Bezirogowan, P., 1998. Autonomy and the right to refuse treatment: patient attitudes after involuntary medication. Hosp. Community Psychiatry 39 (19), 1049–1054.

Shupikai Rinomhota, A., Marshall, P., 2000. Biological Aspects of Mental Health Nursing. Churchill Livingstone, Edinburgh.

Stratton-Powell, H., 2001. PRN lorazepam: the nurse's judgement, the nurse's decision. Unpublished thesis, University of Manchester.

Taylor, D., Paton, C., Kapur, S., 2009. The Maudsley Prescribing Guidelines, tenth ed. Informa Healthcare, London.

Thapa, P., Palmer, S., Owen, R., et al., 2003. PRN (as needed) orders and exposure of psychiatric inpatients to unnecessary psychotropic medications. Psychiatr. Serv. 54 (9), 1282–1286.

Therapeutic Guidelines, 2000. Therapeutic Guidelines: Psychotropic 2000. Therapeutic Guidelines, Melbourne.

Treatment Protocol Project, 2000. Management of Mental Disorders, third ed. World Health Organization Collaborating Centre for Mental Health and Substance Abuse, Sydney.

Usher, K., 2001. Taking neuroleptic medications as the treatment for schizophrenia: a phenomenological study. Aust. N. Z. J. Ment. Health Nurs. 10 (3), 145–155.

Usher, K., Happell, B., 1996. Neuroleptic medication: the literature and implications for mental health nursing. Aust. N. Z. J. Ment. Health Nurs. 5 (4), 191–198.

Usher, K., Happell, B., 1997. Taking neuroleptic medications: a review. Aust. N. Z. J. Ment. Health Nurs. 6 (1), 3–10.

Usher, K., Luck, L., 2004. Psychotropic PRN: a model for best practice management of acute psychotic behavioural disturbance in inpatient psychiatric settings. Int. J. Ment. Health Nurs. 13 (1), 18–21.

Usher, K., Lindsay, D., Sellen, J., 2001. Mental health nurses' PRN psychotropic medication administration practices. J. Psychiatr. Ment. Health Nurs. 8 (5), 383–390.

Usher, K., Lindsay, D., Holmes, C., et al., 2003. PRN psychotropic medications: the need for nursing research. Contemp. Nurse 14 (3), 248–257.

Usher, K., Foster, K., McNamara, P., 2005. Antipsychotic drugs and pregnant or breast feeding women: the issues for mental health nurses. J. Psychiatr. Ment. Health Nurs. 12 (6), 713–718.

Usher, K., Holmes, C., Baker, J., et al., 2007. Enhancing the Understanding of Clinical Decision Making for PRN Medications within Mental Health Facilities. Final report to the Queensland Nursing Council (QNC), Brisbane, Queensland.

Viguera, A.C., Cohen, L.S., 1998. The course and management of bipolar disorder during pregnancy. Psychopharmacol. Bull. 34 (3), 339–353.

Vivian, B.G., Wilcox, J.R., 2000. Compliance communication in home health care: a mutually reciprocal process. Qual. Health. Res. 10 (1), 103–116.

Waddell, L., Taylor, M., 2008. A new self-rating scale for detecting atypical or second-generation antipsychotic side effects. J. Psychopharmacol. 22 (3), 238–243.

Webb, R.T., Howard, L., Abel, K.M., 2004. Antipsychotic drugs for non-affective psychosis during pregnancy and postpartum. Cochrane Database Syst. Rev. 2, CD004411.

Whicher, E., Morrison, M., Douglas-Hall, P., 2002. 'As Required' Medication Regimens for Seriously Mentally Ill People in Hospital (Cochrane Review). Cochrane Library, Issue 3. Update Software, Oxford.

Chapter | 25 |

Physical health

Steve Trenoweth, Deborah Taylor, and Helen Robson

CHAPTER CONTENTS

KEY POINTS

- Good mental and physical health is important to our overall sense of wellbeing.

- People with mental health problems tend to experience poorer physical health, poorer access to healthcare and reduced outcomes compared to the general population, including an increased risk of premature death.

- Mental health nurses must be attentive and responsive to the physical health needs of their client group, which has professional development requirements including developing skills of physical health assessment.

- Lifestyle factors (such as increased rates of smoking, poorer diet, poor uptake of exercise, increased use of substances) can increase the risk of poor physical health among a mental health client group.

- Sleep is compromised when we experience mental distress and physical illness and a lack of sleep has been implicated, in turn, in increasing the risk of both poor physical and mental health.

- Sexual expression is an important part our lives and mental health nurses must be able to promote good sexual health among their client group.

- Mental health problems are a significant cause of morbidity and mortality among women during pregnancy and following childbirth.

KEY TERMS

- ABCDE approach
- annual health check
- auscultation
- AVPU
- breathlessness
- circadian rhythm
- comorbidity
- diet

- dizziness
- drug and alcohol use
- exercise
- Glasgow Coma Scale
- inspection
- lifestyle factors
- medication
- mental health and childbirth
- pain
- palpation
- percussion
- perinatal mental health
- physical health assessment
- premature death
- recovery
- sexuality
- sleep
- sleep hygiene
- smoking
- 'Z drugs'

LEARNING OUTCOMES

The material in this chapter will assist you to:

- consider why there may be inequalities in the access to physical healthcare among people with mental health problems,
- understand the relationship between physical and mental health,
- appreciate the risk, lifestyle and other factors which affect the physical health of people with mental health problems,
- understand the role of the mental health nurse in providing physical healthcare and promoting sexual health and sleep hygiene to mental health service users,
- understand how to conduct a physical health assessment,
- discuss the maternal mental health and perinatal healthcare needs of people with mental health problems,
- respond to physical health emergencies in mental health settings.

INTRODUCTION

Good mental and physical health is of course an important contributory factor in our overall sense of health and wellbeing (Department of Health, 2011). The physical healthcare of people with mental health problems has been an important strategic issue in recent years for successive UK governments. Most recently, the Coalition Government's mental health policy *No Health without Mental Health* (Department of Health, 2011) has a strategic aim of improving the physical health of people with mental health problems so that fewer people with mental health problems will die prematurely. It also aims to ensure that more people with physical ill health will have better mental health. In Chapter 10 we looked at the components of an holistic and comprehensive model of assessment which gathers information based on psychiatric, physical, spiritual and cultural data. In this chapter we look more in depth at physical health and how it might impact on the care, treatment and experience of mental health service users. We look at the contemporary role of the mental health nurse and how nurses can address the health inequalities that people with mental health problems often face. For example, people with severe and ongoing mental health problems often have an increased vulnerability to serious physical illnesses, such as coronary heart disease, diabetes and respiratory diseases, and appear to have poorer access to medical care and treatment compared with the general population.

HEALTH INEQUALITIES

There is overwhelming evidence that the physical health and overall quality of life of people with mental health problems is poor compared to the general population (Cohen and Hove, 2001; Mitchell and Malone, 2006; Parish, 2011; Phelan et al., 2001; SCMH, 1997, 2003; Seymour, 2003; Stroup, 2004). However, there has been a healthcare service response to improve the physical health of people with mental health problems (Department of Health, 2006b), and good physical health remains an unmet need for this client group (DRC, 2006; Phelan et al., 2001).

In an extensive literature review mental disorders have been found to lead to an increased risk of premature death, with 60% of deaths due to physical health problems rather than psychiatric issues (Harris and Barraclough, 1998). It is estimated that people diagnosed with schizophrenia can expect to live, on average, 10 years less than someone without such a diagnosis (Allebeck, 1989; Mentality/NIMHE, 2004). Furthermore, physical health problems seem to develop at a much younger age among people with serious mental health problems compared with the general population, which is particularly noticeable in the 25–44-year age range. In 2006, the Disability Rights Commission published an 18-month investigation into the physical health inequalities experienced by people with mental health problems and learning disabilities (DRC, 2006). The report found that people diagnosed with schizophrenia, bipolar disorder and depression are more likely to experience increased rates of diabetes, heart disease, respiratory disease and cerebrovascular disease. It also seemed that those diagnosed with schizophrenia and bipolar affective disorders were more likely to develop breast cancer, hypertension and bowel cancer and people with serious and enduring mental health problems were more likely to die from such conditions within 5 years of diagnosis when compared to the general population. For example, the survival rate for cancer in this client group appears to be 50% lower than for the general population (Halbreich et al., 1996) and people with symptoms of coronary heart disease are less likely to survive them for more than 5 years (DRC, 2006). There is also an increased risk of chronic obstructive pulmonary disease (Himelhoch et al., 2004) and the risk of heart problems leading to sudden death may be three times higher among people diagnosed with schizophrenia compared to the general population (Casey et al., 2004; Jindal et al., 2005).

It has been argued that part of the reason for this is that physical illness among this client group appears to go undetected or is poorly managed (Cohen and Phelan, 2001; Department of Health, 1999, 2006a; Inventor et al., 2005). Furthermore, people with mental health problems tend to have a poorer experience of, and access to, medical services (DRC, 2006; Mentality/NIMHE, 2004) and are less likely to receive hospital inpatient care for their underlying medical conditions (Mentality/NIMHE, 2004). This may be due at least in part to the ability and responsiveness of medical professionals in primary and secondary services. For example, primary care practitioners, and nurses in general hospital settings (Mavundla, 2000) appear to lack expertise and training in mental health issues (Cohen and Hove, 2001; Mentality/NIMHE, 2004; Phelan et al., 2001; Seymour, 2003) and may not engage in the necessary physical health assessments and examinations required to detect physical illness and disease among those with serious mental health problems. Furthermore, the lack of social and communication skills among some service users with ongoing mental health problems and the stigma of a psychiatric diagnosis may reduce the likelihood that this client group receives appropriate medical healthcare (Phelan et al., 2001).

Some authors have suggested that there exists a professional development deficit among specialist mental health practitioners leading to their inattentiveness and inability to identify and respond to the physical health needs of service users (Dean et al., 2001; Department of Health, 2006b; Phelan et al., 2001). Osborn and Warner (1998) argue that a significant number of inpatients are not given a physical examination and an assessment of the physical health effects experienced from the use of prescribed antipsychotic medication or an adequate assessment of their medical history.

It also seems that some people with mental health problems tend to have more frequent contact with health services; they were found to be less likely to report physical healthcare symptoms spontaneously, may avoid contact with primary care health services and may be less willing to report or discuss concerns about their health or to request physical health checks (Goldman, 1999; SCMH, 2003). There are many suggested reasons for this. For example, people with serious mental health problems may be unaware of their physical health problems due to impaired cognitive functioning (Goldman, 1999) and issues such as social isolation and suspicion may contribute to them not seeking care or adhering to treatment (Phelan et al., 2001). Furthermore, the symptoms of physical disease or illness may be masked by antipsychotic medications, which may dampen down pain, for example (Lambert et al., 2003).

There is much evidence that psychiatric diagnoses may lead to a person's physical health needs being overlooked or ignored or taking second place to their mental healthcare (Dean et al., 2001; Friedli and Dardis, 2002). This 'diagnostic overshadowing' (DRC, 2006) involves the misinterpretation of possible symptoms of physical illness or disease in psychiatric terms (Seymour, 2003) such that complaints of physical health problems by service users may be thought of as psychosomatic or 'irrational' in nature. Furthermore, it seems that the more severe the mental health problem is, the less likely it is that the person's underlying physical health problems will be detected or treated (Jeste et al., 1996). Better medical screening, via comprehensive annual physical health checks (DRC, 2006; Mentality/NIMHE, 2004), can lead to the early identification of physical health problems affording timely interventions where necessary (DRC, 2006). See Box 25.1.

There are also, it seems, assumptions made by many mental health practitioners, such as the belief that people with serious mental health problems are unconcerned about their physical needs and do not attend appointments or are noncompliant with prescribed treatment (Department of Health, 2006b; Mentality/NIMHE, 2004). There is also evidence which suggests that professionals are reluctant to place great emphasis on these aspects of care, due perhaps to perceived poor success rates and the belief that people with serious mental health problems have enough to worry about without asking them to, for example, stop smoking (Robson and Gray, 2005). However, Seymour (2003) found that mental health service users do have concerns about their physical health and that health promotion advice and support would be seen as valuable and helpful.

According to Lester et al. (2003) the success or failure of primary healthcare for those living in the community with a diagnosis of schizophrenia, for example, lies with the quality and consistency of the relationship with their GP (Lester et al., 2003). They carried out semistructured interviews on 45 randomly selected people diagnosed with schizophrenia to establish their perspective on the provision of primary care. The first element of their perceived satisfaction was that of the 'exceptional potential' of each consultation. This referred to the interpersonal competencies of the GP to portray kindness, patience or to inspire confidence in their patient. Other specific competencies identified were those of the importance of listening and the perceived respect afforded to them by GPs who offered the empowerment of explanation and information. The ability to access services with relative ease was also felt to be of significant importance: to obtain an emergency appointment and to request a home visit in particular. Alongside this was the potential for a long-term relationship with the person's GP with the added benefit of continuity of care and the opportunity for the GP to earn the trust of the person, and for him or her to feel that he or she was known as an individual by his or her doctor. The majority of the younger respondents, below the age of 55 years, felt that the doctor–patient relationship was significantly enhanced when they were treated as an equal and were involved in any decision making, specifically in relation to medication. They were, however, realistic about the need to act paternalistically

during a crisis episode of their mental health problem, which may necessitate the skill and expertise of the GP to navigate their way through the medical system. These findings would fully support the recovery focus of the strategy for mental health services and would facilitate the opportunity for health promotion interventions and early identification of health problems, and would arguably demonstrate the gold standard for effective holistic mental healthcare in the community.

COMORBIDITY

The underlying reasons for the increased morbidity and mortality rates in people who have serious mental health problems are undoubtedly very complex. In modern day healthcare provision health and social care are generally dichotomized into physical healthcare and mental healthcare services, which often act independently of each other, and as such people requiring both mental and physical care tend to fall between two stools. This situation lends itself to further enhance the stigma associated with mental health problems, ironically by the very healthcare systems developed to care for and support those individuals. However, modern concepts of holism reflect the notion that it is not minds or bodies that develop illnesses, but *people* who develop illnesses, and it is the overall personal experiences of illness, both physical and mental, that should be the focus of healthcare (Kendell, 2009). Despite the emerging 'holistic' view of health and the modern-day emphasis on community-based service provision, healthcare services remain artificially distinct in the care and treatment of those with mental health problems, as opposed to those with other illnesses (Nash, 2010).

ROLE OF THE MENTAL HEALTH NURSE

The opportunity to reduce the risks of developing physical health problems must be grasped from the outset with proactive health promotion delivered and subsequently supported by ongoing professional input. The aim must be to minimize the risks before damage to physical health occurs. The timeframe for this opportunity is too often missed and professional input to work with the clients to reduce their risk factors occurs at the point where the risk is already present, rather than putting their efforts in at an earlier stage to prevent the risk ever being present (Nash, 2010). It is clear that mental health nurses, due to their breadth and depth of contact, have a significant role here in supporting proactive health promotion strategies, in improving the physical wellbeing of people with mental health problems and in ensuring the equality of access to medical services for mental health service users (Department of Health, 2006a).

In the policy *Choosing Health: Supporting the Physical Health Needs of People with Severe Mental Illness* (Department of Health, 2006b) there was a focus on supporting health promotion programmes for people with severe mental health problems. It cited areas of good practice, such as the employment of a lead mental health nurse practitioner to coordinate health improvement programmes, such as healthy walking groups, smoking cessation and dieting programmes, and ensuring appropriate referral and access to medical services for people with mental health problems and physical health issues.

However, it appears that this potential may remain untapped as there may be a general lack of confidence and uncertainty of their role in relation to meeting physical health needs of mental health service users (Dean et al., 2001). Additionally, there may be a lack of clinical leadership and organizational strategic vision which may result in the quality of physical healthcare varying within nursing teams (Dean et al., 2001; SCMH, 2003; Seymour, 2003).

The *recovery approach* could be a truly pivotal aspect of ensuring the physical health needs of people with serious mental illness are addressed. This approach recognizes that:

> *At the heart of recovery is a set of values about a person's right to build a meaningful life for themselves, with or without the continuing presence of mental health symptoms. Recovery is based upon ideas of self determination and self management. It emphasises the importance of hope in sustaining motivation and supporting expectations of an individually fulfilled life.*

(Shepherd et al., 2008, p. 1)

The foundations of this approach are firmly built upon the principle that the service user must be in the driving seat of his/her recovery, and the starting point for professionals must be an understanding of that person's perception of recovery. The aim would be to facilitate the person to regain control of their life, and active engagement by the service user is seen as an essential aspect of the process of recovery, and the personal process of recovery is viewed as equally important as the clinical outcomes (NIMHE, 2005).

FACTORS AFFECTING PHYSICAL HEALTH

Much of the excess levels of illness and mortality among people with mental health problems are due to factors which may be unconnected with their mental health

problems(s) (Department of Health, 1999). Unhealthy lifestyles, such as higher incidences of smoking, poor exercise and poor nutrition, as discussed below (Mentality/NIMHE, 2004), are compounded by social deprivation, social exclusion, poverty, poor housing and unemployment which have all been implicated as contributory factors to ill health (DRC, 2006; Mentality/NIMHE, 2004). Indeed, people with serious and enduring mental health problems tend to be housed in poorer areas where there are high levels of crime, unemployment and drug misuse and they are significantly more at risk of being, or becoming, homeless (Repper, 2000), which can have a significant impact on the development and maintenance of mental distress. Furthermore, healthy eating and exercise often require financial and motivational resources from the individual concerned, but living on benefits, with poor self-esteem and little social support, and the sedating effects of medication, can impact on an individual's ability to promote and maintain their own health.

McCreadie (2003) examined the lifestyle factors which appear to most influence the physical health of individuals with serious mental health problems. It was found that those people diagnosed with schizophrenia had significantly poorer lifestyles in health terms than even those from the poorest groups in society. However, it appears that it is not one but several 'lifestyle' factors which combine to contribute to the poorer physical health of people with serious mental health problems. That is, while each risk factor is known to individually contribute to health problems, the compounded effects of many such factors within an individual may account for such higher mortality rates. Likewise, the risk of physical ill health is considerably reduced by a multidimensional response, such as a healthy diet and exercise (Mann, 2002). It is therefore necessary for mental health nurses to be aware of a wide range of risk factors to fully respond to both the physical and mental health needs of this client group.

Smoking

Smoking rates have consistently been shown to be higher among people with serious mental health problems (McCloughen, 2003), with this client group also smoking more heavily (20 cigarettes per day or more) than other members of the population (Brown et al., 1999). Kelly and McCreadie (1999) reported that 68% of people diagnosed with schizophrenia who smoked were classified as being heavy smokers (that is, smoking in excess of 25 per day) compared with only 11% of the general population. While people in general tend to smoke out of routine and habit offering a form of relaxation, pleasure and social contact (Robson and Gray, 2005), there have been many explanations for this disparity in smoking rates between this client group and the general population. For example, McCloughen (2003) suggests that smoking may constitute a form of 'self-medication', as the nicotine may help to alleviate some of the symptoms of mental distress and the side effects of medication.

Despite the evidence that smoking has a damaging effect on physical health (such as increased risks of cardiovascular disease, respiratory diseases, cancers and diabetes; Department of Health, 1998, 2004), Stubbs and Gardner (2004) reported that smoking is seen positively by mental health professionals with 54% of mental health workers believing that smoking is helpful in terms of creating therapeutic relationships.

Diet

A poor dietary intake is, of course, a major contributory factor in the development of serious physical illness such as cardiovascular disease, obesity, diabetes and some forms of cancer (Department of Health, 1994). However, a number of research studies have shown that those with serious mental health problems tend to eat a poorer diet compared to the general population (Brown et al., 1999; McCreadie et al., 2003) and consume higher rates of saturated fat and lower levels of fruit and vegetables. Brown et al. (1999) found, in assessing the diets of 102 people diagnosed with schizophrenia, that none of them were eating the levels of fruit and vegetables recommended by the Food Standards Agency (at least five portions of fruit or vegetables each day and at least one portion of oily fish per week) (Food Standards Agency, 2001). McCreadie (2003) reported that in a sample of people diagnosed with schizophrenia 53% demonstrated raised cholesterol levels.

There is also some suggestion that a poorer diet may adversely affect the trajectory of mental health problems. In *Feeding Minds* the Mental Health Foundation highlighted changes in diet over the last 60 years, such as decline in eating vegetables and foods rich in omega-3 fatty acids (such as oily fish, walnuts and flax seeds). They suggest that this has may have had an impact on mental ill health (Mental Health Foundation, 2006). For example, a diet high in saturated fat, low in polyunsaturated fat and high in sugar may impact on the clinical outcome of schizophrenia (Peet, 2004) and negative correlations have been found between dietary intakes of omega-3 fatty acids and the symptoms of both schizophrenia and 'tardive dyskinesia' (Mellor et al., 1996). Furthermore, a deficiency of vitamin B_9 (folic acid) and vitamin B_3 (niacin) has been linked with depression and a deficiency in vitamin B_{12} may be linked to psychotic disorders, whereas vitamin B_1 (thiamine) deficit is a possible precursor to Korsakoff's syndrome (symptoms of which include severe memory loss, confusion, apathy and repetitive behaviour arising from brain damage following long-term excessive alcohol use). Vitamin B_9 appears to reduce the risk of dementia (Abayomi and Hackett, 2004; Godfrey et al., 1990; Gold, 1996; Goodwin et al., 1983).

The Mental Health Foundation (2006) report suggests that an overall positive sense of wellbeing can be promoted by ensuring that attention is paid to promoting a healthy diet among people with mental health problems, such as recommending adequate amounts of complex carbohydrates, essential fats, amino acids, vitamins and minerals and water. However, it is important to recognize that a direct cause-and-effect link between diet and mental disorder has not been established thus far (Abayomi and Hackett, 2004).

Exercise

Obesity is a significant risk factor in the health of this group of people resulting from an apparent lack of physical exercise and a diet rich in saturated fats and sugar (McCreadie, 2003). Some 40–62% of people diagnosed with schizophrenia are overweight or obese compared to 27% of the general population, and this appears more prevalent in females (Kendrick, 1996). Inactivity increases the risks associated with a poor diet whereas exercise reduces the risk of cardiovascular disease, improving lung capacity and reducing the risk of many forms of cancer. There are many positive gains associated with physical exercise such as improving body strength, posture and flexibility. It has also been found to improve self-esteem, encourage social contact and improve sleep patterns (Daley, 2002). However, Brown et al. (1999) found that people with serious mental health problems exercised significantly less than the general population, whereas approximately one-third took no exercise.

Medication

The long-term use of antipsychotic medication for those diagnosed with schizophrenia has also been implicated in the development of physical health problems (Department of Health, 1999; NICE 2002a, 2002b) and may exacerbate existing physical conditions, such as diabetes (Mentality/NIMHE, 2004). Antipsychotic medication appears to compound the risks of a poor diet. Weight gain is often associated with the use of newer (atypical) antipsychotic medication (Allison et al., 2003) which may compound the risk for several physical disorders, such as Type 2 diabetes (Citrome and Yeomans, 2005; Dixon et al., 2004). Koro et al. (2002), furthermore, found that olanzipine increased the likelihood of developing hyperlipidaemia by five times (and other neuroleptic medication increased the likelihood three times) when compared with those not taking any antipsychotic medication. However, this group of people are often less likely than the general population to be prescribed cholesterol-lowering medications (Redelmeier et al., 1998).

An assessment of the risks associated with the use of medication which might undermine the physical health of a person with mental health problems must be balanced against the possible gains for the individual in terms of their overall mental health and wellbeing.

Drug and alcohol use

Alcohol misuse in the UK is a serious social and public health problem and it has a significant impact on the physical and mental health of individuals. Such problems also seem to be increasing. For example, in 2007, the World Health Organization (WHO) found a doubling of deaths in the UK from cirrhosis of the liver, at 10.88 per 100 000 population, an increase from 4.5 per 100 000 compared to the previous 27 years. For mental health service users the use of drugs and/or alcohol may be associated with a poorer recovery from mental health problems. People may also experience an increase in the side effects of neuroleptic medication, as well as an increased risk of violent behaviour and suicide (Vose, 2000). It is estimated that 36% of people with serious mental health problems will have some form of substance abuse problem over the course of a year (Primary Care Mental Health and Education, 2005) and possibly 60% of people diagnosed with schizophrenia may abuse psychoactive drugs and other substances (Citrome and Yeomans, 2005).

There are many indications that a person has been misusing alcohol. First, of course, it is important to ask people how much alcohol they consume; however, we must also be mindful that people may under-report their actual alcohol consumption. As such, there are additional assessments of alcohol misuse which the mental health nurse must be aware of. Most obviously, falls and injuries might be signs of heavy drinking. People who have been misusing alcohol regularly for a prolonged period of time may display tremors of the hand or tongue. There may also be discoloration of the skin (such as abnormal capillarization of facial skin and neck and possible yellow blotches on the skin) and eyes (such as burgundy-coloured capillary engorgement of the conjunctival tissue or a greenish-yellow tinge to the sclera). There are more precise assessments of alcohol consumption such as the use of breathalysers to measure blood alcohol concentration (BAC) and biological markers of the alcohol consumption above safe limits. These include mean corpuscular volume (MCV) of red blood cells, serum gamma-glutamyl transferase (GGT), serum aspartate amino transferase (AST) and especially carbohydrate deficient transferrin (CDT), which can indicate recent excessive alcohol consumption (Dawe et al., 2002).

PHYSICAL HEALTH ASSESSMENT

In order to assess a person's physical health it is important to follow a structured approach which allows for the systematic exclusion of serious illness or injury. Many

physical ailments can be manifested in atypical ways. This particularly applies to people who may have communication difficulties or illnesses which cause them to present in an unusual manner or not to verbalize any complaints at all despite the presence of a potentially serious organic condition affecting their health.

Although physical assessment can imply a thorough head-to-toe examination of the person, in reality this involves skills that are beyond the scope of the average practitioner; indeed, there are differing opinions over whether it should be a nursing role at all (Lesa and Dixon, 2007; West, 2006). Without undertaking a full physical examination, it is possible to still detect the presence of life-threatening illness with the use of both simple techniques and the assessor's senses. Many cues can be detected by what you see, hear and smell without the need for a verbal report. The mental health nurse needs to be able to recognize these cues to facilitate appropriate treatment in order to optimize the service user's physical health.

Note: it is vitally important whenever dealing with a situation where you feel you are out of your area of expertise to call for appropriate help at the earliest opportunity. Most conditions are treatable and with expert help can be reversed to allow the patient to return to relative health. Always be aware of what the emergency numbers are in your work setting and how they should be used.

Structured assessments

Any physical assessment begins with history taking unless dealing with a person who is unable to give you any history; for example, a confused person, someone who has collapsed or someone with a disability which prevents them from being able to communicate. In this situation it may be appropriate to continue to the physical examination of the patient in order to detect any life-threatening emergencies (see the ABCDE approach, below). As soon as possible an attempt should be made to obtain some collateral history either from other staff, friends and relatives or the service user's notes, or both.

When you become aware of a change in a service user's health or perception of their health it is important to take a thorough history. You need to begin by ascertaining the person's description of their symptoms. It is important at this stage that you allow them to explain how they are feeling without making suggestions or working towards a specific diagnosis. This will limit your findings causing you to potentially miss important information.

Pain

Pain is a subjective, unpleasant sensation indicating actual or potential tissue damage. There may be objective signs present in acute pain including sweating, pallor, grimacing and an increase in respiratory rate, heart rate and blood pressure. Chronic pain frequently has little or no obvious signs for the assessor and relies on the history of the patient. Ask open questions, such as: Are you in pain? What does it feel like? Where is the pain? You will obtain a much more useful history if you do not ask leading questions. If a service user tells you they have pain you will need to ascertain when the pain started, where the pain is, the nature of the pain (i.e. stabbing, burning, squeezing, etc), whether the pain is constant or intermittent and if anything relieves or aggravates the pain. Certain symptoms have specific questions which should be asked, as follows. It may be useful to ask the person if they have taken any analgesia and if so when. The site of the pain can often give valuable clues as to what may actually be wrong with the person. However, most sites have numerous possible causes of pain and need to be investigated in order to reach an accurate diagnosis.

Dizziness

Dizziness is a very nonspecific complaint and can be caused by many conditions, most of which are benign. Despite this, it is necessary for any person complaining of dizziness to be investigated to exclude any serious conditions, such as cerebral events, cardiac events, infections and electrolyte imbalances. In all cases the people will need a baseline set of observations (such as vital signs) including postural blood pressure (taken when the person lies down and then stands, which is then repeated 1 min later), an electrocardiogram (ECG) and a urinalysis. If any of these indicate abnormalities the person will need further urgent investigations.

Breathlessness

The symptom of shortness of breath can be subjective (in that the person feels they are unable to breathe easily but the rate and rhythm of their respirations is normal) or objective (in that the assessor notices the person is short of breath because of their inability to speak in sentences, the use of accessory muscles or an obvious increase in the person's respiratory rate at rest). Both of these warrant further assessment but the latter may require more urgent attention. Important questions to ask here will include: Do you have a history of breathing problems? What was the onset of symptoms? Do you have pain when you breathe and if so where? Causes of acute shortness of breath include chest infection, exacerbation of chronic obstructive pulmonary disease (COPD) or asthma, pneumothorax (collapsed lung), cardiac event and pulmonary embolism (blood clot in the lung) to name just a few. Any person reporting or demonstrating an acute onset of difficulty breathing needs urgent medical attention.

The ABCDE approach

The standardized approach to assessment uses the ABCDE approach as outlined below:

A   airway,
B   breathing,
C   circulation,
D   disability,
E   exposure/environment.

This assessment approach is designed to assess people who are presenting with an acute illness and it is imperative that assessment and simple treatments are done simultaneously. The ABC approach is easy to remember and is vital because it facilitates assessment in a way that identifies the most life-threatening emergencies in the order in which they will result in morbidity and or mortality.

Airway

An assessment of the airway in most situations will take very little time. The airway can be patent, at risk, partially occluded or occluded.

A patent airway will be one in which the person is able to speak. If a service user has a reduced level of consciousness and is consequently unable to speak the assessment of the airway involves opening the person's mouth to check for any potential obstruction. An airway is at risk if the person is unconscious deeply enough to prevent them from maintaining their own airway. With a reduction in conscious level comes a relaxation in tone of the tongue and muscles associated with the mouth and jaw. This leads to impairment of the gag reflex which would normally protect the airway from any potential blockage. The presence of a partially obstructed airway may be indicated by associated abnormal sounds including snoring, stridor or gurgling. Snoring, frequently present in a deep sleep or impaired level of consciousness, generally indicates the tongue has fallen back, causing a partial obstruction to airflow. Simple airway-opening manoeuvres including chin lift and head tilt should address this problem. Stridor is an abnormal noise heard on inspiration as a result of a narrowed upper airway. The airway can be partially obstructed by foreign bodies (e.g. broken/false teeth, food bolus, vomit, secretions, blood) or swelling due to allergy, injury, postoperative swelling or disease process. If this swelling continues or the foreign body moves to a smaller area of the airway it can cause a complete occlusion. A person with an obstructed airway will be unconscious and not breathing, indicating a respiratory arrest requiring initiation of basic life support (or BLS) until expert assistance arrives. Delays in instigating basic life support will result in tissue damage as a result of ischaemia (reduction of blood supply) and lead, ultimately, to tissue death. The areas that have the highest oxygen requirements will be damaged first, including the brain, heart and kidneys (Adam et al., 2009).

Breathing

Once your assessment of the airway is complete you then proceed to assess the person's breathing. This involves viewing the person's chest for movement, counting their respirations and observing the depth of respiration, signs of inadequate breathing and work of breathing. The respiratory rate needs to be measured for one full minute. While counting the rate it is a good idea to observe the character of the respirations including the depth and the rhythm.

Some illnesses are characterized by abnormal breathing patterns which if detected at this stage can inform the rest of the assessment and indicate the severity of the condition; examples of this include Kussmaul's and Cheyne–Stokes respirations. The significance of hypo- and hyperventilation needs also to be explored if present as both may be due to serious physiological conditions.

- Kussmaul's respirations are characterized by laboured and deep respirations associated with metabolic acidosis, for example diabetic ketoacidosis and renal failure.
- Cheyne–Stokes respirations are an irregular breathing pattern with alternating rapid shallow breaths followed by periods of apnoea. This type of respiration is a poor prognostic sign usually associated with end of life.
- Hypoventilation is breathing that is not adequate to meet the needs of the body, involving a respiratory pattern that is either too shallow or too slow. This can be caused by drugs that suppress the respiratory centre including opiates, resulting in increased blood carbon dioxide levels and a reduction in oxygen levels. Other causes include neuromuscular diseases and neurological conditions including tumours, injuries, infections and strokes. Patients with severe COPD can also develop a hypoventilatory breathing pattern usually as a result of dangerously high carbon dioxide blood levels. Due to low oxygen levels these patients will typically have a reduced level of consciousness, making respiratory arrest a possibility unless urgent treatment is implemented.
- Hyperventilation is an increase in the respiratory rate and can result in abnormally low levels of carbon dioxide in the blood, leading to dizziness, weakness, tingling around the mouth and fingertips and in extreme cases muscle spasms in the hands and feet. Causes can include anxiety, metabolic disturbances and toxins, for example overdose of aspirin. Tachypnoea (rapid breathing) can also be a sign of increased oxygen requirements in a critically ill patient. It is vitally important that respiratory rate be measured and documented on initial assessment and recorded frequently after that, to establish a trend that will aid in the recognition of any changes or deteriorations. The first vital sign that changes to indicate deterioration in health and which can predict increased patient acuity is the respiratory rate (Goldhill et al., 1999, 2005; Jonsson et al., 2011).

The respiratory assessment includes recognition of increased work of breathing: in a normal healthy adult respiration should be effortless. In an unwell patient with breathing difficulties there are often tell-tale signs that the patient is working hard to maintain adequate oxygenation to the tissues. These signs include the use of accessory muscles (that is, neck and abdominal muscles), an inability to complete a sentence in one breath, increased respiratory rate, posture (such as adopting an upright position to allow for optimal expansion of lungs), noises (wheeze, rails, rhonchi) and an increase in other vital signs including heart rate and blood pressure. It is not possible for patients to continue these compensatory mechanisms indefinitely and they will eventually tire, resulting in hypoventilation and ultimately respiratory arrest unless the work of breathing is reduced. Patients with increased work of breathing need urgent medical attention.

Signs of inadequate breathing include agitation, reduced level of consciousness, cyanosis, and abnormal rate and rhythm of breathing, identified by counting the respiratory rate and a reduction in the patient's oxygen saturation level. Oxygen saturations measure the amount of oxygen bound to circulating haemoglobin; anything below a reading of 95% may be a potentially serious sign and needs to be investigated further. If a person demonstrates signs of inadequate breathing they need urgent treatment to prevent further deterioration.

Circulation

The circulatory system includes the heart and blood vessels. To assess this system it is necessary to measure the heart rate. The most common site to do this is at the radial artery; however, depending on a person's condition it may be necessary to use an alternative pulse such as on the carotid or femoral arteries. When you palpate the pulse it is important to not only make note of the rate but also the character and quality. To facilitate identification of any abnormalities of the pulse you should measure it for a full minute. If the heart rate is fast you may note that it is 'thready', meaning weak or difficult to feel. If a person's heart is beating very hard you may notice that the pulse is 'bounding' indicating increases in the strength of cardiac contractions. This type of pulse is frequently associated with sepsis and is very easy to feel and possibly even visible.

Blood pressure is also an important part of the circulation assessment and needs to be measured, recorded and interpreted in line with normal parameters, bearing in mind that normal variations can occur and that other factors can contribute to raised blood pressure (hypertension) including stress, anxiety, pain and 'white-coat syndrome' (Jhalani et al., 2005).

Another measure of circulation is capillary refill time (CRT). This can be measured by applying pressure to the person's skin for 5 s and then releasing and observing how many seconds it takes for the person's normal skin colour to return. Anything longer than 2 s is prolonged and may indicate inadequate circulation. For an accurate assessment it is recommended to perform CRT measurement as centrally as possible, preferably on the person's sternum, which will have already been exposed to allow for adequate assessment of the patients breathing. If performed peripherally CRT needs to be taken into context with regards to other possible causes of impaired peripheral circulation; for example, the environment, as cold temperatures will cause vasoconstriction resulting in reduced capillary refill. If a person has an abnormal pulse, reduced capillary refill or abnormal blood pressure (deviating from their own normal) they require further urgent investigations including an ECG, possibly blood tests and review/examination by a medical practitioner.

Signs of inadequate circulation can include changes in skin colour, such as a pale, waxy, grey appearance. It is important to manually feel a person's pulse as this will allow you to also take note of the patient's skin. You may also discover the patient is hot, indicating a fever, or clammy and cool, or you may notice signs of an irregular heartbeat like skipped beats or an irregular pulse. In this situation the person may complain of palpitations, difficulty breathing or chest pain. People with inadequate circulation may also be breathless, confused or have a reduced level of consciousness due to increased oxygen requirements and reduced circulating oxygen.

Disability

Disability refers to a person's neurological assessment including their level of consciousness, pupil reaction and blood glucose levels. It is important to note that, as previously mentioned when assessing airway, breathing and circulation, problems with any of them can result in an alteration in a person's mental state or level of consciousness. For this reason it is vitally important that any issues with A, B or C are identified and treatment commenced prior to moving on to D.

In assessing the level of consciousness there are two different commonly used measurement tools which allow the assessor to establish the seriousness of the patient's condition. The first one, AVPU, takes a matter of moments and is useful as part of the initial brief assessment. When the patient is being continuously monitored the Glasgow Coma Scale (GCS) will then also be used. As with any other measurement tool it is vital that the measurements are repeated to identify trends and patterns over time, allowing for the recognition of potentially serious changes in the patient's condition.

AVPU

AVPU is a scoring system that looks at the person's responsiveness level:

A   alert,
V   responds to verbal stimulus,
P   responds to painful stimulus,
U   unresponsive.

If the patient has their eyes open and is able to take in their surroundings they are alert (A), meaning they have sufficient oxygenation to allow for at least some cerebral

functioning, which also indicates a presently patent airway. Verbal responsiveness (V) indicates the patient has a slight reduction in conscious level but is easily roused; they may be drowsy and unable to remain alert without stimulation or they may be sleeping. Responsiveness to pain (P) indicates the patient has a further reduced level of consciousness. Responses to pain may vary from localization to pain to withdrawing from pain; any response to pain would score P on the AVPU score. In order to illicit a response the assessor needs to apply a painful stimulus to the patient, which would only be done after establishing whether the patient responds to voice; for example, a simple shake may then be used followed by a more painful stimulus if the patient remains unresponsive. There are a number of accepted methods of eliciting a pain response, including nail-bed pressure, supraorbital pressure, sternal rub, trapezium squeeze and earlobe pressure. Although any one of these may elicit a response they need to be used with caution. Nail-bed pressure has been reported to elicit a spinal response making it potentially unreliable. Sternal rub, though possibly the easiest, can appear quite brutal if witnessed by relatives or other bystanders; it can also commonly cause bruising if used repeatedly, which may make CRT difficult to elicit. Arguably the best method is the trapezium squeeze, which involves squeezing the muscle between the neck and the shoulder, this can appear more gentle to nonmedical bystanders while still being a painful enough procedure to illicit a response unless the patient is deeply unconscious. A score of unresponsive (U) is a very serious sign indicating that the patient does not respond in any way to any stimulus.

People with a score of P or U are in danger of being unable to maintain their own airway and need urgent attention by critical care personnel. If you are assessing this patient you must call for help as soon as possible and then return to your ABC assessment to ensure they have an adequate airway until help arrives.

The AVPU scale is a simple technique which allows for a baseline level of consciousness assessment. If, however, there is any reduction in consciousness it must be followed up as soon as possible by a full GCS assessment and closely monitored for any changes.

Glasgow Coma Scale

The Glasgow Coma Scale (GCS) is the most widely used assessment tool to evaluate level of consciousness and has been adopted worldwide. It was originally designed in 1974 by Teasdale and Jennett, professors of neurosurgery at the University of Glasgow's Institute of Neurological Sciences. Originally it was a score from 3 to 14 but it has since been developed into the score used today which is from 3 to 15. The scale measures the patient's best eye (E), verbal (V) and motor (M) responses. Each is scored separately and then added up to a potential total of 15. The minimum possible score is 3 which is the equivalent of no response to any stimulus in each category (deep coma or death) and the maximum 15 (a fully alert person). It does take some skill to accurately use the scale, and has potential for variations in score depending on the user's interpretation of the results. This has caused the tool to come into criticism for poor inter-rater reliability with studies recently exploring the use of other scoring systems, including the Full Outline of Responsiveness (FOUR) score. A study by Kevric et al. (2011) indicated greater reliability in the use of the FOUR scale than with the GCS. The study was on a relatively small sample (200 patients) with recommendation made for further study. Until such times, however, the GCS is still the method of choice for assessing level of consciousness and head injury, but the literature agrees that the inter-rater reliability is greatly increased when the GCS is used by experienced clinicians (see Box 25.2).

As well as the above scale the GCS chart includes measurement of pupil size, shape and reactivity and power of upper and lower limbs. When measuring pupil reaction the clinician uses a pen torch and with a sweeping motion shines the light into the patient's eyes one at a time. They observe each pupil's diameter and whether it reacts briskly, slowly or is unreactive to light. It is important to note that some drugs may affect pupil size, including opiates and benzodiazepines.

Lastly the clinician assesses the patient's power in their limbs. It is important to note whether the patient has any injuries that may affect the ability to move the injured limb (see also Box 25.3).

Blood glucose

The final part of the disability assessment is a blood glucose measurement. This is a very simple procedure which can identify the presence of hypo- or hyperglycaemia. Hypoglycaemia can occur without a history of diabetes with symptoms including dizziness, confusion, seizures or collapse. If untreated it can lead to death, although the condition is easily treated and can result in almost instantaneous return to consciousness. Hyperglycaemia occurs in diabetic patients and is sometimes part of the initial presentation of a newly diagnosed diabetic. Symptoms include increased thirst, dehydration, abdominal pain, vomiting, stupor and loss of consciousness and is often associated with other metabolic disturbances/electrolyte imbalances. People with a high blood glucose level need urgent treatment to correct any imbalances, which will return the patient to a normal conscious level.

Exposure/environment

After completing your ABCD assessment the next step is to perform a full examination of the patient to identify the presence of any rashes, bruises, injuries or other marks on the skin which would provide insight into the nature of their illness. Care needs to be taken to ensure the person's dignity is preserved throughout this stage of the assessment. It is at this time that you would also measure the person's temperature to assess for the possibility of hypo- or hyperthermia. In the older person hypothermia can indicate sepsis, which needs to be excluded in an acutely confused patient. If the temperature is found to be abnormal further investigations are warranted. This is classified as a septic screen and would include such things as blood tests, urinalysis, ECG, chest X-ray and others (lumbar puncture, head CT scan) depending on the history and any relevant findings.

Box 25.2 **The Glasgow Coma Scale**

Score response:

Eye opening (E)
- 4 Spontaneous
- 3 To speech
- 2 To pain
- 1 None

Verbal response (V)
- 5 Orientated conversation
- 4 Confused speech
- 3 Inappropriate words
- 2 Incomprehensible sounds
- 1 None

Motor response (M)
- 6 Obeys commands
- 5 Localizes to pain
- 4 Withdraws from pain (normal flexion)
- 3 Abnormal flexion
- 2 Extension
- 1 None

Box 25.3 **Comparing AVPU and GCS**

A Scottish study (Kelly et al., 2004) identified the way in which the AVPU score corresponds to the GCS after observing and comparing their use for more than 1300 poisoned patients.

A is equivalent to GCS 15.
V is equivalent to GCS 12–14.
P is equivalent to GCS 7–9.
U is equivalent to GCS 3.

Anyone with a response of P or U will be at risk of airway obstruction due to an inability to maintain their own airway. These people need urgent assessment and interventions to secure their airway by a critical care clinician, anaesthetist, paramedic or whichever is the first available depending on the setting of the emergency. Initially airway adjuncts, e.g. oral or nasopharangeal airway devices, would be used; however, it may be necessary for the patient to be intubated in order to secure a definitive airway.

Clinical skills

Skills required to perform an ABCDE assessment include inspection, palpation, auscultation and percussion.

Inspection refers to the observations the assessor can make with their own eyes. The whole assessment will involve inspection and you must document what you can see.

Palpation refers to feeling something or the use of touch during an assessment. This is required during measurement of the pulse: for more experienced clinicians it will also involve examination of injured or painful areas to elicit tenderness which will aid in diagnosis.

Auscultation is the use of hearing, specifically using a stethoscope. You may, if able, auscultate the blood pressure using a stethoscope. When assessing the respiratory system (breathing) the clinician will use a stethoscope to assess air entry into each lung and observe breath sounds and any extra noises, such as wheeze. When assessing the cardiovascular system they will listen to the heart sounds and be able to measure the apical heart rate and when assessing the gastrointestinal system they will be able to listen to bowel sounds.

Percussion involves short, sharp taps of the examiners fingers to determine the size, position and density of underlying structures by the sound obtained. This technique is most commonly used in the physical examination of the chest and back (looking at the respiratory system) and the abdomen (the gastrointestinal system).

Vital signs

The value of recording patient observations both on initial assessment and subsequent to that is to identify trends and recognize changes in patient condition. The introduction of Early Warning Score (EWS) charts has facilitated the identification of a patient who is deteriorating, indicating when there is a need to call for expert help (either medical or rapid response team) (Groarke et al. 2008) (see Box 25.4).

> **Box 25.4 Normal parameters for an adult**
>
> - Temperature 36.1–37.9°C
> - Pulse 60–90 beats/min
> - Respiratory rate 12–18 breaths/min
> - Blood pressure 100–139 mmHg (systolic)/60–89 mmHg (diastolic)
> - Oxygen saturation >95% on room air
>
> Keep in mind that patients with COPD can function normally with oxygen saturation levels as low as 90% and do not necessarily need any treatment unless they are experiencing new symptoms or are either subjectively or objectively short of breath.

> **CASE STUDY 1**
>
> Miss M is a 22-year-old West-African female brought into the accident and emergency department with a history of bizarre behaviour. No one accompanies her to hospital: she has been found in the street wandering and behaving strangely, and she was uncooperative with the ambulance staff. The initial assessment is that she is suffering from an acute psychotic episode and she is triaged to the minor injuries part of the department assuming she will need referral to psychiatry. The triage nurse in minor injuries does a set of observations, finding the following: temperature 39°C, pulse 120 beats/min, respirations 24 breaths/min, blood pressure 110/60 mmHg, blood glucose 4.5 mmol/L.
>
> Are these normal? What would you do? What investigations may Miss M require?
>
> Miss M is clearly confused and appears unwell: she is showing signs of hallucinating and is unable to give any history. She has identification on her which is used to discover the lack of any previous mental health diagnosis or any other significant medical condition.
>
> Routine blood tests are performed which indicate a severe infection. A malaria screen is done which is positive for *falciparum* malaria and the eventual diagnosis of encephalitis from malaria is diagnosed. The patient requires admission to the intensive treatment unit due to the severity of her condition.
>
> This case highlights the need for a thorough physical examination including laboratory investigations on anyone presenting acutely with abnormal behaviour, particularly in the presence of abnormal observations.

> **CASE STUDY 2**
>
> Mr P, 55 years old, is admitted to the mental health unit with acute confusion. His family express concerns about his aggressive behaviour. After 2 weeks on the ward he is not improving. In fact he is becoming worse: he is also not eating and is losing weight as a result. The nurse caring for him has some concerns and decides to do a brief physical assessment.
>
> A Clear, patient able to speak, shouting frequently.
> B Respiration rate 22 breaths/min; patient appears to get acutely short of breath on exertion.
> C It is difficult to perform pulse and blood pressure as the patient is noncompliant.
> D Mr P is agitated, non-cooperative and disinhibited.
> E Mr P appears to have lost weight, his clothes appear too big for him and he has a waxy, gaunt countenance.
>
> How would you proceed? Is Mr P's behaviour completely explainable by a psychiatric diagnosis? What, if any, investigations does he need?

Mr P is brought to accident and emergency for medical investigations. He has blood tests which are essentially normal, an ECG which is also normal and a chest X-ray which shows a possible mass. A CT scan of the head is performed which confirms the presence of a secondary brain tumour within his frontal lobe which is now credited for his change in behaviour. He is referred to oncology and will require radiotherapy in the hope of reducing the size of the tumour and reversing some of his behavioural problems.

CASE STUDY 3

Mr B is a 50-year-old male who has been diagnosed with depression. He has a history of alcohol dependence although he has recently undergone a detoxification programme and has so far abstained from further alcohol use. He has a history of deliberate self-harm including overdoses, although usually of low toxicity medications. He has just returned from a period of weekend leave from the ward. You enter Mr B's room to give him his medication and find him unresponsive on his bed. How do you react? What are your priorities?

You call his name and he doesn't respond so you go on to assess ABC and you also shout for help.

A. Mr B is not alert, he is lying on his back and making snoring sounds. You perform a chin lift and straight away the snoring sound stops.

B. Respiratory rate is 8 breaths/min; slow, deep respirations.

C. Pulse is 130 beats/min, blood pressure is 90/50 mmHg.

D. Unresponsive, pupils dilated.

What would you do next?

Ensure help is on its way, dial 999 or enact the medical emergency procedure for your particular service. Keep monitoring the patient while waiting for the ambulance, ensuring the airway is maintained. The most likely diagnosis is tricyclic antidepressant overdose; however, all other possibilities will be investigated by the accident and emergency department team. It is likely the patient will require intubation and admission to an intensive treatment unit.

SLEEP

Sleep is a very important part of our daily lives. It can be compromised when we experience mental distress and physical illness and a lack of sleep has been implicated, in turn, in increasing the risk of both poor physical and mental health (Collier et al., 2003; MHF, 2011).

Sleep is a complex phenomenon and seems to have a restorative function for us as human beings, helping us to improve our psychological and physical health. Everyone differs in the amount of sleep that they need, that is there is no universal optimum period of time which we need to spend asleep. Most people tend to sleep between 7 and 8 h a night, but the overall range between people can be 5–11 h (MHF, 2011). What does appear crucial, however, is that the sleep we do have is of high 'quality'; that is, that we have the appropriate amount of sleep that allows us to awaken feeling refreshed and able to lead our lives without excessive tiredness. Without sleep, our concentration and energy levels tends to be poor and a lack of sleep has implications for our mood and interpersonal relationships (MHF, 2011).

Human beings, along with most animals, have a *circadian rhythm* or a 'biological clock' which governs the natural sleep–wake cycle. Our sleep–wake cycle is regulated by a complex process, involving physiological factors within the body (such as levels of serotonin) and external factors (such as light). When it gets dark, the pineal gland secretes *melatonin* a hormone which regulates our circadian rhythm and which makes us feel drowsy (Gross, 2005).

During sleep we alternate between stages characterized by different depths of sleep (light or deep sleep) and levels of rapid eye movements (REM). REM sleep is characterized by dreaming and it appears that people who experience symptoms of depression tend to dream more (MHF, 2011).

Sleep problems

An in-depth discussion of sleep disorders is not possible here; however, it is important to recognize that there are a number of sleep problems which can seriously disrupt a person's social, psychological and emotional life.

Insomnia is the inability to fall, or remain, asleep and is associated with the feeling that we have had insufficient quality of sleep. Insomnia can be transient and intermittent or chronic and ongoing. Initial insomnia refers to the inability to fall asleep, while midnocturnal (or middle) insomnia refers to waking up in the middle of the night with an associated difficulty of returning to sleep within 30 min. Late (or terminal) insomnia refers to the ability of a person to fall asleep initially but then to awaken in the early morning with an inability of returning to sleep (early morning wakening).

Hypersomnia tends to refer to excessive tiredness and excessive daytime sleepiness, which may be related to obesity and symptomatic of depression, drug and alcohol misuse, side effects of medication (such as antidepressants, anticonvulsants and benzodiazepines), underlying physical illness (such as fibromyalgia [pain in the fibrous tissues in the body with accompanying fatigue and sleep problems], head injuries or other neurological problems or sleep disorders such as narcolepsy [a neurological condition characterized by excessive sleepiness and falling asleep suddenly]) and sleep apnoea. Sleep apnoea tends to occur mostly during REM sleep and refers to a disruption to a person's breathing pattern when asleep, where a person will stop breathing for a short period of time. This can impact on the person's quality of sleep. Risk factors include age (with older people experiencing this problem more than younger people), obesity, smoking and alcohol misuse. Treatment can involve respiratory ventilation via continuous positive airway pressure (CPAP), where a stream of compressed air is delivered via a nasal or face mask (NICE, 2008).

Parasomnias are disruptive sleep problems including nightmares and sleep walking/talking. Nightmares are intense, frightening dreams (MHF, 2011) and tend to occur during REM sleep. People may re-experience past traumas in their nightmares and recurrent nightmares may be associated with periods of anxiety (MHF, 2011). Sleep bruxism (teeth grinding during sleep) can be associated with anxiety or stress, and the use of nicotine, caffeine and alcohol. Bruxism may be improved by treating the underlying psychological cause and the use of a mouth guard may protect against dental problems associated with teeth grinding.

Improving sleep

Promoting healthy sleep is an important function of the mental health nurse (de Niet et al., 2011). *Sleep hygiene* refers to the nonpharmacological steps that can be taken to improve the quality of one's sleep. Below is some general advice which can assist in the promotion of sleep.

- Reduce the amounts of stimulants (tea, coffee, nicotine, cola, chocolate) consumed, particularly prior to bed.
- Increase exercise as this can promote healthy sleep, but avoid vigorous exercise prior to bedtime.
- Try relaxing exercises such as yoga or relaxation techniques such as progressive muscle relaxation or guided visual imagery before bed.
- Alcohol can initially promote sleep but can lead to wakefulness during the night as the body begins to metabolize the alcohol.
- Avoid eating large meals prior to bedtime.
- Ensure exposure to natural light during the day as this helps to promotes a healthy sleep–wake cycle.
- Try to establish a routine before bedtime that helps to promote sleep and try to make sure that the bedroom is relaxing, warm, dark, quiet and comfortable.

For people who have persistent anxieties about sleep and those who have chronic insomnia, cognitive behavioural therapy (CBT) may be used to assist the person in challenging ideas and beliefs which interfere with their sleep (MHF, 2011). However, there is a need for more research into the efficacy of nonpharmacological treatments for insomnia.

Medication (usually hypnotics such as the benzodiazepines and the newer so-called 'Z drugs': zaleplon, zolpidem and zopiclone) is only considered appropriate for the short-term treatment of severe insomnia (see Ch. 24) and where other nonpharmacological techniques (such as those described above) have been unsuccessful (NICE, 2004). There is also some evidence that while benzodiazepines may increase sleep duration they may also lead to increased daytime drowsiness, dizziness and light-headedness (Holbrook et al., 2000).

Assessing sleep

In assessing sleep it is important to remember that the quality of sleep is often subjectively defined. So, while it may be appropriate for a record to be made of the *quantity* or amount a person sleeps during the night (along with sleeping/waking patterns), any assessment must also include the individual's subjective views of the *quality* of their own sleep. The following questions may be helpful in assessing sleep quality.

- On a scale of 1 to 10 how would you rate the quality of your sleep currently? (where 1 is very poor and 10 is very good).
- How many hours per night do you normally sleep? Do you normally sleep throughout the night without interruption, or awaken periodically?
- Has there been any disruption to your normal sleep pattern recently? If yes, in what ways? How do you account for this?
- How easy do you find it to get to sleep? Has this changed recently?
- Do you ever wake up during the night or in the early morning and then find it difficult to fall asleep again?
- Do you experience nightmares? How distressing are they for you? Do you have recurrent nightmares? Can you tell me about them?
- Do you ever wake up feeling tired?
- Do you feel compelled to sleep or nap during the day due to fatigue or tiredness?
- Have you ever had any treatment for sleep problems? If so, what treatment did you receive? Was it helpful?

SEXUAL HEALTH

The issues of sexual health, sexuality and sexual expression and that of mental disorder are often considered to be 'taboo' subjects in society and each are rarely addressed without any form of embarrassment or discomfort. There may also be a lack of the necessary honesty and openness required to ensure that people are fully informed and empowered to attend to these aspects of their health. There is clear evidence that in mental health services specifically it is routine for the issue of sexual healthcare to be attended to inadequately, and it is often simply ignored (Volman and Landeen, 2007). This is despite the recent emphasis on holistic care and more specifically the physical aspects of health within mental health settings (Department of Health, 2006a) and the rise of the profile of sexual health clinics and services in mainstream primary healthcare (Department of Health, 2009). This situation is made all the more unacceptable when we consider the association between sexual health difficulties and increased risks to mental health in addition to the issues around mental disorder and how that can influence a negative impact on the expression of an individual's sexuality.

In 2002 as a result of a WHO consultation on sexual health a working definition of sexual health was determined (WHO, 2002). The opening statement of this definition considered sexuality a central aspect of being human throughout life and encompasses sex, gender identities and roles, sexual orientation, eroticism, pleasure, intimacy and reproduction.

Sexual identity is a major factor which influences many aspects of contemporary social life and is developed throughout life from the gender identities ascribed to us from birth in every society. Early childhood experiences of unpleasant name calling and stigmatization are used to categorize, offend and hurt before children even understand what these terms really mean. This socialization serves to create an environment whereby these behaviours are associated with shame and stigma and are therefore not disclosed or hidden to avoid the unpleasant consequences. Children receive some sexual education in schools, which is often viewed as a contentious issue with the 'rights' and 'wrongs' of it being hotly debated among parents and other social groups, further giving the message to young people that this is a dark, deeply private aspect of our lives that should not be discussed openly and honestly. These facts integral to the human condition serve to create an environment whereby addressing the sexual needs of service users is inherently difficult.

In addition to the very private nature of sexual health, different cultures have very different attitudes to sexuality and the sexual rights of individuals. Within the workforce of mental health services in the UK there is a very diverse representation of cultures and nationalities, each of whom bring their own cultural values to their working relationships. The age of consent for sex varies widely across cultures from 13 to 18 years and homosexuality is illegal in many African countries and Islamic states, and as a consequence the values of the workforce may be in stark contrast to those to whom they provide care (Tummey and Evans, 2008). Thus despite the evidence that the vast majority of mental health workers view the promotion of sexual health as being a part of their role, and fully support the notion that people with mental disorders should not be discouraged from having sex (Hughes and Gray, 2008), there is also compelling evidence that mental health nurses have a lack of knowledge about sexuality alongside conservative attitudes and a recognized anxiety when discussing sexual issues (Quinn and Browne, 2009).

In adulthood, sexuality is an integral and defining feature of who we are, how we form relationships and how we are viewed socially. Social norms dictate that the majority of people marry someone of the opposite sex and then go on to have children and it is accepted that adults have engaged in meeting their sexual needs, although again this is rarely discussed openly or in public. There are many barriers to meeting this integral human need experienced by people with mental health problems, which then impact on their chances of fulfilling social norms and thus enhancing their social status. Barriers to those people who experience mental health problems include issues of social isolation and often the deterioration of social skills which may be as a consequence of this isolation or as a more direct impact of the mental disorder they are experiencing. Added to this many people with mental health problems have a lack of confidence, poor self-esteem and generally a negative self-perception, which further impact on their ability to engage in social situations with ease and their chances of establishing a rapport with someone they find sexually attractive. The experience of having a diagnosis of schizophrenia and the stigma associated with this mental health problem, alongside the perceptions of lay people around what schizophrenia actually means, make the task of forming and maintaining intimate relationships all the more difficult. For example, at what point would it be best to disclose this information to the person you are starting a relationship with, given the effect that this might have on the fledgling relationship? The fear that they may get emotionally hurt, the resulting sense of distress and further damage to their self-esteem may cause the person diagnosed with schizophrenia to repress their need to a sexual aspect to their life. As a consequence of these difficulties, people with mental health problems may not become sexually active, or experience intimacy, until later in life. This may impact on their opportunities to gain the skills and knowledge required to form sexual relationships and to fulfil sexual roles.

The lack of care and attention apportioned to the sexual needs of service users may serve to increase an unspoken belief that they are 'asexual' in the eyes of health professionals. McInnes (2003) reported finding that in many cases it was assumed that any discussion around sexual health is irrelevant as people with chronic illnesses are unlikely to form a relationship, and that society in general is uncomfortable with the notion that people who have a disability or illness might want to have sex.

These attitudes are clearly identifiable historically, as people with mental disorders were desexualized by services. The notion that people with severe mental health problems might want to marry each other has long been met with resistance and disapproval by health professionals.

It would appear therefore that there is a need to address sexual health issues firstly among healthcare professionals, in an effort to increase self-awareness of their own values, prejudice and beliefs around sexuality and mental health and to address their understanding of the need for sexual healthcare to be routinely provided for service users in a truly holistic care package. Given that sexuality and sexual behaviour are not discussed openly or in public by most people, it should not necessarily be anticipated that this would form part of a conversation around health and social wellbeing that is being led by a service user. Sexuality and sexual health require a sensitive yet explicit exploration to be introduced by the health professional as part of an overall assessment of the service user's holistic health needs. By introducing the subject in the context of a trusting and warm therapeutic relationship it may be possible for the service user to open up and discuss any sexual health concerns and to disclose sexual health behaviours to the health professional so that any areas of risk might be identified and health promotion strategies employed in an effort to minimize these. Any such assessment should also routinely focus upon the service user's level of awareness and personal knowledge of sexual health and risk-taking behaviours, as there is an increasing concern that people with mental health problems may not be fully aware of the facts around issues such as HIV acquisition and transmission and other sexually transmitted infections (STIs) (Ngwena, 2011).

Mental health problems can have very deep-rooted and negative effects on sexual relationships and sexual satisfaction in both the service users and their partners. It affects not only their self-image and physical health but also emotional intimacy and reproductive decision making. In many cases it is assumed that any discussion around sexual health is irrelevant as people with chronic illnesses are unlikely to form a relationship. However, this situation leads us to a position of neglecting this health need, despite increasing evidence that people with mental illness are more likely to engage in high-risk sexual behaviour. Higgins et al. (2006) identified that people experiencing serious mental disorders were more likely to have sex with high-risk groups, to have casual sexual encounters and to trade sex for some kind of material gain but were also less likely to use condoms while engaging in these high-risk behaviours. Sexual impulsivity as a result of a manic episode can increase the chances of a person exposing themselves to sexual practices that are inconsistent with their usual standards of personal sexual behaviour and may constitute that person being at increased risk of contracting HIV or STI for the duration of that episode of illness. The impact of this element of the illness can be catastrophic to their social relationships and ultimately have a profound impact on their self-esteem and self-image, causing increased stress at a time of vulnerability. In addition there may be personality deficits – for example, a lack of assertiveness – which may expose this group to being more at risk of sexual exploitation and less able to negotiate safe sexual practices with a partner, and there may be coexisting drug or alcohol problems that may exacerbate the increased exposure to irresponsible and high-risk sexual practices.

Attention to sexual health in mental health settings has often focused upon the impact of psychotropic medication on sexual functioning rather than the overall effects of institutionalization, risk-management initiatives and social exclusion. There is no doubt that many of the medications offered as treatment for mental disorders have adverse side effects that can severely impact on the quality of life experienced by those taking them. These medications often have a negative effect on the person's sexual function and there is evidence that this is one of the most frequent reasons that many service users decide not to take their prescribed medication (Higgins et al., 2006). In addition to neuroleptic medication, many of the antidepressants, specifically those of the selective serotonin-reuptake inhibitor (SSRI) type (see Ch. 24), are known to decrease sexual desire, alongside other sexual dysfunction side effects like erectile dysfunction, delayed ejaculation and anorgasmia. When these unpleasant effects are considered alongside the typical symptomatology of decreased libido within a depressive episode, the situation may be considered to be compounded by the cure. In addition to these physical aspects, service users also identify that the weight gain associated with many psychiatric medications has a negative effect on their self-image and sense of sexual identity. Howard et al. (2002) identified that women with psychotic disorders have significantly lower rates of fertility from around the age of 25 than is seen in the general population. This age-related finding may be in part due to the effects of neuroleptic medication associated with a treatment of psychosis, and its effect on increasing the concentration of prolactin in the blood which would naturally reduce female fertility rate. Howard et al. (2002) found that younger women were more likely to be treated with low doses of medication, which could account for this finding, but also noted that the picture is very unclear as other studies have demonstrated lower fertility rates in women with first-onset schizophrenia, which suggests that the side effects of medication were not the cause of the lower fertility in that group. Whatever the cause, the implications for young women with a mental health problem can be very distressing, and damaging to self-perception and personal goals and ambitions. The desire to have a family and fulfil the role of being a mother could quite naturally place a woman in direct opposition to receiving antipsychotic medication for an illness. The fear among health professions could quite conceivably be around the potentially stressful and negative effects of pregnancy on a woman's mental health. In addition to this, both a woman and her care team may have many anxieties about the longer-term prognosis and the service user's ability to be a 'good mother', and the potential for the damage that 'failing' within that role could cause to all parties.

Inpatient settings afford little or no privacy for sexual intimacy with a partner or for self-masturbation, with regular room checks being undertaken by staff required to manage and minimize potential risks to those in their care. Clearly staff have a responsibility to safeguard vulnerable clients who could be at risk of exploitation from others, or who could engage in risk-taking behaviours due to a lack of capacity to understand the potential for harm, including STIs, false or real allegations of rape and unwanted pregnancy. However, these considerations need to be worked with and the risks minimized rather than adhering to a blanket policy of prevention and intolerance. Sexuality and sexual activity are considered to be a basic human right, but there is evidence that when a service user raises the issue of sexuality and sexual behaviour it is regarded as a clinical problem by mental health professionals caring for them (Buckley and Hyde, 1997).

Where nurses strive to embrace the philosophy of recovery and holism in their practice it would appear that some of the very essence of individual identity is being sidelined, ignored or medicalized in the vast majority of service users. Nurses routinely support service users in maintaining their social roles and functions in the sound knowledge that good, supportive relationships are one of the cornerstones of good mental health and therefore are integral to recovery for those experiencing mental distress. It seems counterintuitive therefore that the role of husband, wife, lover or partner should be left without attention and supportive exploration in this helping relationship at times of greatest need. Volman and Landeen (2007) found that when service users were able to deal with their sexual issues in the same context as their mental health issue they regained their sense of self, which included their sexual sense of self. In addition to this, service users did not restrict the issue of their sexuality to it merely being concerned with their sexual self-concept and identity. They held a much wider view of this aspect of their health, viewing it as an essential and integral part of their overall wellbeing and sense of self. In this research, Volman and Landeen found that sexuality was not limited to the physical aspects by service users. They identified the emotional, intellectual social and psychological aspects of sexuality as being important contributors to an overall sense of wellbeing. This again demands the healthcare worker to offer attention to the 'whole person' in the context of the healthcare relationship as it has a profound effect on the sense of satisfaction of service users.

For sexual health promotion strategies to be effective requires healthcare professionals to offer far more than information to their service users. Training should provide workers with skills to deliver interventions as well as the necessary knowledge around the risks. Studies have demonstrated that although mental health nurses have a generally positive attitude to sexual health and HIV prevention, there is little emphasis on these aspects of care in practice. Hughes and Gray (2008) reported that 70% of mental health workers in their study did not routinely discuss sexual health issues with service users and 81% reported that they did not assess for sexual dysfunction as a side effect of medication. The study also identified that many healthcare workers favoured the use of specialists in providing sexual health promotion and HIV-prevention work with their service users. Perhaps this feature illustrates the social 'discomfort' around discussing sexuality and sexual health in our society. It is essential that nurses and other healthcare professionals have a good understanding of the risks of HIV and other blood-borne infections, alongside all STIs, if they are to be able to assess and support service users in this aspect of their being. Assessment and identification of high-risk behaviours are the cornerstones of sexual health interventions being successful in reducing HIV and STIs in this client group. Interventions must offer the motivation and strategies for the service user to reduce any high-risk behaviours and mental health services must facilitate better links with specialist sexual health services, to learn from their expertise and develop individualized packages of care that serve the specific needs of their service users.

Mental health nurses are often in a unique position with service users by virtue of their close, therapeutic relationship with them. As discussed, talking openly about sexuality is not how we are socialized from a very young age, as a consequence of social taboos. Service users and mental health nurses alike must find ways to overcome the discomfort they feel in discussing sexuality, and acknowledge that this is an integral part of each of our being, and that it is equally understood and experienced in a unique way for each individual. The role of the mental health nurse is to reach an understanding of how this is experienced by their service users and to facilitate an honest assessment of the sexual health needs of that person. This relationship must provide the necessary 'safe' environment for the person to talk openly without fear of being judged, patronized or at worst ignored. The national charity Rethink Mental Illness recommends that mental health staff should receive training on how to promote safe sex, helping people to overcome sexual dysfunction and on protecting service users from sexual harassment (Took, 2002). Conversation should be facilitated by offering the service user to use the vocabulary that they are comfortable with at a level that they understand, rather than the healthcare professional 'hiding behind' the use of medical terminology, socially polite phrases or ambiguous innuendo. Discussion should also be offered around initiating and maintaining intimate relationships and identifying the social skills required for such circumstances, alongside practical advice like the provision of condoms and help with safe-sex principles, in addition to how to overcome potential barriers to protecting their sexual health (Took, 2002). Open discussion of sexual health concerns should offer the opportunity for the person to make sense of their experiences and can assist in them being viewed as a person in an holistic sense, rather than as a product of their mental health issue. It could also be hypothesized that this would ultimately have a positive impact on longer-term commitment to treatment and engagement with services for people with mental health problems. Without sensitive, supportive exploration of sexual health and health issues with service users these problems will continue to impact upon their lives and relationships and could ultimately impact negatively on the person's continued engagement with, and commitment to, treatment.

MENTAL HEALTH AND CHILDBIRTH

Mental health problems are a significant cause of morbidity and mortality among women during pregnancy and following childbirth (Centre for Maternal and Child Enquiries, 2011), with Sullivan and King (2006) suggesting that 15–25% of women will develop a significant mental health problem during pregnancy and the first year postpartum. The spectrum of mental health problems experienced in this period of a woman's life ranges from sadness, or baby blues, which occurs within a few days following childbirth and is experienced by the vast majority of women, to the extremes of infanticide, which is very rare, around three cases per year, but which has a catastrophic impact for all involved (Dalton, 2001). In between these two extremes both postnatal depression and puerperal psychosis are serious affective disorders which demonstrate relatively consistent prevalence rates across nations and across time. These mental health problems can have far-reaching consequences for women's longer-term and ongoing mental health and the development of the infant, alongside the potentially devastating effect on a family. In recent years there has also been an increased awareness of the prevalence of antenatal depression in women, with an incidence rate of between 10 and 17% of birthing women (McCauley et al., 2011). Alongside these specifically perinatal mental health problems (perinatal refers to the period from 28 weeks' gestation to up to 4 weeks following birth) the incidence of childbearing women with a pre-existing mental disorder is increasing, as are the rates of anxiety problems and post-traumatic stress disorder which can occur specifically in relation to childbirth, particularly where the experience

has been complicated or has resulted in a stillbirth (Hadwin, 2007).

Perinatal psychiatric disorders are cared for and managed by multiple teams, including primary care, maternity services and mental health, with all of the complexities of interagency professional working impacting on each case, and the well-acknowledged pitfalls and lack of coordination these circumstances often illustrate. Once the presence or history of a mental problem in a pregnant woman is known to the obstetric care team, this will affect her care pathway from that point onwards. She will be referred by the midwifery team to the obstetrician, her pregnancy being viewed as lying outside of the boundaries of a 'normal' pregnancy which would and could be managed by midwifery care alone. This can be very reassuring to the woman as she may feel that her referral onwards will result in her receiving more supportive and intensive care during her pregnancy and birth. Conversely, the woman may view this referral onwards as her being subjected to more scrutiny and as being viewed as 'abnormal' even within an obstetric setting, due to a mental health problem. Her complication is already the mental health issue and the antenatal care given in response is predetermined by this fact. Midwives routinely ask specific mental health screening questions during the 'booking' of a pregnant woman, and GPs are required to inform maternity services of any history when making a referral (NICE, 2007). These considerations may result in the woman choosing not to accept routine antenatal care or moving to another GP or area in an effort to not disclose a personal history, or family history, of mental health problems and, as a consequence, having the opportunity to be treated as 'normal' by obstetric services. Unfortunately, this may increase the likelihood of late recognition of an increased risk of complications in relation to her pregnancy. National Institute for Health and Clinical Excellence (NICE) guidelines (2007) recommend that a written care plan is developed with the woman and her family within the first trimester (3 months) by all those agencies working with her. The care plan should identify clear care pathways so that all involved know how to access assessment and treatment, and staff should have training and supervision to enable them to follow care pathways. However, even where these considerations are identified and shared by the different agencies caring, there remain concerns about the sharing of confidential information between services as well as fears about litigation should professionals get the balance wrong (McConachie and Whitford, 2009).

It is known that this group of women do have a higher incidence of risk factors for obstetric complications, such as unplanned pregnancy, antenatal hypertension, preterm birth, low birth weight and intrauterine growth retardation as well as higher incidences of emergency Caesarean section and increased vulnerability to foetal and neonatal death (Bennesdsen et al., 2001). Women with a serious mental health disorder often do not present for antenatal care until much later in their pregnancy, perhaps due to fear of stigma and judgemental attitudes from healthcare professions, or fear that the healthcare professionals do not have sufficient training or knowledge of what to do in these circumstances (Edwards and Timmons, 2005). This fear may be well founded as McCauley et al. (2011) found evidence that more than 60% of 161 midwives identified negative responses in their midwifery teams to women with mental disorders, and an overwhelming feeling that many midwives avoided working with women who were known to have a mental health problem. Delayed uptake of antenatal care may also be due to a later recognition of the pregnancy because of an irregular menstrual cycle caused by antipsychotic medication. The implications for this delay in seeking care may be that the woman has continued to take her antipsychotic medication throughout the essential early stages of foetal development, which could have implications for normal development of the foetus in this critical period. Conversely, the decision to withdraw from her medication could significantly increase the woman's risk of relapse, particularly given that this is an anxiety-provoking, stressful and life-changing period in one's life. A subsequent experience of relapse may also present the additional risks of difficulties parenting the child and of losing custody, which would further impact negatively on the woman's mental state.

Screening and early identification of mental health problems in the antenatal period are therefore essential, as the consequences of poor detection methods or lack of early interventions where problems are arising may have a detrimental impact on the health of the mother, her baby and her wider family network. Due to difficulties around the contraindications between many medications used for mental health problems and pregnancy or breastfeeding it is essential that interventions are in place as a matter of priority. Early intervention may offer the opportunity to significantly reduce the need for any such medication further along the line, by successfully utilizing psychosocial interventions or brief psychological interventions in a timely manner. More holistic interventions, such as providing the woman with information about identifying with a local supportive social group (for example, a National Childbirth Trust group, a local antenatal group, or mother-and-baby group), encouraging gentle exercise, undertaking a Wellness Recovery Action Plan or discussing the benefits of a good balanced diet rich in specifically helpful nutrients, such as omega 3, and containing five daily portions of fruit and vegetables. It would also be anticipated that the prognosis for the woman would be improved as a result of earlier intervention and that the potential for any longer-term negative implications for the family unit would also be reduced by prompt identification and action on the part of the healthcare professionals.

Women need support and help with balancing the risks related to decisions surrounding their treatment and care, as well as the reassurance that clinicians are very well placed to assess and identify any manifestations of these risks to both her and her pregnancy in a timely and supportive manner. This multifaceted expertise, however, may not be available from one clinician. There is evidence that midwives do not feel adequately skilled to care for women with underlying mental health problems and that mental healthcare workers do not feel confident that they have the necessary experience, skills or specific knowledge to care for a pregnant woman. In addition to this they report feeling that they do not have the expertise to be able to give adequate consideration to the needs and rights of the unborn child or to the needs of a breast-feeding mother.

The main screening tool utilized to identify women who are at risk of developing postnatal depression is the Edinburgh Postnatal Depression Scale (EPDS), which is a self-assessment rating scale often routinely administered by a health visitor around 6 weeks postnatally. Postnatal depression refers to nonpsychotic depression which occurs up to 1 year following the birth of a baby. It is important to be aware that the vast majority of women who are diagnosed with postnatal depression are cared for by primary care teams and do not require a referral to specialist mental health services. Postnatal depression typically occurs at 8–12 weeks following the birth, although the more severe cases are often identified a little earlier, at 4–6 weeks postnatally (Oates, 2006). Puerperal psychosis occurs within the puerperium, which is defined as the period following childbirth during which the woman's anatomical and physiological changes brought about by the pregnancy are resolved, and the period is considered to last for around 6 weeks. This is arguably the most serious perinatal mental health problem, affecting around 1–2 per 1000 women (Oates, 2006). It usually manifests itself within 2 weeks of the birth and is a severe and often dramatic psychosis, which may develop very rapidly over the course of only a few hours and may be the first psychotic episode the woman has ever experienced. Typical symptoms of this psychosis are hallucinations, delusional ideas, often pertaining to the infant, and a perplexity which is more pronounced than in many other psychotic-type illnesses. The risk of suicide in the perinatal period is a significant issue for practitioners, with suicide being the second most common cause of maternal death (Lewis, 2007). Where suicide occurs within 1 month postnatally the means of committing suicide are often more violent than are generally seen in women at other times of their life. Methods such as shooting, drowning or hanging are not uncommon, which is in contrast to the often more passive methods more commonly used by women at other periods of their lives. There is a paradox here, however, as the rates of suicide during the perinatal period are lower than those of the general population, despite the fact that this is a period of intense emotional and physical stress for the woman, which supports the notion that there may be a protective feature for the woman attached to the early experiences of the role of motherhood.

There is some debate about the nature of perinatal mental health problems, and whether they represent a distinct clinical diagnosis, or whether they are as other mental health problems, but occur around the intensely stressful period around the birth of a child. The *Diagnostic and Statistical Manual of Mental Disorders*, 4th edition (text revision) (American Psychiatric Association, 2000), does not include a diagnostic category for puerperal psychosis, but includes it in other categories. The *International Statistical Classification of Diseases and Related Health Problems*, however, classifies puerperal disorders as those which occur within 6 weeks of birth that cannot be classified elsewhere (WHO, 1992). There is some argument, however, that the clinical features of these illnesses are unusually specific to the timeframe and the influence of the birth of a child.

If a woman requires admission to hospital due to the severity or risks associated with her clinical presentation it is recommended that it should occur in a specialist mother-and-baby mental health setting, unless there are specific reasons for not doing so (NICE, 2007). However, in 2006 the national charity Mind published a report identifying that fewer than 50% of mental health trusts had any specialist perinatal service and only 5% of trusts at that time had any plans for developing any such specialist service. The report also identified that 67% of women who needed admission postnatally were admitted to a general psychiatric ward; the vast majority of these admissions occurred without their babies (Mind, 2006).

There have been concerns raised regarding the attitudes and expertise of generic mental health nurses in relation to their understanding of the specific care and treatment required by a new mother and her baby, due to the lack of consistent exposure they would experience in dealing with these circumstances. In 2009 McConachie and Whitford published a small study into the attitudes of mental health nurses towards severe perinatal mental health problems and reported that participants believed that the symptoms of perinatal disorders were the same as those of any other mental disorders, and therefore they felt confident and competent to deal with the mothers. However, they also reported finding that the presence of a baby in the generic mental health setting made a significant difference to the attitudes of the nurses. Some felt frightened about looking after a baby and did not feel competent to carry out the necessary interaction assessments between mother and baby that were required by the clinical situation, and could not offer the necessary expertise to advise mothers about perinatal medication. The nurses in the study felt that this compromised their ability to advocate for the women in their care (McConachie and Whitford, 2009).

The best-case scenario would be for a woman to be under the care of a good supportive primary care team, who can develop a trusting and close relationship, and for the team to have well-established links with specialist mental health services. The woman could therefore discuss her desire to have a baby with a member of the primary care team or mental health key worker, and make proper, well-informed and adequate preparation for a pregnancy. Advice regarding which psychiatric medications are 'safe' in pregnancy could be offered, and the woman could choose to alter her medication, if necessary, in preparation for pregnancy. This premeditated and well-prepared approach offers the woman the best chances of reducing the risks of stress associated with her pregnancy, which will also reduce her risk of relapse in terms of her mental health and the risks of obstetric complications from the use of medications in the early stages of pregnancy or other stress-related complications. In addition to this, an open and honest approach from all parties involved – the mental health team, the woman, her family and the primary care team, and later the obstetric team – facilitates a more coordinated and holistic response to the pregnancy and any potential complications. It also gives an excellent opportunity for healthcare practitioners to educate, advise and support the woman and her family in terms of what symptoms might be indicative of potential problems and what action they should take in an effort to receive prompt and efficient support should problems arise.

CONCLUSION

Everyone can get physically ill and mental health can at times mask physiological complaints. Whenever a person demonstrates a change in their normal behaviour or an alteration in their appearance (weight loss, pallor, jaundice, etc.) they require a thorough physical assessment. This can be instigated by the mental health team following the described structured approach which should enable the identification of any life-threatening emergencies. Any deviation from the person's normal presentation needs to be investigated further to exclude an organic cause. It is important to remember that many mental health service users may have physical comorbidities, making it vital that mental health staff have an understanding of how to recognize a physically ill patient and the treatment priorities (i.e. ABCDE assessment).

REFERENCES

Abayomi, J., Hackett, A., 2004. Assessment of malnutrition in mental health clients: nurses' judgement vs. a nutrition risk tool. J. Adv. Nurs. 45 (4), 430–437.

Adam, S., Odell, M., Welch, J., 2009. Rapid Assessment of the Acutely Ill Patient. Wiley-Blackwell, Oxford.

Allebeck, P., 1989. Schizophrenia: a life shortening disease. Schizophr. Bull. 15, 81–89.

Allison, D.B., Mackell, J.A., Mcdonnell, D.D., 2003. The impact of weight gain on quality of life among persons with schizophrenia. Psychiatr. Serv. 54 (4), 565–567.

American Psychiatric Association, 2000. Diagnostic and Statistical Manual of Mental Disorders, fourth ed., text rev. American Psychiatric Association, Washington DC.

Bennesdsen, B.E., Mortensen, P.B., Olesen, A.V., et al., 2001. Congenital malformations, stillbirths, and infant deaths amongst children of women with schizophrenia. Arch. Gen. Psychiatry 52, 189–192.

Brown, S., Birtwistle, J., Roe, L., Thompson, C., 1999. The unhealthy lifestyle of people with schizophrenia. Psychol. Med. 29 (3), 697–701.

Buckley, P.F., Hyde, J.L., 1997. State hospitals' responses to the sexual behaviour of psychiatric inpatients. Psychiatr. Serv. 48 (3), 398–399.

Casey, D.E., Haupt, D.W., Newcomer, J.W., et al., 2004. Anti-psychotic induced weight gain and metabolic abnormalities; implications for increased mortality in patient with schizophrenia. J. Clin. Psychiatry 65 (Suppl. 7), 257–269.

Centre for Maternal and Child Enquiries, 2011. Saving mothers' lives: reviewing maternal deaths to make motherhood safer. 2006–2008. BJOG: Int. J. Obstet. Gynaecol. 118 (Suppl. 1), 1–203.

Citrome, L., Yeomans, D., 2005. Do guidelines for severe mental illness promote physical health and well-being? J. Psychopharmacol. 19 (6), 102–109.

Cohen, A., Hove, M., 2001. Physical Health of the Severe and Enduring Mentally Ill: A Training Pack for GP Educators. <http://www.centreformentalhealth.org.uk/pdfs/gp_training_pack.pdf>.

Cohen, A., Phelan, M., 2001. The physical health of patients with mental illness: a neglected area. Ment. Health Promot. Update 2, 15–16.

Collier, E., Skitt, G., Cutts, H., 2003. A study on the experience of insomnia in a psychiatric inpatient population. J. Psychiatr. Ment. Health Nurs. 10, 697–704.

Daley, A.J., 2002. Exercise therapy and mental health in clinical populations; is exercise therapy a worthwhile intervention? Adv. Psychiatr. Treat. 8, 262–270.

Dalton, K., 2001. Depression After Childbirth; How to Recognize, Treat and Prevent Postnatal Depression, fourth ed. Oxford University Press, Oxford.

Dawe, S., Loxton, N., Hides, L., Kavanagh, D., Mattick, R., 2002. Review of Diagnostic Screening Instruments for Alcohol and other Drug Use and other Psychiatric Disorders, second ed. Commonwealth Department of Health Ageing, Brisbane, Queensland.

Dean, J., Todd, G., Morrow, H., Sheldon, K., 2001. Mum, I used to be good looking...look at me now: the physical health needs of adults with mental health problems: the perspectives of users, carers and front-line staff. Int. J. Ment. Health Promot. 3 (4), 16–24.

de Niet, G., Tiemens, B., van Achterberg, T., Hutschemaekers, G., 2011. Applicability of two brief evidence-based interventions to improve sleep quality in inpatient mental health care. Int. J. Ment. Health Nurs. 20, 319–327.

Department of Health, 1994. Nutritional Aspects of Cardiovascular Disease. HMSO, London.

Department of Health, 1998. Smoking Kills: Executive Summary. <http://www.dh.gov.uk/en/Publicationsandstatistics/Publications/PublicationsPolicyAndGuidance/DH_4008708>.

Department of Health, 1999. National Service Framework for Mental Health: Modern Standards and Service Models. <www.dh.gov.uk/en/Publicationsandstatistics/Publications/PublicationsPolicyAndGuidance/DH_4009598>.

Department of Health, 2004. Scientific Committee on Tobacco and Health. Secondhand Smoke. Review of Evidence Since 1998. <http://www.dh.gov.uk/en/Publicationsandstatistics/Publications/PublicationsPolicyAndGuidance/DH_4101474>.

Department of Health, 2006a. From Values to Action: The Chief Nursing Officer's Review of Mental Health Nursing. <www.dh.gov.uk/en/Publicationsandstatistics/Publications/PublicationsPolicyAndGuidance/DH_4133839>.

Department of Health, 2006b. Choosing Health: Supporting the Physical Needs of People with Severe Mental Illness - Commissioning Framework. <http://www.dh.gov.uk/en/Publicationsandstatistics/Publications/PublicationsPolicyAndGuidance/DH_4138212>.

Department of Health, 2009. Moving Forward: Progress and Priorities – Working Together for High Quality Sexual Health. Department of Health, London.

Department of Health, 2011. No Health Without Mental Health: A Cross-Government Mental Health Outcomes Strategy for People of all Ages. <http://www.dh.gov.uk/en/Publicationsandstatistics/Publications/PublicationsPolicyAndGuidance/DH_123766>.

Dixon, L.B., Kreyenbuhl, J.A., Dickerson, F.B., et al., 2004. A comparison of Type 2 diabetes outcomes among persons with and without severe mental illnesses. Psychiatr. Serv. 55 (8), 892–900.

DRC (Disability Rights Commission), 2006. Equal Treatment: Closing the Gap. <http://www.drc.gov.uk/library/health_investigation.aspx>.

Edwards, E., Timmins, S., 2005. A qualitative study of stigma among women suffering from postnatal illness. J. Ment. Health 14 (5), 471–481.

Food Standards Agency, 2001. The Balance of Good Health. <http://www.food.gov.uk/multimedia/pdfs/bghbooklet.pdf>.

Friedli, L., Dardis, C., 2002. Smoke gets in their eyes. Ment. Health Today Jan, 18–21.

Godfrey, P.S., Toone, B.K., Carney, M.W., et al., 1990. Enhancement of recovery from psychiatric illness by methylfolate. Lancet 336, 392–395.

Gold, M.S., 1996. The risk of misdiagnosing physical illness as depression. In: Gold, M.S. (Ed.), The Hatherleigh Guide to Managing Depression, vol. 3. Hatherleigh Publications, New York.

Goldhill, D.R., White, S.A., Summer, A., 1999. Physiological values and procedures in the 24 h before ICU admission from the ward. Anaesthesia 54 (6), 529–534.

Goldhill, D.R., McNarry, A.F., Mandersloot, G., McGinley, A., 2005. A physiologically-based early warning score for ward patients: the association between score and outcome. Anaesthesia 60 (6), 547–553.

Goldman, L.S., 1999. Medical illness in patients with schizophrenia. J. Clin. Psychiatry 60, 10–15.

Goodwin, J.S., Goodwin, J.M., Garry, P.J., 1983. Association between nutritional status and cognitive functioning in a healthy elderly population. J. Am. Med. Assoc. 249, 2917–2921.

Groarke, J.D., Gallagher, J., Stack, J., et al., 2008. Use of an admission early warning score to predict patient morbidity and mortality and treatment success. Emerg. Med. J. 25 (12), 803–806.

Gross, R., 2005. Psychology; The Science of Mind and Behaviour, fifth ed. Hodder Arnold, Abingdon.

Hadwin, P., 2007. Common mental health disorders. In: Price, S. (Ed.), Mental Health in Pregnancy and Childbirth. Churchill Livingstone, Edinburgh, pp. 79–103.

Halbreich, U., Shen, J., Panaro, V., 1996. Are chronic psychiatric patients at increased risk for developing breast cancer? Am. J. Psychiatry 153, 559–560.

Harris, E.C., Barraclough, B., 1998. Excess mortality of mental disorder. Br. J. Psychiatry 173, 11–53.

Higgins, A., Barker, P., Begley, C., 2006. Sexual health education for people with mental health problems: what can we learn from the literature? J. Psychiatr. Ment. Health Nurs. 13, 687–697.

Himelhoch, S., Lehman, A., Kreyenbuhl, J., et al., 2004. Prevalence of chronic obstructive pulmonary disease among those with serious mental illness. Am. J. Psychiatry 161, 2317–2319.

Holbrook, A., Crowther, R., Lotter, A., et al., 2000. Meta-analysis of benzodiazepine use in the treatment of insomnia. Can. Med. Assoc. J. 162, 225–233.

Howard, L.M., Kumar, C., Thornicroft, G., 2002. The general fertility rate in women with psychotic disorders. Am. J. Psychiatry 159 (6), 991–997.

Hughes, E., Gray, R., 2008. HIV prevention for people with serious mental illness: a survey of mental health workers attitudes, knowledge and practice. J. Clin. Nurs. 18, 591–600.

Inventor, B., Henricks, J., Rodman, L., et al., 2005. The impact of medical issues in inpatient geriatric psychiatry. Issues Ment. Health Nurs. 26 (1), 23–46.

Jeste, D.V., Gladsjo, J.A., Lindamer, L.A., et al., 1996. Medical comorbidity in schizophrenia. Schizophr. Bull. 22, 413–430.

Jhalani, J., Goyal, T., Clemow, L., et al., 2005. Anxiety and outcome expectations predict the white-coat effect. Blood Press. Monit. 10 (6), 317–319.

Jindal, R., Mackenzie, E.M., Baker, G.B., Yeragani, V.K., 2005. Cardiac risk and schizophrenia. J. Psychiatry Neurosci. 30, 393–395.

Jonsson, T., Jonsdottir, H., Moller, A.D., Baldursdottir, L., 2011. Nursing documentation prior to emergency admission to the intensive care unit. Nurs. Crit. Care 16 (4), 164–169.

Kelly, C., McCreadie, R.G., 1999. Smoking habits current symptoms and premorbid characteristics of schizophrenia patients in Nithsdale, Scotland. Am. J. Psychiatry 156, 1751–1757.

Kelly, C.A., Upex, A., Bateman, D.N., 2004. Comparison of consciousness level assessment in the poisoned patient using the Alert/Verbal/Painful/Unresponsive Scale and the Glasgow Coma Scale. Ann. Emerg. Med. 44 (2), 108–113.

Kendell, R.E., 2009. The distinction between mental and physical illness. In: Reynolds, J. (Ed.), Mental Health Still Matters, second ed. Palgrave Macmillan, Basingstoke.

Kendrick, T., 1996. Cardiovascular and respiratory risk factors and symptoms amongst general practice patients with long term mental illness. Br. J. Psychiatry 169, 733–739.

Kevric, J., Jelinek, G.A., Knott, J., Welland, T.J., 2011. Validation of the Full Outline of Responsiveness (FOUR) scale for conscious state in the emergency department: comparison against the Glasgow Coma Scale. Emerg. Med. J. 28 (6), 486–490.

Koro, C.E., Fedder, D.O., L'Italien, G.J., et al., 2002. An assessment of the independent effects of olanzipine and risperidone exposure on the risk of hyperlipidaemia in schizophrenic patients. Arch. Gen. Psychiatry 59, 1021–1026.

Lambert, T.J.R., Velakoulis, D., Pantelis, C., 2003. Medical co-morbidity in schizophrenia. Med. J. Aust. 178, S67–S70.

Lesa, R., Dixon, A., 2007. Physical assessment: implications for nurse educators and nursing practice. Int. Nurs. Rev. 54 (2), 166–172.

Lester, H., Tritter, J.Q., England, E., 2003. Satisfaction with primary care: the perspectives of people with schizophrenia. Fam. Pract. 20 (5), 508–513.

Lewis, G. (Ed.), 2007. The Confidential Enquiry into Maternal and Child Health (CEMACH). Saving mothers' lives: reviewing maternal deaths to make motherhood safer 2002–2005. The Seventh Report on Confidential Enquiries into Maternal Deaths in the United Kingdom. CEMACH, London.

McCauley, K., Elsom, S., Muir-Cochrane, E., Lyneham, J., 2011.

Midwives and assessment of perinatal mental health. J. Psychiatr. Ment. Health Nurs. 18, 786–795.

McCloughen, A., 2003. The association between schizophrenia and cigarette smoking: a review of the literature and implications for mental health nursing practice. Int. J. Ment. Health Nurs. 12, 119–129.

McConachie, S., Whitford, H., 2009. Mental health nurses' attitudes towards severe perinatal mental illness. J. Adv. Nurs. 65 (4), 867–876.

McCreadie, R., 2003. Diet, smoking and cardiovascular risk in people with schizophrenia. Br. J. Psychiatry 151, 362–367.

McCreadie, R.G., Scottish Schizophrenia Lifestyle Group, 2003. Diet, smoking and cardiovascular risk in people with schizophrenia: descriptive study. Br. J. Psychiatry 183, 534–539.

McInnes, R.A., 2003. Chronic illness and sexuality. Med. J. Aust. 179 (5), 263–266.

Mann, J.I., 2002. Diet and risk of coronary heart disease and Type 2 diabetes. Lancet 360, 783–789.

Mavundla, T., 2000. Professional nurses' perception of nursing mentally ill people in a general hospital setting. J. Adv. Nurs. 32 (6), 1569–1578.

Mellor, J.E., Laugharne, J.D.E., Peet, M., 1996. Omega-3 fatty acid supplementation in schizophrenic patients. Hum. Psychopharmacol. 11, 39–46.

Mentality/NIMHE, 2004. Healthy body and mind: promoting health living for people who experience mental distress. <http://www.neyh.csip. org.uk/silo/files/hbhmprimarycare. pdf>.

MHF (Mental Health Foundation), 2006. Feeding minds: the impact of food on mental health. <http://www. mentalhealth.org.uk/campaigns/ food-and-mental-health/>.

MHF (Mental Health Foundation), 2011. Sleep matters: the impact of sleep on health and wellbeing. <http://www.mentalhealth.org.uk/ publications/sleep-report/>.

Mind, 2006. Out of the Blue? Mind Publications, London.

Mitchell, A., Malone, D., 2006. Physical health and schizophrenia. Curr. Opin. Int. Med. 5 (5), 524–529.

Nash, M., 2010. Physical Health and Wellbeing in Mental Health Nursing: Clinical Skills for Practice. Open University Press, Maidenhead.

Ngwena, J., 2011. HIV/AIDS awareness in those diagnosed with mental illness. J. Psychiatr. Ment. Health Nurs. 18 (3), 213–220.

NICE (National Institute for Health and and Clinical Excellence), 2002a. Guidance on the use of newer (atypical) antipsychotic drugs for the treatment of schizophrenia. Technology appraisal guidance no. 43. <http://guidance.nice.org.uk/ TA43/guidance/pdf/English>.

NICE (National Institute for Health and and Clinical Excellence), 2002b. Schizophrenia: core interventions in the treatment and management of schizophrenia in primary and secondary care. <http://guidance. nice.org.uk/CG1/guidance/pdf/ English>

NICE (National Institute for Health and and Clinical Excellence), 2004. Zaleplon, zolpidem and zopiclone for the short-term management of insomnia. <http://www.nice.org.uk/ nicemedia/live/11530/32846/32846. pdf>.

NICE (National Institute for Health and and Clinical Excellence), 2007. Antenatal and Postnatal Mental Health: Clinical Management and Service Guidance 45. National Institute for Health and Clinical Excellence, London.

NICE (National Institute for Health and and Clinical Excellence), 2008. Continuous positive airway pressure for the treatment of obstructive sleep apnoea/hypopnoea syndrome. <http://www.nice.org.uk/nicemedia/ live/11944/40085/40085.pdf>.

NIMHE (National Institute for Mental Health In England), 2005. NIMHE guiding statement on recovery. <www.psychminded. co.uk/news/news2005/feb05/ nimherecovstatement.pdf>.

Oates, M., 2006. Perinatal psychiatric syndromes: clinical features. Psychiatry 5 (1), 5–9.

Osborn, D.P.J., Warner, J., 1998. Assessing the physical health of

psychiatric patients. Psychiatr. Bull. 22, 695–697.

Parish, C., 2011. Mental illness reduces life expectancy, research finds. Ment. Health Pract. 14 (10), 5.

Peet, M., 2004. Diet, diabetes and schizophrenia: review and hypothesis. Br. J. Psychiatry 184 (Suppl. 47), S102–S105.

Phelan, M., Stradins, L., Morrison, S., 2001. Physical health of people with severe mental illness. Br. Med. J. 322, 443–444.

Primary Care Mental Health and Education, 2005. Running on Empty: Building Momentum to Improve Well-Being in Severe Mental Illness. <http://www.sane. org.uk/public_html/News/pdfs/ RoE_Report_FINAL.pdf>.

Quinn, C., Browne, G., 2009. Sexuality of people living with a mental illness: a collaborative challenge for mental health nurses. Int. J. Ment. Health Nurs. 18, 195–203.

Redelmeier, D.A., Tan, S.H., Booth, G.L., 1998. The treatment of unrelated disorders in patients with chronic medical diseases. N. Engl. J. Med. 338, 1516–1520.

Repper, J., 2000. Social inclusion. In: Thompson, T., Mathias, P. (Eds.), Lyttle's Mental Health and Disorder. Elsevier, London.

Robson, D., Gray, R., 2005. Can we help people with schizophrenia to stop smoking? Ment. Health Pract. 9 (4), 15–18.

Robson, H., Margereson, C., Trenoweth, S., 2008. Co-morbidity in physical and mental ill-health. In: Lynch, J., Trenoweth, S. (Eds.), Contemporary Issues in Mental Health Nursing. Wiley, Chichester.

SCMH (Sainsbury Centre for Mental Health), 1997. Pulling Together: The Future Roles and Training of Mental Health Staff. <http://www.scmh. org.uk/80256FBD004F6342/vWeb/ pcPCHN6FTHWE>.

SCMH (Sainsbury Centre for Mental Health), 2003. Primary Solutions. An Independent Policy Review on the Development of Primary Care Mental Health Services. Sainsbury Centre for Mental Health, London.

Seymour, L., 2003. Not all in the mind: the physical health of mental health service users. <www.scmh.

org.uk/80256FBD004F3555/
vWeb/flKHAL6PQLA9/$file/
not+all+in+the+mind.pdf>.

Shepherd, G., Boardman, J., Slade, M.,
2008. Making Recovery a Reality.
Sainsbury Centre for Mental Health,
London.

Stroup, T.S., 2004. Antipsychotic drug
treatment of schizophrenia: update
on the Catie trial. In: NCDEU
Abstracts from the 44th Annual
Meeting. 1–4 June 2004, Phoenix,
AZ.

Stubbs, J., Gardner, L., 2004. Survey of
staff attitudes to smoking in a large
psychiatric hospital. Psychiatr. Bull.
28, 204–207.

Sullivan, E.A., King, J.F., 2006. Maternal
Deaths in Australia 2000–2002.
AIHW National Perinatal Statistics
Unit, Sydney.

Took, M., 2002. Mental breakdown
and recovery in the UK. J. Psychiatr
Ment. Health Nurs. 9, 635–637.

Tummey, R.J., Evans, D.T., 2008.
Sexuality. In: Tummey, R., Turner,
T. (Eds.), Critical Issues in Mental
Health. Palgrave-Macmillan,
Basingstoke.

Volman, L., Landeen, J., 2007.
Uncovering the sexual self in people
with schizophrenia. J. Psychiatr.
Ment. Health Nurs. 14, 411–417.

Vose, C.P., 2000. Drug abuse and
mental illness: psychiatry's next
challenge! In: Thompson, T.,
Mathias, P. (Eds.), Lyttle's Mental
Health and Disorder. Elsevier,
London.

West, S.L., 2006. Physical assessment:
whose role is it anyway? Nurs. Crit.
Care 11 (4), 161–167.

WHO (World Health Organization),
1992. ICD-10: International
Statistical Classification of Diseases
and Related Health Problems, tenth
rev. World Health Organization,
Geneva.

WHO (World Health Organization),
2002. Gender and reproductive
rights. <http://www.who.int/
reproductive-health/gender/sexual_
health.html>.

WHO (World Health Organization),
2007. European Health for all
Database (HFA-DB): World Health
Organization Regional Office for
Europe, updated January 2007.
<http://data.euro.who.int/hfadb/>.

Glossary

activity groups Part of psychosocial rehabilitation programmes where organised activities such as art, walking and discussion are designed to engage clients to construct a therapeutic milieu and to help with socialising techniques and imitative behaviour.

absolute neutrophil granulocyte count Total count of the neutrophils in the blood, which provides an indication of a person's ability to fight infection

ACE inhibitor Angiotensin-converting-enzyme inhibitors (ACE inhibitors) are a class (group) of drugs that are used in the treatment of various disorders such as kidney disease and heart conditions.

acute dystonic reaction One of the side effects of traditional antipsychotic medication. Can include the patient having painful muscle spasms in the head, back and torso, which can last minutes or hours; these occur suddenly and can cause fear in the patient.

adjustment disorder An exaggerated emotional or behavioural response to a significant life change or stressor such as a relationship break-up, bereavement, divorce or illness.

adulthood A series of cognitive, social, psychological and physical changes that occur after adolescence until the final stages of one's life.

advanced practice A level of nursing aimed at maximising the nursing contribution to healthcare and improving health outcomes.

affect The observable behaviours associated with changes in a person's mood, such as crying and looking dejected. Some types of affect are blunted, flat, inappropriate, labile and restricted.

ageism The systematic stereotyping of and discrimination against people because of their age alone; making assumptions about how people are viewed throughout the lifespan.

agenda-setting When the client is allowed to control the therapeutic relationship and the treatment regimen.

aggression Actions or behaviours ranging from violent physical acts such as kicks or punches, through to verbal abuse, insults and nonverbal gestures. The overall feeling projected is an attempt to dominate.

agitation (also known as psychomotor agitation) Excessive nonproductive, repetitive motor activity associated with a feeling of inner tension (pacing, hand wringing, fidgeting).

agoraphobia Anxiety about being in places or situations from which escape might be difficult (or embarrassing) or in which help might not be available.

agonist A drug that binds to a receptor of a cell and triggers a response by the cell. An agonist often mimics the action of a naturally occurring substance. An antagonist produces an action. It is the opposite of an agonist, which acts against and blocks an action.

agranulocytosis A blood disorder characterised by severe depletion of white blood cells, rendering the body almost defenceless against infection.

akathisia One of the side effects of traditional antipsychotic medication; involves the person not being able to stay or remain still, being restless and suffering from leg aches.

alogia Impoverished thinking that is observable and indicated by brief, concrete replies to questions, a restricted amount of spontaneous speech or vague, abstract repetitive speech.

ambivalence An individual's tendency to hold conflicting views and feelings such as love and hate, making meaningful decision making difficult.

amnesia An inability to remember events from a particular period. There are a number of different amnesias, including localised amnesia, selective amnesia, generalised amnesia and systematised amnesia.

anhedonia Loss of the feelings of pleasure previously associated with favoured activities.

Glossary

anorexia nervosa A disorder characterised by a refusal to maintain minimal, normal body weight for age and height; an intense fear of gaining weight; disturbed perception of body shape and size and amenorrhoea in postmenarcheal females.

anti-anxiety medication Medication used when anxiety for the individual becomes debilitating. Benzodiazepines are the drug of choice for short-term treatment of anxiety states.

anticholinergic Side effects of traditional antipsychotic medication, including dry mouth, blurred vision, orthostatic hypotension, tachycardia, urinary retention and nasal congestion.

antidepressant medication Medication that enhances the transmission of neurochemicals, particularly serotonin and noradrenaline (norepinephrine), by blocking the reuptake of the neurotransmitters at the synapse, inhibiting their metabolism and destroying and/or enhancing the activity of the receptors.

antipsychotic medication Also known as neuroleptic and typical antipsychotics, these drugs were introduced in the 1950s and revolutionised the treatment of mental illness. Traditional antipsychotics are dopamine antagonists that reduce the 'positive' symptoms of schizophrenia and can affect the 'negative' symptoms.

anxiety A common human experience that is a normal emotion felt in varying degrees by everyone; also a state in which individuals experience feelings of uneasiness, apprehension and activation of the autonomic nervous system in response to a vague, nonspecific threat.

aphasia Impairment in the understanding or transmission of ideas by language in any form (writing, reading, speaking) due to impairment of the brain centres involved in language.

aphonia The inability to produce speech sounds.

arrhythmia An arrhythmia is a disorder of the heart rate (pulse) or heart rhythm, such as beating too fast (tachycardia), too slow (bradycardia) or irregularly.

assertiveness A communication skill that enhances one's interpersonal effectiveness and allows one the choice of how to respond to others. The assertive person protects the rights of each party and achieves goals without hurting others. This results in self-confidence and the ability to express oneself appropriately in emotional and social situations.

asthenia Weakness; lack of energy and strength; loss of strength.

ataxia The partial or complete loss of voluntary muscular movement and coordination.

ataxia A group of neurological disorders that affect balance, coordination and speech. There are many different types of ataxia that can affect people in different ways.

attachment The strong bond or connection one feels for particular people in one's life; usually associated with the primary bond between infant and mother, which can influence one's self-concept, relationships and life experiences.

autism An individual's tendency to retreat into an inner fantasy world, resulting in socially isolating or withdrawing behaviours and loss of contact with reality.

avolition Loss of motivation resulting in impairment in goal-directed activities.

behavioural theories Theories that emphasise the importance of the environment in shaping and changing behaviour in individuals.

behavioural therapy Therapy used to determine what causes and maintains certain behaviours and to develop treatment plans with specific goals; identifies what will be done to achieve goals, how goal achievement will be measured and a timeline for goal achievement.

beta-noradrenergic receptor Any of various cell membrane receptors that can bind with adrenaline (epinephrine) and related substances that activate or block the actions of cells containing such receptors. These cells initiate physiological responses such as increasing the rate and force of contraction of the heart as well as relaxing bronchial and vascular smooth muscle

biomedical model A model based on the idea that normal behaviour occurs because of equilibrium within the body and that abnormal behaviour results from pathological bodily or brain function.

biopsychosocial model of assessment A comprehensive assessment of all aspects of information concerning the consumer: biological, psychological, sociological, developmental, spiritual and cultural information.

bipolar disorder A diagnosis outlined in DSM-IV-TR (*which see*) when a person has previously experienced at least one manic episode and a depressive episode.

body image assessment Assessment of components of body image, including body image distortion, body image avoidance and body image dissatisfaction.

body image avoidance A disturbance of cognition and affect that leads to repetitive body checking and avoidance of social situations that provoke anxiety about the body.

body image dissatisfaction A disturbance of cognition and affect that leads to a negative evaluation of physical appearance.

body image distortion A disturbance of perception in which clients describe their body or parts of it as large or fat despite concrete evidence to the contrary.

body mass index (BMI) A mathematical formula, based on the height and weight of an individual, which is used to help determine the degree of starvation.

bromocriptine A drug used in the treatment of neuroleptic malignant syndrome.

bulimia nervosa A disorder characterised by binge-eating behaviour: eating much larger amounts of food than would normally be eaten in one sitting, and inappropriate, compensatory weight loss behaviours such as self-induced vomiting and purging.

burnout A syndrome in which healthcare workers lose concern and feeling for clients/consumers under their care, becoming detached and distancing themselves from the client/consumer; characterised by emotional exhaustion, depersonalisation and decreased personal accomplishment.

case management Assessing, planning, linking, monitoring and evaluating services with the client, with caseloads shared among the multidisciplinary team.

catastrophising When a person feels inappropriate guilt and thinks of self as incompetent, faulty, unlovable and a failure.

catatonia A severe and debilitating condition with disorganisation of motor behaviour and inability to relate to external stimuli; one of the subtypes of schizophrenia.

catatonia A state of apparent unresponsiveness to external stimuli in a person who is apparently awake.

challenging behaviour Unusual or disturbed, maladaptive behaviours which can include stereotypical or repetitive behaviours (e.g. body rocking), 'acting out' behaviours (e.g. yelling out), self-injurious behaviours (e.g. scratching at one's own skin) or aggression towards others.

Child and Adolescent Mental Health Services Comprehensive services including specialist assessment and treatment options, usually only available in main centres.

childhood The early years of life in which foundations are laid for future development and outcomes.

cimetidine A drug that reduces acid production in the stomach.

circumstantiality A disturbance in form of thought, in which speech is indirect and longwinded.

clanging A disturbance in form of thought, in which words are chosen for their sounds rather than their meanings; includes puns and rhymes.

classification of mental disorders Classification enables information to be provided concerning the patterns of behaviour, thoughts and emotions of consumers.

clinical supervision A positive process that involves reflection of clinical interactions and interventions by one clinician to another more experienced clinician for support, professional development, education and development of clinical practice skills.

code of ethics Guidelines for members of professional groups as to the nature of proper ethical conduct and their obligations to the public.

coexisting disorder Having more than one disorder at the same time, most commonly a mental health disorder and a substance use disorder. Similar terms are comorbidity and dual diagnosis.

cognitive behavioural therapy (CBT) Therapy that aims to help people develop more efficient coping mechanisms by equipping them with strategies that promote logical ways of thinking about and responding to everyday situations.

cognitive restructuring A collaborative nurse–client intervention that aims to monitor and reduce distressing negative cognitions (thoughts), especially in people who are depressed.

collusion When the client attempts to persuade individual staff members to endorse their way of behaving.

community care Health services available from community mental health centres and emphasising the multidisciplinary team; includes services such as counselling, follow-up treatment, referrals and supported accommodation.

comorbidity Having more than one disorder at the same time, most commonly a mental health disorder and a substance use disorder. Similar terms are coexisting disorder and dual diagnosis.

competency When a patient can or should decide and/or be permitted to decide for themselves; beyond this point another or others will need to, or should, decide for the patient.

competency skills In order to protect the public, a specific framework that describes the expected skill base of all practitioners within a specific discipline is set by regulatory bodies and professional nursing organisations.

compulsions Repetitive behaviours (e.g. hand washing, checking) or mental acts (e.g. praying, counting), the goal of which is to prevent or reduce anxiety or distress, not to provide pleasure or gratification.

confabulation Filling in gaps in memory with imaginary experiences.

confidentiality A primary principle of the therapeutic relationship; involves maintaining confidential information about a consumer within the treatment team.

consumer Someone who has the lived experience of mental distress and who has received care from mental health professionals.

containment To provide a place of safety, the hospital and confinement can be seen as a refuge from self-destructiveness and an opportunity to reassure the client and others that illness will not overwhelm them.

continuous care Long-term, ongoing, supportive care of clients with access to a range of services, usually commenced by committed staff and in the discharge planning process.

Glossary

coping The way one deals with change, conflict and demands in life, which can be influenced by factors such as our feelings, thoughts, beliefs and values.

counter-transference The response of the therapist to the patient. Having strong feelings for the patient, either negative or positive, might be a cue that one is experiencing counter-transference.

creatine phosphokinase An enzyme present in muscle, brain and other tissues of vertebrates. When found in very high levels in the blood it indicates injury or stress to muscle tissue.

crisis An event(s) that changes one's day-to-day existence and creates a sense of one's life being out of control, feeling that one is vulnerable and that events are unpredictable; can involve a significant loss for the person involved.

crisis intervention Involvement of assessment, planning, intervention and resolution of a crisis.

cultural competence A model developed from transcultural nursing to describe the role of culture in nurse–patient dynamics and to attempt to understand these cultural dynamics.

cultural respect Allows the individual mental health nurse to value the contribution that culturally appropriate interventions can make to the therapeutic environment.

cultural safety Goes beyond describing the practices of other ethnic groups to nurses learning about their own attitudes and values in their own culture, rather than just learning about the cultures of their clients.

cultural sensitivity Being informed about the 'legitimacy of difference' and allowing oneself to be open to self-exploration.

culture A body of learned behaviours that is used to interpret individual experience and shape individual behaviour, emotion and social responses.

dantrolene A muscle relaxant used for muscle cramps and spasm.

decanoate esters The chemical form in which traditional antipsychotic drugs may be given as long-lasting depot preparations.

defence mechanisms Unconscious processes whereby anxiety experienced by the individual's ego is reduced.

deinstitutionalisation Closure of major psychiatric hospitals and expansion of community-based care for consumers, including relocation of inpatient psychiatric beds into general hospitals.

delirium A syndrome that constitutes a characteristic pattern of signs and symptoms that reduce clarity of awareness and impair the client's ability to focus, sustain or shift attention; tends to develop quickly and fluctuates during the course of the day.

delirium tremens (DTs) A major withdrawal syndrome in which the client presents with a number of complaints, which can include agitation, disorientation, high fever, paranoia, visual hallucinations, coarse tremors and seizures.

delusion A false belief, based on incorrect inference about external reality, that is firmly sustained despite what almost everyone else believes and despite incontrovertible and obvious proof or evidence to the contrary. Types of delusion include bizarre, jealous, erotomanic, grandiose, control, reference, persecution, somatic, thought broadcasting and thought insertion.

dementia A progressive illness that involves cognitive and noncognitive abnormalities and disorders of behaviour; presents as a gradual failure of brain function. It is not a normal part of life or ageing.

democratisation Creating an environment in which staff and clients feel free to express themselves without fear of rejection and to participate in decision making to the extent of one's abilities.

dependence A maladaptive pattern of substance abuse leading to significant impairment or distress and manifested in tolerance, withdrawal and increasing consumption, to the point where obtaining the substance becomes the main focus for the individual; can be physical and/or psychological.

depersonalisation A sense of personal reality being lost or altered, of being estranged from oneself, as if in a dream, or that one's actions are mechanical or otherwise detached from the body or mind.

depot antipsychotic medication Long-acting, injectable forms of traditional antipsychotic medication, used when the patient is unable to take oral medication, if intestinal absorption is questioned or when there might be a medication adherence or compliance problem.

depression A disorder characterised by depressed mood, with feelings of hopelessness and helplessness, lack of pleasure or interest, appetite disturbance, sleep disturbance and fatigue.

derailment A disturbance in form of thought, in which thoughts do not progress logically and ideas are unconnected, shifting between subjects; also known as loosening of association.

derealisation A phenomenon in which the person's sense of the object world is altered. The person might perceive objects to be bigger or smaller than they really are, or once-familiar objects may now seem strange.

detoxification The process by which an alcohol- or drug-dependent person recovers from intoxication in a supervised manner so that withdrawal symptoms are minimised.

developmental theories Theories that highlight the importance of the early months and years of one's life in laying a solid foundation for mental health and wellbeing in adulthood.

dialectical behaviour therapy (DBT) Similar to cognitive behavioural therapy but actively incorporates social skills training; moves between validation and acceptance of the person.

disability An individual's impairment in one or more areas of functioning.

disability services A variety of services for people with intellectual disabilities, including living at home with relatives, shared accommodation, group homes, community-based services, nongovernment organisation service provision and residential institutions.

dissociation Being focused on one's own internal thoughts, and being unaware of the external environment. For example, daydreaming is considered a mild form of dissociation.

distractible speech A disturbance in form of thought, in which nearby stimuli cause repeated changes in the topic of speech.

diuretic Diuretics are medicines that remove water from the body by increasing the amount of urine the kidneys produce.

DSM-IV-TR *Diagnostic and Statistical Manual of Mental Disorders*, 4th edition (text revised), published by the American Psychiatric Association (2000). This classification system assesses the patient across five domains, which help with treatment planning and outcome.

dual diagnosis Having more than one disorder at the same time, most commonly a mental health disorder and a substance use disorder. Similar terms are coexisting disorder and comorbidity.

dual disability Having a comorbid intellectual or developmental disability.

dualism A philosophical position derived from the Cartesian idea that there is a mind–body duality, the body being separate from the soul or moral features (mind).

duty of care The taking of reasonable care by a nurse to avoid acts or omissions which one can reasonably foresee would be likely to injure another.

dysarthria A disorder of speech.

dyscrasia An abnormal state or disorder of the body, especially of the blood.

dystonia Dystonia is characterised by involuntary and uncontrollable muscle spasms which can force affected parts of the body into abnormal, sometimes painful, movements or postures.

eating disorders Complex and serious disorders that involve physical, psychological, social, family and individual factors characterised by serious disturbance of eating behaviours; include anorexia nervosa, bulimia nervosa and eating disorders not otherwise specified.

echolalia A disturbance in form of thought, in which other people's words or phrases are echoed, often in a 'mocking' tone; not the same as repetition of the person's own words (perseveration).

echopraxia Repetition by imitation of the movements of another person. The actions are involuntary and semi-automatic.

egocentrism Focusing on oneself to the degree that other people's needs are beyond one's awareness.

ego-dystonic When a patient's symptoms are experienced as distressing to the individual.

electroconvulsive therapy (ECT) The application of metal electrodes to the head, through which an electric current is delivered. The electrodes can be placed unilaterally or bilaterally. ECT remains a controversial intervention in psychiatry, although it is widely accepted as an effective intervention in the treatment of severe depression.

empathy Observing, listening, understanding and attending; 'being' with the person physically, cognitively and emotionally, understanding their story, thoughts, feelings, beliefs and emotions.

engagement The process of establishing rapport with a client through interactions based on acknowledging and developing a relationship based on trust.

ethical conduct Principles for the practice of ethical conduct by health professionals, including issues of autonomy, beneficence, nonmaleficence and justice.

ethnocentrism The belief that one's own cultural values constitute the human norm and that difference is deviant and wrong.

externalising problems Problems that include antisocial or under-controlled behaviour, such as delinquency or aggression.

extrapyramidal side effects Side effects of antipsychotic drugs on the extrapyramidal motor system; include acute dystonia, parkinsonism, akathisia and tardive dyskinesia.

family therapy An approach to treatment based on the idea that when a family member has a problem, it usually involves the whole family. Family therapists aim to effect change in the entire family system.

fear A response to a known threat; manifests in the same way as anxiety.

flight of ideas A disturbance in form of thought, in which the person's ideas are too rapid for them to express, and so their speech is fragmented and incoherent.

forensic patient A person who has committed a crime while mentally ill and is remanded in custody in an approved mental health service, within a prison, remand centre or forensic psychiatric hospital.

form of thought The amount and rate of production of thought, continuity of ideas and language. Disturbances in form of thought include circumstantiality, clanging, derailment (loosening of associations), distractible speech, echolalia, flight of ideas, illogicality, incoherence, irrelevance, neologisms, perseveration, tangentiality, thought blocking, thought disorder and word approximations. For descriptions of each, see individual entries in this Glossary.

fugue In a long-term dissociative state; the person is unable to remember the past and may also be confused about their identity, unable to remember their name or their occupation.

generalised anxiety disorder (GAD) Excessive anxiety and worry concerning events or activities (apprehensive expectation), occurring more days than not for a period of at least 6 months, and the individual finds it difficult to control.

Geriatric Depression Scale (GDS) Assessment tool designed to assist in making a diagnosis of depression, referral for treatment and to provide a baseline assessment with which to measure the outcome of treatments.

Gillick competence The ability of young people to consent to medical treatment or seek medical consultation as seen in their cognitive ability to make an informed judgement to give consent for treatment.

Glasgow Coma Scale (GCS) A standardised system for assessing the degree of conscious impairment in the critically ill and for predicting the duration and ultimate outcome of coma, primarily in clients with head injury.

grandiosity An inflated appraisal of one's worth, power, knowledge, importance or identity.

grief A natural process that can be experienced after loss, and can be an emotional response of distress, pain and disorganisation.

group cohesion An important component in creating a climate of support and involvement. Sharing among the staff and patients of daily duties and unit resources helps communalism and cohesion to occur.

group therapy The engagement of two or more people in therapy at the same time. Interactions with others in a group situation, especially people who come together with others who experience the same or similar difficulties, have been shown to have positive and beneficial effects.

hallucination A sensory perception that seems real but occurs without external stimulation (unlike an illusion, which is a misinterpretation of real phenomena; see *illusion*). Types of hallucination include auditory, gustatory, olfactory, somatic, tactile and visual.

harm reduction The guiding principle used to identify a range of strategies that target the consequences of drug use rather than the drug itself.

hazardous substance use A repetitive pattern of use that poses a risk of harmful physical and psychological consequences.

Health of the Nation Outcome Scales (HoNOS) Designed in Britain, this scale is used to gather information concerning key areas of mental health and social functioning for service monitoring and outcome measurement.

helping relationship A therapeutic interaction facilitating exploration of responses following a major and significant personal loss leading to a client experiencing grief.

holism Healing of the whole person by recognising the importance of the interrelationships between biological, psychological, social and spiritual aspects of a person.

hope A state of mind that anticipates positive expectations of personally meaningful goal achievement.

'humours' The humoural theory was based on the belief that the body contained four humours – blood, phlegm, yellow bile and black bile – and disease developed when internal or external factors disturbed the balance of the humours and produced injurious effects such as mental illness.

hypersomnia Excessive sleepiness; prolonged nocturnal sleep, difficulty in staying awake during the day and/or undesired daytime sleep episodes.

hyperpyretic Having an extremely elevated temperature.

hypochondriasis A disorder in which the person is intensely preoccupied with their bodily functions and can report any of a wide range of symptoms. The client focuses on what the symptoms might signify and can misinterpret ordinary bodily functions as symptoms of a serious physical illness.

hypomania A form of elevated mood less severe than mania.

ICD-10-AM *International Statistical Classification of Diseases and Related Health Problems*, 10th revision, published by the World Health Organization (1992); provides a comprehensive listing of clinical diagnoses, each with its own numerical code.

ideas of reference Belief that an insignificant or incidental object or event has special significance or meaning for that individual.

identity Part of one's self-concept; develops over time and contributes to one's overall sense of self.

illicit drugs Drugs that are classified as illegal.

illogicality A disturbance in form of thought in which the conclusions reached in a person's speech are illogical.

illusion A misperception or misinterpretation of a real external stimulus, such as seeing a shadow on the wall as a person, or hearing rustling leaves as people speaking.

incoherence A disturbance in form of thought, in which there is verbal rambling with no clear main idea.

incongruent affect A mismatch between a person's thoughts and their emotional expression in a given situation.

informed consent Consent that is (among other requirements) voluntary and specific and comes from a competent person.

insane Coming from the Latin word *insana* meaning not of right mind; the equivalent Greek term is *mania*.

insight The client's ability to understand the reason for and the meaning of their behaviour, feelings and life events.

internalising problems Problems that include inhibited or over-controlled behaviours, such as anxiety or depression.

interpersonal therapy (IPT) Therapy that targets relationships as a key factor in the contribution and maintenance of eating disorders.

intoxication A reversible state that occurs when a person's intake exceeds their tolerance and produces behavioural and/or physical changes.

involuntary admission Compulsory or involuntary detention in an approved psychiatric institution in the best interests of the individual, for treatment that will alleviate the individual's symptoms of mental illness.

irrelevance A disturbance in form of thought, in which a person's replies to questions are not related to the topic being discussed.

JOMAAC A client assessment tool based on observation of the client's judgement, orientation, memory, affect, attitude and cognition.

la belle indifference 'beautiful indifference', where the client shows a marked indifference to or unconcern about their symptoms, even if the symptom is blindness or paralysis.

labile Having rapidly shifting or unstable emotions.

learned helplessness Both a behavioural state and personality trait of one who believes their control over a situation has been lost. It can also relate to hopelessness and powerlessness: an inability to escape an intolerable situation, leading to the ultimate mode of adaptation: subjugation and acceptance.

least-restrictive alternative The option of least restriction for the individual (e.g. community-based care or institution-based treatment), with consideration of the person's level of autonomy, their acceptance and cooperation, and potential for harm to self and to others.

lifespan The sequence of events and experiences in a person's life from birth until death.

limit-setting Explaining to clients what behaviours are acceptable and what is unacceptable, and informing them of the consequences of breaking the rules; aims to offer the client a degree of control over their behaviour by setting firm, fair and consistent limits or rules.

mad A middle-English, pre-twelfth-century word which means having lost reason and judgement.

magical thinking The erroneous belief that one's thoughts, words or actions will cause or prevent a specific outcome in some way that defies the laws of cause and effect.

major depressive disorder A condition involving seriously depressed mood and other symptoms defined by DSM-IV-TR that affect all aspects of a person's bodily system and interfere significantly with their daily living activities.

malingering The intentional production of symptoms in order to avoid some specific duty or responsibility; the incentive to become sick is clearly identifiable.

mania A state of euphoria that results in extreme physical and mental overactivity.

medication adherence/compliance The taking of medication for ongoing treatment of the client's illness. Failure to take medication is often the cause of relapse and readmission to hospital, and can be caused by factors such as the medication having an adverse impact on the patient's life, side effects, insight into the illness and lack of education about the medication.

mental health A state in which an individual has a positive sense of self, personal and social support with which to respond to life's challenges, meaningful relationships with others, access to employment and recreational activities, sufficient financial resources and suitable living arrangements.

mental health assessment and outcome measures Standardised measures in mental health for more reliable, valid and consistent measures of initial assessment and of change that occurs with treatment.

mental health disorders Conditions in which an individual cannot cope and function as previously, causing considerable personal, social and financial distress and affecting healthcare funding, implementation of service provision and community resources.

mental health policy Health policy based on the World Health Organization (WHO) guiding principles of access, equity, effectiveness and efficiency for all people with mental health issues.

mental health promotion A population-health approach to mental health, which attends to the mental health status and needs of the whole population, emphasising a continuum of care from universal prevention to long-term, individual care with early intervention and treatment.

mental illness A condition of impairment and disorganisation of mental function for an individual.

mental retardation A disability typified by major limitations in intellectual functioning and in conceptual, social and practical adaptive skills, that originates before the age of eighteen.

Mental Status Examination (MSE) A semi-structured interview with a consumer to assess the person's current neurological and psychological status using several dimensions, such as perception, affect, thought content, form of thought and speech.

mentoring Process aimed at promoting growth and development in clinicians by means of partnerships with other clinicians in the workplace, involving problem-solving, feedback, support and relationship building.

milieu A physical environment including the social, emotional, interpersonal, professional and managerial elements that comprise a particular setting.

milieu therapy Therapy that involves the environment in the treatment process, the participation of patients and staff in decision making, the use of a multidisciplinary team, open communication and individualised goal-setting with patients.

Mini Mental Status Examination (MMSE) An abbreviated form of the Mental Status Exam; based on observable behaviour in a client assessment interview.

Mini Psychiatric Assessment Schedule for Adults with Developmental Disabilities (Mini PAS-ADD) An accessible assessment tool based on a life events checklist and the client's symptoms.

misconceptions Misinformation and misunderstanding about the origins, course and treatment of mental health problems and mental disorders.

monotherapy Treatment through use of a single drug.

mood A pervasive emotion that colours the person's perception of the world (in contrast to affect, which is the observable behaviours associated with mood, or the visible expression of emotions; see *affect*).

motivational interviewing Basically an adaptation of the Socratic style of interviewing; proceeds from the assumption that change is produced collaboratively and cannot be imposed from outside.

mourning A process needed to help overcome grief, involving the person extricating themselves from their relationship with the deceased person (or object or part of their person).

multidisciplinary team (MDT) A team of individuals from multiple disciplines, such as nurses, psychologists, psychiatrists, social workers and occupational therapists, working together to provide a holistic team approach to care.

myoglobinaemia Damage to muscle cells.

nature-versus-nurture debate A continuing discussion concerning the effects of biological phenomena and inheritance (nature) and the individual's environment and experiences in the world (nurture) and

whether both are vital, inseparable, interdependent components of personality development that influence human behaviour.

necrolysis An exfoliative skin disease in which erythema spreads rapidly over the body, followed by blisters much like those seen in a second-degree burn.

negative symptoms of schizophrenia Tend to include signs and symptoms such as blunting of affect, avolition and anhedonia.

neologisms Disturbance in form of thought, in which a person creates new words or expressions that have no meaning to anyone else.

neuroleptic malignant syndrome A rare disorder that resembles a severe form of parkinsonism with coarse tremor and catatonia, fluctuating in intensity, accompanied by signs of autonomic instability and stupor; risk of death is high.

neuroleptic medication See also *antipsychotic medication*; the term 'neuroleptic' is used to indicate the movement and posture disorder caused as part of the extrapyramidal side effects of some antipsychotic drugs. Antipsychotic medication is the preferred term because the atypical antipsychotics have very little extrapyramidal action.

neuropsychological disorders Disorders, such as schizophrenia, in which the origin of the psychological disturbance lies in the neurological structure and function of the brain.

neurosis A term of mainly historical interest that was used in reference to madness caused by nervous system disease. Since Freud's time, 'neurosis' has been used to refer to nonpsychotic disorder characterised mainly by anxiety.

neurotransmitter A chemical that is released from a nerve cell which thereby transmits an impulse from a nerve cell to another nerve, muscle, organ or other tissue. A neurotransmitter is a messenger of neurologic information from one cell to another.

nongovernment organisations Services that operate outside mainstream government authority and at a community level to support consumers and carers with a range of special needs, e.g. Age UK, Rethink Mental Illness, Mind.

normalisation A humanistic model of care in which people with an intellectual disability are given the same rights and opportunities as any other person, even if the support of appropriate services is needed.

nurse practitioner An advanced practitioner with a high degree of autonomy, who has extended education in a defined scope of practice and is licensed to practise within an extended role.

observation When experienced staff maintain a continuous watchful presence in a nonthreatening, non-intrusive manner to set reasonable limits on behaviour.

obsessions Recurrent persistent thoughts, impulses, images that are intrusive and inappropriate and cause marked anxiety or distress in an individual.

obsessive-compulsive disorder Recurrent obsessions or compulsions that are severe enough to be time-consuming or cause marked distress or significant impairment in an individual.

panic attack A discrete period of intense fear or discomfort in the absence of real danger.

panic disorder The presence of recurrent, unexpected panic attacks followed by concern about having another panic attack or significant behavioural change related to the attacks.

Parkinson's syndrome One of the side effects of traditional antipsychotic medication, with the person exhibiting a rigid, mask-like facial expression, shuffling gait and drooling.

perseveration A disturbance in form of thought, in which the individual persistently repeats the same word or ideas; often associated with organic brain disease.

personality Expression of our feelings, thoughts and patterns of behaviour that evolve over time.

personality disorder A diagnosis that occurs when manifestations of personality in an individual start to interfere negatively with the individual's life or with the lives of those close to them.

personality traits Aspects of our personality that make us unique and interesting and differentiate us from each other.

pharmacokinetics The study of the actions of drugs within the body, including the mechanisms of absorption, distribution, metabolism and excretion.

positive symptoms of schizophrenia Tend to include signs and symptoms such as delusions, hallucinations and motor disturbance.

polypharmacy The use of a number of different drugs, possibly prescribed by different doctors and filled in different pharmacies, by a patient who may have one or several health problems.

polyuria The excessive passage of urine (at least 2.5 L/day for an adult) resulting in profuse urination and urinary frequency (the need to urinate frequently).

postsynaptic Situated behind or occurring after a synapse.

potentiation A synergistic action in which the effect of two drugs given simultaneously is greater than the sum of the effects of each drug given separately.

preceptoring A preceptoring relationship is usually based in the clinical environment and occurs when someone is new to an area (e.g. a new employee or student) and a preceptor is allocated. This is usually an experienced clinician who has been prepared for the preceptoring role, which involves guidance, helping to develop confidence and skills, and facilitates the new person becoming a member of the team.

pressure of speech Speech that is increased in amount, accelerated and difficult or impossible to interrupt.

primary gain Results in relief from psychological pain, anxiety and conflict. For example, having physical symptoms gives legitimacy to feeling unwell.

primary healthcare Strategies and interventions for reducing the prevalence and impact of mental health problems in the community; includes increasing detection, promotion, prevention, early intervention and effective treatment.

prodrome An early or premonitory sign or symptom of a disorder.

professional boundaries Limitations that need to be agreed upon in therapeutic relationships between the client/consumer and the nurse. These boundaries define acceptable and expected behaviour for both the nurse and the client that ensure a 'safe' environment based on ethical practice.

protective factors A number of aspects that guard a person against mental health problems or mental illness; can include, for example, positive relationships, support from peers and a sense of humour.

psychiatric diagnosis A tool designed to describe psychiatric criteria for the behaviour of an individual for purposes of treatment and care.

psychoanalytic theory Developed by Freud, this theory places strong emphasis on the role of the unconscious in determining human behaviour. Mental illness is seen as a state of being fixated at a developmental stage or conflict that has not been resolved.

psychoeducation Education concerning the mental health status and treatment given for the client's mental illness. It is aimed at promoting wellness and providing an opportunity for the young person to gain insight into their condition.

psychosis A condition in which a person has impaired cognition, emotional, social and communicative responses and interpretation of reality.

psychotherapy A form of therapy that is concerned with the nature of the human experience; has a number of interpersonal models with individual philosophy and set techniques, such as cognitive behavioural therapy, motivational interviewing and planned short-term psychotherapy.

psychotropic Exerting an effect on the mind or modifying mental activity.

psychotropic medications A collection of pharmacological agents in current psychiatric use: anti-anxiety sedatives, antidepressants, mood-stabilising, neuroleptic and antipsychotic drugs.

reality confrontation Reflecting an individual's behaviour back to them; a form of giving information and sharing of feelings in an acceptable way.

Glossary

recovery Begins as soon as a person develops mental health problems; emphasises hope and positive mental health and wellness, and focuses on the person being able to live well with or without the illness.

reflective practices Processes that allow the nurse to examine both their practice (actions) and the accompanying cognitions (thoughts) and affective meanings (feelings) in relation to his or her values, biases and knowledge, in the context of a particular situation.

regulation System whereby authorities set and monitor standards in the interests of the public and the professions, and maintain registers of individuals licensed to practise nursing.

rehabilitation Working with mentally ill people to reintegrate them back into the community.

relapse prevention Programmes that aim to teach consumers a set of cognitive and behavioural strategies to enhance their capacity to cope with high-risk situations that could otherwise precipitate relapse.

residual phase The phase of an illness that occurs after remission of the florid symptoms or the full syndrome.

resilience An individual's innate ability to achieve good outcomes in spite of adversity, serious threats and risks.

resocialisation Re-establishing social support networks and peer support through group therapy and individual goal-setting.

risk assessment/management Identifying and estimating risk so that structured decisions can be made as to how best to manage a risk behaviour.

risk factors Factors that influence adolescent development and can change ongoing development; can include, for example, school factors, poverty and peer friendships.

risk/harm assessment Questioning a client about risk of harm to self, risk of harm to others, risk of suicide, risk of absconding and vulnerability to exploitation or abuse.

rumination Repetitive and increasingly intrusive negative thoughts and ideas, which can eventually interfere with other thought processes.

schizophrenia A disorder characterised by major disturbance in thought, perception, thinking and psychosocial functioning; a severe mental illness.

seclusion Method of managing difficult behaviour, based on the therapeutic principles of containment, isolation and decrease in sensory input; usually instigated when other methods, such as talking and medication, have failed.

secondary gain The attention and support provided by others for a physical illness; can involve any benefit other than relief from anxiety.

self-awareness The process of becoming aware of and examining one's own personal beliefs, attitudes and motivations and recognising how these may affect others.

self-disclosure Making knowledge about oneself known to others; to publicly divulge information about one's own life.

self-efficacy The person's expectation that they can cope with and master life events effectively, and that their efforts will achieve satisfactory outcomes.

self-harm Behaviour occurring along a continuum, from pulling one's own hair out, cutting, piercing and burning oneself through to suicide. These behaviours are a mode of self-regulation for the client, and can be comforting and confirming in a world that is out of control from their perspective.

self-help Listening to one's own self-wisdom; can also involve seeking assistance and support from others who have had similar experiences to learn coping skills, tap into resources and find useful information.

set-point theory Argues that weight is largely stable over time and that changes to increase or decrease weight are opposed by the body's internal mechanisms.

sociological theories Theories that examine the influence of societal factors on the behaviour of individuals.

socratic questioning A common technique for encouraging motivation, which helps the client to come to an alternative belief of their own.

somatisation A psychological process whereby anxiety or psychological conflict is translated into physical complaints, although no mechanism has been found.

spiritual assessment Undertaking questions that can provide a deeper understanding of the patient, their social setting and possible origins of the problem. Questions concerning the client's concept of God, sources of strength and hope, religious practices and meaning and purposes in the client's life would be considered.

splitting staff An attempt by the client to split the treatment team by appealing to individual members, by sharing 'secrets' and suggesting that the staff member is the 'only one' who understands or is approachable.

stage theories Theories developed from Darwin's work on evolution that are based on measuring and monitoring a person's individual development against a set of expected 'norms' as certain age milestones are achieved.

standards of practice Standards that describe the expected performance of nurses providing mental healthcare; represent the commitment to accountability of mental health nurses. Mental health nursing standards of practice include a rationale and attributes for each standard, performance criteria and clinical indicators of practice.

Steven–Johnsons syndrome A serious systemic (bodywide) allergic reaction with a characteristic rash involving the skin and mucous membranes, including the buccal mucosa (inside of the mouth). The disease is due to a hypersensitive (allergic) reaction to one of a number of immunological stimuli including drugs and infectious agents.

stigma A notion that mental illness is something to be avoided, hidden away or shameful.

strengths A person's resilience, aspirations, talents and uniqueness; what a person can do and do well.

stress A psychological response to any demand or stressor; can be experienced as negative (distress) or positive. Individuals can respond differently to the same stressor.

stress-diathesis model A model used to understand how mental illness occurs; individuals are exposed to stressful events in the course of their lives and these events may precipitate symptoms in some people who have a predisposition to mental illness.

stress management Managing the effects of the stress one is experiencing by changing the situation, increasing one's ability to deal with the situation, changing one's perception of the situation, and/or changing one's behaviour.

substance abuse The use of drugs or alcohol in a way that disrupts prevailing social norms; these norms vary with culture, gender and generations.

sundowning effect An increase in behavioural problems for the client, occurring in the evening hours and beginning around sunset.

tangentiality A disturbance in form of thought, in which the individual gives irrelevant or oblique replies to questions. The reply might refer to the topic but not be a complete answer.

tardive dyskinesia Stereotypical involuntary movement of the tongue, lips and feet; results from prolonged use of traditional antipsychotics.

telephone counselling Method of crisis counselling that usually involves a single session and affords anonymity to the caller at a time when the person may be feeling vulnerable. The counsellor helps the person cope with the crisis by working through feelings and problem-solving.

teratogenic effect The combined consequences of consuming a harmful substance, such as a drug, on a developing foetus; may manifest itself as growth deficiency and/or mental retardation.

theophylline An alkaloid derived from tea or produced synthetically; it is a smooth-muscle relaxant used chiefly for its bronchodilator effect in the treatment of chronic obstructive pulmonary emphysema, bronchial asthma, chronic bronchitis and bronchospastic distress.

therapeutic alliance The development of the trusting, beneficial and understanding partnership that needs to exist between the nurse and the client/consumer for a therapeutic relationship to develop.

therapeutic community An environment in which the emphasis is on normal functioning rather than on a psychiatric illness or disability. In this community, the people who are being treated are referred to as consumers or residents.

therapeutic relationship An enabling relationship that supports the needs of the patient; is based on rapport and differs from social and intimate relationships.

thought blocking A disturbance in form of thought, in which there are abrupt gaps in the individual's flow of thoughts; not caused by anxiety, poor concentration or being distracted.

thought disorder A disturbance of the form in which an individual expresses their thoughts (structure, grammar, syntax, logic), or sometimes the content of their thoughts.

thriving Where a person is better off after an adverse situation than before; can be seen as a positive response to the adverse situation.

tic An involuntary, sudden, rapid, recurrent, nonrhythmic, stereotyped motor movement or vocalisation.

transference When a person transfers beliefs, feelings, thoughts or behaviours that occurred in one situation, usually in their past, to a situation that is happening in the present. Traditionally referred to the patient with unconscious feelings or beliefs about someone in their past transferring these feelings or beliefs onto the therapist.

triage assessment A process for decision making that occurs when alternatives for acute care are being considered. A comprehensive assessment is undertaken, including the person's symptoms and current situation.

tyramine A substance found in some foods. Too much tyramine can trigger migraines and hypertensive crisis.

unipolar Often used to describe a major depressive episode, whereby the mood remains low, as opposed to bipolar where the mood can shift between high and low.

victim A person who has endured a form of physical and/or psychological or emotional harm at another's hand, e.g. a person who has suffered sexual assault, domestic violence and/or rape.

violence A serious physical attack where the intent is to cause harm to an individual or object.

voluntary admission Admission of individuals, with their full permission, who require treatment in an approved mental health setting because of the severity of their mental illness, and also for individuals suffering from an acute episode of a mental illness.

withdrawal Usually but not always associated with substance dependence. Most individuals going through withdrawal have a craving to readminister the substance to reduce the symptoms. The development of a substance-specific syndrome due to the cessation of (or reduction in) substance use that has been heavy and prolonged.

word approximations A disturbance in form of thought, in which the individual strings words together in new and unconventional ways to create a particular meaning; often associated with organic brain disease.

Index

Note: Page numbers followed by "*f*", "*t*", and "*b*" refers to figures, tables, and boxes respectively.